The M. D. Anderson Surgical Oncology Handbook

Fourth Edition

M. D. Anderson Cancer Center
Department of Surgical Oncology
Houston, Texas

Editors

Barry W. Feig, M.D.
David H. Berger, M.D.
George M. Fuhrman, M.D.

Lippincott Williams & Wilkins
a Wolters Kluwer business
Philadelphia • Baltimore • New York • London
Buenos Aires • Hong Kong • Sydney • Tokyo

Acquisitions Editor: Brian Brown
Managing Editor: Julia Seto
Project Manager: Dave Murphy
Manufacturing Manager: Benjamin Rivera
Associate Director of Marketing: Adam Glazer
Cover Designer: Stephen Druding
Compositor: TechBooks
Printer: R.R. Donnelley, Crawfordsville

530 Walnut Street
Philadelphia, PA 19106 USA
LWW.com

Printed in the USA

Library of Congress Cataloging-in-Publication Data

The M. D. Anderson surgical oncology handbook / edited by Barry W. Feig, David H. Berger, and George M. Fuhrman.—4th ed.
p. ; cm.
Includes bibliographical references and index.
ISBN 0-7817-5643-X (pbk. : alk. paper)
1. Cancer—Surgery—Handbooks, manuals, etc. I. Feig, Barry W., 1959– II. Berger, David H., 1959– III. Fuhrman, George M. IV. University of Texas M. D. Anderson Cancer Center. Dept. of Surgical Oncology. V. Title: Surgical oncology handbook.
[DNLM: 1. Neoplasms–surgery–Handbooks. QZ 39 M111 2006]
RD651.M17 2006
616.99′4059—dc22

2006013941

To purchase additional copies of this book, call our customer service department at (800) 638-3030 or fax orders to (301) 223-2320. International customers should call (301) 223-2300.

Visit Lippincott Williams & Wilkins on the Internet: at LWW.com. Lippincott Williams & Wilkins customer service representatives are available from 8:30 am to 6:00 pm, ET.

10 9 8 7 6 5 4 3 2 1

To our wives (Barbara, Adrianne, and Laura) and families, for their support, enthusiasm, and patience through our many years of training and continued long hours spent in the care of patients with cancer.

Contents

Contributors

Eddie K. Abdalla, MD, FACS *Assistant Professor, Department of Surgical Oncology, The University of Texas M. D. Anderson Cancer Center, Houston, Texas*

Syed A. Ahmad, MD *Assistant Professor of Surgery, Division of Surgical Oncology, Department of Surgery, University of Cincinnati Medical Center, Barrett Cancer Center, Cincinnati, Ohio*

Daniel Albo, MD, PhD *Assistant Professor of Surgery, Michael E. DeBakey Department of Surgery, Baylor College of Medicine, Chief, Section of General Surgery and Surgical Oncology, Department of Surgery, Michael E. DeBakey VA Medical Center, Houston, Texas*

Waddah B. Al-Refaie, MD *Fellow, Division of Surgery, Department of Surgical Oncology, The University of Texas M. D. Anderson Cancer Center, Houston, Texas*

Keith D. Amos, MD *Fellow, Department of Surgical Oncology, The University of Texas M. D. Anderson Cancer Center, Houston, Texas*

Robert H. I. Andtbacka, MD, CM *Fellow and Clinical Specialist, Department of Surgical Oncology, The University of Texas M. D. Anderson Cancer Center, Houston, Texas*

Gildy V. Babiera, MD, FACS *Assistant Professor, Department of Surgical Oncology, The University of Texas M. D. Anderson Cancer Center, Houston, Texas*

Chad M. Barnett, PharmD *Clinical Pharmacy Specialist, Division of Pharmacy, The University of Texas M. D. Anderson Cancer Center, Houston, Texas*

David H. Berger, MD *Professor and Vice Chair, Michael E. DeBakey Department of Surgery, Baylor College of Medicine, Operative Care Line Executive, Michael E. DeBakey VA Medical Center, Houston, Texas*

Shanda H. Blackmon, MD, MPH *Instructor, Thoracic & Cardiovasc Surgery Department, The University of Texas M. D. Anderson Cancer Center, Houston, Texas*

Richard J. Bold, MD *Associate Professor of Surgery, Department of Surgery, University of California Davis, Chief, Division of Surgical Oncology, University of California Davis Cancer Center, Sacramento, California*

Michael Bouvet, MD *Professor, Department of Surgery, University of California San Diego, La Jolla, California*

George J. Chang, MD *Assistant Professor, Department of Surgery Oncology, The University of Texas M. D. Anderson Cancer Center, Houston, Texas*

Judy L. Chase, PharmD, FASHP *Coordinator, Clinical Pharmacy Services, Division of Pharmacy, The University of Texas M. D. Anderson Cancer Center, Houston, Texas*

Eugene A. Choi, MD *Fellow, Department of Surgical Oncology, The University of Texas M. D. Anderson Cancer Center, Houston, Texas*

Janice N. Cormier, MD, MPH *Assistant Professor, Department of Surgical Oncology, The University of Texas M. D. Anderson Cancer Center, Houston, Texas*

Keith A. Delman, MD *Assistant Professor, Division of Surgical Oncology, Department of Surgery, Winship Cancer Institute, Emory University, Atlanta, Georgia*

Colin P. N. Dinney, MD *Professor, Departments of Urology and Cancer Biology, Chairman, Department of Urology, The University of Texas M. D. Anderson Cancer Center, Houston, Texas*

Barry W. Feig, MD, FACS *Professor of Surgery, Department of Surgical Oncology, The University of Texas M. D. Anderson Cancer Center, Houston, Texas*

Jules A. Feledy, Jr., MD *Department of Reconstructive and Microvascular Surgery, The Metropolitan Institute For Plastic Surgery, Washington, DC*

Wayne A. I. Frederick, MD *Associate Professor, Department of Surgery, Howard University, Associate Director, Howard University Cancer Center, Howard University Hospital, Washington, DC*

George M. Fuhrman, MD *Program Director General Surgery Residency, Atlanta Medical Center, Atlanta, Georgia*

Jeffrey E. Gershenwald, MD *Associate Professor, Departments of Surgical Oncology and Cancer Biology, The University of Texas M. D. Anderson Cancer Center, Houston, Texas*

Ricardo J. Gonzalez, MD *Fellow, Department of Surgical Oncology, The University of Texas M. D. Anderson Cancer Center, Houston, Texas*

Ana M. Grau, MD *Assistant Professor, Department of Surgery, Meharry Medical College and Vanderbilt University, Department of Surgery, Nashville General Hospital at Meharry and Vanderbilt University Medical Center, Nashville, Tennessee*

Mouhammed A. Habra, MD *Fellow, Department of Endocrine Neoplasia and Hormonal Disorders, The University of Texas M. D. Anderson Cancer Center, Houston, Texas*

Matthew M. Hanasono, MD *Assistant Professor, Department of Plastic Surgery, The University of Texas M. D. Anderson Cancer Center, Houston, Texas*

Kelly L. Herne, MD *Volunteer facilty, Department of Dermatology, The University of Texas Houston Medical School, Houston, Texas*

Wayne L. Hofstetter, MD *Assistant Professor of Surgery, Department of Thoracic and Cardiovascular Surgery, The University of Texas M. D. Anderson Cancer Center, Houston, Texas*

F. Christopher Holsinger, MD, FACS *Assistant Professor, Department of Head and Neck Surgery, The University of Texas M. D. Anderson Cancer Center, Houston, Texas*

Kelly K. Hunt, MD *Professor of Surgery, Chief, Surgical Breast Section, Department of Surgical Oncology, Associate Medical Director, Nellie B. Connally Breast Center, The University of Texas M. D. Anderson Cancer Center, Houston, Texas*

Rosa F. Hwang, MD *Assistant Professor of Surgery, Department of Surgical Oncology, The University of Texas M. D. Anderson Cancer Center, Houston, Texas*

Sharon Renae Hymes, MD *Associate Professor, Department of Dermatology, The University of Texas M. D. Anderson Cancer Center, Houston, Texas*

Jeffrey E. Lee, MD, FACS *Professor of Surgery, Department of Surgical Oncology, The University of Texas M. D. Anderson Cancer Center, Houston, Texas*

Jeffrey T. Lenert, CDR, MC, USNR *Assistant Professor, Department of Surgery, Uniformed Services University of Health Sciences, Staff Surgical Oncologist, Department of Surgery, National Naval Medical Center, Bethesda, Maryland*

Paul F. Mansfield, MD, FACS *Professor of Surgery, Division of Surgery, Department of Surgical Oncology, The University of Texas M. D. Anderson Cancer Center, Houston, Texas*

Funda Meric-Bernstam, MD *Associate Professor, Department of Surgical Oncology, The University of Texas M. D. Anderson Cancer Center, Houston, Texas*

Kenneth A. Newkirk, MD *Assistant Professor, Department of Otolaryngology-Head and Neck Surgery, MEDSTAR-Georgetown University Medical Center, Washington, DC*

Alexander A. Parikh, MD *Assistant Professor of Surgery, Division of Surgical Oncology, Vanderbilt University Medical Center, Nashville, Tennessee*

Timothy M. Pawlik, MD, MPH *Assistant Professor, Department of Surgery, Johns Hopkins School of Medicine, Johns Hopkins Hospital, Baltimore, Maryland*

Nancy D. Perrier, MD *Associate Professor of Surgery, Department of Surgical Oncology, The University of Texas M. D. Anderson Cancer Center, Houston, Texas*

James A. Reilly, Jr., MD, FACS *Surgical Oncologist, Director—Breast Care Center, Department of Surgery, Nebraska Methodist Hospital, Omaha, Nebraska*

Geoffrey L. Robb, MD, FACS *Professor and Chair, Department of Plastic Surgery, The University of Texas M. D. Anderson Cancer Center, Houston, Texas*

Emily K. Robinson, MD *Associate Professor, Department of Surgery, The University of Texas M. D. Anderson Cancer Center, Medical Director, Memorial Hermann Cancer Center, Memorial Hermann Hospital Texas Medical Center, Houston, Texas*

Steven E. Rodgers, MD, PhD *Fellow, Department of Surgical Oncology, The University of Texas M. D. Anderson Cancer Center, Houston, Texas*

Jorge E. Romaguera, MD *Professor, Department of Lymphoma and Myeloma, The University of Texas M. D. Anderson Cancer Center, Houston, Texas*

Brian M. Slomovitz, MD, MS *Clinical Fellow, Department of Gynecologic Oncology, The University of Texas M. D. Anderson Cancer Center, Houston, Texas*

Pamela T. Soliman, MD *Clinical Fellow, Department of Gynecologic Oncology, The University of Texas M. D. Anderson Cancer Center, Houston, Texas*

Carmen C. Solorzano, MD *Assistant Professor, Department of General Surgery, Rush University, Director, Department of Endocrine Surgery Fellowship, Rush University Medical Center, Chicago, Illinois*

Francis R. Spitz, MD *Assistant Professor of Surgery, Department of Surgery, Hospital of University of Pennsylvania, Philadelphia, Pennsylvania*

Jeffrey J. Sussman, MD, FACS *Assistant Professor of Surgery, Department of Surgery, University of Cincinnati, Cincinnati, Ohio*

Eva Thomas, MD *Assistant Professor, Department of Breast Medical Oncology, The University of Texas M. D. Anderson Cancer Center, Houston, Texas*

George P. Tuszynski, PhD *Professor, Department of Neuroscience, Temple University, Philadelphia, Pennsylvania*

Douglas S. Tyler, MD *Professor of Surgery, Chief Surgical Oncology, Vice Chairman (VA Services), Department of Surgery, Duke University Medical Center, Durham, North Carolina*

Ara A. Vaporciyan, MD *Associate Professor, Department of Thoracic & Cardiovascular Surgery, The University of Texas M. D. Anderson Cancer Center, Houston, Texas*

Gauri R. Varadhachary, MD *Assistant Professor, Department of Gastrointestinal Medical Oncology, The University of Texas M. D. Anderson Cancer Center, Houston, Texas*

Thomas N. Wang, MD, PhD *Associate Professor, Attending Physician, Department of Surgery, Medical College of Georgia, Augusta, Georgia*

Jeffrey D. Wayne, MD *Assistant Professor of Surgery, Department of Surgery-Surgical Oncology, Northwestern University Feinberg School of Medicine, Attending Physician, Department of Surgery, Northwestern Memorial Hospital, Chicago, Illinois*

Judith K. Wolf, MD *Associate Professor, Department of Gynecologic Oncology, The University of Texas M. D. Anderson Cancer Center, Houston, Texas*

Christopher G. Wood, MD *Associate Professor, Departments of Urology and Cancer Biology, The University of Texas M. D. Anderson Cancer Center, Houston, Texas*

Jonathan Scott Zager, MD *Fellow, Department of Surgical Oncology, The University of Texas M. D. Anderson Cancer Center, Houston, Texas*

Foreword

What are the components of contemporary surgical care for the patient burdened by cancer? The answer to this question is to be found in the discipline of surgical oncology, which is arguably more of a cognitive than a technical surgical specialty. Other than several surgical procedures that are only infrequently performed outside of cancer centers (such as trisegmentectomy, hemipelvectomy, and regional pancreatectomy), the specialty of surgical oncology focuses on integrating surgery with other modalities of cancer treatment such as radiation oncology and systemic chemotherapy approaches. This integration is achieved via the crucible of prospective clinical trials that have emerged as the hallmark of clinical scientific research in oncology. To be effective, the surgical oncologist must understand the natural biology of solid tumors including their inception, proliferation, and dissemination. Such an understanding also implies a more than passing awareness of the underlying basic and translational science that is currently pushing the frontiers of our understanding in oncology further and further.

In addition to knowledge about the natural biology of tumors, the surgical oncologist must be intimately aware of the diagnostic options in the initial evaluation of the tumor and the staging systems by which a given tumor can be described, prognosis ascertained, and therapeutic algorithms accessed. The applicable treatments and their indications, risks, and benefits are critically important as part of this cognitive armamentarium. Moreover, in this era of managed care and cost containment, outcomes and research-defined surveillance strategies are also a part of the knowledge base of the practicing surgical oncologist.

The targeted audience of *The M. D. Anderson Surgical Oncology Handbook*, now in its fourth edition, includes surgeons-in-training as well as surgeons of all specialties who are in practice. Other healthcare professionals will no doubt find this concise manual to be of use as a ready reference as well, in much the same manner as the first and second editions of this book has been utilized by the oncology community at large. The credit for this current handbook belongs to the present and former surgical oncology fellows at The University of Texas M. D. Anderson Cancer Center. These efforts, coupled with your own interest, will help ensure that the solid tumor oncology patient receives the best possible multimodality care available. We hope that you find this handbook useful in this critical effort.

Raphael E. Pollock, M.D., Ph.D.
Head, Division of Surgery
Professor and Chairman
Department of Surgical Oncology
M. D. Anderson Cancer Center
Houston, Texas

Preface

The *M. D. Anderson Surgical Oncology Handbook* was written in an attempt to document the philosophies and practices of the Department of Surgical Oncology at the M. D. Anderson Cancer Center. The purpose of the book is to outline basic management approaches based on our experience with surgical oncology problems at M. D. Anderson. The book is intended to serve as a practical guide to the established surgical oncology principles for treating cancer as it involves each organ system in the body. This fourth edition has included new chapters on basic science and the treatment of tumors of unknown primary origin. In addition, updated information has been added on new treatments and procedures including lymphatic mapping for breast cancer and melanoma, hyperthermic isolated limb perfusion for extremity melanoma and sarcoma, cryosurgery for liver tumors, as well as many other new advances in treatment.

This book is written by current and former surgical oncology fellows at M. D. Anderson. Although the target audience for the first edition was the surgical house staff and surgical oncology trainees, we found that there was a significantly wider appeal for the book across multiple disciplines and at various levels of training and experience. We have, therefore, widened the scope of the fourth edition to reach this broader group. The authors represent various training programs, and they have spent at least two years at the M. D. Anderson Cancer Center studying only surgical oncology. The diversity of authors allows us to present the current opinions and practices of the M. D. Anderson Department of Surgical Oncology, along with other opinions and treatment options practiced in our far-ranging surgical training. Although there is no "senior" well-known name associated with the book, the authors represent 160 years of surgical training; we have not, however, become dogmatic and unyielding in our medical practices.

This handbook is not meant to encompass all aspects of oncology in minute detail. Rather, it is an attempt to address commonly encountered as well as controversial issues in surgical oncology. While other authors present their opinions and approaches as firmly established, we have tried to point out controversies and show alternative approaches to these problems besides our own.

We would like to thank the surgical staff at the M. D. Anderson Cancer Center for their assistance with the content of this book and for their devoted teaching in the hospital clinics, wards, and operating rooms. In addition, we would particularly like to thank the patients seen and treated at M. D. Anderson for their warmth and appreciation of our care, as well as for their patience and understanding of the learning process.

B.W.F.
D.H.B.
G.M.F.

1

Noninvasive Breast Cancer

Robert H. I. Andtbacka, Funda Meric-Bernstam, Emily K. Robinson, and Kelly K. Hunt

Noninvasive breast cancer comprises two separate entities: ductal carcinoma in situ (DCIS) and lobular carcinoma in situ (LCIS). DCIS is defined as a proliferation of epithelial cells confined to the mammary ducts, whereas LCIS is defined as a proliferation of epithelial cells confined to the lobules. Neither DCIS nor LCIS has demonstrable evidence of invasion through the basement membrane. Because they are noninvasive, DCIS and LCIS do not pose a risk of metastasis.

DUCTAL CARCINOMA IN SITU

Epidemiology

Before the introduction of screening mammography, most cases of DCIS remained undetected until they formed a palpable mass. Widespread use of routine screening mammography has resulted in a 10-fold increase in the reported incidence of DCIS since the mid-1980s. In the United States, the incidence is now 10 to 20 per 100,000 woman-years, and some have estimated that more than 58,000 new cases of DCIS will be diagnosed in 2006. The reported prevalence of DCIS has increased as the quality and sensitivity of mammography have improved, and DCIS currently accounts for 20% to 44% of all new screen-detected breast neoplasms in North America, with 1 case of DCIS detected per 1,300 screening mammograms.

The median age reported for patients with DCIS ranges from 47 to 63 years, similar to that reported for patients with invasive carcinoma. Some studies have reported a trend toward a lower median age when DCIS is detected during screening examinations. The frequency of a family history of breast cancer among first-degree relatives of patients with DCIS (i.e., 10%–35%) is the same as that reported for women with invasive breast malignancies. Other risk factors for DCIS are the same as those for invasive breast cancer and include older age, proliferative breast disease, nulliparity, and older age at the time of first full-term pregnancy.

Pathology

DCIS is a proliferation of malignant cells that have not breached the ductal basement membrane and arise from ductal epithelium in the region of the terminal lobular-ductal unit. DCIS probably represents one stage in the continuum of histologic progression from atypical ductal hyperplasia to invasive carcinoma. DCIS comprises a heterogeneous group of lesions with variable histologic architecture, molecular and cellular characteristics, and clinical behavior. Malignant cells proliferate to obliterate the ductal lumen, and there may be an associated breakdown of the myoepithelial cell layer of the basement membrane surrounding the ductal lumen. Also, DCIS has been linked with changes in the surrounding stroma resulting in fibroblast proliferation, lymphocyte infiltration, and angiogenesis. Although the process is poorly understood, most invasive ductal carcinomas are believed to arise from DCIS.

Classification of Ductal Carcinoma In Situ

DCIS is generally classified as one of five subtypes—comedo, solid, cribriform, micropapillary, and papillary—based on differences in the architectural pattern of the cancer cells and nuclear features. Cribriform, comedo, and micropapillary are the most common subtypes, although two or more patterns coexist in up to 50% of cases.

The identification of factors indicative of aggressive biology has led to a fundamental change in the way noninvasive breast cancer is classified. The old classification system, a strictly descriptive histologic nomenclature, has been abandoned in favor of a system that incorporates these prognostic factors and stratifies lesions based on their likelihood of recurrence. Lagios et al. (1989) identified high nuclear grade and comedo necrosis as factors predictive of local recurrence. At 8 years, patients whose tumors had a high nuclear grade and comedo necrosis had a 20% local recurrence rate after breast conservation surgery and irradiation, compared with 5% for those patients whose tumors did not have necrosis and were a lower nuclear grade. Subsequently, Silverstein et al. (1995) developed the Van Nuys classification in which three risk groups were distinguished based on the presence or absence of high nuclear grade and comedo-type necrosis: (1) non–high-grade DCIS without comedo-type necrosis, (2) non–high-grade DCIS with comedo-type necrosis, and (3) high-grade DCIS with or without comedo-type necrosis. Silverstein et al. found 31 cases of local recurrence among 238 patients who underwent breast-conserving surgery; the local recurrence rate was 3.8% in group 1, 11.1% in group 2, and 26.5% in group 3. The 8-year actuarial disease-free survival rate was 93% for group 1, 84% for group 2, and 61% for group 3. Other classification systems have also been proposed; however, no single classification system has been universally accepted.

Multifocality

Multifocal DCIS is generally defined as DCIS present in two or more foci separated by 5 mm in the same breast quadrant. Most investigators believe that multifocal disease in fact represents intraductal spread from a single focus of DCIS. By careful serial subsectioning, Holland et al. (1990) demonstrated that multifocal lesions that appeared to be separate using traditional pathological techniques actually originated from the same focus in 81 of 82 mastectomy specimens.

Multicentricity

Multicentric DCIS is defined as DCIS presenting as a separate focus outside the index quadrant. The reported incidence of multicentricity may depend on the extent of the pathological review and therefore varies from 18% to 60%, but is more likely to be around 30% to 40%. Because mammary lobules are not constrained by the artificially imposed quadrant segregations, cursory pathological examination may incorrectly interpret contiguous intraductal spread as multicentricity. Approximately 96% of all local recurrences after treatment of DCIS occur in the same quadrant as the index lesion, implicating residual untreated disease rather than multicentricity, and raising questions about the importance of multicentricity. The incidence of detection of DCIS is higher in autopsy studies than in the general population, suggesting that not all DCIS lesions become clinically significant.

Microinvasion

The American Joint Committee on Cancer (AJCC) staging system (Singletary et al., 2002) defines microinvasion as invasion of breast cancer cells through the basement membrane at one or more foci, none of which exceeds a dimension of 1 mm. A breast cancer with microinvasion is classified as a "T1mic" tumor, whereas DCIS is classified as "T0." Microinvasion upstages the cancer from stage 0 to stage 1 in the AJCC staging system.

The incidence of microinvasion in DCIS varies according to the size and extent of the index lesion. Lagios et al. (1989) reported a 2% incidence of microinvasion in patients with DCIS measuring less than 25 mm in diameter, compared with a 29% incidence of microinvasion in index lesions larger than 26 mm. The incidence of microinvasion is also higher in patients with high-grade or comedo-type DCIS tumors with necrosis and in patients with DCIS tumors who present with a palpable mass or nipple discharge. Some investigators have questioned whether it is useful to distinguish pure DCIS from DCIS with microinvasion. By definition, DCIS does not have the ability to metastasize to axillary lymph nodes or distant sites, whereas DCIS with microinvasion does. Axillary metastasis has been reported in 0% to 20% of patients with microinvasive DCIS. In addition, patients with microinvasive DCIS have been shown to have a worse prognosis. Mirza et al. (2000) reported the long-term results of breast-conserving therapy in DCIS and early-stage (T1) breast cancer and noted that the 20-year disease-specific survival rates were better among patients with DCIS than among patients with DCIS with microinvasion or T1 invasive tumors. Patients with microinvasion and those with T1 tumors had similar survival rates. In a retrospective study of 1,248 serially sectioned DCIS tumors, de Mascarel et al. (2002) reported a 10.1% incidence of axillary metastases in cases of DCIS with a cluster of microinvasive cells. Patients with DCIS had a better 10-year distant metastasis-free survival rate than patients with microinvasive DCIS (98% and 91%, respectively). The overall survival rate was also better in patients with DCIS (96.5% vs. 88.4%). The metastasis-free and overall survival rates were worse in patients with invasive ductal carcinoma than in patients with microinvasive DCIS. These results suggest that DCIS with microinvasion should be characterized as a small invasive tumor with a good outcome and that the therapeutic approach for these patients should be similar to that for patients with invasive cancer. However, further study is needed to investigate the biology of microinvasion.

Diagnosis

Clinical Presentation

Before the advent of routine mammography, most patients with DCIS presented with a palpable mass, nipple thickening or discharge, or Paget disease of the nipple. Occasionally, DCIS was an incidental finding in an otherwise benign biopsy specimen. The palpable lesions were large, and up to 25% demonstrated associated foci of invasive disease. Now that screening mammography is more prevalent, most cases of DCIS are diagnosed with of the aid of mammography alone when the tumor is still clinically occult. Patients with abnormalities detected by mammography should also undergo imaging of the contralateral breast because 0.5% to 3.0% of patients have synchronous occult abnormalities or cancers in the contralateral breast. Mammographic images should be compared with previous images, if available, to establish interval changes.

Mammographic Features

On a mammogram, DCIS can present as microcalcifications, a soft-tissue density, or both. Microcalcifications are the most common mammographic manifestation of DCIS (80%–90%). DCIS accounts for 80% of all breast carcinomas presenting with calcifications. Any interval change from a previous mammogram is associated with malignancy in 15% to 20% of cases and most often indicates in situ disease. Holland et al. (1990) described two different classes of microcalcifications: (1) linear branching-type microcalcifications, which are more often associated with high–nuclear-grade, comedo-type lesions; and (2) fine, granular calcifications, which are primarily associated with micropapillary or cribriform lesions of lower nuclear grade that do not show necrosis. Although the mammographic morphology of microcalcifications suggests the architectural type of DCIS, it is not always reliable. Holland et al. also demonstrated that the mammographic findings significantly underestimated the pathological extent of disease, particularly in cases of micropapillary DCIS. Lesions were more than 2 cm larger by histologic examination than by mammographic estimation in 44% of cases of micropapillary lesions, compared with only 12% of cases of the pure comedo subtype. However, when magnification views were used in the mammographic examination, the extent of disease was underestimated in only 14% of cases of micropapillary tumors. Hence, magnification views increase the image resolution and are better able to detect the microcalcification shape, number, and extent when compared with mammography alone and should be used routinely in the evaluation of suspicious mammographic findings.

Other Imaging Modalities

Mammography remains the standard for radiographic evaluation of DCIS. The role of other imaging modalities, such as ultrasound and magnetic resonance imaging (MRI), has yet to be established for DCIS. Ultrasound is beneficial in the evaluation of a palpable lesion and the assessment of regional lymph node basins, but it is not as reliable in routine breast screening. Contrast-enhanced MRI is also very sensitive in the detection of DCIS and invasive cancer, but it lacks specificity. DCIS has a nonspecific appearance and nonspecific kinetic enhancement curves that can mimic fibrocystic changes and other benign findings. The cost and accessibility of MRI also make it less feasible as an effective screening method. However, there is evidence that patients at high risk for breast cancer or those women with very nodular breasts may benefit from screening with MRI.

Diagnostic Biopsy

Stereotactic core-needle or vacuum-assisted biopsy is the preferred method for diagnosing DCIS. Calcifications that appear faintly on mammograms or that are deep in the breast and close to the chest wall may be difficult to target with stereotactic biopsy. In addition, use of stereotactic biopsy in patients above the weight limit of the stereotactic system (about 135 kg [297 lb]) and in patients with small breasts may be impossible. Patients who cannot remain prone or who cannot cooperate for the duration of the procedure are also not good candidates for stereotactic biopsy. Bleeding disorders and the concomitant use of anticoagulants are relative contraindications. Biopsy specimens should be radiographed to document the sampling of suspicious microcalcifications. Care should be taken to mark the biopsy site with a metallic clip in the event that all microcalcifications are removed with the biopsy procedure.

Because stereotactic core-needle and vacuum-assisted biopsy specimens represent only a sample of an abnormality observed on mammography, the results are subject to sampling error. Invasive carcinoma is found on excisional biopsy in 20% of patients in whom DCIS was diagnosed by a stereotactic core-needle biopsy. If the core-needle biopsy results are discordant with the findings of imaging studies, an excisional biopsy should be performed to confirm the diagnosis. After diagnosis using stereotactic core-needle biopsy, 30% to 50% of patients with atypical ductal hyperplasia and 20% of patients with radial scar are found to have a coexistent carcinoma near the site of the biopsy. Therefore, when the final pathological studies from core-needle biopsy procedures indicate either of these diagnoses, this should be followed by a surgical excisional biopsy.

Patients who are not candidates for stereotactic biopsy or who have stereotactic biopsy results that are inconclusive or discordant with the mammographic findings should undergo excisional biopsy. This technique is performed with the assistance of preoperative needle localization of the mammographic abnormality or of the previously placed metallic clip marking the biopsy site. Specimen radiography is essential to confirm the removal of microcalcifications of interest. The excisional biopsy should be performed with the aim of obtaining a margin-negative resection that can serve as a definitive surgery.

Treatment

The diagnosis of DCIS is followed by a mastectomy or breast-conserving surgery (also referred to as segmental mastectomy, lumpectomy, or wide local excision) performed with needle localization. Most patients who undergo breast-conserving surgery receive postoperative radiation therapy to improve local control.

Postoperative endocrine therapy with tamoxifen should also be considered for those patients whose tumors are estrogen receptor positive.

Mastectomy Versus Breast-conserving Therapy

Traditionally, DCIS has been treated with mastectomy. However, because breast-conserving techniques for invasive disease have been shown to be effective local therapy, the practice of treating a noninvasive condition with a surgical procedure more radical than that used to treat its invasive counterpart has been questioned. The rationale for performing total mastectomy in patients with DCIS is based on the high incidence of multifocality and multicentricity, as well as on the risk of occult invasion associated with the disease. Thus, mastectomy remains the standard with which other proposed therapeutic modalities should be compared. However, no prospective trials have compared outcomes after mastectomy with those after breast-conserving surgery in patients with DCIS. A retrospective review by Balch et al. (1993) documented a local relapse rate of 3.1% and a mortality rate of 2.3% after mastectomy for DCIS. The cancer-related mortality rate following mastectomy for DCIS was 1.7% in a series reported by Fowble (1989) and ranged from 0% to 8% in a review by Vezeridis and Bland (1994).

In one of the largest studies comparing breast-conserving therapy with mastectomy, Silverstein et al. (1992) examined 227 cases of DCIS without microinvasion. In this nonrandomized study, patients with tumors smaller than 4 cm with microscopically clear margins underwent breast-conserving surgery and radiation therapy, whereas patients with tumors larger than 4 cm or with positive margins underwent mastectomy. The rate of disease-free survival at 7 years was 98% in the mastectomy group compared with 84% in the breast-conserving surgery group ($p = 0.038$), with no difference in overall survival rates. In a meta-analysis, Boyages et al. (1999) reported a recurrence rate of 22.5%, 8.9%, and 1.4% following breast-conserving surgery alone, breast-conserving surgery with radiation therapy, and mastectomy, respectively. In patients who underwent breast-conserving surgery alone, approximately 50% of the recurrences were invasive cancers. Although recurrence rates are higher in patients who undergo breast-conserving surgery than in patients who undergo mastectomy, no survival advantage has been shown for the latter group.

Technique of Breast-conserving Surgery

The goal of breast-conserving surgery is to remove all suspicious calcifications and obtain negative surgical margins. Because DCIS is usually nonpalpable, breast-conserving surgery is most often performed with mammographic needle localization. Intraoperative orientation of the specimen with two or more marking sutures is critical for margin analysis. In addition, specimen radiography is essential to confirm the removal of all microcalcifications. In patients with extensive calcifications, bracketing of the calcifications with two or more wires may assist in the excision of all suspicious calcifications.

After whole-specimen radiography, the specimen should be inked and then serially sectioned for pathological examination to evaluate the margin status and extent of disease. Chagpar et al. (2003) demonstrated that intraoperative margin assessment with the use of sectioned-specimen radiography enabled re-excisions to be performed at the same surgery if the microcalcifications extended to the cut edge of the specimen, minimizing the need for second procedures for margin control. After the intraoperative margins are deemed adequate, the boundary of the resection cavity is marked with radiopaque clips to aid in the planning of postoperative radiation therapy and in mammographic follow-up.

The intraoperative goal of breast-conserving surgery is to obtain tumor-free margins of 1 cm if possible. This goal is based on the data provided by Holland et al. (1990), which demonstrated that up to 44% of lesions extended more than 2 cm further on histologic examination than that estimated by mammography. However, in most women, a 1-cm margin is not cosmetically feasible. Therefore, what constitutes an adequate margin for DCIS remains controversial. Most surgeons advocate re-excision for positive surgical margins, and many surgeons advocate re-excision for close margins, using varying thresholds of less than 1, 2, or 5 mm. Neuschatz et al. (2002) reported that residual tumor was found on re-excision in 41% of patients with DCIS with 0- to 1-mm margins, 31% of patients with 1- to 2-mm margins, and 0% of patients with greater than 2-mm margins. Lesion size was another predictor of residual DCIS.

Radiation Therapy

Most patients with DCIS who undergo breast-conserving surgery receive postoperative radiation therapy. Three prospective randomized studies have evaluated the role of radiation therapy following breast-conserving surgery for DCIS. In the National Surgical Adjuvant Breast and Bowel Project (NSABP) B-17 trial, 818 women with localized DCIS were randomized to breast-conserving surgery or breast-conserving surgery plus radiation therapy after margin-negative resections. At a follow-up time of 12 years, radiation therapy was associated with a reduction in the cumulative incidence of noninvasive ipsilateral breast tumors from 14.6% to 8.0% and with a reduction in the incidence of invasive ipsilateral breast tumors from 16.8% to 7.7%. There was no difference in the 12-year overall survival rate in the two groups, with 86% of women alive in the breast-conserving surgery group and 87% alive in the breast-conserving surgery plus radiation therapy group. However, 58% of all deaths occurred before any breast cancer event, and the death of 12 patients (3.0%) in the breast-conserving surgery group and 15 patients (3.6%) in the breast-conserving surgery plus radiation therapy group was attributed to invasive breast cancer.

The overall benefit of radiation therapy for patients with DCIS was also observed in the European Organization for Research and Treatment of Cancer 10853 trial (Julien et al., 2000). In this trial, 1,010 women with DCIS were randomized to breast-conserving surgery or breast-conserving surgery plus radiation therapy. At a median follow-up time of 4.25 years, radiation therapy was associated with a reduction in the incidence of noninvasive ipsilateral breast tumors from 8.8% to 5.8% and with a reduction in the incidence of invasive ipsilateral breast tumors from 8.0% to 4.8%. The lower recurrence rates in this trial when compared with those in the NSABP B-17 were attributed to the shorter follow-up time.

A third trial, which was conducted by the United Kingdom Coordinating Committee on Cancer Research, also confirmed the benefits of radiation therapy for local control (Houghton et al., 2003). After a median follow-up time of 4.4 years, there was a reduction in the incidence of noninvasive ipsilateral breast tumors from 7% to 3% and a reduction in the incidence of invasive ipsilateral tumors from 6% to 3%. The conclusion from these three prospective randomized trials is that the addition of radiation therapy following breast-conserving therapy for DCIS results in an approximately 50% relative reduction in breast cancer recurrence.

Breast-conserving surgery alone (i.e., without radiation therapy) has been suggested to be sufficient in a select subgroup of patients with DCIS. Initial data that supported the use of breast-conserving surgery alone in the treatment of DCIS came from a study by Lagios et al. (1989) in which 79 patients with mammographically detected DCIS underwent margin-negative excision alone. After a follow-up time of 124 months, the local recurrence rate was 16% overall—33% for the subgroup of patients with high-grade lesions and comedo necrosis versus only 2% for the patients with low- or intermediate-grade lesions.

Subsequently, Silverstein et al. (1996) developed the Van Nuys Prognostic Index (VNPI) by combining three statistically significant predictors of local recurrence: tumor size, margin width, and pathological classification. This index was recently modified to include patient age as a statistically significant predictor of local recurrence and is now referred to as the University of Southern California (USC)/VNPI (Silverstein, 2003). Numerical values ranging from 1 (best prognosis) to 3 (worst prognosis) are assigned for each of the four predictors. A size score of 1, 2, and 3 is given to small tumors (≤15 mm), intermediate tumors (16–40 mm), and large tumors (≥41 mm), respectively. Margin width is assigned a score of 1 if 10 mm or greater, 2 if 1 to 9 mm, and 3 if less than 1 mm. The pathological classification is 1 for non–high-grade DCIS without necrosis, 2 for non–high-grade DCIS with necrosis, and 3 for high-grade DCIS with or without necrosis. Patient age is assigned a score of 1 for greater than 60 years, 2 for 40 to 60 years, and 3 for less than 40 years. The sum of these results is the USC/VNPI score, with 4 being the lowest possible score and 12 the highest possible score. The USC/VNPI scores of 706 patients with DCIS treated with breast-conserving therapy with or without radiation therapy were retrospectively determined, and outcomes were compared by using local recurrence as the endpoint. Among patients with a USC/VNPI score of 4, 5, or 6, the addition of radiation therapy did not appear to confer an advantage over excision alone for local recurrence-free survival. In contrast, for patients with a USC/VNPI score of 7, 8, or 9, the absolute 12-year local recurrence-free survival rate was 12% higher among those who underwent radiation therapy and excision than among those who underwent excision alone (73% vs. 61%). Although patients with a USC/VNPI score of 10, 11, or 12 showed the greatest benefit with the addition of radiation therapy, local recurrence rates still exceeded 40% in 8 years regardless of irradiation. Based on the USC/VNPI score, Silverstein (2003) proposed the following treatment schema for DCIS: wide local excision alone for patients with a USC/VNPI score of 4 to 6, excision plus radiation therapy for patients with a USC/VNPI score of 7 to 9, and mastectomy for patients with a USC/VNPI score of 10 to 12. The USC/VNPI score may be a useful adjunct in therapeutic decision making; however, its validity has yet to be tested prospectively.

As indicated by the USC/VNPI score, margin width is an independent prognostic factor for recurrence. Silverstein et al. (1999) evaluated the role of postoperative radiation therapy for patients with margin-negative resections in a retrospective analysis of 469 patients. This study compared patients with DCIS treated with breast-conserving surgery with and without radiation therapy. They found that postoperative radiation therapy did not lower the local recurrence rate among patients with margins that were at least 10 mm. In contrast, even on reanalysis of the NSABP B-17 data, all patient cohorts benefited from radiation therapy, regardless of the clinical or mammographic tumor characteristics. Furthermore, Wong et al. (2003) reported that a prospective single-arm trial of no radiation therapy in patients with grade 1 to 2 DCIS that was no more than 2.5 cm and excised with 1 cm or greater margins conducted at the Dana-Farber/Harvard Cancer Center was terminated after a median follow-up of 3.3 years because of the number of local recurrences observed, 2.5% per patient-year corresponding to a 5-year rate of 12.5%.

Two prospective studies are currently investigating the role of observation, tamoxifen, and radiation therapy after breast-conserving therapy in good-risk patients. In the Eastern Cooperative Oncology Group E-5194 trial, patients with DCIS no more than 2.5 cm and low or intermediate grade, or DCIS no more than 1 cm and high grade and margins of at least 3 mm, undergo breast-conserving surgery alone. Tamoxifen use is allowed for 5 years postoperatively. In the Radiation Therapy Oncology Group 9804 trial, patients with DCIS no more than 2.5 cm, low or intermediate grade, and margins of at least 3 mm are randomly assigned to postoperative radiation therapy or observation with the option of tamoxifen use in each group. In both of these trials, the primary outcome will be local recurrence. These trials will provide valuable information about observation alone in patients who undergo breast-conserving surgery for good-risk DCIS.

Some have estimated that approximately 20% of all women undergoing breast-conserving surgery who would benefit from radiation therapy do not receive it as part of their treatment. The rates of radiation therapy use have been shown to vary, depending on the region of the country that the patient lives in and the age of the patient. Also, many patients choose mastectomy over breast-conserving surgery for DCIS because they are not able to complete 6 weeks of daily radiation therapy because of social considerations. Other patients who are candidates for breast-conserving surgery choose to undergo a mastectomy because of concerns about postirradiation complications. In patients not receiving radiation therapy, local recurrences in the breast tend to occur in the immediate vicinity of the breast-conserving cavity. Hence, the impact of whole breast irradiation in reducing local recurrence may be limited to the immediate surrounding area of initial involvement. Based on this, some have suggested that equivalent local control can be achieved by radiating only the tissue surrounding the resection cavity. Accelerated partial breast irradiation is a technique where high-dose radiation is delivered only to the area at highest risk for recurrence. The treatment is completed over 4 to 5 days, whereas conventional whole breast external beam radiation therapy requires 5 to 6 weeks. Several methods of accelerated partial breast irradiation have been described, including brachytherapy via multiple catheters placed in the breast parenchyma, localized conformal external beam radiation therapy, brachytherapy via bead or seed implants, single-dose intraoperative radiation therapy, and brachytherapy via a balloon catheter inserted into the cavity after breast-conserving surgery. The NSABP recently initiated the B-39 trial, in which patients with no more than 3-cm invasive stage I or II breast cancer or DCIS will be randomized to adjuvant whole breast external beam radiation therapy or accelerated partial breast irradiation after undergoing margin-negative breast-conserving surgery. Patients will receive chemotherapy and endocrine therapy when appropriate. The primary endpoint will be local tumor control, and the secondary endpoints are disease-free and overall survival, cosmetic results, and treatment toxicity. This trial will provide valuable information about the potential role for accelerated partial breast irradiation.

Endocrine Therapy

Two prospective randomized trials have evaluated the effect of tamoxifen on outcome in patients treated with breast-conserving surgery for DCIS. In the NSABP B-24 trial, 1,804 women with DCIS were randomly assigned to breast-conserving surgery and radiation therapy followed by either tamoxifen at 20 mg per day or a placebo for 5 years. Sixteen percent of the women in this study had positive resection margins. Women who received tamoxifen had fewer breast cancer events at 7 years' follow-up than did the placebo group (10.0% vs. 16.9%). Among those who received tamoxifen, the rate of ipsilateral invasive breast cancer was 2.6% at 7 years compared with 5.3% in the control group. Tamoxifen also decreased the 7-year cumulative incidence of contralateral breast neoplasms (invasive and noninvasive) to 2.3% compared with 4.9% in the control group. The benefit of tamoxifen therapy also extended to patients with positive margins or margins of unknown status. There was no difference in the 7-year overall survival rate, which was 95% in both the tamoxifen and the placebo groups. Most deaths occurred before recurrence developed and were not necessarily related to breast cancer. A subanalysis based on estrogen receptor status indicated that women with estrogen receptor-positive DCIS who received tamoxifen had a 59% reduction in their relative risk of breast cancer events when compared with those who received the placebo. Among patients with estrogen receptor-negative DCIS, there was no added benefit from tamoxifen.

In a second prospective randomized trial (United Kingdom Coordinating Committee on Cancer Research), patients underwent breast-conserving surgery and were randomized to no adjuvant treatment, adjuvant radiation therapy or tamoxifen, or adjuvant radiation therapy plus tamoxifen. Patients with positive margins were excluded from this trial, and only 10% of the women were younger than 50 years old, compared with 33% in the NSABP B-24 trial. After a median follow-up time of 4.4 years, Houghton et al. (2003) reported that radiation therapy had the greatest impact on reducing ipsilateral breast cancer events, whereas tamoxifen added to radiation therapy did not result in a significant additional benefit. The relatively short follow-up time and complex design of this trial makes interpretation of the results in direct comparison to the NSABP B-24 trial difficult.

The decision of whether to use adjuvant tamoxifen for patients with DCIS should be made on an individual basis. The use of tamoxifen has been associated with vasomotor symptoms, deep vein thrombosis, pulmonary embolus, and increased cataract formation. The risk of endometrial cancer among patients who receive the drug is two to seven times the norm. Tamoxifen may be associated with increased rates of stroke and benign ovarian cysts. Therefore, the effects of tamoxifen to reduce ipsilateral breast tumors and to prevent contralateral breast disease should be weighed against the risk of tamoxifen use in each patient. In addition, tamoxifen should be reserved for patients with estrogen receptor-positive tumors.

Aromatase inhibitors have been shown to be beneficial in the adjuvant treatment of invasive breast cancer in postmenopausal women. These agents have fewer cardiovascular side effects than tamoxifen and may be beneficial in the adjuvant treatment of patients with DCIS following breast-conserving surgery. Two ongoing randomized prospective clinical trials—NSABP B-35 and the International Breast Cancer Intervention Study (IBIS-II)—are comparing tamoxifen with anastrozole following breast-conserving surgery in patients with a diagnosis of DCIS. Results from these trials should determine the role of aromatase inhibitors in the adjuvant treatment of DCIS.

Axillary Node Staging

Because DCIS is a noninvasive disease, lymph node involvement is not expected. Thus, the role for axillary lymph node dissection is limited, and node dissection should not be performed on a routine basis. In cases where patients have large tumors (>4 cm) or extensive microcalcifications, a focus of invasion can be missed because of limited pathological sampling, and such patients are at risk for lymph node metastasis. Hence, patients who undergo mastectomy for large, high-grade DCIS should be considered for intraoperative lymphatic mapping and sentinel lymph node dissection because it is not possible to perform lymphatic mapping after a mastectomy if invasive cancer is found in the mastectomy specimen. Patients with large, high-grade, or palpable DCIS who are undergoing breast-conserving surgery are also potential candidates for intraoperative lymphatic mapping and sentinel lymph node dissection (discussed in detail in Chapter 2). Diagnosis of DCIS with the use of stereotactic core-needle biopsy is associated with a 20% rate of concomitant invasive cancer on final pathological examination, further emphasizing the importance of sentinel lymph node dissection at the time of mastectomy for large, high-grade lesions. In a study by Cox et al. (1998), the combination of hematoxylin-eosin staining and immunohistochemistry revealed that 6% of patients with newly diagnosed DCIS had metastatic disease in the sentinel nodes. Klauber-DeMore et al. (2000) found that sentinel lymph nodes were positive for cancer among 12% of patients with DCIS considered to be at high risk for invasion and among 10% of patients who had DCIS with microinvasion. This risk must be weighed against the risk of lymphedema associated with sentinel node dissection in each patient.

Predictors of Local Relapse

There are several features of DCIS that are associated with a less favorable clinical course. Traditional pathological variables, such as large tumor size (>3 cm), high nuclear grade, comedo-type necrosis, and involved margins of excision, are associated with a greater risk of local recurrence, as previously discussed. Involved margins of resection constitute the most important independent prognostic variable for predicting local relapse. As described previously, the USC/VNPI combines four significant predictors of local recurrence: tumor size, margin width, pathological classification, and patient age. In addition to a young patient age (<50 years of age), a family history of breast cancer is associated with an increased risk of local recurrence; however, these factors are not considered contraindications for breast-conserving therapy. Molecular markers, such as overexpression of HER-2/*neu*, nm23, heat shock protein, and metallothionein; low expression of p21 Waf1 and Bcl2; and DNA aneuploidy have been associated with high-grade comedo lesions, but their importance as independent prognostic variables in DCIS has not been clarified.

Treatment and Outcome of Local Recurrence

The overall survival rate in patients with DCIS is excellent. In the NSABP B-17 trial, only 27 deaths (3.3%) attributable to breast cancer had occurred after a median follow-up time of 12 years. In the NSABP B-24 trial, 0.8% of the patients died as a consequence of their breast cancer after 7 years of follow-up. In both trials, and in other studies, approximately 50% of all local recurrences were invasive cancers. The management of local recurrence depends on the therapy the patient received for the primary cancer. In cases of local recurrence in patients who underwent breast-conserving surgery without radiation therapy, re-excision with negative margins and postoperative radiation therapy constitute treatment options. For patients who have recurrent breast cancer after receiving breast-conserving surgery and radiation therapy, mastectomy is usually the preferred treatment. If the recurrent tumor is invasive, staging of the axillary nodes is performed with lymphatic mapping and sentinel lymph node dissection or with axillary lymph node dissection.

The prognosis after treatment of local recurrence depends on whether the recurrence is invasive or noninvasive. Silverstein et al. (1998) found that among patients with invasive recurrent disease, the 8-year disease-specific mortality rate was 14.4%, and the distant disease probability was 27.1%. In a follow-up study, Romero et al. (2004) reported a 10-year disease-specific mortality rate of 15% in patients with invasive recurrent disease. Although most patients with recurrent disease after DCIS do survive, an invasive recurrence is a serious event. Patients with DCIS should undergo long-term follow-up for both recurrent disease and development of new ipsilateral or contralateral primary tumors.

Surveillance

Following breast-conserving surgery, a mammogram should be obtained to detect residual microcalcifications. In addition, a mammogram should be obtained 4 to 6 months after the completion of radiation therapy to establish a new baseline. Follow-up of patients after breast-conserving surgery with or without radiation therapy should include annual or biannual physical examination and annual mammography for the first 5 years, with an annual physical examination and mammogram thereafter. Both patients who undergo breast-conserving therapy and those who undergo mastectomy should be monitored closely for new primary cancers in the contralateral breast. The risk of development of a new primary cancer in the contralateral breast after treatment of DCIS is two to five times greater than the risk of development of a first primary breast cancer and is approximately the same as the risk of development of a new contralateral primary cancer after invasive cancer.

Current Management of Ductal Carcinoma In Situ at The University of Texas M. D. Anderson Cancer Center

An algorithm for the current treatment of DCIS at M. D. Anderson Cancer Center is outlined in Figure 1.1. Patients diagnosed with a mammographic abnormality undergo contralateral mammography, and the mammograms are compared with previous images, if available. In cases in which DCIS is suspected, magnification views are routinely used to delineate the abnormality further. Ultrasound is also frequently used to assess tumor size, multicentricity, and nodal status. Diagnostic biopsy is performed by using a vacuum-assisted stereotactic core-needle biopsy technique. When DCIS is diagnosed, the pathological evaluation details the tumor type and grade, as well as any evidence of microinvasion. The status of both the estrogen and the progesterone receptors is determined and reported.

The choice of surgical therapy is based on several factors, including tumor size and grade, margin width, mammographic appearance, and patient preference. The benefits and risks of breast-conserving surgery and mastectomy should be discussed in detail with each patient. Most patients with DCIS are candidates for breast-conserving therapy, and the choice of this local treatment does not influence their overall survival. Mastectomy is indicated in patients with diffuse, malignant-appearing calcifications in the breast and persistent positive margins after attempts at surgical excision. Although tumor size is not an absolute indication for

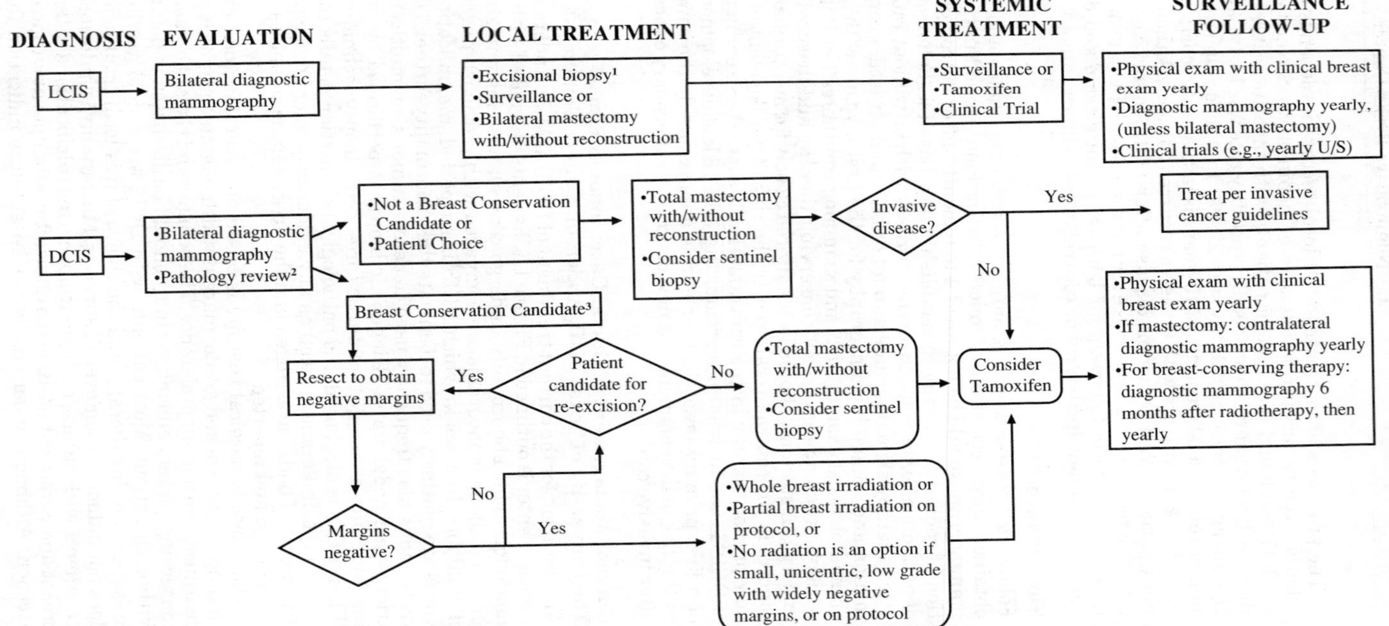
DIAGNOSIS
EVALUATION
LOCAL TREATMENT
SYSTEMIC TREATMENT
SURVEILLANCE FOLLOW-UP
LCIS
Bilateral diagnostic mammography
•Excisional biopsy[1]
•Surveillance or
•Bilateral mastectomy with/without reconstruction
•Surveillance or
•Tamoxifen
•Clinical Trial
•Physical exam with clinical breast exam yearly
•Diagnostic mammography yearly, (unless bilateral mastectomy)
•Clinical trials (e.g., yearly U/S)
DCIS
•Bilateral diagnostic mammography
•Pathology review[2]
•Not a Breast Conservation Candidate or
•Patient Choice
•Total mastectomy with/without reconstruction
•Consider sentinel biopsy
Invasive disease?
Yes
Treat per invasive cancer guidelines
No
Breast Conservation Candidate[3]
Resect to obtain negative margins
Yes
Patient candidate for re-excision?
No
•Total mastectomy with/without reconstruction
•Consider sentinel biopsy
Consider Tamoxifen
•Physical exam with clinical breast exam yearly
•If mastectomy: contralateral diagnostic mammography yearly
•For breast-conserving therapy: diagnostic mammography 6 months after radiotherapy, then yearly
No
Yes
Margins negative?
•Whole breast irradiation or
•Partial breast irradiation on protocol, or
•No radiation is an option if small, unicentric, low grade with widely negative margins, or on protocol

mastectomy, mastectomy is often preferred for patients with large (>4 cm in diameter), high-grade DCIS. There are few data available on the efficacy of breast-conserving surgery for DCIS with index lesions greater than 4 cm in diameter. Mastectomy may also be a better choice when a patient's anxiety over the possibility of recurrence outweighs the impact a mastectomy would have on her quality of life. Immediate breast reconstruction should be considered for all patients who require or elect mastectomy. Intraoperative margin assessment with sectioned-specimen radiography is used for most patients undergoing breast-conserving surgery and for patients with extensive calcifications undergoing skin-sparing mastectomy. Re-excision is usually recommended for patients who have margins less than 2 mm on final pathological examination after breast-conserving surgery.

Patients who undergo mastectomy for DCIS routinely undergo intraoperative lymphatic mapping and sentinel lymph node dissection. In patients who undergo breast-conserving surgery, sentinel lymph node dissection is performed on an individual basis and primarily reserved for cases where the DCIS is palpable or high grade or exhibits comedo-type necrosis.

Adjuvant radiation therapy is recommended to reduce the risk of local recurrence in patients who undergo breast-conserving surgery. Breast-conserving surgery alone (without radiation therapy) is considered for selected patients with small (<1 cm in diameter), low-grade lesions that have been excised with margins of at least 5 mm and who can be observed diligently for recurrence. Partial breast irradiation is offered on protocol only. Tamoxifen is offered for 5 years to women with estrogen receptor-positive DCIS who do not have a history of venous thromboembolism or stroke.

Following surgical resection, patients undergo annual physical and clinical breast examinations. Other organizations, such as the National Comprehensive Cancer Network, recommend a physical examination every 6 months for 5 years and annually thereafter. Whether this improves the detection of recurrence and outcome is not known. Patients who receive breast-conserving surgery and radiation therapy undergo a diagnostic mammogram 6 months after the completion of radiation therapy and annual bilateral mammograms thereafter. If a mastectomy is performed,

Figure 1.1. Management of lobular carcinoma in situ (LCIS) and ductal carcinoma in situ (DCIS) at M. D. Anderson. [1]Excisional biopsy is performed for patients with LCIS detected by core-needle biopsy analysis. Excision is performed with the intent of achieving negative margins in patients with pleomorphic LCIS. [2]A pathology review is performed, which includes determining the tumor size, histologic type, and nuclear grade; ruling out an invasive component; determining the lymph node status if lymph node surgery was performed; and determining the estrogen and progesterone receptor status. [3]Candidates for breast-conserving surgery are those with unicentric disease, whose ratio of tumor size to breast size allows for an acceptable cosmetic result with resection margins greater than or equal to 2 mm. *Note:* Clinical trials are considered the preferred treatment options for eligible patients. U/S, ultrasound.

the patient is followed with an annual diagnostic contralateral mammogram.

All patients with DCIS are considered for clinical trials, which are the preferred treatment options for eligible patients.

LOBULAR CARCINOMA IN SITU

LCIS was first described as a distinct pathological entity in 1941. During the era that followed, the treatment of LCIS was the same as that of invasive carcinoma—radical mastectomy. Haagensen is credited with altering the treatment philosophy for LCIS. In their review of 211 cases, Haagensen et al. (1978) noted a 17% incidence of subsequent invasive carcinomas among women in whom disease was diagnosed as LCIS and treated by observation alone (without surgery). The risk of developing a subsequent carcinoma was equal for both breasts, and only six patients died of breast cancer. Haagensen concluded that close observation for LCIS allowed for early detection of subsequent malignancy, with associated high cure rates. Haagensen's rationale for observation as a treatment philosophy for LCIS was based on his view that patients with LCIS were at increased risk for invasive breast cancer but that LCIS itself did not progress into a malignancy. However, more recent work has indicated that certain types of LCIS may be indolent precursors of infiltrating cancer and that surgical resection should be considered in selected subtypes of LCIS.

Epidemiology

The incidence of LCIS is difficult to estimate because the diagnosis is most often made following a purely incidental finding. LCIS is often not detectable by palpation, gross pathological examination, or mammography. Evaluation of mammographic abnormalities has found LCIS to be present in 0.5% to 1.3% of breast core-needle biopsy specimens and 0.5% to 3.9% of excisional breast biopsy specimens.

Traditionally, LCIS has been more commonly reported in premenopausal women than in postmenopausal women. In Haagensen's series described previously, 90% of the patients were premenopausal. In a review of the Surveillance, Epidemiology, and End Results program database, Li et al. (2002) reported that from 1978 to 1998 the incidence of LCIS increased in all age groups, but that it increased the most in women 50 to 79 years old. The increase in incidence in women 40 to 49 years old continued to the 1987 to 1989 time period and then stabilized, whereas the incidence in women age 50 years or older increased throughout the study period. During the 1996 to 1998 time period, the incidence of LCIS was the highest in women 50 to 59 years old (11.47/100,000 person-years) followed by women 60 to 69 years old (8.14/100,000 person-years). The reason for this increase in LCIS is believed to be multifactorial and partially the result of increased use of screening mammography; therefore, an increased number of biopsies were performed for mammographically detected breast abnormalities. Estrogen has been hypothesized to play an important role in the pathogenesis of LCIS; thus, the increased use of hormone replacement therapy in postmenopausal women may also account for the increased incidence of LCIS in women age 50 years or older.

The theory that LCIS represents a marker of increased risk of invasive breast carcinoma has traditionally been supported by the fact that the mean age at diagnosis is 10 to 15 years younger than that for invasive cancer. However, as the incidence of LCIS has increased in women 50 years of age and older, the incidence of infiltrating lobular carcinoma in this age group has increased concurrently, whereas women younger than 50 years old have not experienced an increase in invasive lobular carcinoma. Recently, some have suggested that LCIS is morphologically and biologically more heterogeneous than previously reported. Although classic LCIS may not be associated with invasive lobular carcinoma, cases of larger, more pleomorphic LCIS lesions may represent clonal proliferation of cells that may progress to invasive lobular carcinoma. Molecular analysis of LCIS and invasive lobular carcinoma has revealed loss of or decreased expression of the cell surface adhesion molecule E-cadherin in both tumor types. This contrasts with ductal carcinoma, in which E-cadherin expression is usually maintained. LCIS and invasive ductal carcinoma have also been shown to exhibit similar loss of heterozygosity. In addition, in an analysis of 180 patients with LCIS treated with breast-conserving therapy, Fisher et al. (2004) reported that eight of nine patients (89%) with invasive ipsilateral breast carcinoma recurrence had a recurrence of the lobular type. These data further strengthen the theory that LCIS is not only a marker for increased risk of invasive breast cancer, but also a direct precursor of invasive lobular carcinoma.

Pathology

LCIS is characterized by an intraepithelial proliferation of the terminal lobular-ductal unit. The cells are slightly larger and paler than those that line the normal acini, but the lobular architecture remains intact. The cells have a homogeneous morphology and do not display prominent chromatin. The cytoplasm-to-nucleus ratio is normal, with infrequent mitoses and no necrosis. The proliferating cells do not penetrate the basement membrane. Recently, a pleomorphic variant of LCIS with larger nuclei, central necrosis, and calcifications was described. This variant may be more prone to progressing to invasive lobular carcinoma.

The diagnosis of LCIS involves the differentiation of LCIS from other forms of benign disease and from invasive lesions. In the absence of complete replacement of the lobular unit, "atypical lobular hyperplasia" is the designated pathological term. Papillomatosis in the terminal ducts may resemble LCIS but lacks the characteristic involvement of the acini. DCIS may extend retrograde into the acini, but it has a more characteristic anaplastic cell morphology and generally expresses E-cadherin. LCIS is contained within the basement membrane and is thus distinguished from invasive lobular carcinoma.

Numerous studies have documented that LCIS is multifocal and multicentric. If diligently sought, foci can be found elsewhere in the breast in almost all cases. In addition, LCIS is identified in the contralateral breast in 50% to 90% of cases. Thus, the presence of LCIS reflects a phenotypic manifestation of a generalized abnormality present throughout both breasts. As a result, the treatment of LCIS should be directed not only at the index lesion, but also at both breasts.

Diagnosis

Clinical Presentation

Because LCIS is usually not detectable by physical examination or mammography, it is most commonly diagnosed as an incidental finding in a breast biopsy specimen. Therefore, the clinical presentation of patients with LCIS is similar to that of patients requiring breast biopsy for fibroadenoma, benign ductal disease, DCIS, or invasive breast cancer. Patients diagnosed with LCIS should undergo bilateral diagnostic mammography to exclude other mammographic abnormalities. Ultrasound is also useful in evaluating suspicious findings.

Treatment

Surgery

The optimal clinical management of patients diagnosed with LCIS with the use of a core-needle biopsy remains controversial. In the past, many surgeons opted to observe such patients because a diagnosis of LCIS was considered a marker for increased risk of breast cancer rather than a precursor of invasive cancer. However, recent studies by Arpino et al. (2004) and others have reported a 0% to 10% risk of synchronous invasive breast cancer and a 0% to 50% risk of synchronous DCIS in patients diagnosed with LCIS by core-needle biopsy specimens. Hence, patients with LCIS diagnosed by core-needle biopsy specimens are now recommended to undergo surgical excision to rule out synchronous invasive cancer and DCIS.

In contrast with DCIS, there is a lack of prospective randomized trials evaluating adjuvant treatment following surgical excision of LCIS. Most of the patients diagnosed with LCIS since the mid-1970s have undergone clinical observation alone based on the recommendations of Haagensen et al. (1978). In a study of patients who underwent observation alone after margin negative surgical excision of LCIS, Fisher et al. (2004) reported an overall 14.4% ipsilateral and 7.8% contralateral breast cancer recurrence rate after 12 years. Nearly 85% of ipsilateral breast tumor recurrences were detected by mammography, and the risk of ipsilateral recurrence was approximately 1.6% per year. More than 96% of all ipsilateral recurrences occurred in the same quadrant as the original LCIS. Nine of 26 (34.6% [5.0% of the total]) patients with ipsilateral recurrence had an invasive tumor, an incidence that was similar to that in patients with contralateral breast tumor recurrence (5.6% of the total). However, the contralateral recurrences occurred later. Only 2 of the 180 patients in the study died from breast cancer, resulting in a breast cancer-specific mortality rate of 1.1% at 12 years of follow-up time. The free excision margins were believed to have contributed to the low rate of invasive ipsilateral recurrence. In another study of 100 patients with LCIS, Ottesen et al. (2000) reported a 13% invasive ipsilateral breast cancer recurrence rate and a 16% overall recurrence rate. In this study, margin status was not evaluated, and the invasive ipsilateral breast tumor recurrence rate was more than double that observed by Fisher et al. (2004). Hence, complete excision of LCIS with negative margins may result in decreased occurrence of invasive breast cancer. However, at the present time, the data are insufficient to recommend re-excision to achieve negative margins for LCIS. Further study of the various LCIS subtypes is needed to determine whether patients with some subtypes would indeed benefit from re-excision.

Contralateral mirror-image breast biopsy, a procedure advocated for patients with LCIS in the past, has fallen out of favor because a mirror-image biopsy negative for LCIS does not eliminate the need for close observation of the remaining breast tissue in the contralateral breast. A viable therapeutic option for LCIS is bilateral prophylactic mastectomy. This approach is usually reserved for patients who have additional risk factors for breast cancer or who experience extreme anxiety regarding the observation and/or chemoprevention options. Because LCIS poses no risk of regional metastasis, axillary node dissection is not required. Immediate breast reconstruction should be offered for patients who undergo prophylactic mastectomy for LCIS.

Endocrine Therapy and Chemoprevention

Another treatment option for patients with a diagnosis of LCIS is chemoprevention with tamoxifen. In the NSABP P-1 breast cancer prevention trial, Fisher et al. (1998) observed a 56% decrease in the incidence of invasive breast cancers in a subset of women with LCIS who received tamoxifen as compared with women with LCIS who underwent observation alone. The annual hazard rate of invasive cancer was 5.69 per 1,000 women who received tamoxifen compared with 12.99 per 1,000 women who did not. Postmenopausal women with LCIS were eligible to be randomized between tamoxifen and raloxifene in the NSABP P-2 trial, which closed to accrual in 2004 (the Study of Tamoxifen And Raloxifene). The first results from this trial are expected in 2006.

Radiation Therapy

Adjuvant radiation therapy has not been evaluated specifically for the treatment of LCIS, and data are currently insufficient to recommend this treatment on a routine basis. If synchronous DCIS or invasive breast cancer is found in an excised LCIS specimen, the patient will benefit from radiation therapy and should receive treatment according to the guidelines for DCIS or invasive breast cancer.

Surveillance

Following breast-conserving therapy for LCIS, patients should undergo annual or biannual physical examinations with bilateral breast examinations. They should also undergo annual bilateral diagnostic mammography. Use of screening ultrasound in patients with LCIS is being evaluated. Also, patients who undergo a bilateral mastectomy with or without reconstruction should undergo an annual physical examination, and any suspicious lesions should be evaluated with ultrasound and biopsy analysis.

Current Treatment of Lobular Carcinoma In Situ at M. D. Anderson Cancer Center

The algorithm for treatment of patients with LCIS at M. D. Anderson is outlined in Figure 1.1. Patients found to have LCIS by biopsy analysis are evaluated with bilateral diagnostic mammography if not performed prior to obtaining the biopsy specimen. The new mammograms are compared with previous images, if available. Suspicious lesions are further evaluated with ultrasound, and additional core-needle biopsy specimens are obtained when appropriate.

Patients found to have a suspicious abnormality on mammography or ultrasound undergo breast-conserving therapy with excision of the abnormality under needle localization. If they are found to have synchronous DCIS or invasive breast cancer, subsequent treatment is administered according to the guidelines for these tumors. Re-excision to attain negative margins is not routinely performed in patients found to have isolated classical LCIS in an excised specimen. If necessary, re-excision is performed to achieve negative margins in patients with a diagnosis of pleomorphic LCIS. Bilateral prophylactic mastectomy is reserved for patients with additional risk factors for breast cancer and patients who experience extreme anxiety regarding the observation and/or chemoprevention options.

Patients who undergo breast-conserving therapy for LCIS do not routinely receive radiation therapy but are offered tamoxifen if they are suitable candidates for antiestrogen therapy.

After breast-conserving surgery, patients undergo annual physical examinations and bilateral diagnostic mammography. Following a bilateral prophylactic mastectomy with or without reconstruction, patients are also evaluated with the use of annual physical examinations, and any suspicious lesions are investigated by using ultrasound and biopsy analysis when appropriate.

All patients with LCIS are considered for clinical trials, which are the preferred treatment options for eligible patients.

RECOMMENDED READING

Arpino G, Allred CG, Mohsin SK, et al. Lobular neoplasia on core-needle biopsy—clinical significance. *Cancer* 2004;101:242.

Balch CM, Singletary SE, Bland KI. Clinical decision-making in early breast cancer. *Ann Surg* 1993;217:207.

Boyages J, Delaney G, Taylor R. Predictors of local recurrence after treatment for ductal carcinoma in situ—a meta-analysis. *Cancer* 1999;85:616.

Chagpar A, Yen T, Sahin A, et al. Intraoperative margin assessment reduces reexcision rates in patients with ductal carcinoma in situ treated with breast conserving surgery. *Am J Surg* 2003;186:371.

Cox CE, Pendas S, Cox JM, et al. Guidelines for sentinel node biopsy and lymphatic mapping of patients with breast cancer. *Ann Surg* 1998;227:645.

de Mascarel I, MacGrogan G, Mathoulin-Pélissier S, et al. Breast ductal carcinoma in situ with microinvasion: a definition supported by a long-term study of 1248 serially sectioned ductal carcinomas. *Cancer* 2002;94:2134.

Fisher B, Costantino J, Redmond C, et al. Lumpectomy compared with lumpectomy and radiation therapy for the treatment of intraductal breast carcinoma. *N Engl J Med* 1993;328:1581.

Fisher B, Costantino JP, Wickerham DL, et al. Tamoxifen for

prevention of breast cancer: report of the National Surgical Adjuvant Breast and Bowel Project P-1 study. *J Natl Cancer Inst* 1998; 90:1371.

Fisher B, Dignam J, Wolmark N, et al. Tamoxifen in treatment of intraductal breast cancer: National Surgical Adjuvant Breast and Bowel Project B-24 randomised controlled trial. *Lancet* 1999;353:1993.

Fisher B, Land S, Mamounas E, et al. Prevention of invasive breast cancer in women with ductal carcinoma in situ: an update of the National Surgical Adjuvant Breast and Bowel Project Experience. *Semin Oncol* 2001;28:400.

Fisher ER, Costantino J, Fisher B, et al. Pathological findings from the National Surgical Adjuvant Breast Project (NSABP) Protocol B-17. *Cancer* 1995;75:1310.

Fisher ER, Land SR, Fisher B, et al. Pathologic findings from the National Surgical Adjuvant Breast and Bowel Project: twelve-year observations concerning lobular carcinoma in situ. *Cancer* 2004;100:238.

Fowble B. Intraductal noninvasive breast cancer: a comparison of three local treatments. *Oncology* 1989;3:51.

Haagensen CA, Lome N, Lattes R, et al. Lobular neoplasia (so-called lobular carcinoma in situ) of the breast. *Cancer* 1978;42:757.

Holland R, Hendricks JH, Verbeek AL, et al. Extent, distribution, and mammographic/histological correlations of breast ductal carcinoma in situ. *Lancet* 1990; 335:519.

Houghton J, George WD, Cuzick J, et al. Radiotherapy and tamoxifen in women with completely excised ductal carcinoma in situ of the breast in the UK, Australia, and New Zealand: randomised controlled trial. *Lancet* 2003; 362:95.

Julien J-P, Bijker N, Fentiman IS, et al. Radiotherapy in breast-conserving treatment for ductal carcinoma in situ: first results of the EORTC randomised phase III trial 10853. *Lancet* 2000;355:528.

Klauber-DeMore N, Tan LK, Liberman L, et al. Sentinel lymph node biopsy: is it indicated in patients with high-risk ductal carcinoma-in-situ and ductal carcinoma-in-situ with microinvasion? *Ann Surg Oncol* 2000;2:636.

Lagios MD, Margolin FR, Westdahl PR, et al. Mammographically detected duct carcinoma in situ. *Cancer* 1989;63:618.

Li CI, Anderson BO, Daling JR, et al. Changing incidence of lobular carcinoma in situ of the breast. *Breast Cancer Res Treat* 2002; 75:259.

Mirza NQ, Vlastos G, Meric F, et al. Ductal carcinoma-in-situ: long-term results of breast-conserving therapy. *Ann Surg Oncol* 2000;7:656.

Neuschatz AC, DiPetrillo T, Steinhoff M, et al. The value of breast lumpectomy margin assessment as a predictor of residual tumor burden in ductal carcinoma in situ of the breast. *Cancer* 2002;94:1917.

Nielson M, Thomsen JL, Primdahl U, et al. Breast cancer and atypia among young and middle-aged women: a study of 110 medicolegal autopsies. *Br J Cancer* 1987; 56:814.

Ottesen GL, Graversen HP, Blichert-Toft M, et al. Carcinoma in situ of the female breast. 10 year follow-up results of a prospective nationwide study. *Breast Cancer Res Treat* 2000; 62:197.

Page DL, Dupont WD, Rogers LW, et al. Continued local recurrence of carcinoma 15–25 years after a diagnosis of low grade ductal carcinoma in situ of the breast treated only by biopsy. *Cancer* 1995;76:1197.

Romero L, Klein L, Wei Y, et al. Outcome after invasive recurrence in patients with ductal carcinoma in situ of the breast. *Am J Surg* 2004;188:371.

Silverstein MJ. The University of Southern California/Van Nuys prognostic index for ductal carcinoma in situ of the breast. *Am J Surg* 2003;186:337.

Silverstein MJ, Cohlan BF, Gierson ED, et al. Ductal carcinoma in situ: 227 cases without microinvasion. *Eur J Cancer* 1992;28:630.

Silverstein MJ, Lagios MD, Craig PH, et al. A prognostic index for ductal carcinoma in situ of the breast. *Cancer* 1996;77:2267.

Silverstein MJ, Lagios MD, Groshen S, et al. The influence of margin width on local control of ductal carcinoma in situ of the breast. *N Engl J Med* 1999; 340:1455.

Silverstein MJ, Lagios MD, Martino S, et al. Outcome after invasive local recurrence in patients with ductal carcinoma in situ of the breast. *J Clin Oncol* 1998;16:1367.

Silverstein MJ, Poller DN, Waisman JR, et al. Prognostic classification of breast ductal carcinoma in situ. *Lancet* 1995;345:1154.

Singletary SE, Allred C, Ashley P, et al. Revision of the American Joint Committee on Cancer staging system for breast cancer. *J Clin Oncol* 2002;20:3628.

Vezeridis MP, Bland KI. Management of ductal carcinoma in situ. *Surg Oncol* 1994;3:309.

Wong JS, Gadd MA, Gelman R, et al. Wide resection alone for ductal carcinoma in situ (DCIS) of the breast. *Proc Am Soc Clin Oncol* 2003;22:12.

Invasive Breast Cancer

Jonathan S. Zager, Carmen C. Solorzano, Eva Thomas, Barry W. Feig, and Gildy V. Babiera

EPIDEMIOLOGY

Breast cancer is a leading health concern in the United States because it is the second most common cause of death among American women (after lung cancer) and the leading cause of death among women ages 40 to 50 years. In 2005, approximately 212,930 new cases will be diagnosed, and nearly 40,870 breast cancer-related deaths will occur. In the United States, white females have the highest incidence of breast carcinoma, and the incidence increases with increasing age. For an American woman, the lifetime risk of being diagnosed with breast cancer is 1 in 7 or 14%, and the lifetime risk of dying from breast cancer is approximately 3.4%.

According to the National Cancer Institute's Surveillance, Epidemiology, and End Results Program, the incidence of breast cancer increases rapidly during the fourth decade of life. After menopause, the incidence continues to increase but at a much slower rate, peaking in the seventh and eighth decades of life and slowly leveling off after 80 years of age. The overall incidence of breast cancer in all races has increased over the last two decades from approximately 110 to 130/100,000 patients (all races) to 114 to 140/100,000 patients from 1990 to 2000. From 1990 to 2001, survival rates improved steadily and significantly for women with locoregional disease in all age groups, and the age-adjusted breast cancer mortality rate for white women in the United States dropped. However, for African American women, the 5-year relative survival rates are lower than those for white women for localized disease (90% vs. 97%), regional disease (66% vs. 79%), and metastatic disease (15% vs. 23%).

The rate of diagnosis of regional disease decreased in the late 1980s in the United States among women older than 40 years. This decrease likely reflects the increased use of mammography in the early 1980s. In contrast, the increase in survival rates in the same time period, particularly for women with regional disease, likely reflects improvements in systemic adjuvant therapy. Therefore, both screening mammography and improved therapy have probably contributed to the recent decline in breast cancer mortality rates in the United States.

RISK FACTORS

The most important risk factor for the development of breast cancer is gender. The female-to-male ratio for breast cancer is 100:1. Therefore, this chapter focuses on risk factors among women. Singletary nicely summarized risk factors for breast cancer in a 2003 review article, and a simplified version is provided in Table 2.1.

Table 2.1. Risk factors for breast cancer and associated relative risks

Risk Factor	Category at Risk	Relative Risk
Germline mutations	BRCA-1 and younger than 40 years old	200
	BRCA-1 and 60–69 years old	15
Proliferative breast disease	Lobular carcinoma in situ	16.4
	Ductal carcinoma in situ	17.3
Personal history of breast cancer	Invasive breast cancer	6.8
Ionizing radiation exposure	Hodgkin disease	5.2
Family history	First-degree relative with premenopausal breast cancer	3.3
	First-degree relative with postmenopausal breast cancer	1.8
Age at first childbirth	Older than 30 years	1.7–1.9
Hormone replacement therapy with estrogen and progesterone	Current user for at least 5 years	1.3
Early menarche	Younger than 12 years	1.3
Late menopause	Older than 55 years	1.2–1.5

Singletary SE. Rating the risk factors for breast cancer. *Ann Surg* 2003;237: 474.

Genetic alterations predisposing individuals to breast and ovarian cancer have received much attention recently. Although these gene mutations are inherited, only 5% to 10% of breast cancers are believed to result from an inherited mutated gene. Autosomal dominant conditions associated with an increased risk of breast cancer include Li-Fraumeni syndrome, BRCA-1 and BRCA-2 mutations, Muir-Torre syndrome, Cowden disease, and Peutz-Jeghers syndrome (Table 2.2). Although autosomal dominant, these conditions do not always exhibit 100% penetrance. Another inherited condition that may be associated with breast cancer is the autosomal recessive disorder ataxia-telangiectasia.

The most common genetic anomalies associated with an increased risk of breast cancer are the BRCA-1 and BRCA-2 genes. The BRCA-1 gene is found on the long arm of chromosome 17q, and the BRCA-2 gene is found on chromosome 13. Both BRCA-1 and BRCA-2 mutations are associated with an increased risk of ovarian cancer, but the risk is higher in BRCA-1. The risk of developing breast or ovarian cancer differs with the exact site of

Table 2.2. Autosomal dominant conditions associated with possible development of breast cancer

Syndrome	Defect	Associated Condition or Increased Risk for . . .
BRCA-1	Mutation of chromosome 17q	Malignancies of the breast, ovaries, and possibly prostate and colon
BRCA-2	Mutation of chromosome 13q	Malignancies of the breast (including male), ovaries, prostate, larynx, and pancreas
Li-Fraumeni	Mutation in the p53 gene on chromosome 17p	Malignancies of the breast, brain, and adrenal glands; soft-tissue sarcomas
Muir-Torre	Mutation in DNA mismatch repair genes (*hMLH1* and *hMSH2*) on chromosome 2p	Malignancies of the breast and gastrointestinal (GI) and genitourinary tracts; sebaceous tumors (i.e., hyperplasia, adenoma, epithelioma, carcinoma), keratoacanthoma
Cowden disease	Mutation in the *PTEN* gene on chromosome 10q	Malignancies of the breast, colon, uterus, thyroid, lung, and bladder; hamartomatous polyps in GI tract
Peutz-Jeghers	Mutation in the *STK11* gene on chromosome 19p	Malignancies of the breast and pancreas; mucocutaneous melanin deposition, hamartomas of the GI tract

the BRCA-1 mutation on chromosome 17q but ranges from 37% to 87% by age 70 for breast cancer and from 11% to 42% by age 60 for ovarian cancer.

A personal history of breast cancer is a significant risk factor for the development of cancer in the contralateral breast. The incidence of contralateral breast cancer is 0.5% to 1.0% per year of follow-up.

Exposure to ionizing radiation for the treatment of Hodgkin disease has been associated with a markedly increased risk of breast cancer if the exposure was before age 30 (relative risk is 5.2). The risk is less in the first 15 years after treatment than after 15 years.

Nonproliferative breast diseases such as adenosis, fibroadenomas, apocrine changes, duct ectasia, and mild hyperplasia carry no increased risk of breast cancer. However, proliferative breast diseases are associated with breast cancer to various degrees.

Moderate or florid hyperplasia without atypia, papillomas, and sclerosing adenosis carry a slightly increased risk of breast cancer (1.5 to 2 times that of the general population). Atypical ductal or lobular hyperplasia is associated with a moderately increased risk of developing breast cancer (4 to 5 times). Lobular carcinoma in situ is associated with a high risk of breast cancer (8 to 10 times). These risks apply equally to both breasts, even if the breast disease was unilateral.

Age is an important risk factor for the development of breast cancer. The risk that breast cancer will develop in a white American woman in a single year increases from 1:207 at less than age 39 years to 1:13 between ages 60 and 79.

A family history of breast cancer increases a woman's risk of breast cancer. The highest risk is associated with the presence of breast cancer in a young first-degree relative with bilateral breast cancer. The overall risk depends on the number of relatives with cancer, their ages at diagnosis, and whether the disease was unilateral or bilateral. For example, a 30-year-old woman whose sister had bilateral breast cancer before age 50 has a cumulative probability of breast cancer by age 70 of 55%. This probability decreases to 8% for a 30-year-old woman whose sister developed unilateral breast cancer after age 50.

A number of endogenous endocrine factors have also been implicated as risk factors in breast cancer. The risk of breast cancer for women who experience menopause after age 55 is twice that of women who experience menopause before age 44. Although age at menarche is important, age at onset of regular menses may have a larger effect on risk. Women who began to have regular ovulatory cycles before age 13 have a fourfold greater risk than those whose menarche occurred after age 13 and who had a 5-year delay to the development of regular cycles. The cumulative duration of menstruation may also be important. Women who menstruate for more than 30 years are at greater risk than those who menstruate for less than 30 years. Age at first childbirth has a greater effect on risk than the number of pregnancies. For example, a woman who had her first child before age 19 has half the risk of a nulliparous woman. Women who have their first child between 30 and 34 years of age have the same risk as nulliparous women, and women who have their first child after age 35 have a greater risk than nulliparous women. These observations indicate that the hormonal milieu at different times in a woman's life may affect her risk of breast cancer.

Exogenous hormone replacement therapy is known to increase a woman's risk of breast cancer (relative risk after 5 years of treatment is 1.3). However, the benefits associated with hormone replacement therapy include increased bone density and fewer postmenopausal symptoms. Therefore, treating physicians should thoroughly discuss with their patients the risks and benefits of this therapy.

PATHOLOGY

Invasive carcinomas of the breast tend to be histologically heterogeneous tumors. The vast majority of these tumors are adenocarcinomas that arise from the terminal ducts. There are five common histologic variants of mammary adenocarcinoma:

1. *Infiltrating ductal carcinoma* accounts for 75% of all breast cancers. This lesion is characterized by the absence of special histologic features. It is hard on palpation and gritty when transected. It is associated with various degrees of fibrotic response. Often there is associated ductal carcinoma in situ (DCIS) within the specimen. Infiltrating ductal carcinomas commonly metastasize to axillary lymph nodes. The prognosis for patients with these tumors is poorer than that for patients with some of the other histologic subtypes (i.e., mucinous, colloid, tubular, and medullary). Distant metastases are found most often in the bones, lungs, liver, and brain.
2. *Infiltrating lobular carcinoma* is seen in 5% to 10% of breast cancer cases. Clinically, this lesion often has an area of ill-defined thickening within the breast. Microscopically, small cells in a single- or Indian-file pattern are characteristically seen. Infiltrating lobular cancers tend to grow around ducts and lobules. Multicentricity and bilaterality are observed more frequently in infiltrating lobular carcinoma than in infiltrating ductal carcinoma. The prognosis for lobular carcinoma is similar to that for infiltrating ductal carcinoma. In addition to metastasizing to axillary lymph nodes, lobular carcinoma is known to metastasize to unusual sites (e.g., meninges and serosal surfaces) more often than do other forms of breast cancer.
3. *Tubular carcinoma* accounts for only 2% of breast carcinomas. The diagnosis of tubular carcinoma is made only when more than 75% of the tumor demonstrates tubule formation. Axillary nodal metastases are uncommon with this type of tumor. The prognosis for patients with tubular carcinoma is considerably better than that for patients with other types of breast cancer.
4. *Medullary carcinoma* accounts for 5% to 7% of breast cancers. Histologically, the lesion is characterized by poorly differentiated nuclei, a syncytial growth pattern, a well-circumscribed border, intense infiltration with small lymphocytes and plasma cells, and little or no DCIS. The prognosis for patients with pure medullary carcinoma is favorable; however, mixed variants with invasive ductal components will have prognoses similar to invasive ductal carcinoma.
5. *Mucinous or colloid carcinoma* constitutes approximately 3% of breast cancers. It is characterized by an abundant accumulation of extracellular mucin surrounding clusters of tumor cells. Colloid carcinoma is slow growing and tends to be bulky. If a breast carcinoma is predominantly mucinous, the prognosis is favorable.

Rare histologic types of breast malignancy include papillary, apocrine, secretory, squamous cell and spindle cell carcinomas, and carcinosarcoma. Infiltrating ductal carcinomas occasionally have small areas containing one or more of these special histologic types. Tumors with these mixed histologic appearances behave similarly to pure infiltrating ductal carcinomas.

STAGING

Typically, breast cancer is staged using the American Joint Committee on Cancer (AJCC) guidelines. The AJCC TNM breast cancer staging system was updated in 2003 and published in the sixth edition of the *AJCC Cancer Staging Manual*. The most recent TNM classifications and stage groupings for breast cancer are summarized in Table 2.3.

DIAGNOSIS

History and Physical Examination

The diagnosis of breast cancer has undergone a dramatic evolution since the mid-1980s. Previously, 50% to 75% of all breast cancers were detected by self-examination. Subsequent to the widespread availability of mammographic screening programs, there has been a shift toward the diagnosis of clinically occult, nonpalpable lesions. Despite this trend, evaluation of a woman for breast cancer continues to be based on a careful history and physical examination.

The history is directed at assessing cancer risk and establishing the presence or absence of symptoms indicative of breast disease and should include age at menarche, menopausal status, previous pregnancy, and use of oral contraceptives or postmenopausal replacement estrogens. A personal history of breast cancer and other cancers treated with radiation or chemotherapy (e.g., Hodgkin disease) is important. In addition, the family history of breast cancer or ovarian cancer in first-degree relatives (i.e., mother or sister) should be established. After the risk for breast cancer has been determined, the patient should be assessed for specific symptoms. Breast pain and nipple discharge are often, but not always, associated with benign processes such as fibrocystic disease and intraductal papilloma. Malaise, bony pain, and weight loss are rare but may indicate metastatic disease.

Physical examination by the health care provider must constantly take into consideration the comfort and emotional well-being of the patient. Examination is initiated by careful visual inspection with the patient sitting upright. Nipple changes, gross asymmetry, and obvious masses are all noted. The skin must be carefully inspected for subtle changes; these can range from slight dimpling to the more dramatic *peau d'orange*, warm or erythematous appearance associated with locally advanced or inflammatory breast cancer. In large or ptotic breasts, the breasts should be lifted to facilitate inspection of the inferior portion of the breast and inframammary fold. After careful inspection and with the patient remaining in the sitting position, the periclavicular regions are examined for potential nodal disease. Both axillae are then carefully palpated. If palpable, nodes should be characterized as to their number, size, and mobility. Examination of the axilla always includes palpation of the axillary tail of the breast; assessment of this area is often overlooked once the patient is placed in a supine position. Palpation of the breast parenchyma itself is accomplished with the patient supine and the ipsilateral arm placed over the head. The subareolar tissues and each quadrant of both breasts are systematically palpated. Masses are

(Text continues on page 32.)

Table 2.3. Current AJCC TNM classification and stage grouping for breast carcinoma

Classification and Stage Grouping	Definition
Primary tumor (T)	
TX	Primary tumor cannot be assessed
T0	No evidence of primary tumor
Tis	Carcinoma in situ
Tis (DCIS)	Ductal carcinoma in situ
Tis (LCIS)	Lobular carcinoma in situ
Tis (Paget)	Paget disease of the nipple with no tumor
	Note: Paget disease associated with a tumor is classified according to the size of the tumor.
T1	Tumor 2 cm or less in greatest dimension
T1mic	Microinvasion 0.1 cm or less in greatest dimension
T1a	Tumor more than 0.1 cm but not more than 0.5 cm in greatest dimension
T1b	Tumor more than 0.5 cm but not more than 1 cm in greatest dimension
T1c	Tumor more than 1 cm but not more than 2 cm in greatest dimension
T2	Tumor more than 2 cm but not more than 5 cm in greatest dimension
T3	Tumor more than 5 cm in greatest dimension
T4	Tumor of any size with direct extension to (a) chest wall or (b) skin, only as described as follows
T4a	Extension to chest wall, not including pectoralis muscle
T4b	Edema (including peau d'orange) or ulceration of the skin of the breast, or satellite skin nodules confined to the same breast
T4c	Both T4a and T4b
T4d	Inflammatory carcinoma
Regional lymph nodes (N)	
NX	Regional lymph nodes cannot be assessed (e.g., previously removed)
N0	No regional lymph node metastasis
N1	Metastasis in movable ipsilateral axillary lymph node(s)
N2	Metastases in ipsilateral axillary lymph nodes fixed or matted, or in clinically apparent ipsilateral internal mammary nodes in the *absence* of clinically evident axillary lymph node metastasis
N2a	Metastasis in ipsilateral axillary lymph nodes fixed to one another (matted) or to other structures

(*continued*)

Table 2.3. (*Continued*)

Classification and Stage Grouping	Definition
N2b	Metastasis only in clinically apparent ipsilateral internal mammary nodes and in the *absence* of clinically evident axillary lymph node metastasis
N3	Metastasis in ipsilateral infraclavicular lymph node(s), or in clinically apparent ipsilateral internal mammary lymph node(s) and in the *presence* of clinically evident axillary lymph node metastasis; or metastasis in ipsilateral supraclavicular lymph node(s) with or without axillary or internal mammary lymph node involvement
N3a	Metastasis in ipsilateral infraclavicular lymph node(s) and axillary lymph node(s)
N3b	Metastasis in ipsilateral internal mammary lymph node(s) and axillary lymph node(s)
N3c	Metastasis in ipsilateral supraclavicular lymph node(s)
Regional lymph nodes (pN)	
pNX	Regional lymph nodes cannot be assessed (e.g., previously removed, not removed for pathological study)
pN0	No regional lymph node metastasis histologically, no additional examination for isolated tumor cells
pN0(i−)	No regional lymph node metastasis histologically, negative IHC
pN0(i+)	No regional lymph node metastasis histologically, positive IHC, no IHC cluster greater than 0.2 mm
pN0(mol−)	No regional lymph node metastasis histologically, negative molecular findings (RT-PCR)
pN0(mol+)	No regional lymph node metastasis histologically, positive molecular findings (RT-PCR)
pN1mi	Micrometastasis (greater than 0.2 mm, none greater than 2.0 mm)
pN1	Metastasis in 1 to 3 axillary lymph nodes, and/or in internal mammary nodes with microscopic disease detected by sentinel lymph node dissection but not clinically apparent
pN1a	Metastasis in 1 to 3 axillary lymph nodes
pN1b	Metastasis in internal mammary nodes with microscopic disease detected by sentinel lymph node dissection but not clinically apparent

(*continued*)

Table 2.3. (*Continued*)

Classification and Stage Grouping	Definition
pN1c	Metastasis in 1 to 3 axillary lymph nodes and in internal mammary lymph nodes with microscopic disease detected by sentinel lymph node dissection but not clinically apparent
pN2	Metastasis in 4 to 9 axillary lymph nodes, or in clinically apparent internal mammary lymph nodes in the *absence* of axillary lymph node metastasis
pN2a	Metastasis in 4 to 9 axillary lymph nodes (at least one tumor deposit greater than 2.0 mm)
pN2b	Metastasis in clinically apparent internal mammary lymph nodes in the *absence* of axillary lymph node metastasis
pN3	Metastasis in 10 or more axillary lymph nodes, or in infraclavicular lymph nodes, or in clinically apparent ipsilateral internal mammary lymph nodes in the *presence* of 1 or more positive axillary lymph nodes; or in more than 3 axillary lymph nodes with clinically negative microscopic metastasis in internal mammary lymph nodes; or in ipsilateral supraclavicular lymph nodes
pN3a	Metastasis in 10 or more axillary lymph nodes (at least one tumor deposit greater than 2.0 mm), or metastasis to the infraclavicular lymph nodes
pN3b	Metastasis in clinically apparent ipsilateral internal mammary lymph nodes in the *presence* of 1 or more positive axillary lymph nodes; or in more than 3 axillary lymph nodes and in internal mammary lymph nodes with microscopic disease detected by sentinel lymph node dissection but not clinically apparent
pN3c	Metastasis in ipsilateral supraclavicular lymph nodes
Distant metastasis (M)	
MX	Distant metastasis cannot be assessed
M0	No distant metastasis
M1	Distant metastasis

DCIS, ductal carcinoma in situ; LCIS, lobular carcinoma in situ; IHC, immunohistochemistry; RT-PCR, reverse transcriptase-polymerase chain reaction. Adapted from American Joint Committee on Cancer (AJCC). *AJCC Cancer Staging Manual*. 6th ed. 2002.

noted with respect to their size, shape, location, consistency, and mobility.

Critical analysis of physical examinations has shown that the exams are often inadequate for differentiating benign and malignant breast masses. Various series have identified a 20% to 40% error rate, even among experienced examiners. Because of the high rate of inaccuracy, any persistent breast mass requires additional evaluation. Furthermore, for the differentiation of a locally advanced or inflammatory breast carcinoma, a multidisciplinary team consisting of a medical oncologist, surgeon, and radiation oncologist should be consulted to obtain a consensus as to the patient's clinical presentation and the most appropriate treatment regimen.

Evaluation of Palpable Lesions

The choice of initial diagnostic evaluation after the detection of a breast mass should be individualized for each patient according to age, perceived cancer risk, and characteristics of the lesion. For most patients, mammographic evaluation is an important initial step. Mammography in this setting serves two purposes, to assess the risk of malignancy for the palpable lesion and to screen both breasts for other nonpalpable lesions. Bilateral synchronous cancers occur in approximately 3% of all cases; at least half of these lesions are nonpalpable.

For a palpable lesion, mammograms may reveal the stellate or spiculated appearance typical of malignancy. Calcifications, nipple changes, and axillary adenopathy may also be visualized. The presence or absence of these mammographic findings can predict malignancy with an accuracy of 70% to 80%. Mammography is least accurate in younger patients with dense breasts; for this reason, it is rarely used in patients younger than the age of 30 years for screening.

After mammographic evaluation, palpable masses suspected to be malignant should undergo fine-needle aspiration (FNA) biopsy or, preferably, core-needle biopsy. Some clinicians advocate needle biopsy at the time of initial evaluation (i.e., before mammography). For most patients being treated at M. D. Anderson Cancer Center (MDACC), biopsy is deferred until after mammographic examination is completed because a needle-puncture hematoma will occasionally obscure future radiographic evaluation. For young patients with dense breasts for whom mammography is not ideal, needle biopsy with or without the aid of ultrasonography is the primary mode of evaluation. However, if the lesion can be visualized under ultrasound, it is preferable to perform needle biopsy with ultrasound guidance to confirm that the needle is within the abnormality.

FNA with a 22-gauge needle allows for accurate differentiation between cystic and solid masses and provides material for cytologic examination but does not establish an invasive component if a breast cancer diagnosis is made. Cystic lesions cannot be differentiated from solid lesions by mammography but are very well characterized by ultrasonography. Benign breast cysts typically yield nonbloody fluid and become nonpalpable after aspiration. Bloody or serous fluid should be submitted for cytologic analysis. The incidence of malignancy among breast cysts is approximately 1% and is limited almost exclusively to cysts that yield bloody or serous fluid or have a residual mass after aspiration. Aspiration is often curative; only one in five breast cysts will recur, and most of these are obliterated with a second drainage. If persistent, however, excision is usually recommended.

For solid lesions, several passes through the lesion with the syringe under constant negative pressure will typically yield ample material for cytologic evaluation. The material is evacuated onto a microscopic slide and immediately fixed in 95% ethanol. Multiple studies have demonstrated that FNA is simple, safe, and accurate in evaluating benign and malignant breast masses. However, for lesions interpreted as malignant, cytologic evaluation is unable to differentiate between in situ and invasive carcinoma. Core-needle biopsy allows the pathologist to distinguish invasive and in situ carcinoma by providing a core of tissue for histopathological evaluation.

Although physical examination, mammography, and needle biopsy all carry a risk of error when used alone, the combination of these three modalities is extremely accurate in predicting whether a palpable lesion is benign or malignant. For lesions with equivocal or contradictory results, open biopsy is the definitive test. The MDACC approach to palpable and nonpalpable breast masses are outlined in Figures 2.1 and 2.2.

Evaluation of Nonpalpable Lesions

Because of the increasing availability of mammographic screening programs, the diagnostic rate of nonpalpable breast cancer has risen rapidly in the United States. Since 1997, the American Cancer Society, the National Cancer Institute, and the American College of Radiology have released updated guidelines for breast cancer screening that are in large part based on new data published in 1997. Each organization recommends that women begin regular screening mammography in their forties.

Mammographic signs of malignancy can be divided into two main categories: microcalcifications and density changes. Microcalcifications can be clustered or scattered. Density changes include discrete masses, architectural distortions, and asymmetries. The most predictive mammographic findings of malignancy are spiculated masses with associated architectural distortion, clustered microcalcifications in a linear or branching array, and microcalcifications associated with a mass. The American College of Radiology developed the Breast Imaging Reporting and Data System, which categorizes mammographic findings as follows: I = negative (no findings); II = benign appearance; III = probably benign appearance (<2% chance of malignancy); IV = findings suspicious for breast cancer (further divided into IVa, mildly suspicious, and IVb, moderately suspicious); and V = findings highly suspicious for breast cancer (>90% chance of breast cancer).

Once screening mammography demonstrates a suspicious lesion, further evaluation is necessary for diagnosis. For lesions interpreted as "probably benign" (i.e., well-defined, solitary masses), careful counseling and repeat mammography in 6 months may be undertaken in patients at low risk for breast cancer. For certain lesions, ultrasonography may identify a subset

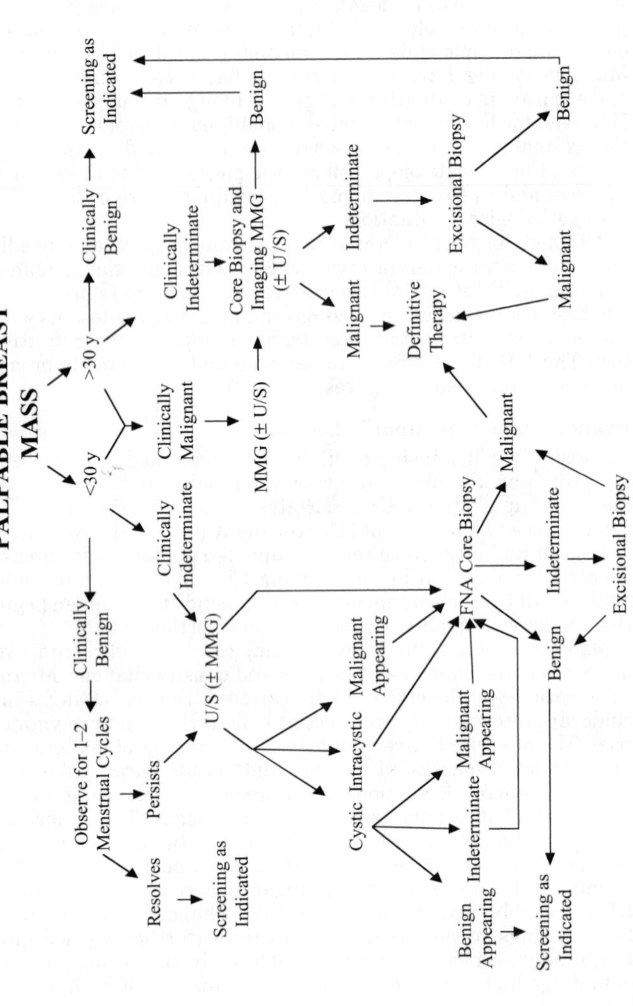
PALPABLE BREAST MASS
<30 y
>30 y
Clinically Benign
Observe for 1–2 Menstrual Cycles
Resolves
Screening as Indicated
Persists
Clinically Indeterminate
Clinically Malignant
U/S (± MMG)
MMG (± U/S)
Clinically Benign
Screening as Indicated
Clinically Indeterminate
Core Biopsy and Imaging MMG (± U/S)
Benign
Malignant
Indeterminate
Excisional Biopsy
Definitive Therapy
Malignant
Benign
Cystic
Intracystic
Malignant Appearing
Benign Appearing
Indeterminate
Malignant Appearing
FNA Core Biopsy
Benign
Indeterminate
Malignant
Excisional Biopsy
Screening as Indicated

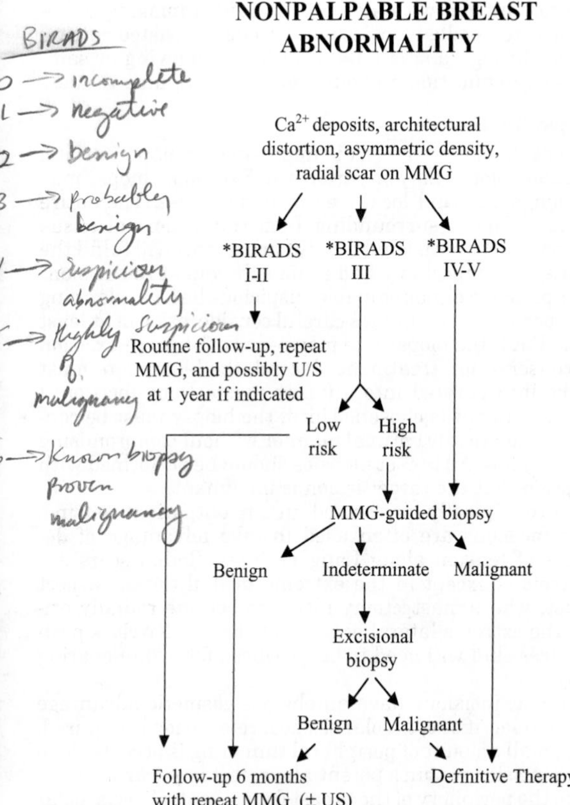

Figure 2.2. University of Texas M. D. Anderson Cancer Center algorithm for the workup of a nonpalpable breast mass. BIRADS, Breast Imaging Reporting and Data System.

of cystic lesions that will not require biopsy. Ultrasonography may also be used to guide fine-needle or core-needle biopsy. For suspicious lesions, some form of biopsy is required. Ultrasound-guided biopsy is not useful for evaluating microcalcifications because they are typically not sonographically visible. However, mammography-guided stereotactic breast biopsy is a useful technique for obtaining tissue for diagnosis from nonpalpable lesions and microcalcifications. The MDACC approach to nonpalpable breast masses is outlined in Figure 2.1.

Tissue sampling can be obtained with the Mammotome (Ethicon Endo Surgery, Cincinnati, OH) device, which is used at

Figure 2.1. University of Texas M. D. Anderson Cancer Center algorithm for the workup of a palpable breast mass.

MDACC in conjunction with stereotactic guided imaging to obtain multiple core-needle biopsies via a vacuum-assisted cutting device placed through a small 1/4-in incision removing or sampling the lesion in question and often some surrounding tissue.

Breast Biopsy Technique

When core-needle biopsy or FNA is impossible or inappropriate, excisional breast biopsy may be performed. Excisional biopsy may serve both diagnostic and local treatment purposes. The entire suspicious mass and a surrounding 1-cm rim of normal tissue should be excised. An excisional biopsy such as this will fulfill the requirements for lumpectomy and avoid subsequent re-excision.

For either palpable or nonpalpable suspicious lesions, planning an optimal open biopsy mandates careful consideration of at least three issues. First, the biopsy site may require future re-excision for breast conservation treatment. Second, the biopsy site must be able to be incorporated into a future mastectomy incision if this form of treatment is chosen. Third, the biopsy must be constructed in a cosmetically optimal manner without compromising oncologic principles. All breast biopsies should be performed with the assumption that the target lesion is malignant.

Biopsies are typically performed in an outpatient setting. Curvilinear incisions are often used to take advantage of decreased lines of tension along Langer's lines. Radial scars are generally avoided except in the extreme medial (lower) aspect of the breast, where mastectomy incisions become radially oriented or in the extreme lateral position at the 2 or 3 o'clock position, where less skin will need to be sacrificed for a skin-sparing mastectomy.

Circumareolar incisions have an obvious cosmetic advantage but may lead to sacrifice of areolar tissue if re-excision is required. Although a small amount of peripheral tunneling is acceptable to maintain an incision within a potential mastectomy scar, extreme tunneling to the periphery of the breast from a central periareolar incision must be avoided. Situating the incision well away from the abnormality for cosmetic reasons not only makes it virtually impossible to identify the tumor bed if re-excision is required, but also results in the removal of an inordinate amount of breast tissue. Therefore, the incision should generally be placed directly over the malignant lesion to avoid excessive tissue removal that may compromise cosmetic outcome or to prevent being unable to locate the tumor bed if re-excision is required. Patients who undergo breast-conserving surgery should have a separate axillary incision that is not contiguous with the breast incision. Separating these incisions provides a better cosmetic outcome (the axillary drain will cause the biopsy cavity to become distorted if they are not separated).

For nonpalpable lesions, preoperative needle localization with a self-retaining hook wire is required. This procedure requires careful communication between the radiologist and the surgeon. For most lesions, the localizing needle is placed under mammographic guidance into the breast via the shortest direct path to the lesion. The self-retaining wire is placed through the needle, and then the needle may or may not be removed at the discretion of the surgeon. Postlocalization mammograms of the wire are reviewed to confirm that the wire is within the targeted area. Excisional biopsy is then performed by excising breast tissue around the wire tip. For superficial lesions, an ellipse of skin at the point of wire insertion may be removed en bloc with the underlying breast tissue. Postexcision specimen radiographs are essential to confirm the localized target was removed. Often, the entry site of the wire is not directly over the targeted lesion, and this trajectory should be accounted for when the incision is placed on the breast.

Once the biopsy specimen has been excised, it must be handled carefully. The surgeon should note the orientation of the excised breast tissue and then hand deliver the specimen to the pathology department. The lateral, medial, superior, inferior, superficial, and deep margins should be inked in a color-coded manner. Material should be processed for receptor analysis and flow cytometry.

Closure of the biopsy incision requires meticulous hemostasis. Deep parenchymal sutures often cause cosmetically unpleasing distortion of the residual breast and should be avoided. Drains are not used in the breast. The skin is closed with a subcuticular suture, and a light dressing is placed.

PRETREATMENT EVALUATION

Once the diagnosis of breast cancer has been made, appropriate treatment planning involves evaluating the extent of disease both locally in the breast and regional nodes and of distant sites (typically to the lung, liver, and bone). For patients with stage I or stage II breast cancer, this evaluation is usually limited to a complete history and physical examination, a chest radiograph, and evaluation of serum liver chemistries. The routine use of bone scans in asymptomatic patients with apparent early-stage breast cancer carries an extremely low yield; several studies have demonstrated only a 2% incidence of positive scan results in this setting. In contrast, up to 25% of asymptomatic patients with apparent stage III cancer have positive bone scan results; thus, routine scanning in this population appears worthwhile. In the absence of increased serum liver chemistries or palpable hepatomegaly, liver imaging is not used routinely in the preoperative evaluation of patients with early-stage disease.

Ultrasound is routinely used at MDACC to evaluate the axillary nodal basin and any suspicious infraclavicular, supraclavicular, or internal mammary adenopathy. Suspicious nodes can be sampled by ultrasound-guided FNA. Positive results influence the decision on how to proceed with further therapy. Patients with positive axillary nodal FNAs can be scheduled for an axillary lymph node dissection (ALND) at the time of lumpectomy or mastectomy, therefore avoiding sentinel lymph node (SLN) biopsy and a second surgery, or they can be referred to the medical oncologist for systemic neoadjuvant chemotherapy.

TREATMENT

Many of the current recommendations regarding therapy for invasive breast cancer have been influenced by the results of randomized, prospective clinical trials performed by the National

Surgical Adjuvant Breast and Bowel Project (NSABP). A summary of selected trials is presented in Table 2.4.

Early-Stage Breast Cancer (T1, T2, N0, N1)

Approximately 75% of patients with breast cancer present with tumors less than 5 cm in diameter and no evidence of fixed or matted nodes. These patients with early-stage breast cancer are generally treated (a) with breast conservation and radiation therapy or total mastectomy with or without reconstruction and (b) with evaluation of the regional nodes in the form of ALND or SNL biopsy.

Breast Conservation Versus Mastectomy

Many patients with breast cancer can be effectively treated with breast-conserving therapy (BCT). Since 1970, seven prospective randomized trials comparing breast conservation strategies with radical or modified radical mastectomy have failed to demonstrate any survival benefit to the more aggressive approach. Among these trials, the two most widely known were conducted by Harris et al. (1992) at the National Cancer Institute in Milan, Italy, and by Fisher et al. (1995) in conjunction with the NSABP in the United States. The Milan trial was limited to patients with stage I breast cancer (tumor less than 2 cm and negative axillary lymph nodes) and compared radical mastectomy with a breast conservation strategy involving quadrantectomy, ALND, and radiation therapy. No significant differences in local control, disease-free survival, or overall survival rate have been noted, even in the most recent follow-up of these studies almost 20 years after their inception.

NSABP B-06 examined women with primary tumors up to 4 cm in diameter and N0 or N1 nodal status. Patients were randomly assigned to modified radical mastectomy, lumpectomy with ALND, or lumpectomy and ALND plus radiation therapy. Histologically negative margins were required in the breast conservation groups. Disease-free and overall survival rates did not differ significantly among the three groups, but the local recurrence rate was markedly reduced at 10 years by radiation therapy (12% with radiation therapy vs. 53% without radiation therapy). These results upheld breast conservation as an appropriate treatment for patients with stage I or stage II breast cancer and made it clear that radiation therapy is required as an integral part of any breast conservation strategy.

The current standard for BCT at MDACC for local control of the breast is excision of the tumor with negative margins followed by radiation therapy at the appropriate time. The use of systemic therapy is based on age, tumor size, nodal involvement, and receptor status and is given before (neoadjuvant) or after (adjuvant) surgery. A radiation oncologist sees the patients after completion of surgery or adjuvant chemotherapy to determine radiation dosimetry and simulation, and radiation therapy is begun 3 to 4 weeks after surgery. A dose of 50 Gy is given to the whole breast, and then 10 Gy is given to the operative site as a boost using tangential ports and computerized dosimetry.

The use of partial breast radiation therapy for BCT instead of whole breast irradiation with a boost to the tumor site is

Table 2.4. Summary of selected NSABP therapeutic trials for invasive breast cancer

Trial	Treatment	Outcome
NSABP B-04	Total mastectomy vs. total mastectomy with XRT vs. radical mastectomy	No significant difference in disease-free or overall survival rates
NSABP B-06	Total mastectomy vs. lumpectomy vs. lumpectomy with XRT	No significant difference in disease-free or overall survival rates; addition of XRT to lumpectomy reduced local recurrence rate from 39% to 10%
NSABP B-13	Surgery alone vs. surgery plus adjuvant chemotherapy in node-negative patients with estrogen receptor-negative tumors	Improved disease-free survival rate for adjuvant chemotherapy group
NSABP B-14	Surgery alone vs. surgery plus adjuvant tamoxifen in node-negative patients with estrogen receptor-positive tumors	Improved disease-free survival rate for adjuvant tamoxifen group
NSABP B-18	Neoadjuvant chemotherapy with doxorubicin, cyclophosphamide, or both for 4 cycles vs. the same regimen given postoperatively	No significant difference in overall survival or disease-free survival rates (53% and 70% at 9 years in the postoperative group and 69% and 55% in the preoperative group)
NSABP B-21	Lumpectomy plus tamoxifen vs. lumpectomy plus tamoxifen plus XRT vs. lumpectomy plus XRT for node-negative tumors <1 cm	Combination of XRT and tamoxifen was more effective than either alone in reducing ipsilateral breast tumor recurrence

(*continued*)

Table 2.4. (***Continued***)

Trial	Treatment	Outcome
NSABP B-27	Neoadjuvant chemotherapy comparing AC × 4 cycles then surgery vs. AC × 4 cycles, docetaxel × 4 cycles then surgery vs. surgery between 4 cycles of AC and 4 cycles of docetaxel	Groups I and III were combined and compared with group II; clinical and pathological complete response rates increased significantly among patients who received preoperative AC and docetaxel
NSABP B-32	SLN biopsy followed by axillary dissection vs. SLN biopsy alone for clinically node-negative patients	SLN identification rate was similar in both groups, accuracy was high for both, negative predictive value was high for both

NSABP, National Surgical Adjuvant Breast and Bowel Project; XRT, radiation therapy; AC, doxorubicin (Adriamycin), cyclophosphamide; SLN, sentinel lymph node.

currently being investigated. Advantages of partial breast irradiation include shorter treatment (5 days vs. 6 weeks); less scatter radiation to the lungs, heart, and coronary vessels; and less skin burning and desquamation. Numerous studies are in progress to evaluate the dosimetry, side effect profiles, and efficacy of partial breast irradiation. Until the results of these studies are known, partial breast irradiation should be considered experimental and be performed under protocol only. The delivery methods for partial breast irradiation currently under investigation are radiation therapy through brachytherapy catheters placed intraoperatively or postoperatively and three-dimensional conformal radiation given externally to the breast postoperatively.

Although BCT and mastectomy result in equivalent survival rates for patients with stage I or stage II disease, the decision to conserve the breast must be made individually. Of utmost importance for the success of BCT is the patient's motivation and commitment to preserve the breast and prevent advanced recurrences: daily outpatient radiation treatments over 5 to 6 weeks are required. More important is long-term follow-up of the preserved breast to detect breast cancer recurrences. Other factors that must be considered in making the choice between mastectomy and breast conservation surgery, are outlined in Table 2.5.

For extremely small breasts, the cosmetic result may be unacceptable following local excision, especially for patients with sizeable tumors. For large or pendulous breasts, lack of uniformity in radiation dosing may result in unattractive fibrosis and retraction. Patients may benefit from mastectomy plus reconstruction and perhaps surgical augmentation or reduction of the

Table 2.5. Absolute and relative contraindications to breast-conserving therapy

Absolute contraindications
Prior radiotherapy to the breast or chest wall
Radiotherapy use during pregnancy
Diffuse suspicious or malignant-appearing microcalcifications
Multicentric disease
Positive pathologial margin after multiple attempts to obtain negative margins
Relative contraindications
Multifocal disease requiring two or more separate surgical incisions
Active connective tissue disease involving the skin (especially scleroderma and lupus)
Tumor size >5 cm (controversial)
Focally positive margins after multiple attempts to obtain negative margins

Adapted from *National Comprehensive Cancer Network Guidelines*, 2005.

contralateral breast. Patients with larger tumors might also be best served by mastectomy because of the poor cosmetic outcome that results when a large area of the breast and the defect are removed. Very little data exist in a prospective randomized setting for the feasibility of BCT in patients with large tumors. Khanna et al. investigated the outcomes for 68 patients who underwent BCT without the use of preoperative (neoadjuvant) chemotherapy for 4- to 12-cm tumors. The mean tumor diameter was 5 cm, and the median follow-up was 48 months. The actuarial locoregional recurrence rate was 8.5%, and no recurrence occurred in patients who had negative surgical margins. No significant difference in disease-free survival rates was noted for patients who underwent BCT and those who underwent mastectomy. Ninety-four percent of the patients who underwent BCT reported a favorable cosmetic outcome. Alternatively, a more attractive approach to treating T3 tumors, or for patients with unfavorable breast–tumor ratios, may be neoadjuvant chemotherapy, which may shrink the tumor to the point where breast conservation is feasible or cosmetically optimal.

Although, there does not appear to be any difference in overall survival for patients who undergo mastectomy or BCT for early-stage breast cancer. There does appear to be a difference in recurrence rates between the two surgical treatment options. Attempts have been made to identify patients with a high rate of local recurrence after BCT on the basis of the histology of the primary tumor. To date, there have been no documented significant differences in local recurrence by histologic subtype. The risk of local recurrence has been shown to be higher for women younger than 35 years and for women whose tumors are greater than 2 cm in diameter, regardless of lymph node status. For patients with positive lymph nodes, nuclear grade is also significantly correlated with recurrence. The local recurrence rates for BCT quoted in the major published studies (notably, the Milan study, NSABP B-06, and the Danish Breast Cancer Cooperative Group study) range from 2.6% to 18%, which is slightly higher than the range quoted for mastectomy (2.3% to 13%). In the Milan study, the 20-year crude incidence rate for recurrence was significantly higher for BCT than for mastectomy (8.8% vs. 2.3%) ($p < 0.001$). However, there was no significant difference in overall survival rates between BCT and mastectomy in any of these studies. The ultimate goal of BCT for patients with early-stage breast cancer is to provide an optimal cosmetic result without compromising local control. Clearly, a multidisciplinary effort coupled with careful patient selection is critical for the successful outcomes of BCT.

LOCALLY ADVANCED BREAST CANCER

Locally advanced breast cancer encompasses tumors with a broad range of biological behaviors. This category includes tumors that are large or have extensive regional lymph node involvement without evidence of distant metastatic disease at initial presentation. These tumors fall into the category of stage III disease according to the AJCC system. Approximately 10% to 20% of all patients with breast cancer have stage III disease, which includes T3 tumors with N1, N2, or N3 disease; T4 tumors with any N classification; or any T classification with N2 or N3 regional lymph node involvement. Approximately 25% to 30% of stage III breast cancers are inoperable at the time of diagnosis.

Many locally advanced breast cancers are discovered by a patient or her spouse. The remaining are discovered during routine physical examination. On occasion, a discrete mass may not be present; rather, there is a diffuse infiltration of the breast tissue. These patients present with a breast that is asymmetric, immobile, and different in consistency from the contralateral breast. Seventy-five percent of patients with stage III disease will have clinically palpable axillary or supraclavicular lymph nodes at the time of diagnosis. This clinical finding is confirmed on pathological examination in 66% to 90% of patients. Of the patients with positive nodes, 50% will have more than four nodes involved. When appropriate staging is performed, 20% of patients with stage III disease are found to have distant metastases at presentation. Distant metastases are also the most frequent form of treatment failure and usually appear within 2 years of the initial diagnosis.

Both FNA and core-needle biopsy can be used to confirm breast cancer in these patients. These procedures are usually easily performed because of the large tumor size at presentation. The Halsted radical mastectomy, which was initially believed to be the treatment of choice for locally advanced breast cancer, has been proven to be inadequate for local control and long-term patient survival. In 1942, Haagensen reported a 53% local recurrence rate and a 0% 5-year overall survival rate among 1,135 patients with stage III breast cancer who had undergone a Halsted radical mastectomy.

The failure of surgery alone to control stage III breast cancer led to the use of radiation therapy as a single-agent treatment modality in this group of patients. However, the results with radiation therapy were in some cases inferior to those seen with surgery alone. The 5-year overall survival and local recurrence rates seen with radiation therapy alone have ranged from 10% to 30% and from 25% to 70%, respectively.

Surgery plus radiation therapy for locally advanced breast cancer also results in poor overall results. The lack of efficacy of the combination of two local treatment modalities confirmed that stage III breast cancer is a systemic disease. Although local control increased slightly (but insignificantly) with surgery plus radiation therapy, the 5-year overall survival rate was unchanged, and patients continued to die of distant metastases.

In the early 1970s, systemic combination chemotherapy was added to the local treatments for locally advanced breast cancer. Initial protocols were designed to administer the chemotherapy after local treatment, but this sequence of treatment does not allow for assessment of the efficacy of the chemotherapy because all measurable disease is removed before administration of the drugs. The current practice is to administer induction chemotherapy before any local treatment. This sequence allows for reduction of the initial tumor burden before surgery, treatment of the potential systemic disease without delay, and assessment of the response of the tumor to the treatment being rendered.

Several cancer treatment centers have reported experiences with combined modality therapy for locally advanced disease. Although the protocols differ among institutions with respect to the specific chemotherapy regimens and the type of local treatment, the studies have used induction neoadjuvant chemotherapy followed by local treatment (i.e., surgery, radiation therapy, or both) and subsequent adjuvant chemotherapy. Many patients with locally advanced breast cancer are now being treated with this chemotherapy sandwich approach.

Patients with locally advanced breast cancer are typically treated with an anthracycline-based regimen and a taxane before surgery or sandwiched around surgery. If postoperative chemotherapy is planned, it should precede radiation therapy to avoid interrupting the treatment of systemic disease because distant metastases are the most frequent form of treatment failure. Adjuvant hormonal therapy is routinely offered to all patients with receptor-positive tumors once they have completed systemic and locoregional therapy.

INFLAMMATORY BREAST CANCER

Inflammatory breast cancer is a rare, virulent form of locally advanced breast cancer. It represents 1% to 6% of all breast cancers and presents as erythema, warmth, and edema of the breast. Rapid onset of symptoms (within 3 months) is necessary to make the diagnosis of inflammatory carcinoma. The time course distinguishes it from locally advanced breast cancer with secondary lymphatic invasion, which usually progresses slowly over more than 3 months. Pain is also present in half of patients with inflammatory breast cancer. Confusion of the physical findings as symptoms of an infectious process often results in delays in diagnosis and treatment. Tumor emboli are often seen in the subdermal lymphatics on microscopic examination. Biopsy for diagnosis should include a segment of involved skin because a dominant mass is usually not palpable on physical examination. Ultimately, the diagnosis of inflammatory breast carcinoma is based on the clinical evaluation, which includes the timeframe for which the signs and symptoms appear.

Inflammatory carcinoma, similar to other forms of locally advanced breast cancer, is a systemic disease. In a study of inflammatory carcinoma, local therapy as the only treatment modality resulted in poor outcomes; the median survival was less than 2 years, and the 5-year overall survival rate was 5%. The use of multimodality therapy in these patients has improved local control and overall survival rate over local therapy alone. Standard treatment is anthracycline and then taxane-based chemotherapy, either both before surgery or sandwiched around surgery. Radiation is administered after completion of all surgery and systemic therapy. Patients whose disease progresses during chemotherapy proceed to preoperative radiation therapy or, if the cancer is operable, surgery.

Axillary Lymph Node Dissection

ALND is still the gold standard of care when evaluating the draining nodal basin for lymph node metastases. Although ALND appears to contribute little to overall patient survival, it is important for staging and local control. ALND provides information with prognostic and treatment implications for women undergoing breast conservation surgery or modified radical mastectomy. The role of the routine use of ALND has been redefined in the past decade by the widespread use and development of the SLN biopsy technique. Nevertheless, an ALND is still considered appropriate as a first line of treatment for local control and staging of the axillary lymph nodes, particularly in certain situations such as (a) FNA biopsy-proven axillary lymph node metastases or (b) when there are suspicious and palpable nodes in the axilla.

The incidence of axillary lymph node metastases increases as the primary tumor grows. A substantial proportion of patients with apparent early-stage breast cancer present with axillary nodal metastases. In one study, 17% of patients with clinically staged T1N0 disease had histologically positive nodes; this figure rose to 27% for patients with clinically T2N0 staged disease. Other studies have found that 10% of patients with tumors smaller than 0.5 cm have positive axillary lymph nodes. Tumors 0.5 to 1.0 cm are associated with positive axillary lymph nodes in 13% to 22% of patients, and 1.1- to 2.0-cm tumors are associated with lymph node metastases in up to 30% of patients.

The contribution of ALND to local control is small but measurable. In NSABP B-04, which compared radical mastectomy with simple mastectomy (without ALND) with and without irradiation, 40% of patients with clinically negative axillae had positive nodes at radical mastectomy, and 1% of these patients eventually experienced recurrence in the axilla. In patients with unoperated axillae (simple mastectomy group), 18% eventually developed clinical adenopathy that required delayed ALND; four of these patients eventually experienced recurrence in the axilla despite delayed ALND. No survival disadvantage was seen for patients undergoing delayed versus immediate ALND. Radiation was less effective than ALND in preventing eventual recurrence in the axilla, especially among patients with clinically positive nodes.

In addition to contributing to local control, ALND provides staging and prognostic information because nodal status is a major predictor of outcome. For all patients with node-negative cancer, a 10-year survival rate of at least 70% may be anticipated. For patients with 1 to 3 positive nodes this rate drops to 40%, and for patients with 4 to 10 positive nodes the rate drops to less than 20%. Micrometastatic nodal disease (less than 2 mm in diameter) carries a better prognosis than macrometastatic disease.

The current standard of care is an anatomic level I or level II ALND for all patients with stage I or stage II breast cancer. For patients with invasive breast cancer who are undergoing BCT, ALND should be performed via a separate axillary incision that does not extend anterior to the pectoralis fold. ALND should consist of en bloc removal of levels I and II nodal tissue, and if level III nodes are grossly or pathologically involved, removal of these nodes should be included in the ALND. However, removal of clinically negative level III lymph nodes is of little benefit with respect to staging because only 1% to 3% of stage I or stage II patients show level III involvement in the absence of level I or level II disease. Level III dissections carry a substantially higher risk of subsequent lymphedema, especially if radiation therapy is also used. The level I or level II ALND should preserve the long thoracic and thoracodorsal nerves and avoid stripping of the axillary vein. A closed-suction drain is placed and removed after the drainage has sufficiently decreased.

Patients with early-stage disease with a low risk of axillary lymph node involvement may not require a full ALND, and SLN biopsy may be the best way to stage the axillary lymph node in these patients. The best approach for patients with T1 tumors might be SLN biopsy to detect lymph node metastases because SLN biopsy provides prognostic information with presumably less morbidity and helps formulate a treatment strategy. Although this approach may seem reasonable, no national consensus has currently been reached regarding the use of SLN biopsy.

Sentinel Lymph Node Biopsy

Identifying patients with metastases in the axillary lymph nodes with ALND is extremely important for prognosis, regional treatment, and local control. But because breast cancer size on presentation has become progressively smaller due to the widespread use of screening mammography, the probability of nodal involvement has also decreased. In addition, the complications associated with the routine use of ALND to determine axillary metastases has made it increasingly hard to justify this procedure in certain patient populations. The challenge is to use ALND only in patients with nodal metastases. A newer approach that enables selective lymphadenectomy is lymphatic mapping and SLN biopsy. The SLN is often defined as the first lymph node to receive lymphatic drainage from a primary breast cancer and, therefore, the node most likely to contain metastatic tumor cells. When SLN biopsy is performed by an experienced team consisting of a surgeon, nuclear medicine physician, pathologist, and operating room nurses and technicians, the finding of a tumor-free SLN almost invariably indicates that the patient has node-negative breast cancer and need not undergo further axillary dissection. However, SLN biopsy should not be undertaken until the team has consistently documented a high rate of SLN identification and low rate of false-negative SLNs.

SLN biopsy is an unstandardized standard of care. Controversy exists as to whether the dye or radioisotope should be injected intraparenchymally, intradermally, or subareolarly; whether it should be injected the day before or the day of surgery; the dose of the radioisotope; and whether blue dye, radioisotope, or both should be used. The plethora of literature on SLN biopsy in breast cancer and the techniques and idiosyncrasies of this method exist. Most reported studies state: successful SLN detection in 94% to 98% of patients, an accuracy rate of 97% to 100%, and a false-negative rate of 0% to 15%.

SLN biopsy can be performed using radiolabeled colloid, vital blue dye, or both. Preoperative lymphoscintigraphy, although not mandatory, can be used to identify the SLN and document patterns of lymphatic drainage. A handheld gamma counter, the aid of visible blue dye, or both can be used intraoperatively to locate the SLN.

SLN biopsy may be unsuccessful in patients with certain clinical presentations: (a) palpable axillary adenopathy, (b) medial hemisphere location of the primary tumor where preoperative lymphoscintigraphy did not identify an axillary SLN, (c) previous axillary surgery because the lymphatic drainage from the primary may be distorted, and (d) large biopsy cavity (larger than 6 cm) because the lymphatic drainage from the surrounding breast tissue may not be the same as that of the primary tumor.

An important question is the clinical significance of SLN positivity as indicated by immunohistochemical analysis but not by routine hematoxylin and eosin staining. A better understanding of the natural history of the disease would help determine whether subsequent axillary dissection, axillary radiation therapy, or adjuvant chemotherapy is needed in patients with micrometastasis in the SLN. Several regional and national studies (American College of Surgeons Oncology Group Z0010/Z0011) are being conducted to address the issues associated with this new technique. The NSABP B-32 is a prospective randomized phase III trial to assess whether SLN biopsy results in the same prognosis, regional control, and overall survival rate as does ALND for invasive breast cancers. Patients with clinically negative nodes were randomly assigned to SLN biopsy with immediate ALND or to SLN biopsy alone. In both groups, a SLN was identified in 97% of patients, 26% of whom were SLN positive. In 61.5% of the SLN-positive patients, the positive SLNs were the only positive nodes. In the groups assigned to SLN biopsy with immediate ALND, the false-negative rate was 9.7%, the negative predictive value was 96.1%, and the accuracy was 97.2%. The investigators concluded that the rate of SLN identification was similar in both groups and that overall accuracy and the negative predictive value were high in both groups.

Two other groups of patients that might be considered for SLN biopsy at the time of their definitive surgery, but that are still rather controversial, are those receiving total mastectomy for noninvasive cancer and high-risk patients receiving prophylactic mastectomy. These two groups of patients may be at high risk for harboring an occult invasive cancer. Performing an SLN biopsy at the time of mastectomy may preclude the patient from having to undergo a second operation and an axillary lymph node dissection in the event that an occult invasive cancer is discovered after histopathological evaluation of the mastectomy specimen.

BREAST RECONSTRUCTION

For patients not undergoing breast conservation, breast reconstruction should be considered a standard option of cancer therapy. Reconstruction may involve autologous tissue, synthetic implants, or both. Although satisfactory results can be obtained with either immediate or delayed reconstruction, MDACC physicians favor immediate reconstruction for most patients, particularly those unlikely to undergo postmastectomy radiation therapy. Immediate reconstruction carries a substantial psychological benefit for many women and often allows a better cosmetic result. The initiation of adjuvant chemotherapy is not significantly delayed, and concerns that local recurrence may go undetected in a reconstructed breast are not well founded, especially for T1 and T2 lesions. However, if the patient is known to require postmastectomy radiation, the patient is often counseled to delay the reconstruction. Chapter 24 expands on the technical details and potential options for breast reconstruction.

At MDACC, almost half of the patients with breast cancer treated with mastectomy undergo immediate reconstruction. Although the method of reconstruction is individualized, pedicled or free transverse rectus abdominis myocutaneous flaps are the most commonly used. Contralateral augmentation or reduction may be performed to maximize symmetry. For patients with bilateral breast cancer who desire mastectomy or patients with a perceived high risk for a contralateral second primary lesion, simultaneous contralateral prophylactic mastectomy with bilateral immediate reconstruction is a viable option. Counseling regarding the possibility of postmastectomy radiation and its subsequent complications to the reconstructed breast should always be discussed with the patient.

MDACC physicians typically perform a skin-sparing mastectomy in patients undergoing immediate breast reconstruction because preservation of breast skin allows for a more natural contour to the reconstructed breast. No increased risk of local recurrence has been observed for patients treated with skin-sparing techniques.

CURRENT TREATMENT STANDARDS FOR SYSTEMIC ADJUVANT THERAPY

For node-positive and node-negative breast cancer patients, decisions regarding adjuvant chemotherapy must be individualized. Current standards are based largely on patient age, level of estrogen receptors expressed by the tumor, size of the primary tumor, and histologic status of the axilla. Other factors to consider are overall health status, *HER-2/neu* oncogene amplification, and nuclear grade. General guidelines regarding the use of adjuvant chemotherapy are presented in Table 2.6.

Table 2.6. Adjuvant chemotherapy recommendations for patients with invasive breast carcinoma on the basis of axillary nodal status, menopausal status, estrogen receptor expression, and tumor size

Nodal, Menopausal, and ER Status	Tumor Size	Therapy	Comments
Positive node			
Premenopausal			
Negative	Any	Multidrug combination chemotherapy (CMF, CAF, or AC; AC + T[a])	Four to 8 cycles of anthracyclines and taxanes in combination or sequence are the standard for all node-positive patients, regardless of ER or menopausal status; this adjuvant therapy has been shown to prolong overall survival
Positive		Multidrug combination chemotherapy (CMF, CAF, or AC; AC + T) + tamoxifen	Addition of tamoxifen to chemotherapy prolongs overall survival
Postmenopausal			
Negative		Multidrug combination chemotherapy (CMF, CAF, or AC; AC + T)	Twenty percent reduction in recurrence and 11% reduction in mortality in patients ages 50 to 69; minimal data for patients age ≥ 70
Positive		Tamoxifen 20 mg QD with or without multidrug combination chemotherapy (CMF, CAF, or AC; AC + T)	Combination chemotherapy and tamoxifen results in longer overall survival than tamoxifen alone

Negative node			
Pre- or postmenopausal			
Positive or negative	<1 cm	None; consider tamoxifen or AI for contralateral risk reduction	Overall survival after local treatment alone is >90%; low toxicity and beneficial effects of tamoxifen or AI may justify its use
Negative	≥1 cm and <2 cm	Consider multidrug combination chemotherapy (CMF, CAF, or AC)	Prognostic factors, such as grade and HER 2/neu status may be useful in selecting patients for chemotherapy
	≥2 cm	Multidrug combination chemotherapy (CMF, CAF, or AC)	Reduction in risk of recurrence is equal to that observed in node-positive disease
Positive	≥1 cm	Tamoxifen with or without multidrug combination chemotherapy (CMF, CAF, or AC)	Chemotherapy is recommended for women with high-grade tumors or T2 lesions; tamoxifen or AI therapy is recommended for tumors 1 to 2 cm; decisions about the addition of cytotoxic therapy for pre- or postmenopausal women should be made on the basis of estrogen receptor levels, performance status, and tumor factors

ER, estrogen receptor; CMF, cyclophosphamide, methotrexate, 5-fluorouracil; CAF; cyclophosphamide, doxorubicin (Adriamycin), 5-fluorouracil; AC, doxorubicin (Adriamycin), cyclophosphamide; T, taxane; QD, every day; AI, aromatase inhibitor.

[a] Addition of the taxane paclitaxel to 4 cycles of AC as treatment alternative.

Current standards favor the use of multidrug combination chemotherapy in all patients except those with the most favorable presentation (i.e., node negative and primary tumor less than 1 cm). Results from the Early Breast Cancer Trialists' Collaborative Group (EBCTCG) in 1995 and again in 2000 indicated that multidrug chemotherapy significantly reduces disease recurrence and death in both node-positive and node-negative patients, regardless of stage, menopausal status, receptor status, or patient age.

Numerous chemotherapy regimens are effective in the adjuvant setting. The EBCTCG has shown that combination chemotherapy is more effective than single agents. Six months of CMF (cylcophosphamide, methotrexate, and 5-fluorouracil) was the standard for many years and is still used by some oncologists. The anthracyclines doxorubicin and epirubicin have become the mainstay of adjuvant chemotherapy. Three months of the anthracycline regimen AC (adriamycin and cyclophosphamide) was shown to be equivalent to 6 months of CMF and is therefore a commonly used regimen in the United States. However, the three-drug anthracycline regimens FAC (5-fluorouracil, adriamycin, and cyclophosphamide) and FEC are superior to CMF and are thus probably superior to AC. Hence, the three-drug regimens are preferred at MDACC. For node-negative patients, acceptable effective adjuvant chemotherapy options include CMF, AC, FAC, and FEC.

The taxanes paclitaxel and docetaxel plus anthracyclines have been compared with anthracyclines alone in node-positive patients. Three large randomized trials have demonstrated a longer disease-free survival time among node-positive patients who received taxane plus anthracycline. Thus, it is widely accepted that node-positive patients should receive AC, FAC, or FEC in sequence or in combination with paclitaxel or docetaxel.

Chemotherapy is typically given every 3 weeks, although emerging data have demonstrated similar efficacy with weekly or every-2-week ("dose dense") chemotherapy. The EBCTCG meta-analysis has shown that less than 3 months of chemotherapy is insufficient and more than 6 months is unnecessary. Stem cell transplant has not been shown to improve the overall survival rate and should be used only in the context of a clinical trial.

Tamoxifen, which was originally recommended for the treatment of postmenopausal women with estrogen receptor-positive breast cancer, is now indicated for a much broader range of patients. Regardless of patient age or menopausal status, when used for the standard 5 years, tamoxifen is associated with a 47% reduction in the risk of breast cancer recurrence and a 26% reduction in the risk of death. Tamoxifen therapy is generally well tolerated; treatment-limiting adverse effects develop in less than 5% of patients. In addition to its antitumor properties, tamoxifen increases bone density and reduces serum cholesterol levels. However, tamoxifen also increases the incidence of endometrial cancer and thromboembolic events. Standard treatment with tamoxifen is 5 years. A meta-analysis of five randomized clinical trials showed that patients who were treated with tamoxifen for 3 to 5 years had a greater reduction in recurrence than did patients treated for 1 to 2 years (22% ± 8% vs. 7% ± 11%). Data from NSABP B-14 indicated that 10 years of tamoxifen use offer no survival advantage over 5 years. Tamoxifen and chemotherapy together achieve an additive survival benefit.

The aromatase inhibitors anastrozole, letrozole, and exemestane work by inhibiting the aromatase enzyme that catalyzes the conversion of adrenal corticosteroids to estrogens and therefore decreases the production of estrogens in postmenopausal women only. The efficacy and side effect profiles of anastrozole and tamoxifen were compared in postmenopausal women in the ATAC (Arimidex, Tamoxifen Alone or in Combination) trial, the largest breast cancer therapeutic trial ever conducted. The results of the trial demonstrated that in adjuvant endocrine therapy for postmenopausal patients with early-stage breast cancer, anastrozole resulted in a higher disease-free survival rate (86.9% vs. 84.5%), longer time to recurrence, and lower incidence of contralateral breast cancer. The results also demonstrated that the incidence of endometrial cancer, vaginal bleeding and discharge, cerebrovascular events, venous thromboembolic events, and hot flashes occurred significantly less frequently with anastrozole, whereas musculoskeletal disorders and fractures occurred less frequently with tamoxifen. As a result of the ATAC trial, anastrozole is now the preferred hormone therapy for postmenopausal patients with receptor-positive breast cancer.

For patients already taking tamoxifen, recent studies have examined the role of switching from tamoxifen to the aromatase inhibitor exemestane after 2 to 3 years of tamoxifen or the aromatase inhibitor, and letrozole after 5 years of tamoxifen. Both trials demonstrated that switching to the aromatase inhibitors increased the disease-free survival rate. It is unclear when an aromatase inhibitor should be initiated, and ongoing trials are comparing the timing and sequence of tamoxifen and aromatase inhibitors.

There is no role for aromatase inhibitors in premenopausal women, and tamoxifen remains the gold standard for these patients. Ongoing trials are examining the usefulness of ovarian ablation in addition to tamoxifen in premenopausal patients, but there is currently no data to support the routine use of ovarian ablation outside of a clinical trial.

SYSTEMIC NEOADJUVANT THERAPY

The use of neoadjuvant chemotherapy has its origins in the management of inoperable locally advanced breast cancer. Further rationale for using neoadjuvant therapy includes the potential to downsize tumors and subsequently be able to offer more patients BCT, the ability to assess the in vivo response to chemotherapeutic agents, and the theoretical early treatment of distant micrometastatic disease. The disadvantages of using neoadjuvant chemotherapy include the possible delay of curative surgery, psychosocial factors, suboptimal clinical and radiologic assessment of the primary tumor, and the potential loss of prognostic information.

The NSABP B-18 trial demonstrated that neoadjuvant chemotherapy for operable primary breast cancer allowed more patients to successfully undergo breast conservation surgery and correlated clinical and pathological response to prognosis.

However, it also demonstrated that there was no survival advantage with neoadjuvant chemotherapy over standard adjuvant chemotherapy. Therefore, if the patient's primary tumor size at initial presentation precludes a good breast conservation outcome, but the primary tumor has the potential to be downsized by neoadjuvant chemotherapy and the woman desires breast conservation surgery rather than mastectomy, neoadjuvant chemotherapy should be offered. There is still potential for a higher risk of recurrence with conservative surgery than with mastectomy, regardless of whether neoadjuvant or adjuvant therapy is used, and this risk should be discussed with the patient.

The effect of different chemotherapy regimens on tumor response can best be measured in the neoadjvuant setting because this may correlate to prognosis and to continued improvement of breast-conserving surgery rates. The results from NSABP B-27 clearly demonstrated that four cycles of AC preoperatively or four cycles of AC followed by surgery with four cycles of docetaxel postoperatively was not as efficacious in obtaining a clinical or pathological complete response as both four cycles of AC followed by four cycles of docetaxel in the neoadjuvant setting. The addition of docetaxel to AC increased the clinical complete response rate by 50% and nearly doubled the pathological complete response rate compared with AC alone.

At MDACC, the use of FAC or paclitaxel in the neoadjuvant setting was evaluated. Patients were randomly assigned to receive neoadjuvant FAC or paclitaxel and then have local therapy followed by additional FAC, XRT, ± (with or without tamoxifen) if they were postmenopausal and had receptor-positive tumors. At 4 years, the disease-free survival rate was not significantly different between the FAC and paclitaxel groups (83% vs. 86%), but the pathological complete response rate was significantly better in the FAC group (16.4% vs. 8.1%).

Another trial examining a different neoadjuvant chemotherapy regimen was the Aberdeen trial. In this trial, the patients received four doses of CVAP (cyclophosphamide, vincristine, doxorubicin, and prednisone) and then were examined for a clinical response. Those without a complete response went on to receive four doses of docetaxel, and those with a complete response were randomly assigned to receive four more doses of CVAP or four cycles of non–cross-resistant chemotherapy docetaxel. This study demonstrated the rate of breast-conserving surgery was improved for those who received the non–cross-resistant docetaxel (CVAP followed by docetaxel) (67%) compared with those who received CVAP followed by more CVAP (48%).

Finally, the use of neoadjuvant chemotherapy provides researchers with opportunities to improve chemotherapy use and patient outcomes based on tumor response. Newer techniques such as microarray gene profiling are being used to develop a method of classifying gene profiles associated with particular tumors that may correlate with pathological complete response. These data may eventually identify which patients will benefit from a particular regimen or which patients can be spared systemic therapy.

TRASTUZUMAB

Trastuzumab (Herceptin) is a monoclonal antibody that targets the *HER-2/neu* oncogene, which codes for a growth factor that is overexpressed in 25% to 30% of breast cancers. The antibody works by binding to the HER-2 growth factor receptors present on the surface of the cancer cells and thereby downregulates the receptors. The effects of trastuzumab are restricted to patients with *HER-2/neu*-overexpressing tumors. Trastuzumab is effective as a single agent, but it acts synergistically with numerous chemotherapeutic agents, including taxanes and vinorelbine. For this reason, trastuzumab plus chemotherapy is the standard of care for patients with *HER-2/neu*-amplified, metastatic tumors. Trastuzumab is now being evaluated in earlier-stage breast cancer.

In the neoadjuvant setting, trastuzumab plus non–anthracycline-containing chemotherapy has been shown in various small trials to induce a complete pathological response in 19% to 35% of patients. One of four ongoing trials currently looking at the effectiveness of an adjuvant regimen containing trastuzumab plus chemotherapy, NSABP B-31 is examining the use of doxorubicin and cyclophosphamide followed by paclitaxel with or without trastuzumab. Researchers at MDACC examined the efficacy of neoadjuvant trastuzumab plus paclitaxel and FEC in treating operable *HER-2/neu*-positive breast cancers and compared these patients with patients who received only paclitaxel and FEC. The results demonstrated that trastuzumab-based neoadjuvant therapy resulted in a significantly higher pathological complete response rate. Because there have been reports of congestive heart failure in patients treated with trastuzumab, neoadjuvant or adjuvant trastuzumab should be used only in the setting of clinical trials until the long-term cardiac safety data are known.

SURGICAL CONSIDERATIONS AFTER NEOADJUVANT CHEMOTHERAPY

There are numerous factors to consider before using neoadjuvant chemotherapy to treat breast cancer. (a) Will administering neoadjuvant chemotherapy convert an otherwise large tumor requiring mastectomy into one manageable by BCT? If not, then neoadjuvant chemotherapy may not be desirable because a mastectomy will need to be performed either way, and much of the information (e.g., tumor size and lymph node involvement with metastases) useful in determining whether there is a role for further treatment with radiation may be lost. (b) The tumor in the breast must be carefully localized with a clip or permanent marker before chemotherapy to ensure proper localization of the tumor during surgery in the event that the chemotherapy produces a complete clinical response. (c) How much tissue should be removed during surgery after chemotherapy is completed? The answer is debatable, but generally all gross disease plus any other suspicious areas with a rim of normal-appearing tissue should be removed. (d) How should the nodal basin after neoadjuvant chemotherapy be managed? One option is to screen the axilla before chemotherapy with ultrasound or SLN biopsy. If there are either clinically suspicious nodes or nodes that appear to harbor disease, SLN biopsy or ultrasound-guided FNA of the nodes in question could be performed before the start of chemotherapy to confirm metastases. If the result of the biopsy is positive, then a formal ALND should be performed during definitive surgery. A negative ultrasound-guided FNA or SLN biopsy result produces more of a dilemma. In this situation, whether to perform SLN biopsy or ALND after chemotherapy is unclear and is currently being investigated by the American College of Surgeons Oncology Group. At MDACC, oncologists routinely perform SLN biopsy after neoadjuvant chemotherapy during definitive surgery if the patients were clinically node negative by physical and ultrasound examinations prior to initiating chemotherapy.

FOLLOW-UP AFTER PRIMARY TREATMENT OF INVASIVE BREAST CANCER

After primary therapy for invasive breast cancer, patients must be made aware of the long-term risk for recurrent or metastatic disease. Although most studies report that recurrences occur within 5 years after primary therapy, recurrences can occur more than 20 years after primary therapy.

The published American Society of Clinical Oncology guidelines for follow-up indicate that there is no survival advantage to routine laboratory and radiographic studies because early detection of metastatic disease rarely affects the overall survival rate. Instead, patients should meet with their doctors for discussion of new symptoms, physical exams, and yearly mammograms. Scheduled follow-up visits should be undertaken every 4 months for years 1 and 2, every 6 months for years 3 through 5, and every 12 months thereafter. Monthly self-examination of the breasts is also recommended. Mammography is done 6 months after the completion of BCT to allow surgery- and radiation-induced changes to stabilize, and then yearly. For patients who have undergone mastectomy, a contralateral mammogram is obtained yearly. Routine bone scans, skeletal surveys, and computed tomographic scans of the abdomen and brain yield an extremely low rate of occult metastases in otherwise asymptomatic patients and is not cost-effective for patients with early-stage breast cancer.

LOCALLY RECURRENT BREAST CANCER

The time course, clinical significance, and prognosis of locally recurrent breast cancer vary dramatically between patients undergoing BCT and those undergoing mastectomy. Local recurrence rates of 5% to 10% at 8 to 10 years have been reported for patients with conserved breasts. Local recurrence typically occurs over a protracted time and is associated with systemic metastases in less than 10% of patients. Local recurrence following lumpectomy is curable in most cases; 50% to 63% of patients with local recurrence will remain disease-free 5 years after salvage mastectomy.

In contrast, local chest wall recurrence following mastectomy typically occurs within the first 2 to 3 years after surgery. It is associated with distant metastases in as many as two thirds of patients and results in eventual death for many. One third of patients with chest wall recurrence will have concurrent distant metastatic disease, and within 1 year, half will have distant disease. The median survival in this setting is 2 to 3 years.

Although unclear, patients with an apparently isolated local recurrence after BCT can often be treated without systemic cytotoxic chemotherapy depending on the stage at presentation. Any patient with a local recurrence, especially chest wall recurrences after mastectomy, should undergo complete restaging after detection of the recurrence. For patients with a purely local recurrence, surgical excision plus radiation therapy provides better local control than does either modality alone.

METASTATIC BREAST CANCER

Metastatic breast cancer generally cannot be cured, and treatment is mainly palliative. The median survival after detection of distant metastases is 2 years, but some patients live for many years. Other than trastuzumab-based chemotherapy, chemotherapy rarely prolongs survival and is directed at improving tumor-related symptoms and slowing the spread of the tumor. The most common site of distant metastatic spread is the osseous skeleton; other common sites are the soft tissues, lymph nodes, lungs, pleura, and liver. Certain subtypes of breast cancer present different patterns of metastases. For example, patients with rapidly growing, hormone receptor-negative, and poorly differentiated tumors are likely to have metastases to visceral organs (e.g., liver, lungs, brain), whereas patients with slowly growing, hormone receptor-positive, and well-differentiated tumors are likely to develop metastases to bone and soft tissues and are less likely to exhibit early life-threatening manifestations.

For patients with metastases, the decision to treat with systemic chemotherapy or hormonal therapy rests on several issues: the site and extent of the disease, hormone receptor status, disease-free interval, age, and menopausal status. Patients with slowly growing, limited, and non–life-threatening metastatic disease and hormone receptor-positive or known hormone-responsive tumors are generally offered hormonal therapy as the first therapeutic modality. Because all hormonal manipulations used today have a better therapeutic ratio than do cytotoxic therapies, the practical result of sequential hormonal therapies is that patients can be actively treated with few systemic side effects. When hormonal therapy is no longer effective, these patients proceed to chemotherapy. For patients with more extensive (i.e., symptomatic) or life-threatening disease and for all patients with hormone receptor-negative breast cancer, combination chemotherapy is the first treatment of choice. Anthracyclines (e.g., doxorubicin) and taxanes (e.g., paclitaxel, docetaxel) are currently the most effective antitumor agents against metastatic breast cancer.

The choice of initial chemotherapy depends on the patient's age, performance status, prior neoadjuvant and adjuvant chemotherapy, and disease-free interval. Anthracyclines or taxanes are options, as are capecitabine, vinorelbine, and gemcitabine. Because metastatic breast cancer is incurable with standard therapies, enrollment in clinical trials is always encouraged. Targeted agents against epidermal growth factor receptor, vascular endothelial growth factor, and other tumor-related proteins are actively under investigation. Trastuzumab-based chemotherapy is the standard of care for those with *HER-2/neu*-amplified tumors; however, for all other patients, combination chemotherapy has not been shown to prolong survival over sequential single agents, and it is associated with more intense side effects. Thus, outside of a clinical trial, patients with metastatic breast cancer are typically treated with sequential single agents.

BREAST CANCER AND PREGNANCY

The incidence of breast cancer, which accounts for 2.8% of breast malignancies, detected during pregnancy is 2 per 10,000 gestations. The diagnosis of breast cancer is typically more difficult in a pregnant woman because of a low level of suspicion based on a generally young patient age, the relative frequency of nodular changes in the breast during pregnancy, and the increase in breast density during pregnancy that renders mammographic imaging less accurate. For these and other reasons, diagnosis of breast cancer during pregnancy is frequently delayed. This delay, rather than specific differences in the biology of breast cancer between pregnant and nonpregnant women, likely explains the relatively poor prognosis for women with breast cancer detected during pregnancy. When matched for tumor stage, pregnant women with breast cancer appear to have a similar prognosis as nonpregnant patients with breast cancer.

Because the accuracy of mammography is limited in this setting, all persistent and suspicious breast masses discovered during pregnancy should undergo evaluation by FNA, core-needle biopsy, or excisional biopsy plus an ultrasound examination. Excisional biopsy under local anesthesia is safe at any time during pregnancy. Incisional biopsy is not recommended for diagnosis because of the possibility of the patients developing a fistula. Although controversial, when cancer is diagnosed, mammography can still be performed in the gravid female when the fetus is shielded adequately. Once a diagnosis of malignancy is established, treatment decisions are influenced by the specific trimester of pregnancy. For women who want to complete their pregnancies, the goal should be curative treatment of the breast cancer without injury to the fetus. Termination of pregnancy in the hope of minimizing hormonal stimulation of the tumor does not alter maternal survival and is not recommended.

Surgical treatment of gestational breast cancer is generally identical to that of nongestational breast cancer. There is no evidence that extra-abdominal surgical procedures are associated with premature labor or that the typically used anesthetic agents are teratogenic. Modified radical mastectomy as primary therapy can be undertaken at any point during pregnancy without undue risk to the mother or fetus. For cancer detected during the third trimester, delaying primary treatment for up to 4 weeks to allow for delivery before surgery is acceptable. If modified radical mastectomy is undertaken during pregnancy, breast reconstruction should not be performed simultaneously; a symmetric result is impossible until the postpartum appearance of the contralateral breast is known.

For women desiring breast conservation, treatment is complicated by the fact that radiation therapy is contraindicated during pregnancy. For cancers detected during the third trimester, lumpectomy and axillary dissection can be performed safely using general anesthesia, and radiation therapy can be delayed until after delivery. Longer delays may be detrimental to maternal outcome, although the time limit within which radiation therapy must be carried out to minimize the risk of local recurrence is unknown.

It may be necessary to administer cytotoxic adjuvant chemotherapy during pregnancy, which may raise fears of congenital malformations. Most studies have demonstrated no increased risk of fetal malformation associated with chemotherapy administered during the second and third trimesters. In contrast, chemotherapy administration during the first trimester is associated with an increased incidence of spontaneous abortion and congenital malformation, especially when methotrexate is used.

CYSTOSARCOMA PHYLLODES

Cystosarcoma phyllodes represents an uncommon fibroepithelial breast neoplasm and accounts for only 0.5% to 1% of breast carcinomas. These tumors can occur in women of all ages, including adolescents and the elderly, but most arise in women between 35 and 55 years of age. Cystosarcoma phyllodes are typically quite large and have a mean diameter of 4 to 5 cm. Because phyllodes tumors and fibroadenomas are mammographically indistinguishable, the decision to perform excisional biopsy is usually based on large tumor size, a history of rapid growth, and patient age. Predicting the behavior of these tumors on the basis of histopathological features such as histiotype (benign vs. indeterminate vs. malignant), margin status, stromal overgrowth, and size has been difficult partly because of their rarity. Common sites of metastases from malignant cystosarcoma phyllodes are lung, bone, and mediastinum.

Appropriate treatment for phyllodes tumors is complete surgical excision. Breast conservation surgery with appropriate margins is the preferred primary therapy. The incidence of local recurrence ranges from 5% to 15% for benign tumors and 20% to 30% for malignant tumors. Local recurrences are typically salvageable with total mastectomy and do not affect the overall survival rate. For all phyllodes tumors, the low incidence of axillary nodal metastases (less than 1%) obviates lymphadenectomy. The reported rates of distant metastasis for patients with malignant tumors range from 25% to 40%. The presence of stromal overgrowth may be the strongest predictor of distant metastasis and ultimate outcome. To date, no role for radiation therapy, chemotherapy, or hormonal therapy has been established for this disease.

RECOMMENDED READING

Anonymous. American Joint Committee on Cancer (AJCC). *AJCC Cancer Staging Manual.* 6th ed. 2002. Springer-Verlag publishers.

Anonymous. Polychemotherapy for early breast cancer: an overview of the randomized trials. Early Breast Cancer Trialists' Collaborative Group. *Lancet* 1998;352:930.

Anonymous. Tamoxifen for early breast cancer: an overview of the randomized trials. Early Breast Cancer Trialists' Collaborative Group. *Lancet* 1998;351:1451.

Barnavon Y, Wallack MK. Management of the pregnant patient with carcinoma of the breast. *Surg Gynecol Obstet* 1990;171:347.

Baum M, Buzdar A, Cuzick J, et al. The ATAC (Arimidex, Tamoxifen Alone or in Combination) Trialists' Group. Anastrozole alone or in combination with tamoxifen versus tamoxifen alone for adjuvant treatment of postmenopausal women with early-stage breast cancer: results of the ATAC (Arimidex, tamoxifen alone or in combination) trial efficacy and safety update analyses. *Cancer* 2003;98:1802.

Braun S, Pantel K, Muller P, et al. Cytokeratin-positive cells in the bone marrow and survival of patients with stage I, II, or III breast cancer. *N Engl J Med* 2000;342:525.

Cady B. A contemporary view of axillary dissection. *Breast Dis Year Book Q* 2001;12:22.

Chaney AW, Pollack A, McNeese MD, et al. Primary treatment of cystosarcoma phyllodes of the breast. *Cancer* 2000;89:1502.

Fisher B, Anderson S, Redmond CK, et al. Reanalysis and results after 12 years of follow-up in a randomized clinical trial comparing total mastectomy with lumpectomy with or without irradiation in the treatment of breast cancer. *N Engl J Med* 1995;333:1456.

Fisher B, Bryant J, Wolmark N, et al. Effect of preoperative chemotherapy on the outcome of women with operable breast cancer. *J Clin Oncol* 1998;16:2672.

Fisher B, Redmond C, Fisher ER, et al. Ten-year results of a randomized clinical trial comparing radical mastectomy and total mastectomy with or without radiation. *N Engl J Med* 1985;312:674.

Giuliano AE. Sentinel lymph node dissection in breast cancer. *Proc Am Soc Clin Oncol* 2001;530.

Greco M, Agresti R, Cascinelli N, et al. Breast cancer patients treated without axillary surgery: clinical implications and biologic analysis. *Ann Surg* 2000;232:1.

Grodstein F, Meir S, Graham C, et al. Postmenopausal hormone therapy and mortality. *N Engl J Med* 1997;336:1769.

Harris JR, Lippman ME, Veronesi U, et al. Breast cancer. *N Engl J Med* 1992;327:319, 390, 473.

Henderson IC. Risk factors for breast cancer development. *Cancer* 1993;71(suppl 6):2128.

Hortobagyi GN. Treatment of breast cancer. *N Engl J Med* 1998; 339:974.

Jemal A, Tiwari RC, Murray T, et al. Cancer Statistics 2004. *CA: Cancer J Clin* 2004;54:8.

Keisch M, Vicini F, Kuske RR, et al. Initial clinical experience with the MammoSite breast brachytherapy applicator in women with early-stage breast cancer treated with breast-conserving therapy. *Int J Radiat Oncol Biol Phys* 2003;55:289.

Khanna MM, Mark RJ, Silverstein MJ, et al. Breast conservation management of breast tumors 4 cm or larger. *Arch Surg* 1992; 9:1038.

Krag D, Weaver D, Ashikaga T, et al. The sentinel node in breast cancer: a multicenter validation study. *N Engl J Med* 1998; 339:941.

Kuerer HM, Hunt KK, Newman LA, et al. Neoadjuvant chemotherapy in women with invasive breast carcinoma: conceptual basis and fundamental surgical issues. *J Am Coll Surg* 2000;190: 350.

McGuire WL, Clark GM. Prognostic factors and treatment decisions in axillary node-negative breast cancer. *N Engl J Med* 1992; 326:1756.

Morrow M, Harris JR, Schnitt SJ. Local control following breast-conserving surgery for invasive cancer: results of clinical trials. *J Natl Cancer Inst* 1995; 87:1669.

Overgaard M, Hansen PS, Overgaard J, et al. Postoperative radiotherapy in high-risk premenopausal women with breast cancer who receive adjuvant chemotherapy. Danish Breast Cancer Cooperative Group 82b Trial. *N Engl J Med* 1997; 337:949.

Singletary SE. Rating the risk factors for breast cancer. *Ann Surg* 2003;237:474.

Singletary SE. Systemic treatment after sentinel lymph node biopsy in breast cancer: who, what, and why? *J Am Coll Surg* 2001;192:220.

SEER cancer registry database. www.seer.cancer.gov

Sonnenschein E, Toniolo P, Terry MB, et al. Body fat distribution and obesity in pre- and postmenopausal breast cancer. *Int J Epidemiol* 1999;28:1026.

Staren ED, Omer S. Hormone replacement therapy in postmenopausal women. *Am J Surg* 2004;188:136.

Melanoma

Timothy M. Pawlik and Jeffrey E. Gershenwald

EPIDEMIOLOGY

The incidence of invasive cutaneous melanoma in the United States has been rising by an average of 3% per year. An estimated 68,780 cases of invasive melanoma will be diagnosed in the United States in 2006. For Americans, the current estimated lifetime risk of developing melanoma is 1 in 74; an estimated 10,710 people will die of melanoma in 2006. The incidence of melanoma has been increasing faster than that of any other cancer. The major environmental risk factor, exposure to ultraviolet B (UV-B) radiation, is reflected in geographic and ethnic patterns of melanoma rates. Although there is some evidence that the increase in melanoma incidence has abated very recently—possibly as a result of increased early detection, changes in recreational behavior, and increased sun protection—it is unclear when the melanoma epidemic will peak and how geographic patterns will change over time. There have been changes in the distribution and stage of melanoma at diagnosis, with an increase in thinner lesions. At present, many melanomas seen at many institutions are less than 1 mm thick.

RISK FACTORS

Identifying risk factors and estimating an individual's risk of developing melanoma are important. Stratifying patients by risk can be clinically useful in determining primary prevention strategies and in directing the level of screening. Patients identified as being at high risk for melanoma should be recruited to prevention trials. Multiple factors can place a patient at risk for developing melanoma:

1. *Skin type:* People with a white racial background have at least ten times the melanoma incidence of African Americans and seven times the melanoma incidence of American Hispanics. In addition, white patients who are fair or who have red hair, light skin, or blue eyes have a particular propensity to be at increased risk for melanoma.
2. *Age:* The incidence of melanoma increases with age. Data have shown that the incidence of melanoma is similar in women and men younger than 50 years and higher in men than in women older than 50 years.
3. *Gender:* In general, the incidence of melanoma is higher in men than in women. Specifically, a man's risk of melanoma development over his lifetime is 1.7 times a woman's risk.
4. *Tanning bed use:* The use of a tanning bed more than ten times per year is associated with a doubling in the risk of melanoma for patients age 30 years or older. Young patients who use tanning booths more than ten times per year have

more than seven times the melanoma risk of patients who do not use tanning booths.

5. *Previous melanoma:* The risk of developing a second melanoma in a patient who has had a melanoma is 3% to 7%; this risk is more than 900 times that of the general population.
6. *Sunlight exposure:* Occasional or recreational exposure to sunlight, especially a history of severe blistering sunburn, has been associated with increased risk of melanoma. There is a correlation between the number of severe and painful sunburn episodes and the risk of melanoma; patients who have a history of ten or more severe sunburns are more than twice as likely to develop a melanoma compared with patients who have no history of sunburns. It is important to note that even sunburns after the age of 20 years may be associated with an increased risk of melanoma. The effects of sunlight have been attributed to exposure to UV-B radiation, which, according to hypothetical mechanisms of melanoma induction, may account for approximately two-thirds of melanomas.
7. *Benign nevi:* Although a benign nevus is most likely not a precursor of melanoma, the presence of large numbers of nevi has been consistently associated with an increased risk of melanoma. Persons with more than 50 nevi, all of which are greater than 2 mm in diameter, have 5 to 17 times the melanoma risk of persons with fewer nevi.
8. *Family history:* A family history of melanoma increases a person's risk of melanoma by three to eight times. Persons who have two or more family members with melanoma are at a particularly high risk for developing melanoma.
9. *Genetic predisposition:* Specific genetic alterations have been implicated in the pathogenesis of melanoma. At least four distinct genes—located on chromosomes 1p, 6q, 7, and 9—may play a role in melanoma. A tumor suppressor gene located on chromosome 9p21 is probably involved in familial and sporadic cutaneous melanoma. Deletions or rearrangements of chromosomes 10 and 11 are also well documented in cutaneous melanoma. More recently, genetic research has identified specific variants that confer susceptibility to cutaneous malignant melanoma. Variants outside the coding region of the *CDKN2A* gene are associated with melanoma predisposition. A mutation in the 5′ untranslated end of *CDKN2A* generates a novel upstream initiation codon that abrogates expression of p16, which is necessary for tumor suppression.

   Another genetic alteration that may play a role is mutation in the B-RAF gene. RAF proteins are a family of serine/threonine-specific protein kinases that form part of a signaling module that regulates cell proliferation, differentiation, and survival. In mammals, there are three isoforms: A-RAF, B-RAF, and C-RAF. Recently, it was shown that the B-RAF isoform is mutated in a high proportion (60%–70%) of melanomas. The majority of the mutations that have been found in B-RAF are somatic changes presumed to be induced by environmental factors. Most studies have concluded that

B-RAF is not a melanoma predisposition gene. Rather, some investigators have proposed a model in which B-RAF plays a key role in protecting against progression in the early stages of the disease. One mutation, a glutamic-acid-for-valine substitution at position 600 (V600E), accounts for more than 90% of the B-RAF mutations in melanoma. This mutation causes activation of downstream effectors of the mitogen-activated protein kinase-signaling cascade, leading to melanoma tumor progression by an unknown mechanism.

10. *Atypical mole and melanoma syndrome:* Previously known as dysplastic nevus syndrome, atypical mole and melanoma syndrome is characterized by the presence of large numbers of atypical moles (dysplastic nevi) that represent a distinct clinicopathological type of melanocytic lesion. They can be precursors of melanoma and/or markers of increased melanoma risk. Although the actual frequency of an atypical mole progressing to melanoma is small, patients with atypical mole and melanoma syndrome should be observed closely, and family members should also be screened.

CLINICAL PRESENTATION

Clinical features of melanoma include variegated color, irregular raised surface, irregular perimeter, and surface ulceration. A biopsy should be performed on any pigmented lesion that undergoes a change in size, configuration, or color. The so-called *ABCDE*s of early diagnosis are an easy mnemonic device to help physicians and laypersons remember the early signs of malignant melanoma. *A* denotes lesion asymmetry, *B* border irregularity, *C* color variegation, *D* diameter greater than 6 mm, and *E* a lesion that is evolving or enlarging.

When a patient presents with a lesion suggestive of melanoma, a thorough physical examination must be performed, with particular emphasis on the skin, all nodal basins, and subcutaneous tissues. Chest radiography and liver function studies should be performed if invasive melanoma is confirmed. Further evaluation is based on pathological findings. In general, we discourage routine extensive evaluation with computed tomography or positron emission tomography (PET) because their yield in the absence of symptoms, abnormal laboratory findings, or abnormal findings on chest radiography is very low in patients with primary melanoma.

MELANOMA BIOPSY

The choice of biopsy technique varies according to the anatomical site, size, and shape of the lesion. Definitive therapy must be considered in choosing a biopsy technique. Either an excisional biopsy or an incisional biopsy using a scalpel or punch is acceptable. An excisional biopsy allows the pathologist to most accurately determine the thickness of the lesion. For excisional biopsies, a narrow margin of normal-appearing skin (1–3 mm) is taken with the specimen. An elliptical incision is used to facilitate closure. The biopsy incision should be oriented to facilitate later wide local excision (e.g., longitudinally on extremities) and minimize the need for a skin graft to provide wound closure. We reserve punch biopsy for lesions that are large, are located on anatomical areas where maximum preservation of surrounding skin is important, or can be completely excised with a 6-mm punch. Punch biopsies should be performed at the most raised or darkest area of the lesion. Full-thickness biopsy into the subcutaneous tissue must be performed to permit proper microstaging of the lesion (see the T Staging section later in this chapter).

Shave biopsies are discouraged if a diagnosis of melanoma is being considered. Fine-needle aspiration biopsy may be used to document nodal and extranodal melanoma metastases but should not be used to diagnose primary melanomas. In general, we send all pigmented lesions for permanent-section examination and perform definitive surgery at a later time.

PATHOLOGY

Although the pathological analysis primarily consists of microscopic examination of hematoxylin-eosin–stained tumor, several melanocytic cell markers may also be useful in confirming the diagnosis of melanoma. Two antibodies widely used in immunohistochemical evaluations are S-100 and HMB-45. S-100 is expressed not only by more than 90% of melanomas, but also by several other tumors and some normal tissues, including dendritic cells. In contrast, the monoclonal antibody HMB-45 is relatively specific (yet not as sensitive) for proliferative melanocytic cells and melanoma. It is therefore an excellent confirmatory stain for neoplastic cells when the diagnosis of melanoma is being considered. Recently, anti-MART-1 staining has also been shown to be useful in the diagnosis of melanoma.

The major types of melanoma are as follows:

1. *Superficial spreading melanomas* constitute the majority of melanomas (approximately 70%) and generally arise in a preexisting nevus.
2. *Nodular melanomas* are the second most common type (15%–30%). Nodular melanomas progress to invasiveness more quickly than other types; however, when depth of the melanoma is controlled for, nodular melanomas are associated with the same prognosis as other lesions.
3. *Lentigo maligna melanomas* constitute a small percentage of melanomas (4%–10%). These lesions occur in sun-exposed areas and are related to sun exposure. Lentigo maligna melanomas are typically located on the faces of older white women. Many years can elapse before a lentigo maligna melanoma becomes invasive. In general, lentigo maligna melanomas are large (>3 cm at diagnosis), flat lesions and are uncommon in individuals younger than 50 years. Although these lesions have traditionally been believed to be less aggressive, the prognosis of patients with lentigo maligna melanoma ultimately depends on the depth of invasion.
4. *Acral lentiginous melanomas* occur on the palms (palmar), soles (plantar), or beneath the nail beds (subungual), although not all palmar, plantar, and subungual melanomas are acral lentiginous melanomas. These melanomas account for only 2% to 8% of melanomas in white patients but for a substantially higher proportion of melanomas (35%–60%) in darker-skinned patients. They are often large, with an average diameter of approximately 3 cm.

5. *Amelanotic melanomas* are melanomas that occur without pigmentation changes. These lesions are uncommon and are more difficult to diagnose because of their lack of pigmentation. Factors such as change in size, asymmetry, and irregular borders suggest malignancy and should prompt a biopsy.

STAGING

The melanoma staging system has been revised numerous times as understanding of the disease has evolved. In 2002, the American Joint Committee on Cancer (AJCC) published a revised staging system for cutaneous melanoma in the sixth edition of the *AJCC Cancer Staging Manual.* The revisions reflect the results of an extensive survival analysis of prognostic factors that was conducted using data from nearly 30,000 melanoma patients. Features of the revised system include new strata for primary tumor thickness, incorporation of primary tumor ulceration as an important staging criterion in both the tumor (T) and node (N) classifications, revision of the N classification to reflect the importance of regional nodal tumor burden, and new categories for stage IV disease (Tables 3.1 and 3.2).

T Classification

Breslow tumor thickness and tumor ulceration serve as the dominant prognostic factors in the T classification. A third prognostic factor—Clark level of invasion—is important for patients with thin (T1) primary lesions.

Breslow tumor thickness, measured in millimeters, is determined by using an ocular micrometer to measure the total vertical height of the melanoma from the granular layer to the area of deepest penetration. Clark level of invasion is determined by using an ocular micrometer to determine the depth of penetration into the dermis. Consistent and uniform data now support the conclusion that measurement of Breslow tumor thickness is more reproducible than measurement of Clark level of invasion and that Breslow tumor thickness is the more accurate predictor of outcome. Moreover, the AJCC Melanoma Task Force has adopted the Breslow depth values of 1, 2, and 4 mm as cut-offs for the T categories (Table 3.1). However, Clark level of invasion remains an important prognostic factor for patients with T1 lesions (Table 3.1).

Primary tumor ulceration is histopathologically defined as the absence of an intact epidermis overlying a portion of the primary tumor. Importantly, ulcerated melanomas are associated with a significantly worse prognosis than nonulcerated melanomas of the same thickness. In the T category of the AJCC staging system, the letter *a* signifies a nonulcerated lesion, while *b* signifies an ulcerated lesion. Ulcerated primary melanomas are classified in the same stage as nonulcerated lesions of the next higher T category (e.g., T1b and T2a lesions are both stage Ib) (Table 3.2).

N Classification

In both the previous version of the AJCC staging system and the new, revised version, regional nodal tumor burden is the most important predictor of survival in patients without distant

Table 3.1. 2002 American Joint Committee on cancer TNM classification for cutaneous melanoma

T Classification	Thickness	Ulceration Status
T1	≤1.0 mm	a: Without ulceration and level II/III b: With ulceration or level IV/V
T2	1.01–2.0 mm	a: Without ulceration b: With ulceration
T3	2.01–4.0 mm	a: Without ulceration b: With ulceration
T4	>4.0 mm	a: Without ulceration b: With ulceration
N Classification	**No. of Metastatic Nodes**	**Nodal Metastatic Mass**
N1	1 node	a: Micrometastasis[a] b: Macrometastasis[b]
N2	2–3 nodes	a: Micrometastasis b: Macrometastasis c: In-transit met(s)/ satellite(s) without metastatic nodes
N3	4 or more metastatic nodes, or matted nodes, or in-transit met(s)/satellite(s) with metastatic node(s)	
M Classification	**Site**	**Serum Lactate Dehydrogenase Level**
M1a	Distant skin, subcutaneous, or nodal metastases	Normal
M1b	Lung metastases	Normal
M1c	All other visceral metastases	Normal
	Any distant metastasis	Elevated

[a]Micrometastases are diagnosed after sentinel or elective lymphadenectomy.
[b]Macrometastases are defined as clinically detectable nodal metastases confirmed by therapeutic lymphadenectomy or nodal metastases that exhibit gross extracapsular extension.
Adapted from Balch CM, Buzaid AC, Soong SJ, et al. Final version of the American Joint Committee on Cancer staging system for cutaneous melanoma. *J Clin Oncol* 2001;19:3635–3648, with permission.

Table 3.2. 2002 American Joint Committee on cancer stage groupings for cutaneous melanoma

	Clinical Staging[a]			Pathological Staging[b]		
	T	N	M	T	N	M
0	Tis	N0	M0	Tis	N0	M0
IA	T1a	N0	M0	T1a	N0	M0
IB	T1b	N0	M0	T1b	N0	M0
	T2a	N0	M0	T2a	N0	M0
IIA	T2b	N0	M0	T2b	N0	M0
	T3a	N0	M0	T3a	N0	M0
IIB	T3b	N0	M0	T3b	N0	M0
	T4a	N0	M0	T4a	N0	M0
IIC	T4b	N0	M0	T4b	N0	M0
III[c]	Any T	N1	M0	—	—	—
		N2				
		N3				
IIIA	—	—	—	T1–4a	N1a	M0
				T1–4a	N2a	M0
IIIB	—	—	—	T1–4b	N1a	M0
				T1–4b	N2a	M0
				T1–4a	N1b	M0
				T1–4a	N2b	M0
				T1–4a/b	N2c	M0
IIIC	—	—	—	T1–4b	N1b	M0
				T1–4b	N2b	M0
				Any T	N3	M0
IV	Any T	Any N	Any M1	Any T	Any N	Any M1

[a]Clinical staging includes microstaging of the primary melanoma and clinical and/or radiologic evaluation for metastases. By convention, it should be used after complete excision of the primary melanoma with clinical assessment for regional and distant metastases.
[b]Pathological staging includes microstaging of the primary melanoma and pathological information about the regional lymph nodes gained after partial or complete lymphadenectomy. Pathological stages 0 and 1A are the exceptions; patients with this stage of disease do not require pathological evaluation of the lymph nodes.
[c]There are no stage III subgroups for clinical staging.
Adapted from Balch CM, Buzaid AC, Soong SJ, et al. Final version of the American Joint Committee on Cancer staging system for cutaneous melanoma. *J Clin Oncol* 2001;19:3635–3648, with permission.

disease. The description of the nodal tumor burden, however, was markedly refined in the latest staging system. This change reflects the increasing use of cutaneous lymphoscintigraphy, lymphatic mapping, and sentinel lymph node biopsy (SLNB), which have significantly enhanced the ability to detect nodal metastases in the regional nodal basin.

In the new staging system, both the actual number of lymph nodes and the tumor burden (microscopic vs. macroscopic) within the node are taken into account. Patients who have clinically negative lymph nodes but pathologically documented nodal metastases are defined as having "microscopic" or "clinically occult" nodal metastases (designated by the letter *a* in the N category of the new staging system). In contrast, patients with clinical evidence of nodal metastases that is confirmed on pathological examination are defined as having "macroscopic" or "clinically apparent" nodal metastases (designated by the letter *b* in the N category of the new staging system). Survival rates for patients with macroscopic nodal disease are significantly worse than rates for patients with microscopic nodal disease. Data from the World Health Organization (WHO) Melanoma Program showed that patients who underwent wide local excision and concomitant elective regional lymph node dissection and were found on pathological review to have microscopic nodal disease fared significantly better than patients who underwent wide local excision followed by therapeutic lymphadenectomy performed when nodal disease became clinically evident (5-year survival rates, 48.2% vs. 26.6%, $p = 0.04$).

Multiple studies have demonstrated that the number of pathologically involved lymph nodes is a dominant and independent predictor of outcome in patients with melanoma. In the analysis on which the new AJCC staging system is based, the best prognostic grouping of positive nodes was one versus two to three versus four or more. These cut-offs for number of positive nodes have therefore been incorporated into the N classification of the AJCC staging system.

Interestingly, the presence of tumor ulceration, a dominant prognostic factor within the T classification system, has also been shown to be an independent adverse prognostic factor in patients with regional nodal disease. In fact, ulceration of the primary tumor was the only primary tumor prognostic feature that independently predicted survival in patients with nodal metastases. As such, patients with an ulcerated primary lesion are upstaged within the N category (as well as the T category) compared with patients with similar nodal tumor burden with a nonulcerated primary lesion (Table 3.3).

The presence of clinically or microscopically detectable satellite metastases around a primary melanoma or in-transit metastases between the primary tumor and regional lymph nodes (see the Management of In-transit Metastases section later in this chapter) portends a poor prognosis. In recognition of this important concept and in view of the similar survival rates among patients with satellite and in-transit metastases, the AJCC Melanoma Task Force omitted "satellitosis" from the T category, in which it was formerly included, and in-transit metastasis or satellite(s) are now assigned a separate classification, N2c. Furthermore, because patients who have both satellites or in-transit metastases and concomitant lymph node metastases have a worse outcome than patients with either disease feature alone, patients with both microsatellites or in-transit metastases and lymph node metastases are classified as N3, regardless of the number of synchronous metastatic lymph nodes.

M Classification

All primary melanomas associated with distant metastatic disease are classified as stage IV. Within the M classification there is

Table 3.3. Affect of ulceration on American Joint Committee on cancer (AJCC) T classification and 5-year survival

T Classification	Thickness	Ulceration Status	5-Year Survival (%)	AJCC Stage Grouping
T1	≤1.0 mm	a: Without ulceration and level II/III	95	IA
		b: With ulceration or level IV/V	91	IB
T2	1.01–2.0 mm	a: Without ulceration	89	IB
		b: With ulceration	77	IIA
T3	2.01–4.0 mm	a: Without ulceration	79	IIA
		b: With ulceration	63	IIB
T4	>4.0 mm	a: Without ulceration	67	IIB
		b: With ulceration	45	IIC

only one group, M1, but there are three subcategories. The subcategories reflect the fact that there are survival differences among patients with metastatic disease, depending on the anatomical sites of metastasis. Distant metastases to the skin, subcutaneous tissue, or distant lymph nodes are designated M1a; they are associated with a better prognosis than metastases at any other anatomical site. Metastases to the lung are associated with an intermediate prognosis and are designated M1b. Visceral metastases are associated with the worst prognosis and are designated M1c. In general, the 1-year survival rates of patients who have M1a, M1b, and M1c disease are 59%, 57%, and 41%, respectively.

Serum lactate dehydrogenase (LDH) level is included in the M category because in the analysis on which the new AJCC staging system is based, serum LDH level was one of the most important predictors of poor prognosis in patients with metastatic disease, even after accounting for site and number of metastases. Patients with distant metastases who have an elevated serum LDH level at the time of staging are assigned to category M1c, regardless of the site of their distant metastases.

Metastatic Melanoma of Unknown Primary Site

One area of clear interest to the surgical oncologist is metastatic melanoma of unknown primary site. Approximately 5% of patients with melanoma present with metastatic disease of the lymph nodes from an unknown primary tumor. Several studies

Table 3.4. Metastatic melanoma of unknown primary: Stringent definition of patient population

Exclude patients with any of the following:
- History of having had a mole, birthmark, freckle, chronic paronychia, or skin blemish previously excised, electrodesiccated, or cauterized
- Metastatic melanoma in one of the node-bearing areas and presentation with a scar indicating previous local treatment in the skin area drained by this lymphatic basin
- No recorded physical examination of anus and genitalia
- Previous orbital enucleation or exenteration

have compared these patients with similar cohorts of patients who have equivalent nodal status and a known primary site in terms of recurrence and survival. Although patients with unknown primary tumors were historically believed to have a worse prognosis, several recent large studies have contradicted these early findings. Patients with metastatic melanoma and an unknown primary tumor must be examined carefully from scalp to toes for a potential primary tumor site. For the purpose of studying this subgroup of patients, strict criteria have been established in the course of retrospective analysis to exclude patients with potential sites of an occult primary tumor that may have been missed Table 3.4. In an important study from Memorial Sloan-Kettering Cancer Center, published by Chang and Knapper in 1982, 166 patients with metastatic melanoma of unknown primary site were reviewed retrospectively. This group comprised 4.4% of all the melanoma cases followed during the review period. These patients were compared on several parameters with a control group of patients who had known primary tumors. All patients had clinical stage II disease according to the older staging criteria in which patients with suggestive palpable lymph nodes were defined as having clinical stage II disease. The distribution of metastases in patients with unknown primary tumors was similar to that in patients with known primary tumors. Most tumors were found in the axillary lymph nodes, and many were found in the groin and cervical regions. Patients with clinical stage II disease had a 46% 5-year survival rate and a 41% 10-year survival rate, a finding similar for men and women. Patients who had residual disease in the lymphadenectomy specimen, indicating the presence of more extensive lymph node involvement, had lower survival rates. Finally, patients who had prompt lymphadenectomy had a substantially better prognosis than those who had a delay in treatment, with a threefold improvement in the 5- and 10-year survival rates. A second large series from the John Wayne Cancer Center reviewed 188 patients with lymph node metastases from unknown primary melanoma and compared these with a group of patients with a known primary tumor. Several variables—such as age, gender, anatomical site, and treatment with adjuvant immunotherapy—were similar in the two groups. In this group of patients with clinical stage II melanoma, those with lymph node metastases from an unknown primary melanoma had no significant improvement in 5- and 10-year survival rates than patients with a known primary melanoma. Recently, a retrospective analysis from the University of Pennsylvania of 40 patients with melanoma of unknown primary site revealed that overall 4-year survival rate for these patients was significantly higher than that for patients with equivalent nodal disease and a known concurrent primary melanoma (57% vs. 19%). Similarly, patients with melanoma of unknown primary site with visceral metastases had longer median survival than those with known primary tumors.

More recently, Cormier et al, from the University of Texas M. D. Anderson Cancer Center conducted a retrospective analysis of consecutive patients with melanoma (from 1990 to 2001) metastatic to regional lymph nodes. Among these patients, 71 patients with MUP and 466 controlled patients who had regional lymph node metastases of a similar stage with a known primary site were identified. The authors found that after they underwent lymph node dissection, patients with MUP were classified with Nib diseases (47%), N2b disease (14%), or N3 disease (39%). With a median follow-up of 7.7 years, the 5-year and 10-year overall survival rate were 55% and 44%, respectively, for patients with MUP, compared to 42% and 32%, respectively, for the control group (P=0.04). By multivariate analyses, age 50 years or older, male gender and N2b or N3 disease status were identified as adverse prognostics factors, and MUP was identified as a favorable prognostic factor (hazard ratio 0.61; 95% confidence interval, 0.42–0.86; P = .006) for overall survival. The authors concluded that the relatively favorable long-term survival of patients with MUP in this study have a natural history that is similar to (if not better than) the survival of many patients with Stage III disease. Therefore, patients with MUP should be treated with an aggressive surgical approach with curative intent and should be considered for stage III adjuvant therapy protocols.

MANAGEMENT OF LOCAL DISEASE

Local control of a primary melanoma requires wide excision of the tumor or biopsy site—down to but not including the deep fascia, and with a margin of normal-appearing skin. The risk of local recurrence correlates more with tumor thickness than with margins of surgical excision. Thus, it is rational to vary surgical margins according to tumor thickness.

Margin Width

Historically, even thin melanomas were excised with wide margins (3–5 cm). Studies have demonstrated, however, that narrower margins are associated with the same recurrence rates as wider margins.

The first randomized study involving surgical margins for melanomas less than 2 mm thick was reported by the WHO Melanoma Group. In an update of the study including 612 patients randomly assigned to a 1-cm or 3-cm margin of excision, there were no local recurrences among patients with primary melanomas thinner than 1 mm. There were four local recurrences among the 100 patients with melanomas 1 to 2 mm thick, and all four occurred in patients with 1-cm margins. There was no significant difference in survival between the 1- and 3-cm surgical margin groups. These results demonstrate that a narrow excision margin (i.e., 1 cm) is safe for thin (<1 mm) melanomas.

A multi-institutional prospective randomized trial from France compared 5- and 2-cm margins in 319 patients with melanomas at least 2 mm thick. There were no differences in local recurrence rate or survival between the two groups. A randomized clinical trial from the United Kingdom compared 1- and 3-cm margins in 900 patients with melanomas at least 2 mm thick. With a median follow-up time of 60 months, a 1-cm margin was associated with a significantly increased risk of locoregional recurrence; however, overall survival was similar in the two groups. A randomized prospective study conducted by the Intergroup Melanoma Committee compared 2- and 4-cm radial margins of excision for intermediate-thickness melanomas (1–4 mm). There was no difference in local recurrence rate between the two groups. Forty-six percent of patients in the 4-cm group required skin grafts, whereas only 11% of patients in the 2-cm group did ($p < 0.001$). Taken together, these data strongly support the use of a 2-cm margin for intermediate-thickness lesions.

The optimal margin width for thick melanomas (>4 mm) is still unknown. A retrospective review of 278 patients with thick primary melanomas demonstrated that the width of the excision margin (≤2 cm vs. >2 cm) did not significantly affect local recurrence, disease-free survival, or overall survival rates after a median follow-up of 27 months.

Based in large part on the data from randomized, prospective trials, several recommendations can be made for margins of excision (Table 3.5). Patients with invasive melanoma less than 1 mm thick can be treated with a 1-cm margin of excision, whereas patients with melanoma 2 to 4 mm thick can be treated with a 2-cm margin. For patients with melanoma 1 to 2 mm thick, a simple recommendation is difficult because this patient population has been studied in several trials evaluating a range of excision margins. In general, a 2-cm margin is preferred if anatomically feasible, and in regions of anatomical constraint (e.g., the face), a 1-cm margin is sufficient. This recommendation is based on the fact that overall survival was similar for patients with 1- and 3-cm margins in the WHO trial. In patients with melanoma thicker than 4 mm, a 2-cm margin is probably safe, although

Table 3.5. Summary of recommendations for excision margins

Tumor Thickness	Excision Margin
≤1 mm	1 cm
1–2 mm	1–2 cm
2–4 mm	2 cm
>4 mm	2 cm[a]

[a]No randomized prospective trials have specifically addressed this cohort.

no prospective randomized trials have specifically addressed this thickness group.

Wound Closure

If there is any question about the ability to achieve suitable wound closure, a plastic or reconstructive surgeon should be consulted. Options for closure include primary closure, skin grafting, and local and distant flaps.

Primary closure is the method of choice for most lesions, but it should be avoided when it will distort the appearance of a mobile facial feature or interfere with function. Many defects can be closed using an advancement flap, undermining the skin and subcutaneous tissues to permit primary closure. Primary closure usually requires that the longitudinal axis of an elliptical incision be at least three times the length of the short axis. Closure of the wound edges is usually performed in two layers—a dermal layer of 3-0 or 4-0 undyed absorbable sutures and either interrupted skin closure using 3-0 or 4-0 nonabsorbable sutures or a running subcuticular skin closure using 4-0 monofilament absorbable sutures. Three layers are sometimes used.

Application of a skin graft is one of the simplest reconstructive methods used for wound closure. Split-thickness skin grafts are used most commonly. For lower-extremity primary lesions, split-thickness grafts should be harvested from the extremity opposite the melanoma. In general, skin grafts should be harvested from an area remote from the primary melanoma and outside the zone of potential in-transit metastasis. A full-thickness skin graft can provide a result that is both more durable and of higher aesthetic quality than a split-thickness graft. Full-thickness grafts have most commonly been used on the face, where aesthetic considerations are most significant. Donor sites for full-thickness skin graft to the face should be chosen from locations that are likely to match the color of the face, such as the postauricular or preauricular skin or the supraclavicular portion of the neck.

Local flaps offer numerous advantages for repair of defects that cannot be closed primarily, especially on the distal extremities and on the head and neck. Color match is excellent, durability of the skin is essentially normal, and normal sensation is usually preserved. Transposition flaps and rotation flaps of many varieties have been used successfully.

Distant flaps should be used when sufficient tissue for a local flap is not available and when a skin graft would not provide adequate wound coverage. Myocutaneous flaps and free flaps can be used. Discussion of such complex methods is beyond the scope of this chapter, but these techniques are familiar to plastic and reconstructive surgeons and are discussed in greater detail in Chapter 24.

Special Anatomical Sites

Fingers and Toes

More than three-fourths of subungual melanomas involve either the great toe or the thumb. A melanoma located on the skin of a digit or beneath the nail should be removed by a digital amputation, with as much of the digit saved as possible. In general, amputations are performed at the middle interphalangeal joint of the fingers or proximal to the distal joint of the thumb. More proximal amputations are not associated with improved survival. For a melanoma located on a toe, an amputation of the entire digit at the metatarsal-phalangeal joint is indicated; for melanomas of the great toe, the amputation can be performed proximal to the interphalangeal joint. Lesions arising between two toes may require amputation of both toes.

Sole of the Foot

Excision of a melanoma on the plantar surface of the foot often produces a sizable defect in a weight-bearing area. If possible, a portion of the heel or ball of the plantar surface should be retained to bear the greatest burden of pressure. Where possible, deep fascia over the extensor tendons should be preserved as a base for skin coverage. A plantar flap, which can be raised either laterally or medially, can provide well-vascularized local tissue for weight-bearing areas, while also providing some sensation. More recently, staged closure of some plantar melanomas, particularly of the heel, have been performed with initial use of a vacuum-assisted closure device to stimulate granulation tissue followed by staged skin graft application. Such an approach may obviate complex reconstruction.

Face

Facial lesions usually cannot be excised with more than a 1-cm margin because of adjacent vital structures. The tumor diameter, the tumor thickness, and the tumor's exact location on the face must all be considered when margin width is planned.

Breast

Wide local excision with primary closure is the treatment of choice for melanoma on the skin of the breast; mastectomy is not generally recommended. As with any trunk lesion, lymphoscintigraphy should be done before selective lymphadenectomy (see the Management of Regional Lymph Nodes section later in this chapter) if selective lymphadenectomy is indicated on the basis of primary tumor factors.

Special Clinical Situations

Giant Congenital Nevi

A giant congenital nevus has been defined as a nevus that measures at least 15 cm in diameter or at least twice the size of the affected person's palm. Patients with giant congenital nevi have an estimated 6% lifetime risk of developing a melanoma. Half of the melanomas that develop in giant congenital nevi develop within the first 5 years of life. Decisions about the management of giant congenital nevi are difficult because such lesions are often so extensive that prophylactic surgical excision is impossible. When the location and size of a lesion permit prophylactic excision, excision should be considered before the age of 2 years.

Mucosal Melanoma

Patients with true mucosal melanoma—including melanoma of the mucosa of the head and neck, vagina, and anal canal—have a generally poor prognosis, regardless of surgical therapy. We usually do not recommend an aggressive surgical approach to patients with clinically localized disease. We reserve extended resection for bulky or recurrent tumors and favor therapeutic lymphadenectomy over elective lymph node dissection (see the Management of Regional Lymph Nodes section later in this chapter). In particular, we recommend local excision of anal melanomas over abdominoperineal resection. Abdominoperineal resection is associated with much greater morbidity, leaves the patient with a permanent colostomy, offers no survival advantage, and does not treat at-risk inguinal nodes unless the procedure is combined with groin dissection. Adjuvant radiation therapy may be administered to patients with mucosal melanoma in an attempt to decrease the risk of locoregional recurrence.

Desmoplastic Melanoma

Desmoplastic melanoma is an uncommon histologic variant of melanoma that is characterized by unusual spindle-cell morphology and the presence of fusiform melanocytes dispersed in a prominent collagenous stroma. Classically presenting as a thick primary tumor, desmoplastic melanoma is associated with a higher incidence of local recurrence than nondesmoplastic melanoma. Histologically, desmoplastic melanoma may display morphologic heterogeneity. Specifically, some desmoplastic melanomas are characterized by a uniform desmoplasia that is prominent throughout the entire tumor ("pure" desmoplastic melanoma), whereas other desmoplastic melanomas appear to arise in association with other histologic subtypes ("mixed" desmoplastic melanoma). Distinguishing the phenotypic heterogeneity of desmoplastic melanomas has been reported to be important for stratifying patients with regard to rate of lymph node metastasis and prognosis. Recent data indicate that patients with pure desmoplastic melanoma have a lower incidence of positive sentinel lymph nodes than do patients with mixed desmoplastic melanoma or nondesmoplastic melanoma. Although some authors have reported a worse prognosis for patients with desmoplastic melanoma, the majority of studies have described a better prognosis for patients with desmoplastic melanoma compared with patients who have nondesmoplastic melanoma of similar stage. In a few studies in which pure desmoplastic melanoma was differentiated from mixed desmoplastic melanoma, patients with mixed desmoplastic melanoma had a greater risk of death or metastatic disease than patients with the pure form.

Pregnancy

The precise influence of pregnancy or hormonal manipulation on the clinical course of malignant melanoma has not been defined. Because historical case reports suggested a poor outcome for pregnant women with melanoma, some investigators suggested that melanoma may be hormonally stimulated and therefore more aggressive in pregnant women. More recently, multiple studies have documented overall good outcomes for women with melanoma during pregnancy.

A WHO study reported that women who were diagnosed during pregnancy had a worse prognosis compared with women diagnosed and treated before pregnancy. The two groups of women in this study were not similar; mean tumor thickness was 2.38 mm in the pregnant women and 1.49 mm in the nonpregnant women. After adjusting for this difference, there was no difference in survival. Other studies have similarly shown that tumors tend to be thicker in pregnant women than in nonpregnant women and that pregnancy at the time of diagnosis is not a significant prognostic factor in multivariate analyses. In a recent large population-based study of pregnant women conducted over a 9-year period in California, there was no evidence of a more advanced stage, thicker tumors, increased risk of metastasis to lymph nodes, or worse survival in pregnant women. Furthermore, maternal and neonatal outcomes were equivalent to those of pregnant women and their newborns without melanoma.

In aggregate, these data support the concept that malignant melanoma is not more common, more aggressive, or more lethal during pregnancy. Surgery is the treatment of choice in pregnant patients with early-stage melanoma. There is no proof that abortion protects the mother from subsequent development of metastases. Although opinions differ on planning pregnancy after a diagnosis of melanoma, the weight of evidence does not demonstrate an increased risk of developing metastatic disease with pregnancy. Furthermore, several studies have found no association between oral contraceptive use and survival in melanoma.

MANAGEMENT OF LOCAL RECURRENCE

True local recurrence is defined as recurrence at the site of the primary tumor, within or continuous with the scar, and is most likely the result of incomplete excision of the primary tumor; it represents a relatively rare pattern of recurrence. In many cases, such "local recurrences" may more appropriately be considered persistence of the primary tumor. The prognosis after a true local recurrence is significantly better than that associated with in-transit disease (see the next section), and therefore the correct classification of local recurrence versus in-transit disease is important in treatment planning. A local recurrence consisting of a single lesion in a patient whose primary melanoma had favorable prognostic features may be appropriately treated with excision alone. Patients with local recurrences consisting of multiple, small and superficial lesions may be treated in a fashion similar to that used to treat patients with in-transit disease (see the next section).

MANAGEMENT OF IN-TRANSIT DISEASE

Traditionally, in-transit disease has been described as recurrent locoregional disease found in the dermis or subcutaneous tissue between the primary melanoma and the regional lymph node basin. This pattern of recurrence is unique to melanoma and is reported to occur in 5% to 10% of melanoma cases. Although the molecular determinants and pathophysiology of in-transit disease are poorly understood, in-transit recurrences are most likely an intralymphatic manifestation of melanoma metastases. Independent predictors of in-transit recurrence include age greater than 50 years, a lower-extremity primary tumor, increasing Breslow depth, ulceration, and positive sentinel lymph node (SLN) status. Regional nodal metastases occur in about two-thirds of patients with in-transit disease and, if present, are associated with lower survival rates. Predictors of distant recurrence among patients with in-transit recurrence include positive SLN status, in-transit tumor size of at least 2 cm, and disease-free interval before in-transit recurrence of less than 12 months. Interestingly, recent data suggest that patients who present with synchronous distant and in-transit disease have a worse disease-specific survival compared with patients who present with only in-transit or distant disease.

Some have suggested that dissection of the regional nodal basin—by either SLNB or complete lymphadenectomy—increases the risk of in-transit metastases. These authors hypothesize that dissection disturbs lymph flow, leading to deposition of metastatic cells in the intervening lymphatic vessels. A critical analysis of the data, however, provides compelling evidence that neither SLNB nor completion lymph node dissection in SLN-positive patients increases the incidence of in-transit metastases. In a recent review of 2,018 patients with primary melanomas at least 1 mm thick treated over a 10-year period at the Sydney Melanoma Unit, there was no significant difference in the rate of in-transit metastases between patients treated with wide local excision alone (4.9%) and those treated with wide local excision and SLNB (3.6%). Because the two groups were similar in terms of median tumor depth, rate of ulceration, and Clark level, these data strongly support the concept that early nodal intervention has little impact on the natural history of in-transit metastases. In a separate study of 1,395 patients from The University of Texas M. D. Anderson Cancer Center, patients with a positive SLN had a significantly higher rate of in-transit metastases (12%) than patients with a negative SLN (3.5%). Taken together, these data indicate that biology—not surgical technique—establishes the risk of in-transit metastases.

For patients with in-transit metastases confined to a limb that are not amenable to standard surgical measures (e.g., patients with recurrent and/or multiple in-transit metastases and patients with large-burden in-transit disease), regional chemotherapy techniques such as isolated limb perfusion or, more recently, isolated limb infusion, may be considered. Amputation is rarely indicated.

Hyperthermic Isolated Limb Perfusion

Hyperthermic isolated limb perfusion with melphalan has been used to treat in-transit metastases of the extremities since the mid-1950s. Melphalan is currently the most active single agent for use in hyperthermic isolated limb perfusion. Overall response rates of 7% to 80% (complete response rate, 46%; partial response rate, 34%) can be achieved, and the median response duration in patients with a complete response ranges from 9 to 19 months. Nonrandomized studies of hyperthermic limb perfusion by Lienard et al. reported a high complete response rate (90%) with a combination of melphalan, tumor necrosis factor-α (TNF-α), and interferon-γ (IFN-γ) and a somewhat lower response rate with melphalan alone (52%). The durability of these responses has not yet been reported. Fraker et al. reported a 100% response rate in patients treated with melphalan alone and a 90% response rate in patients treated with melphalan, IFN-γ, and TNF-α, although the latter combination resulted in a higher complete response rate (80% vs. 61%). A multicenter randomized trial sponsored by the American College of Surgeons Oncology Group comparing melphalan alone with a combination of melphalan and TNF-α for patients who have in-transit metastases was recently closed to accrual because the interim analysis failed to reveal a benefit for TNF-α. As a result, TNF-α is not currently being used in the United States in isolated limb perfusion procedures.

The routine use of hyperthermic isolated limb perfusion in the adjuvant setting has marginal, if any, benefit. Although a randomized multicenter phase III trial showed increased disease-free interval in patients with in-transit metastases and regional lymph node metastasis, this effect was transient and predominantly occurred in patients with a more favorable prognosis (tumor thickness of 1.5 to 2.99 mm). This study showed no benefit of isolated limb perfusion with respect to time to distant metastasis or survival duration.

Although hyperthermic isolated limb perfusion may be effective as primary treatment for in-transit metastases, the isolated limb perfusion technique involves a complex and invasive operative procedure entailing expensive equipment, long operating times, and considerable ancillary staff. In an attempt to achieve similar results using less complex techniques, a new regional chemotherapy technique, isolated limb infusion, has recently been developed for the management of in-transit metastases.

Isolated Limb Infusion

Isolated limb infusion is essentially a low-flow isolated limb perfusion performed via percutaneously inserted catheters, but without oxygenation of the circuit (Fig. 3.1). In general, using standard radiologic techniques, catheters are inserted percutaneously into the main artery and vein of the unaffected limb and delivered intravascularly to the contralateral tumor-bearing extremity. Under general anesthesia, after a pneumatic tourniquet is inflated proximally, cytotoxic agents (generally melphalan and actinomycin-D) are infused through the arterial catheter and "hand-circulated" with a syringe technique for 20 to 30 minutes. Progressive hypoxia occurs because, in contrast to isolated limb perfusion, no oxygenator is used. The hypoxia and acidosis associated with isolated limb infusion are therapeutically attractive because numerous cytotoxic agents, including melphalan, appear to damage tumor cells more effectively under hypoxic conditions. In fact, hypoxia and acidosis have been reported to increase the cytotoxic effects of melphalan in experimental models by a factor of three. The Sydney Melanoma Unit has also shown

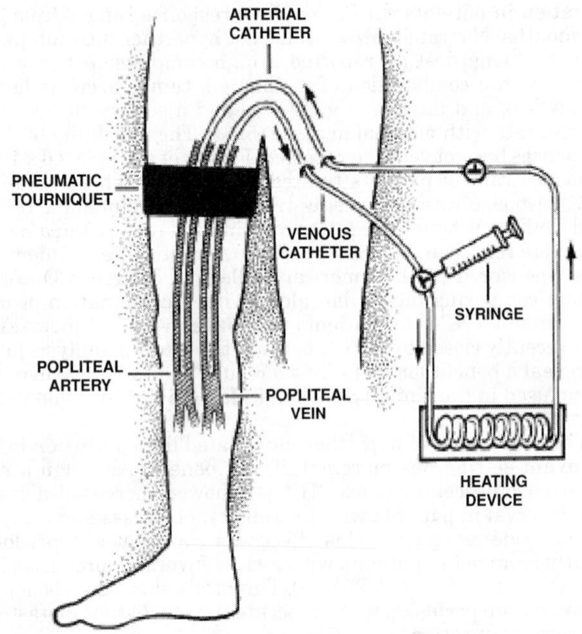

Figure 3.1. Schematic drawing depicting an isolated limb infusion. The catheters are typically placed percutaneously by an interventional radiologist via the contralateral extremity, with the catheter tips positioned in the tumor-bearing extremity just below the inguinal ligament in the superficial femoral artery and vein. After inflation of the tourniquet, chemotherapy is manually infused for 20 to 30 minutes, after which the limb is washed out with 1 liter of normal saline. (Reprinted from Lindner P, Doubrovsky A, Kam PC, et al. Prognostic factors after isolated limb infusion with cytotoxic agents for melanoma. *Ann Surg Oncol* 2002;9:127–136, with permission.)

that isolated limb infusion with fotemustine after dacarbazine chemosensitization can be successful when gross limb disease has not been controlled by one or more isolated limb infusions with melphalan.

At the completion of the drug exposure, the limb vasculature is flushed with a crystalloid solution via the arterial catheter, and the effluent is discarded. Although the limb tissues are exposed to the cytotoxic agent for only a short period (up to 30 minutes), there appears to be adequate cellular uptake for tumor cell killing. Isolated limb infusion has been shown to yield response rates similar to those observed after conventional hyperthermic isolated limb perfusion; overall response rates of 85% (complete response rate, 41%; partial response rate, 44%) have been achieved in at least one study. Because of the simplicity of the isolated infusion technique, it may be a more attractive option for patients with comorbidities or the elderly.

Toxicity and Morbidity

Hyperthermic isolated limb perfusion and isolated limb infusion can be associated with potentially significant regional adverse effects, including myonecrosis, nerve injury, compartment syndrome, and arterial thrombosis, sometimes necessitating fasciotomy or even major amputation. Following isolated limb infusion, regional adverse effects appear to be similar to those reported after conventional hyperthermic isolated limb perfusion, with 41% of patients experiencing grade II toxic effects and 53% experiencing grade III toxic effects. Systemic toxic effects, including hypotension and adult respiratory distress syndrome, have sometimes been seen with the addition of TNF-α to the perfusion or infusion regimen. Because limb perfusion or infusion requires a high degree of technical expertise and is associated with a significant risk of complications, the procedure should be performed only in centers that have experience with the technique. At present, there is little evidence to justify the use of prophylactic perfusion or infusion, except as part of a clinical trial.

MANAGEMENT OF REGIONAL LYMPH NODES

Regional lymph nodes are the most common site of melanoma metastasis. Effective palliation and sometimes cure can be achieved in patients with regional metastases. Fine-needle aspiration or core biopsy can usually yield a diagnosis in patients who develop clinically enlarged regional nodes. Open biopsy is rarely warranted.

The management of clinically negative regional lymph nodes has been the focus of a long and sometimes contentious debate. Historically, some surgeons preferred to perform lymphadenectomy only for clinically demonstrable nodal metastases. This type of excision has been termed *delayed* or *therapeutic lymph node dissection* (TLND). Other surgeons have chosen to excise the nodes even when they appeared normal in patients who are at increased risk of developing nodal metastases. This excision has been termed *immediate, prophylactic,* or *elective lymph node dissection* (ELND). More recently, many surgeons have adopted a selective approach to regional lymph node dissection—the technique of intraoperative lymphatic mapping and SLN identification originally developed by Morton et al.

Therapeutic Lymph Node Dissection

With TLND, only patients with known metastases undergo a major lymphadenectomy; this reduces the number of potentially unnecessary lymphadenectomies and may not reduce the chance for cure. The disadvantage of TLND is that delaying treatment until lymph node metastases are clinically evident may result in many patients having distant micrometastases at the time of lymphadenectomy. Chances for cure may therefore be diminished.

Elective Lymph Node Dissection

ELND has the theoretical advantage of treating melanoma nodal metastases at a relatively early stage in the natural history of the disease. The disadvantage of ELND is that many patients undergo surgery when they do not have nodal metastasis. Advocates of ELND argue that patients with clinically negative, histologically positive lymph nodes at ELND have a better chance for survival (50%–60%) than do patients in whom the regional lymph nodes are not dissected, and clinically apparent metastases develop in the regional lymph nodes during follow-up (15%–35%). None of four randomized, prospective studies assessing ELND have demonstrated an overall survival advantage for this technique. Two trials, one from the WHO and another from the Mayo Clinic, were ultimately criticized because the study populations were at low risk for occult nodal disease, and patients were therefore unlikely to benefit from the proposed surgical treatment.

Although ELND does not offer a survival benefit to all patients, two recently completed prospective randomized trials that targeted higher-risk, clinically node-negative patients suggest that ELND may have some survival benefit in certain patient subgroups. In the WHO ELND Trial, patients with truncal melanoma at least 1.5 mm thick were randomized to wide local excision and ELND versus wide local excision and observation. Updated results from this trial demonstrated that patients in the ELND treatment arm who were found to have microscopic nodal disease at ELND had better overall survival than did patients in whom palpable adenopathy developed after wide excision alone. The long-term results of the Intergroup Melanoma Trial are similar. In this trial, patients with intermediate-thickness melanomas (1.0–4.0 mm) who underwent wide excision and ELND were compared with a similar group of patients who underwent wide excision alone followed by observation of the regional nodal basin. Although this trial did not demonstrate a difference in overall 10-year survival rates, four prospectively selected subgroups were found to have significantly better 10-year survival with ELND than with nodal observation: patients whose primary tumors were without ulceration (84% vs. 77%; $p = 0.03$); patients with primary tumor thickness between 1.0 and 2.0 mm (vs. thicker) (86% vs. 80%; $p = 0.03$); patients with extremity (vs. truncal) melanoma (84% vs. 78%; $p = 0.05$); and patients younger than 60 years (81% vs. 74%; $p = 0.03$). The results of a recently published multicenter trial from Germany also demonstrated an absolute survival advantage, of at least 13%, for patients with positive nodes detected on SLNB compared with patients with positive nodes detected during observation of the nodal basin. Although this analysis was retrospective, the results were consistent with the findings of the WHO study.

Taken together, these data call into question recommendations to delay lymphadenectomy until palpable nodal disease develops; the data also support the use of alternative approaches to permit earlier identification of occult nodal disease. A more rational, selective approach, lymphatic mapping and SLNB, has now been widely adopted. This technique satisfies many proponents of both ELND and TLND.

Intraoperative Lymphatic Mapping and Sentinel Lymph Node Biopsy

Several investigators have proposed intraoperative lymphatic mapping and SLNB as a minimally invasive procedure for identifying the approximately 20% of patients who harbor occult microscopic disease. This approach is sometimes termed *selective lymphadenectomy*.

Several studies have demonstrated that the SLNs are the first nodes to contain metastases, if metastases are present, and thus the pathological status of the SLNs reflects that of the entire regional nodal basin. If the SLN lacks metastasis, the remainder of the regional lymph nodes is unlikely to contain disease, and a completion lymphadenectomy need not be performed. Multiple studies have demonstrated that the false-negative rate for SLNB is less than 4%, with the predictive value of a negative SLN approaching 99%. Other studies have confirmed the validity of the SLN concept and the accuracy of SLNB as a staging procedure. It is imperative, however, that the surgeon employing SLNB have adequate pathology and nuclear medicine support.

Technique

Lymphatic mapping and SLNB is performed at the time of wide excision of the primary tumor or biopsy site. Since the introduction of lymphatic mapping and SLNB, the technique has undergone several refinements that have resulted in improved detection of SLNs.

Use of a vital blue dye (isosulfan blue 1%) to help identify SLNs has been part of the lymphatic mapping and SLNB procedure since its introduction. The blue dye is injected into the patient intradermally around the intact tumor or biopsy site. The blue dye is taken up by the lymphatic system and carried via afferent lymphatics to the SLN. The draining nodal basin is explored, and the afferent lymphatic channels and first draining lymph nodes (the SLNs) are identified by the uptake of the blue dye. With the use of blue dye alone, a SLN is identified in approximately 85% of cases. Although this initial approach was promising, it left 15% of patients unable to benefit from SLNB because no SLN was identified.

Subsequently, two additional techniques have been incorporated that have significantly improved SLN localization: (a) preoperative lymphoscintigraphy and (b) intraoperative injection of technetium-99 (^{99}Tc)-labeled sulfur colloid accompanied by intraoperative use of a handheld gamma probe. Preoperative lymphoscintigraphy using ^{99}Tc-labeled sulfur colloid permits the identification of patients with multiple draining nodal basins and patients with lymphatic drainage to SLNs located outside standard nodal basins, including epitrochlear, popliteal, and ectopic sites (Fig. 3.2). In patients with melanomas that drain to multiple regional nodal basins, the histologic status of one draining basin does not predict the status of other basins. In one study, among

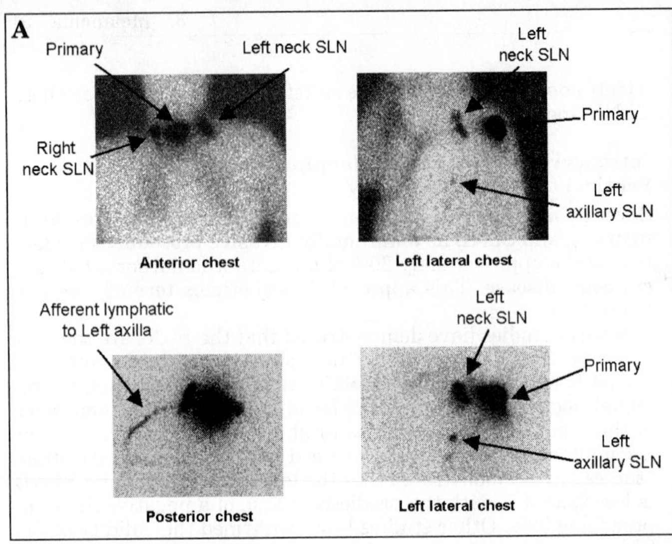
A
Primary
Left neck SLN
Right
neck SLN
Anterior chest
Left
neck SLN
Primary
Left
axillary SLN
Left lateral chest
Afferent lymphatic
to Left axilla
Posterior chest
Left
neck SLN
Primary
Left
axillary SLN
Left lateral chest

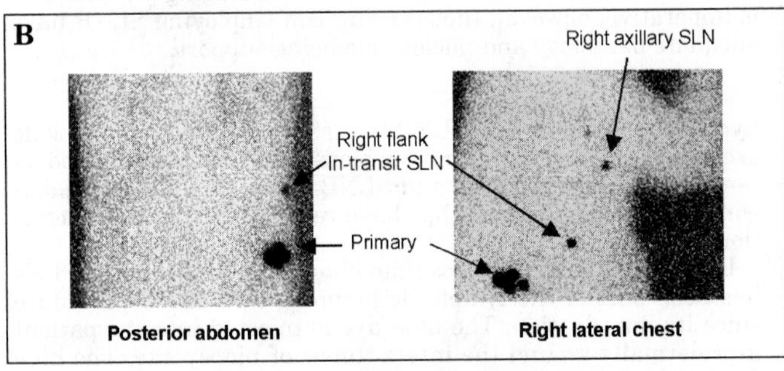
B
Right axillary SLN
Right flank
In-transit SLN
Primary
Posterior abdomen
Right lateral chest

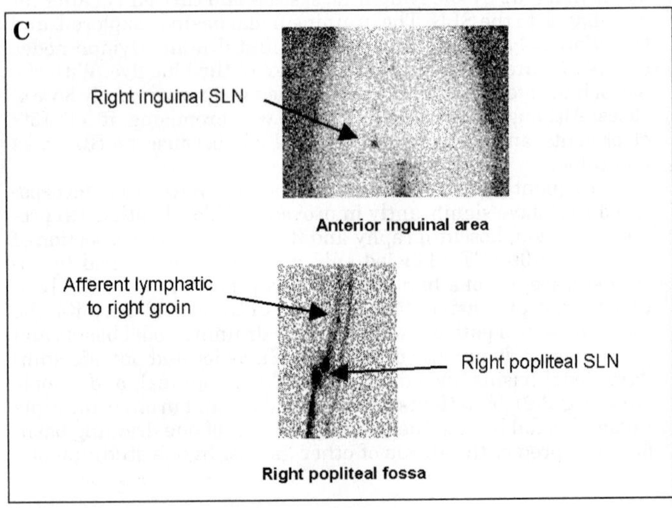
C
Right inguinal SLN
Anterior inguinal area
Afferent lymphatic
to right groin
Right popliteal SLN
Right popliteal fossa

54 patients who underwent an SLNB of an unusual nodal site, 7 (13%) had lymph node metastases in that location. In four of the seven patients, the only positive SLN was from the unusual site. Therefore, it is particularly important to identify and assess all at-risk regional nodal basins to properly stage the disease.

Probably the most important development in the SLNB technique has been the introduction of intraoperative lymphatic mapping using a handheld gamma probe. In this approach, 0.5 to 1.0 mCi of ^{99}Tc-labeled sulfur colloid is injected intradermally 1 to 4 hours before surgery. During surgery, a handheld gamma probe is used to transcutaneously identify SLNs that will be removed. The use of both blue dye and radiocolloid increases the surgeon's ability to identify the SLN (greater than 96% to 99% accuracy) compared with the use of blue dye alone (84% accuracy). Although most clinicians use this combined modality approach, some favor the single-agent strategy of ^{99}Tc-labeled sulfur colloid alone, and they have reported similarly excellent results.

Side Effects

SLNB is associated with substantially fewer postoperative complications compared with ELND, which is characterized by complete regional node extirpation. SLNB is associated with less extensive surgery and thus a lower rate of side effects. Moreover, the SLNB technique itself is associated with substantially fewer postoperative complications than ELND, including lower rates of lymphedema, pain, numbness, and loss of active range of motion. In addition, recent data have shown that the SLNB technique does not increase the incidence of in-transit recurrence compared with wide local excision alone.

Incidence and Predictors of Positive Sentinel Lymph Nodes

Knowledge of the factors predictive of a positive SLN is useful for counseling patients regarding treatment options. In most studies, the incidence of positive SLNs in patients undergoing SLNB ranges from 15% to 20%. However, multivariate analyses have revealed several factors that increase the risk of positive SLNs: increased tumor thickness, ulceration, high mitotic index, age younger than 50 years, and axial tumor location. In one report, the incidence of a positive SLN was 4% among patients with melanomas 1.0 mm or thinner and 44% among patients with melanomas thicker than 4.00 mm (Table 3.6). In the same report, patients with ulcerated primary tumors had a higher incidence of SLN metastases compared with those with nonulcerated lesions (35% vs. 12%, respectively). The incidence of SLN metastases by

Figure 3.2. Preoperative lymphoscintigraphy. After injection of ^{99}Tc-labeled sulfur colloid at the primary cutaneous melanoma site (upper midline back), preoperative lymphoscintigraphy revealed (A) drainage to multiple nodal basins (bilateral neck and left axilla), (B) "in-transit"/ectopic sentinel lymph nodes (SLNs) in the right flank region and right axilla from a primary tumor of the right lateral back, and (C) SLNs in a right lower-extremity popliteal fossa lymph node basin and a right inguinal lymph node basin from a primary tumor of the heel. (Photos courtesy of Jeffrey E. Gershenwald, MD.)

Table 3.6. Effect of ulceration on SLN metastases for a given tumor thickness ($n = 1{,}375$)

Tumor Thickness (mm)	Total Patients (%)	Positive SLN					
			Not Ulcerated		Ulcerated		p Value[a]
		All (%)	(%)	AJCC Stage[b]	(%)	AJCC Stage[b]	Ulcerated vs. Not
≤1.00	28	4	3	IA	16	IB	0.026
1.01–2.00	38	12	11	IB	22	IIA	0.007
2.01–4.00	23	28	25	IIA	34	IIB	0.115
>4.00	11	44	33	IIB	53	IIC	0.021
All Patients	100	17	12		35		<0.0001

SLN, sentinel lymph node; AJCC, American Joint Committee on Cancer.
[a]Fisher exact test for each tumor thickness group.
[b]Stage groupings calculated using tumor thickness and ulceration data only.
Reprinted from Rousseau DL, Jr, Ross MI, Johnson MM, et al. Revised American Joint Committee on Cancer staging criteria accurately predict sentinel lymph node positivity in clinically node-negative melanoma patients. *Ann Surg Oncol* 2003;10(5):569–574, with permission.

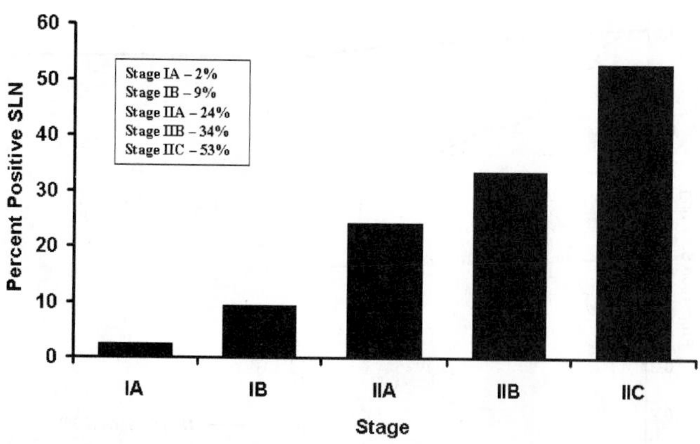

Figure 3.3. Incidence of positive sentinel lymph nodes (SLNs) by American Joint Committee on Cancer disease stage (n = 1,375). The difference between each stage is statistically significant. The *inset* shows the percentage of patients with a positive SLN within each category. (Reprinted from Rousseau DL, Jr, Ross MI, Johnson MM, et al. Revised American Joint Committee on Cancer staging criteria accurately predict sentinel lymph node positivity in clinically node-negative melanoma patients. *Ann Surg Oncol* 2003;10:569–574, with permission.)

AJCC stage is shown in Figure 3.3. The incidences of positive SLNs for stages IA, IB, IIA, IIB, and IIC were 2%, 9%, 24%, 34%, and 53%, respectively.

Prognostic Value of Sentinel Lymph Node Status

The prognostic significance of the pathological status of the SLNs has been convincingly demonstrated. Data from M. D. Anderson Cancer Center demonstrated that SLN status was the most significant clinicopathological prognostic factor with respect to survival in patients with melanoma. In an updated analysis of 1,487 patients who underwent SLNB (median tumor thickness, 1.5 mm), the 5-year survival rate for patients with positive SLNs was 73.3%, compared with 96.8% for patients with negative SLNs (Fig. 3.4) (J. Gershenwald, unpublished data, 2005). Several other multivariate regression analyses have shown that regional lymph node status is the most powerful predictor of recurrence (both regional and distant) and survival, even among patients with thick melanomas. According to a recent analysis of the AJCC database, 5-year survival rates for patients with stage III disease range from 69% for patients with only one microscopically positive lymph node and a nonulcerated primary melanoma to 13% for patients with clinically evident nodal disease with more than three pathologically involved nodes and an ulcerated primary tumor.

The prognostic importance of distinguishing between microscopically and macroscopically positive lymph nodes has been emphasized by incorporation of this criterion into the newly

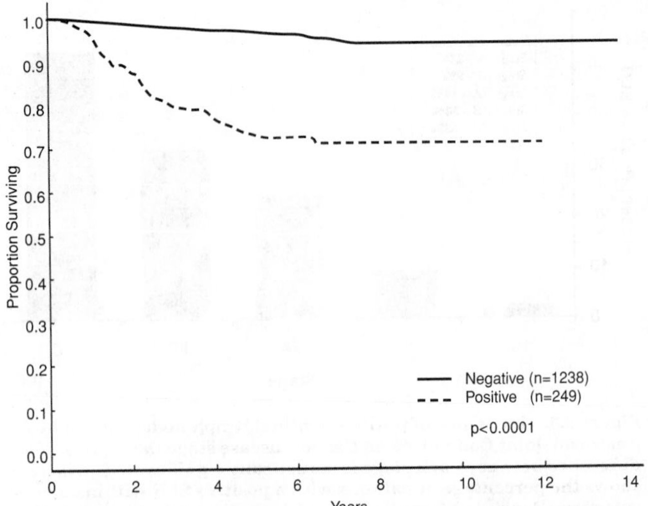

Figure 3.4. Disease-specific survival by sentinel lymph node (SLN) status in 1,487 patients. SLN status was the most significant clinicopathologial prognostic factor with respect to survival. The 5-year disease-specific survival rate was 73.3% for patients with positive SLNs, compared with 96.8% for patients with negative SLNs.

revised melanoma staging system. The concept of tumor burden will likely be important in the era of SLNB as accurate microscopic staging of SLNs becomes even more widespread and patients are better stratified on the basis of microscopic tumor burden into similar risk subgroups. In fact, several studies have shown that the diameter of the largest lymph node tumor nodule and the total lymph node tumor volume are significant predictors of recurrence and survival. In one study, a tumor deposit diameter of 3 mm was identified as a significant cut-off point: The 3-year survival probability was 86% for patients with a largest tumor deposit diameter of 3 mm or less and 27% for patients with a largest deposit diameter greater than 3 mm. In the future, as our understanding of the significance of microscopic nodal tumor burden is refined, clinical decisions regarding the need for and extent of further surgery or adjuvant therapy may also be based on the extent of microscopic nodal tumor burden.

The recently completed Multicenter Selective Lymphadenectomy Trial-I was designed to assess whether a selective approach to regional lymphadenectomy—limiting complete nodal dissection to patients with microscopic disease in SLNs—confers a survival benefit compared with wide local excision of the primary melanoma and observation of the regional nodal basin. Patients with primary cutaneous melanomas at least 1 mm thick or with Clark level IV or V tumors with any Breslow thickness were eligible for the trial. Patients were randomly assigned to wide excision alone plus observation or wide excision plus lymphatic mapping and SLNB, with subsequent completion lymphadenectomy if SLNs were positive. Although this trial has reached target accrual, final results are not yet available. Results from this important study should help define whether selective lymphadenectomy is associated with a survival benefit. Another trial, the Multicenter Selective Lymphadenectomy Trial-II, will explore the impact of completion lymphadenectomy in patients with a positive SLN.

Pathological Evaluation of Sentinel Lymph Nodes

Pathologists have traditionally examined the multitude of lymph nodes obtained from a lymphadenectomy by examining one hematoxylin-eosin–stained section from each paraffin block. This conventional approach, however, can miss disease in SLNs, primarily because of sampling error. In one study, 8 of 10 patients who underwent SLNB and subsequently developed regional nodal failure in nodal basins that were negative for disease according to conventional histologic examination of SLNs had microscopic disease detected when the SLNs were reassessed using specialized pathological techniques. Data from this and other studies suggest that failure to use specialized techniques, rather than failure to correctly identify SLNs, accounts for many cases of false-negative findings on SLNB.

With the SLNB technique, fewer lymph nodes are submitted for analysis than are submitted with complete lymphadenectomy, and the pathologist can therefore focus on only those nodes—the SLNs—that are at the highest risk. Currently, the combination of hematoxylin-eosin assessment of several levels and immunohistochemical analysis is generally considered a standard practice in assessing SLNs. Several antibodies directed against melanoma-associated antigens (S-100, HMB-45, tyrosinase, MAGE3, and MART-1) are routinely used for immunohistochemical evaluation. Because certain antibodies have low specificity (S-100) and others have low sensitivity (HMB-45, MAGE3, and tyrosinase), a panel of antibodies is commonly used. At our institution, this panel includes HMB-45 and MART-1.

Because even the combination of histologic and immunohistochemical examination of SLNs may fail to identify isolated melanoma cells or oligocellular deposits, some have suggested a molecular-based approach to examination of SLNs. With use of the reverse transcriptase-polymerase chain reaction (RT-PCR), it is estimated that one melanoma cell in a background of 1×10^6 to 1×10^7 normal cells can be identified. Some investigators have proposed, however, that this level of diagnostic sensitivity may actually overestimate clinically relevant disease. Positivity rates in studies using RT-PCR to evaluate SLNs for micrometastatic melanoma range from 55% to 73%, compared with a rate of 30%, which would be expected on the basis of known clinicopathological risk factors and patterns of recurrence. Some studies show that the prognosis of patients with an SLN that is positive by RT-PCR but negative by histologic or immunohistochemical analysis is worse than that of patients who have SLNs negative by both techniques.

Although preliminary results have been intriguing, the true clinical significance of positive RT-PCR findings in a histologically negative SLN is still unknown, in part because most studies that have addressed this question to date had short follow-up times and did not compare RT-PCR with current standard histologic techniques. It therefore remains difficult to draw final conclusions about the prognostic significance of SLNs that are positive by RT-PCR but negative by current conventional histologic analysis. Importantly, at least one recent study suggests that patients with submicroscopic disease detected by tyrosinase RT-PCR do not have a higher recurrence risk than patients with RT-PCR–negative SLNs. The relative clinical importance of conventional histologic examination, serial sectioning, immunohistochemical analysis, and molecular staging in patients undergoing lymphatic mapping and SLNB is being evaluated in a large, multicenter, randomized, prospective trial known as the Sunbelt Melanoma Trial.

Prediction of Metastatic Melanoma in Nonsentinel Nodes

Currently, patients who have a melanoma-positive SLN identified on SLNB subsequently undergo completion lymphadenectomy. When the non-SLNs are excised and evaluated by hematoxylin-eosin staining and immunohistochemistry, less than one-third of completion lymphadenectomy specimens contain additional nodes with metastatic disease. Because more than two-thirds of patients have metastatic disease identified only in SLNs, there has been interest in identifying patients who, despite having a positive SLN, have a low probability of metastatic disease in non-SLNs.

In an analysis of primary tumor and SLN characteristics, the relative area of tumor in the SLN and the Breslow thickness of the primary tumor most accurately predicted the presence of tumor in non-SLNs. The density of dendritic leukocytes in the paracortex also predicted the presence of tumor in non-SLNs. These three features alone and in combination were able to predict the presence of tumor in non-SLNs with high accuracy. Although these results are intriguing and warrant further study, decisions regarding completion lymphadenectomy cannot yet be made strictly on the basis of primary tumor or SLN characteristics. Completion lymphadenectomy following identification of a positive SLN remains the current standard of care.

Current Practice Guidelines

In general, patients with cutaneous melanoma are offered SLNB if the primary tumor is at least 1.0 mm thick, or if the primary tumor is less than 1.0 mm thick, if it is at least Clark level IV, is ulcerated, or demonstrates evidence of regression and if the patient has no evidence of metastatic melanoma in regional lymph nodes and distant sites on physical examination and staging evaluation. Evidence of vertical growth phase, a pathological feature that has been associated with an increased risk of lymphatic metastases, has also been adopted as an indication for SLNB. Recently, several groups have offered SLNB to patients whose primary tumors have a high mitotic rate because this factor has also been reported to be a strong predictor of SLN positivity.

When the SLNs are negative, no further surgery is performed, and the remaining regional lymph nodes are left intact. When the SLNs show evidence of metastatic disease, completion lymphadenectomy of the affected nodal basin is the current standard of care. Pathological evaluation of completion lymphadenectomy specimens often reveals no additional disease. However, it is important to remember that completion lymphadenectomy specimens are routinely assessed with standard histologic techniques rather than the more rigorous examination reserved for SLNB specimens. As a result, there may actually be additional disease in the completion nodal specimen that goes undetected. This disease would represent a potential source of subsequent recurrence if it were not removed. Because such recurrences are difficult to treat surgically and may contribute to significant morbidity, completion lymphadenectomy performed for microscopic disease provides the potential for improved regional control. In addition, identifying patients with minimal disease burden by using the SLN approach may help identify the group of patients who may derive an improved survival benefit from early TLND. Furthermore, knowledge of the pathological status of the SLNs allows proper staging and thus facilitates decision making regarding adjuvant treatment.

Technical Considerations

Axillary Dissection

GENERAL. Axillary dissection must be complete and include the level III lymph nodes (Fig. 3.5). The arm, shoulder, and chest are prepared and included in the surgical field.

INCISION. We use a horizontal, slightly S-shaped incision beginning anteriorly along the superior portion of the pectoralis major muscle, traversing the axilla over the fourth rib, and extending inferiorly along the anterior border of the latissimus dorsi muscle.

SKIN FLAPS. Skin flaps are raised anteriorly to the midclavicular line, inferiorly to the sixth rib, posteriorly to the anterior border of the latissimus dorsi muscle, and superiorly to just below the pectoralis major insertion. The medial side of the latissimus dorsi muscle is dissected free from the specimen, exposing the thoracodorsal vessels and nerve. The lateral edge of the dissection then proceeds cephalad beneath the axillary vein. These maneuvers allow the remainder of the dissection to proceed from medial to lateral. The fatty and lymphatic tissue over the pectoralis major muscle is dissected free around to its undersurface, where the pectoralis minor muscle is encountered. The interpectoral groove is exposed.

LYMPH NODE DISSECTION. The medial pectoral nerve is preserved. The interpectoral nodes are dissected free. The upper axilla is exposed by bringing the patient's arm over the chest by adduction and internal rotation. If nodes are bulky, the pectoralis minor muscle may be divided to facilitate exposure. Dissection proceeds from the apex of the axilla inferolaterally. Dissection of the upper axillary lymph nodes should be sufficiently complete that the thoracic outlet beneath the clavicle, Halsted's ligament, and subclavius muscle are seen (Fig. 3.6). Fatty and lymphatic

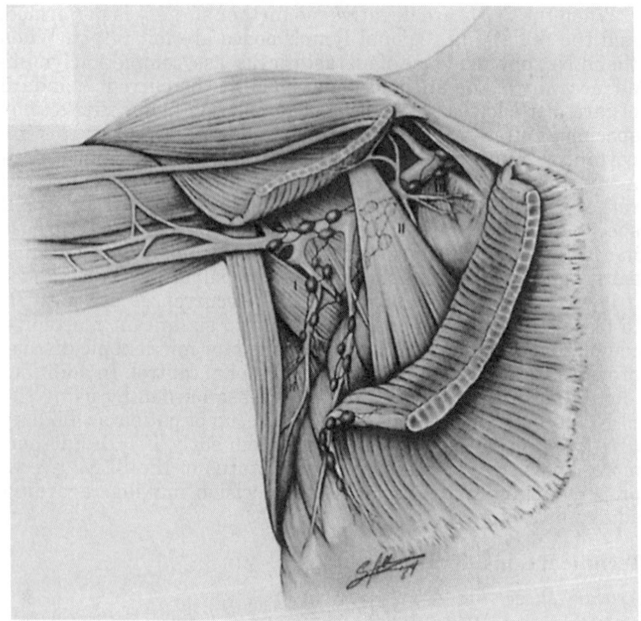

Figure 3.5. Lymphatic anatomy of the axilla showing the three groups of axillary lymph nodes defined by their relationship to the pectoralis minor muscle. The highest axillary nodes (level III) medial to the pectoralis minor muscle should be included in an axillary lymph node dissection for melanoma. (From Balch CM, Milton GW, Shaw HM, et al., eds. *Cutaneous Melanoma*. Philadelphia, Pa: Lippincott; 1985, with permission.)

tissues are dissected downward over the axillary vein. The apex of the dissected specimen is tagged. Dissection then continues until the thoracodorsal vessels and the long thoracic and thoracodorsal nerves are identified. The fatty tissue between the two nerves is separated from the subscapularis muscle. The specimen is removed from the lateral chest wall. Intercostobrachial nerves traversing the specimen are sacrificed. The specimen is swept off the latissimus dorsi and serratus anterior muscles.

WOUND CLOSURE. One 15F closed-suction catheter is placed percutaneously through the inferior flap into the axilla. An additional catheter may be inserted through the inferior flap and placed over the pectoralis major muscle. The skin is closed with interrupted 3-0 undyed absorbable sutures and running 4-0 subcuticular undyed absorbable sutures.

POSTOPERATIVE MANAGEMENT. Suction drainage is continued until output is less than 30 mL per day. By approximately 3 weeks, the suction catheters are removed, regardless of the amount of drainage, to avoid infection. Any subsequent collections of serum are removed by needle aspiration. Mobilization of the arm is discouraged during the first 7 to 10 days after surgery. Over the

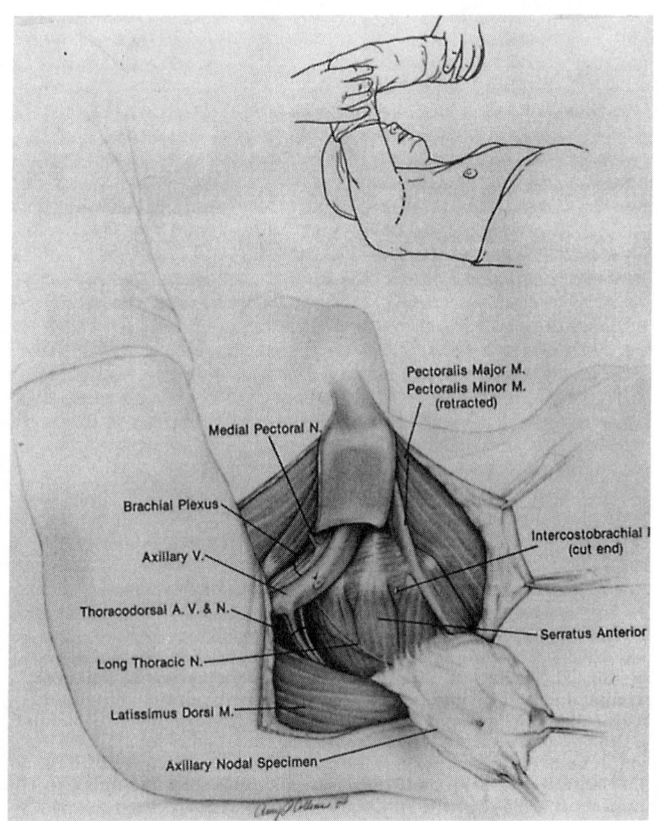

Figure 3.6. Access to the upper axilla. The arm is draped so that it can be brought over the chest wall during the operation. This facilitates retraction of the pectoralis muscles upward to reveal the level III axillary lymph nodes. (From Balch CM, Milton GW, Shaw HM, et al., eds. *Cutaneous Melanoma*. Philadelphia, Pa: Lippincott; 1985, with permission.)

ensuing 4 weeks, gradual mobilization of the arm is encouraged. The complication rate for axillary lymph node dissection is low. The most frequent complication is wound seroma (see the Complications section).

Groin Dissection

For groin dissection, the patient is placed in a slight frog-leg position.

INCISION. A reverse lazy-S incision is made from superomedial to the anterior superior iliac spine, vertically down to the inguinal crease, obliquely across the crease, and then vertically down to the apex of the femoral triangle.

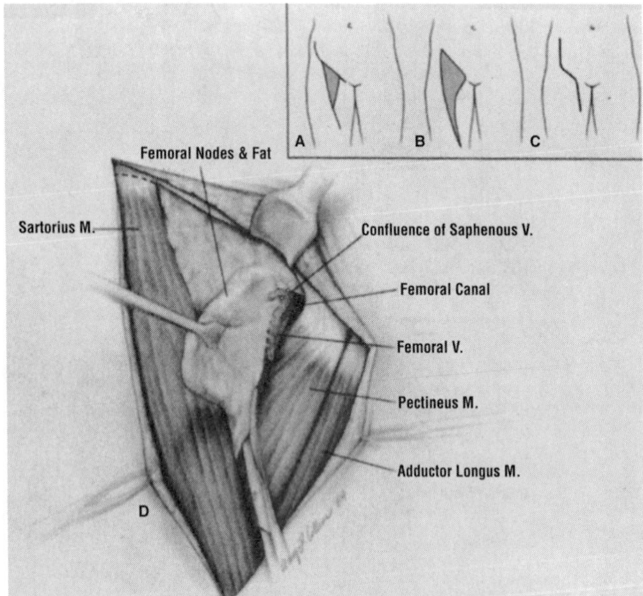

Figure 3.7. Technique of inguinal lymph node dissection. (From Balch CM, Milton GW, Shaw HM, et al., eds. *Cutaneous Melanoma*. Philadelphia, Pa: Lippincott; 1985, with permission.)

SKIN FLAPS. The limits of the skin flaps are medially to the pubic tubercle and the midbody of the adductor magnus muscle, laterally to the lateral edge of the sartorius muscle, superiorly to above the inguinal ligament, and inferiorly to the apex of the femoral triangle. We sometimes incorporate an ellipse of skin with the specimen.

LYMPH NODE DISSECTION. Dissection is carried down to the muscular fascia superiorly (Fig. 3.7). All fatty, node-bearing tissue is swept down to the inguinal ligament and off the external oblique fascia. Medially, the spermatic cord or round ligament is exposed, and nodal tissue is swept laterally. Nodal tissue is swept off the adductor fascia to the femoral vein. At the apex of the femoral triangle, the saphenous vein is divided. Laterally, nodal tissue is dissected off the sartorius muscle and the femoral nerve. With dissection in the plane of the femoral vessels, the nodal tissue is elevated up to the level of the fossa ovalis, where the saphenous vein is suture-ligated at the saphenofemoral junction. The specimen is dissected to beneath the inguinal ligament, where it is divided. Cloquet's node (the lowest iliac node) is sent as a separate specimen for frozen-section examination (Fig. 3.8).

SARTORIUS MUSCLE TRANSPOSITION. The sartorius muscle is divided at its origin on the anterior superior iliac spine (Fig. 3.9). The lateral femoral cutaneous nerve is preserved. The proximal

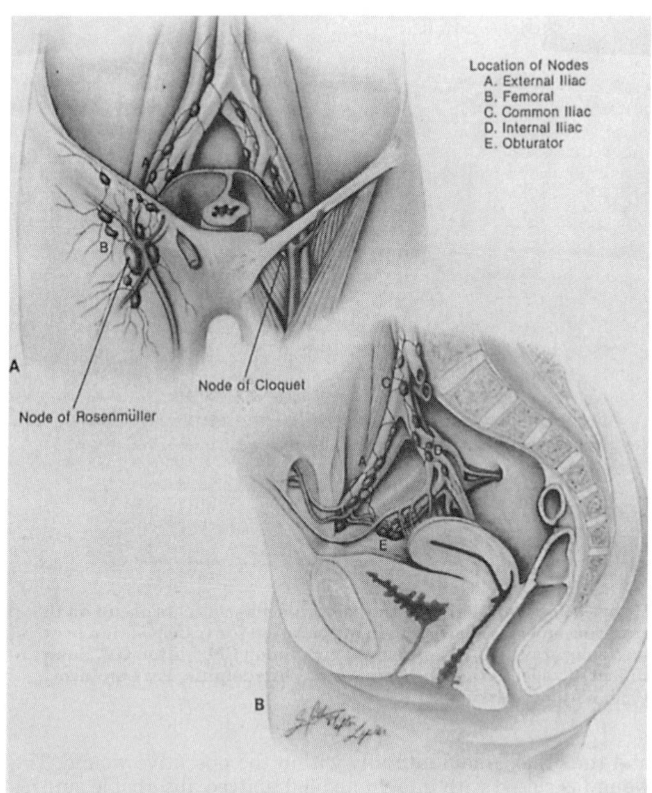

Figure 3.8. A: Lymphatic anatomy of the inguinal area demonstrating the superficial and deep lymphatic chains. Cloquet's node lies at the transition between the superficial and deep inguinal nodes. It is located beneath the inguinal ligament in the femoral canal. B: The iliac nodes include those on the common and superficial iliac vessels and the obturator nodes. Obturator nodes should be excised as part of an iliac nodal dissection. (From Balch CM, Milton GW, Shaw HM, et al., eds. *Cutaneous Melanoma*. Philadelphia, Pa: Lippincott; 1985, with permission.)

two or three neurovascular bundles going to the sartorius muscle are divided to facilitate transposition. The muscle is placed over the femoral vessels and tacked to the inguinal ligament, fascia of the adductor, and vastus muscle groups. Depending on the bulk of disease and patient anatomy, the saphenous vein and sartorius muscles may be preserved.

WOUND CLOSURE. The skin edges are examined for viability and trimmed back to healthy skin, if necessary. Intravenous administration of fluorescein and a Wood's lamp may be used to identify poorly perfused skin edges. Two closed-suction drains are placed through separate small incisions inferiorly. One is laid medially

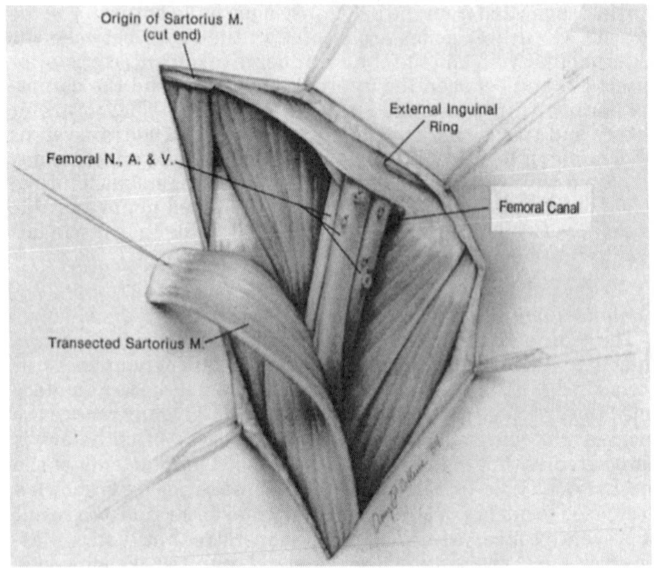

Figure 3.9. Transection of the sartorius muscle at its origin on the anterior superior iliac spine in preparation for transposition over the femoral vessels and nerves. (From Balch CM, Milton GW, Shaw HM, et al., eds. *Cutaneous Melanoma*. Philadelphia, Pa: Lippincott, 1985; with permission.)

and the other is laid laterally within the operative wound. The wound is closed with interrupted 3-0 undyed absorbable sutures in the dermis and followed by skin staples.

POSTOPERATIVE MANAGEMENT. The patient begins ambulating the day following surgery; a custom-fit elastic stocking may be used during the day for 6 months. After this period, the stocking may be discontinued if no leg swelling occurs.

DISSECTION OF THE ILIAC AND OBTURATOR NODES. We generally perform deep dissection—dissection of the iliac and obturator nodes—for the following indications: (a) known involvement of the nodes revealed by preoperative imaging studies, (b) more than three grossly positive nodes in the superficial lymph node dissection specimen, or (c) metastatic disease in Cloquet's node by frozen-section examination. To gain access to the deep nodes, we extend the skin incision superiorly. The external oblique muscle is split from a point superomedial to the anterior superior iliac spine to the lateral border of the rectus sheath. The internal oblique and transversus abdominis muscles are divided, and the peritoneum is retracted superiorly. An alternative approach is to split the inguinal ligament vertically, medial to the femoral vein. The ureter is exposed as it courses over the iliac artery. Dissection continues in front of the external iliac artery to separate the external iliac nodes. The inferior epigastric artery and vein are divided, if necessary. Dissection of the lymph nodes continues to the common iliac artery. Nodes in front of the external iliac vein are dissected to the point at which the internal iliac vein proceeds under the internal iliac artery. The plane of the peritoneum is traced along the wall of the bladder, and the fatty tissues and lymph nodes are dissected off the perivesical fat starting at the internal iliac artery. Dissection is completed on the medial wall of the external iliac vein, and the nodal chain is further separated from the pelvic fascia until the obturator nerve is seen. Obturator nodes are located in the space between the external iliac vein and the obturator nerve (in an anteroposterior direction) and between the internal iliac artery and the obturator foramen (in a cephalad-caudad direction). The obturator artery and vein usually need not be disturbed. The transversus abdominis, internal oblique, and external oblique muscles may be closed with running sutures. The inguinal ligament, if previously divided, is approximated with interrupted nonabsorbable sutures to Cooper's ligament medially and to the iliac fascia lateral to the femoral vessels.

Neck Dissection

Lymph node metastases from melanomas in the head and neck were previously believed to follow a predictable pattern. However, it is now known that lymphatic drainage from melanomas of the head and neck can be multidirectional and unpredictable. ELND or SLNB may be misdirected in as many as 59% of patients if the operation is based on classic anatomical studies without preoperative lymphoscintigraphy. These findings strongly support the use of lymphoscintigraphy in patients with melanomas in the head and neck.

At M. D. Anderson, the treatment of choice for patients with melanoma in the head and neck region and clinically involved nodes is wide local excision of the primary lesion with either modified radical neck dissection or selective neck dissection, followed by adjunctive radiation therapy. In patients with lesions at least 1.5 mm thick who have undergone selective neck dissection and in patients with nodal relapse, adjunctive radiation therapy gives a locoregional control rate of 88%.

Melanomas arising on the scalp or face anterior to the pinna of the ear and superior to the commissure of the lip can metastasize to intraparotid lymph nodes because these nodes are contiguous with the cervical nodes. When intraparotid nodes are clinically involved, it is advisable to combine neck dissection with parotid lymph node dissection and then administer radiation therapy.

Complications

The most common acute postoperative complication of selective lymphadenectomy is wound infection. Rates range from 5% to 19%. In an analysis of data from the Sunbelt Melanoma Trial, the complications associated with SLNB for melanoma were evaluated in 2,120 patients. Overall, 96 (4.6%) of the patients developed major or minor complications associated with SLNB, whereas 103 (23.3%) of 444 patients experienced complications associated with SLNB plus completion lymph node dissection. The authors concluded that the SLNB alone is associated with significantly less morbidity compared with SLNB plus completion lymph node dissection.

Following formal lymphadenectomy, the rate of lymphocele or seroma formation is 3% to 23%. Leaving suction catheters in place until the drainage decreases to 30 to 40 mL per day may reduce the incidence of seroma. However, prolonged use of catheters is associated with a higher rate of infection. Lymphedema is the most serious long-term complication of formal lymphadenectomy. Three series have shown that the incidence of leg edema after groin dissection can be decreased by preventive measures, including perioperative antibiotics, elastic stockings, leg elevation exercises, and diuretics. Prophylactic measures are important because reversing the progression of edema is difficult. Skin flap problems can occur with some frequency. Expectant management of ischemic edges often results in full-thickness necrosis and prolonged hospitalization. Therefore, if skin flap edges are of questionable viability, we return the patient to the operating room early for flap revision. Clinically detectable deep vein thrombosis is uncommon.

ADJUVANT THERAPY

Interferon Alfa-2b

High-dose IFN alfa-2b is approved by the U.S. Food and Drug Administration as adjuvant treatment for patients with melanoma who have a high risk of recurrence. Currently, patients with locally recurrent, nodal, in-transit, or satellite disease should be considered candidates for adjuvant high-dose IFN alfa-2b.

Approval of IFN alfa-2b was based on the results of the Eastern Cooperative Oncology Group (ECOG) E1684 prospective randomized trial, which assigned patients to high-dose IFN alfa-2b or observation after wide local excision. The IFN alfa-2b dosage was 20 million units/m^2/day intravenously for 4 weeks followed by 10 million units per m^2 three times a week subcutaneously for the next 48 weeks. Both node-positive and high-risk node-negative (T4pN0) patients were included; the majority of patients had experienced recurrence of disease in the regional nodes after prior wide local excision. All patients underwent either ELND or TLND. Of the 287 patients enrolled, 89% were node positive. IFN alfa-2b improved median overall survival from 2.8 to 3.8 years and improved 5-year relapse-free survival rates from 26% to 37% at a median follow-up of 7 years. The beneficial effect of IFN alfa-2b was most pronounced in the node-positive patients. Of note, the rate of toxic effects was high: Two patients died, 67% of patients experienced grade 3 toxic effects, and 50% of patients either stopped treatment early or required dose reduction.

A recent updated analysis of E1684, at a median follow-up of 12.6 years, showed a persistent gain in median overall survival (45.8 months for the IFN alfa-2b arm vs. 32 months for observation). The survival difference, however, was no longer statistically significant, possibly because deaths from intercurrent illness on both arms overshadowed melanoma-specific mortality. The updated results did continue to show a highly significant improvement in relapse-free survival.

The E1690 trial, another ECOG trial, was initiated before a significant impact on survival had been noted in E1684. In E1690, designed as a confirmation and extension of E1684, 642 patients with high-risk (stage IIb or III) melanoma were randomized in a three-arm study to receive the E1684 high-dose regimen, low-dose IFN alfa-2b (3 million units per m^2 three times a week for 2 years), or observation only. Seventy-five percent of the patients had nodal metastases (50% had recurrent disease in the regional nodes). Unlike E1684, E1690 allowed entry of patients with T4 primary tumors, regardless of whether lymph node dissection was performed, and 25% of the patients in the trial had deep primary tumors (compared with 11% in E1684).

In E1690, at a median follow-up of 52 months, high-dose IFN alfa-2b demonstrated a relapse-free survival benefit exceeding that of low-dose IFN alfa-2b or observation. The 5-year estimated relapse-free survival rates for high-dose IFN alfa-2b, low-dose IFN alfa-2b, and observation were 44%, 40%, and 35%, respectively ($p = 0.03$). The relapse-free survival benefit was equivalent for node-negative and node-positive patients. As of this writing, neither high-dose nor low-dose IFN alfa-2b has demonstrated an overall survival benefit compared with observation.

An analysis of salvage therapy for patients whose disease relapsed on E1690 demonstrated that a significantly larger proportion of patients in the observation arm than in the high-dose IFN arm received IFN alfa-containing salvage therapy, which may have confounded interpretation of the survival benefit of assigned treatments. Some of the discrepancy between the findings of E1684 and E1690 may be attributable to differences in patient demographic profiles. E1690 included patients with more favorable disease characteristics: Only 75% of patients were node positive, and of these, 51% had nodal recurrence. In E1690, 25% of patients enrolled were clinical stage II; in E1684, 11% were pathological stage II. Presumably, some of the clinical stage II patients in E1690 would have been pathological stage III had lymphadenectomy been required. An updated analysis of E1690 with a median follow-up of 7.2 years has confirmed the study's original conclusions.

ECOG trial E1694 was initiated to compare the efficacy and safety of a ganglioside vaccine with the efficacy and safety of high-dose IFN alfa-2b in patients with stage IIb or stage III melanoma. The ganglioside GM2 is a serologically well-defined melanoma antigen and the most immunogenic ganglioside expressed on melanoma cells. Preliminary studies had suggested that the antibody response to GM2 was correlated with relapse-free and overall survival. In E1694, 774 eligible patients with high-risk melanoma (tumor thickness >4.0 mm or regional lymph node metastasis) were randomized to receive high-dose IFN alfa-2b or GM2 vaccine. The study was closed early by the data safety monitoring board because of the clear superiority of IFN alfa-2b in terms of both disease-free and overall survival. The estimated 2-year relapse-free survival rates were 62% in the high-dose IFN alfa-2b arm and 49% in the GM2 vaccine arm. Furthermore, analysis of the hazard of relapse and death in subgroups based on the number of lymph nodes demonstrated the superiority of IFN alfa-2b over GM2 in all nodal subsets. E1694 also showed a statistically significant benefit for IFN alfa-2b in node-negative high-risk patients.

A recent pooled meta-analysis of primary data from the ECOG/Intergroup trials of high-dose IFN ($n = 1{,}916$) revealed a clear benefit of high-dose IFN alfa-2b in terms of relapse-free survival and a more modest benefit in terms of overall survival (odds ratio = 0.9, $p = 0.05$). Data from an updated analysis of the ECOG database demonstrated that (a) the survival impact of IFN alfa-2b was confined to regimens that incorporated both high-dose induction and high-dose subcutaneous maintenance; (b) reduction of hazard was observed early; and (c) the relapse-free survival advantage was sustained off treatment, in contrast to the more limited relapse-free survival advantage reported by the low-dose trials.

Results of trials investigating low-dose IFN alfa-2b have been disappointing. The previously mentioned E1690 trial, a three-arm trial that included low-dose IFN alfa-2b as one of the treatments, demonstrated a nonsignificant improvement in relapse-free survival in patients with high-risk stage II or stage III melanoma who received low-dose IFN alfa-2b for 2 years. The modest improvement in the low-dose IFN alfa-2b arm compared with the control arm disappeared within 2 years after therapy was stopped. The European Organization for Research and Treatment of Cancer 18871 trial also demonstrated that a regimen of very low-dose IFN alfa-2b (1 million units per m^2) injected subcutaneously on alternate days for 1 year did not affect overall survival for patients with high-risk melanoma. Because of the lack of a demonstrable durable clinical benefit, low-dose IFN alfa-2b has not been approved as adjuvant therapy for melanoma in the United States.

Radiation Therapy

Although surgery remains the primary treatment for patients with localized melanoma, available data indicate a need for improved locoregional control in cases in which complete surgical resection is difficult or high-risk features are noted pathologically. Factors associated with a high risk of subsequent regional basin recurrence include lymph nodes at least 3 cm in size, four or more positive lymph nodes, the presence of extracapsular extension, and recurrent disease after initial surgical resection. Retrospective and phase II prospective studies have revealed that adjuvant radiation therapy can significantly improve the locoregional control rate in these clinical settings. In one study in patients with lymph node metastases from melanoma with high-risk features, adjuvant radiation therapy delivered using a hypofractionated regimen resulted in an 87% 5-year regional nodal basin control rate, superior to the 50% to 70% local control rate achieved with surgery alone. The hypofractionated regimen was well tolerated and is convenient for such patients, in whom survival expectations may be low. The impact of adjuvant radiation therapy on the incidence of distant metastasis and overall survival has yet to be determined. Significant improvements in outcome will require commensurate improvements in systemic disease control. The importance of local control in reducing morbidity, however, should not be underestimated, and future research goals should include randomized clinical trials to further define the role of adjuvant radiation therapy alone or in combination with systemic therapy. In general, patients with multiple involved or matted regional nodes or with extracapsular extension of regional lymphatic metastases should be considered for adjuvant radiation therapy.

Chemotherapy

No confirmed studies have demonstrated a benefit of adjuvant chemotherapy in patients with melanoma who are at high risk for relapse. On the contrary, a randomized trial of adjuvant dacarbazine versus no adjuvant treatment showed a statistically significant decrease in survival in the adjuvant treatment arm. Adjuvant chemotherapy should be considered only in the context of a clinical trial.

MANAGEMENT OF DISTANT METASTATIC DISEASE

Common sites of distant metastasis in melanoma patients are, in order of decreasing frequency, skin and subcutaneous tissues, lung, liver, and brain. Patients with systemic metastases have a poor prognosis. General guidelines for choosing treatment modalities follow, but no treatment for metastatic melanoma has been proven to prolong survival. Experimental treatments are an option for most patients in whom distant metastases are diagnosed.

Surgery

Surgery is a very effective palliative treatment for isolated accessible distant metastases. Examples of accessible lesions include isolated visceral metastases, isolated brain metastases, and occasionally isolated lung metastases.

Lesions Causing Gastrointestinal Tract Obstruction

Gastrointestinal tract obstruction from metastatic melanoma is usually due to large polypoid lesions that mechanically obstruct the bowel or act as a lead point for intussusception. These submucosal lesions are generally removed by bowel resection.

Pulmonary Metastases

The value of resecting pulmonary metastases from malignant melanoma is controversial. In a study examining 65 pulmonary resections performed for histologically proven pulmonary metastases discovered after treatment of the primary melanoma, the postthoracotomy actuarial survival rate was 25% at 5 years (median interval from pulmonary resection to death, 18 months). Survival was not affected by the location, histologic subtype, Breslow thickness, or Clark level of the primary tumor, or by the type of resection. Patients without regional nodal metastases before thoracotomy had a median survival of 30 months, compared with 16 months for all other patients. The authors concluded that patients with isolated pulmonary metastases from melanoma may benefit from resection of metastases.

Liver Metastases

Fifteen to 20% of patients with metastatic melanoma have liver metastases. Historically, the median survival of patients with liver metastases has ranged from 2 to 7 months. Chemotherapy is of limited efficacy against liver metastases, so surgical resection may represent the only potentially curative option for patients with melanoma metastatic to the liver.

Some investigators have suggested that resection of hepatic metastasis is not warranted because of the associated dismal prognosis. Other investigators have suggested that resection may be appropriate only in patients with an ocular primary tumor because their clinical course is better than that of patients with liver metastases from cutaneous primary tumors. In a recent series of 40 patients who underwent resection of liver metastases from melanoma, 75% of the patients developed a subsequent recurrence. Patients with cutaneous melanoma were significantly more likely to have a subsequent recurrence outside the liver, suggesting that the disease is systemic at the time of hepatic resection. No patient with cutaneous melanoma metastatic to the liver was alive at 5 years. Thus, selection of patients for resection of hepatic metastases must be individualized and include an extensive evaluation of the extent of the disease. We currently recommend that patients with limited hepatic metastases who can be rendered surgically free of disease be considered for hepatic resection. However, because recurrence after resection is common, resection should be performed as part of a multidisciplinary approach in conjunction with systemic therapy.

Brain Metastases

Melanoma ranks behind only small-cell carcinoma of the lung as the most common tumor that metastasizes to the brain. An unusual feature of brain metastases is their propensity for hemorrhage, which occurs much more frequently with melanoma brain metastases than with brain metastases from other primary tumors. Hemorrhage occurs in 33% to 50% of patients with brain metastases from melanoma.

Surgical excision (followed in selected cases by cranial irradiation) is the treatment of choice in the case of a solitary, surgically accessible brain metastasis. Tumor excision is relatively safe, alleviates symptoms in most patients, and prevents further neurologic damage. Although long-term disease-free survival is uncommon, a rare patient may live more than 5 years after surgery. Radiation therapy is preferred when the lesions are numerous or are located in areas that preclude a safe operation. Gamma knife radiosurgery is also an option for patients with small to medium brain metastases who have a reasonable life expectancy and no signs of increased intracranial pressure.

Recurrent Distant Metastases

Unfortunately, many patients undergoing complete surgical resection of distant metastatic melanoma (stage IV) develop recurrent disease. A recent study examined whether a second metastasectomy could prolong the survival of patients with recurrent stage IV melanoma. In this study, the recurrent disease affected soft tissue, pulmonary, gastrointestinal, cerebral, skeletal, and gynecologic sites. Median survival following treatment for recurrent stage IV melanoma was 18.2 months after complete metastasectomy, compared with 12.5 months after a palliative surgical procedure and 5.9 months after nonsurgical management. The 5-year survival rate was 20% for patients in the complete metastasectomy group, compared with 7% for those in the palliative surgery group and 2% for those in the nonsurgical group. By multivariate analysis, the two most important prognostic factors for survival following diagnosis of recurrent stage IV melanoma were a prolonged disease-free interval before recurrence and complete surgical removal of the recurrent disease. These findings indicate that metastasectomy can prolong the survival of patients with recurrent stage IV melanoma and should be considered if all clinically evident tumors can be resected.

Radiation Therapy

In the treatment of cutaneous and lymph node metastases with radiation, most authors have observed improved response rates with higher fractional doses of radiation. The appropriate dose fractionation should be based on normal tissue tolerance. Multiple or recurrent skin or subcutaneous lesions may be treated successfully with hypofractionated radiation therapy. Predictors of a response to radiation therapy include primary tumor location in the head and neck region and total radiation dose above 40 Gy; age, gender, and histologic subtype have no impact. External-beam radiation therapy can provide long-term local control and effective palliation. Symptomatic bony metastases from melanoma also frequently respond to external-beam radiation therapy.

Chemotherapy

Single-agent chemotherapy remains the standard of care for systemic chemotherapy in patients with metastatic melanoma. Dacarbazine is the drug of choice, with a response rate of 16%. Other drugs, including cisplatin, paclitaxel, docetaxel, and the dacarbazine analog, temozolomide, have also shown activity in this disease. In a phase II trial of 56 patients treated with temozolomide, a complete response was documented in three patients (all with lung metastases) and a partial response in nine patients (21% overall response rate).

Based on observed single-agent activity, several combination regimens have been investigated, and preliminary results appear promising. The Dartmouth regimen (dacarbazine, cisplatin, carmustine, and tamoxifen) was initially reported to have an overall response rate of 55% and complete response rate of 20%. However, subsequent multicenter trials have failed to corroborate these favorable results. In fact, in randomized phase III trials, the two most active combination chemotherapy regimens, the Dartmouth regimen and cisplatin, vinblastine, and dacarbazine, have not proven to be superior to single-agent dacarbazine in terms of overall survival. Other combinations, such as temozolomide and cisplatin, have not been shown to have clear benefits in terms of response rates but may be associated with a higher incidence of grade 3 or grade 4 emesis.

If no objective response is observed after two or three courses of a particular chemotherapy regimen, it is usually prudent to discontinue that regimen and consider other approaches. In general, even when metastatic melanoma responds to systemic chemotherapy, the duration of the response is usually short, in the range of 3 to 6 months.

Vaccine and Biological Therapies

Morton et al. demonstrated that intralesional injection of viable bacillus Calmette-Guérin (BCG) organisms could lead to the regression of intradermal melanoma metastasis. Even more significantly, uninjected lesions occasionally regressed following BCG therapy. This finding demonstrated the ability of the body's immune system to destroy melanoma when properly stimulated, leading to investigations of BCG as a potential therapy for melanoma. Although several nonrandomized trials using historical controls and two small randomized trials of intralesional or intralymphatic BCG showed a statistically significant overall survival benefit in favor of BCG, multiple other randomized trials failed to substantiate these findings. Nonetheless, interest in modulating the immune system to treat melanoma has persisted.

Monoclonal Antibodies

Monoclonal antibody therapy is generally well tolerated and has shown activity in phase I trials in patients with metastatic melanoma. Monoclonal antibodies have been used to target radiation and potent plant toxins to tumors, and anti-idiotype antibodies have been used to stimulate immune responses.

Tumor Vaccines

Tumor vaccines have been used in the treatment of advanced melanoma and as adjuvant therapy for patients with high-risk melanoma. These vaccines may contain (a) irradiated tumor cells, usually obtained from the patient; (b) partially or completely purified melanoma antigens; or (c) tumor cell membranes from melanoma cells infected with virus (viral oncolysates). Synthetic vaccines containing genes that encode for tumor antigens and the peptide antigens themselves are also being evaluated, as are vaccines containing genes encoding for immune costimulatory signal proteins.

Allogeneic tumor cell vaccines, generally prepared from cultured cell lines or lysates thereof, offer several potential important advantages over autologous tumor cell vaccines: Allogeneic vaccines are readily available and can be standardized, preserved, and distributed in a manner akin to any other therapeutic agent. To date, the majority of studies involving allogeneic tumor vaccines have been small, single-institution studies. None of these have demonstrated an unequivocal benefit for immunotherapy with allogeneic tumor cells administered in conjunction with BCG compared with no treatment or treatment with BCG alone. Two randomized studies have been conducted in which allogeneic melanoma vaccines were administered with or without cyclophosphamide given for 3 days prior to vaccination. The results of these studies have been conflicting, with one suggesting a decrease in suppressor cell activity and one suggesting an increase in suppressor cell activity and augmented antibody response.

Novel vaccine strategies under investigation include administration of synthetic peptides based on known melanoma T-cell antigens, genetic vaccines, and combinations of vaccines with cytokines or costimulatory molecules. Morton et al. conducted nonrandomized studies of a polyvalent melanoma vaccine (Canvaxin) in patients with stage III or stage IV disease. Matched-pair analyses of data from extensive phase 2 trials demonstrated a consistent overall survival benefit for Canvaxin therapy in stage III melanoma (5-year overall survival rate: 49% for Canvaxin vs. 37% for no vaccine; $p = 0.0001$) and stage IV melanoma (5-year overall survival rate: 39% for Canvaxin vs. 20% for no vaccine; $p = 0.0009$). Vaccine-induced immune responses have correlated with improved survival after resection of local, regional, and distant disease. Two seperate phase 3 clinical trials of Canvaxin in patients with stage III or IV melanoma were discontinued in 2005 based on the recommendation of the data safety monitoring board after an interim analysis of the study data. The monitoring board found that the data were unlikely to provide significant evidence of a survival benefit for Canvaxin versus placebo in patients with stage III or stage IV melanoma.

In 2002, the Southwest Oncology Group published the results of a large, randomized trial (S9035) comparing co-administration of an allogeneic melanoma cell lysate (Melacine) and detoxified endotoxin/mycobacterial cell wall skeleton (DETOX) versus no treatment in patients with intermediate thickness, node-negative melanoma. The primary aim of this trial was to determine the effect of the vaccine on relapse-free survival. A major secondary aim was to determine if the effectiveness of the vaccine was based on patients' HLA class I allele expression. At a median follow-up of 4.1 years, there was no difference in overall relapse-free survival between the two groups. The patients in the vaccine arm expressing at least 2 M5 alleles, however, had better disease-free survival than the corresponding patients in the observation arm. Furthermore, vaccine-arm patients expressing at least 2 M5 alleles had better disease-free survival than vaccine-arm patients expressing fewer than 2 M5 alleles.

Cellular Therapies

Cellular therapies also exhibit some promise. Rosenberg et al. at the U.S. National Cancer Institute and others have reported their experiences with adoptive immunotherapy using tumor-infiltrating lymphocytes and, more recently, dendritic cells. An overall response rate of 37% was seen in patients with stage IV disease. Newer forms of cellular-based therapy are being developed, including effector cells from tumor vaccine-primed lymph nodes. Trials using in vitro pulsed dendritic cell infusion are ongoing. In addition, new work is examining whether preferential induction of apoptosis by sequential 5-Aza-2 deoxycytidine-depsipeptide (FR901228) treatment in melanoma cells to improve recognition of specific targets by cytolytic T lymphocytes may serve as a useful adjunct to immunotherapy.

Immunotherapy

Immunotherapy with either interleukin (IL)-2 or IFN has demonstrated response rates of 10% to 15% in appropriately selected patients. In patients who have a complete response, responses can be of greater durability than those with chemotherapy. IL-2 promotes the proliferation, differentiation, and recruitment of T, B, and NK cells and initiates cytolytic activity in a subset of lymphocytes. In patients who had a complete response to IL-2, the majority (86%) remained in ongoing complete remission from 39 to more than 148 months. In patients with a partial response, median response duration has been 36 to 45 months. Although the overall response rate is low (10%–15%), the durability of the responses led the U.S. Food and Drug Administration to approve high-dose IL-2 for metastatic melanoma. However, IL-2 and IFN administration are associated with multiple side effects; therefore, these agents should be administered only by physicians experienced in the management of such therapies. One major systemic toxic effect with high-dose IL-2 administration is "capillary leak syndrome." This toxic effect is, fortunately, uncommon, but it can be life threatening.

Biochemotherapy

Multiple trials have been conducted to investigate the benefit of combining biological therapy with chemotherapy (so-called biochemotherapy). These trials indicate that biochemotherapy is associated with higher response rates and longer median survivals than chemotherapy alone. Specifically, phase I and II studies have evaluated combinations of IL-2, IFN, and chemotherapy (cisplatin, dacarbazine, or cyclophosphamide). Preliminary results from a series of small studies using combinations of IL-2, IFN alfa, and cisplatin have indicated overall response rates of 40%. Recently, a phase III trial was completed at M. D. Anderson that compared inpatient sequential biochemotherapy with traditional outpatient chemotherapy with respect to response, time to progression, overall survival rate, and toxicity. All patients had either stage IV or inoperable stage III disease, an ECOG performance status of 0 to 3, no symptomatic brain metastases, no prior chemotherapy, and adequate cardiac, hematologic, and renal reserves. The response rate was 48% with biochemotherapy and 25% with standard chemotherapy (p = 0.0001). The time to progression was 4.6 months with biochemotherapy and 2.4 months with standard chemotherapy (p = 0.0007). The median survival was 11.8 months with biochemotherapy and 9.5 months with standard chemotherapy (p = 0.055). Biochemotherapy did induce severe constitutional toxic effects—myelosuppression, infections, and hypotension—but all of these were found to be manageable on the general ward. In a more recent phase II trial by the same group, the addition of IFN alfa-2a to IL-2 was examined. Although the response rate for this regimen was low, durable responses with median survival durations of 30+ months were seen in selected patients. However, several phase III trials have not consistently demonstrated an improvement in either response rates or overall survival.

Adoptive immunotherapy combining nonmyeloablative chemotherapy with high-dose IL-2 is another potentially promising therapeutic strategy currently under investigation.

FOLLOW-UP

Melanoma has a more variable and unpredictable clinical course than almost any other human cancer. At M. D. Anderson, the schedule of follow-up evaluations for patients with melanoma varies according to the risk of recurrence. In general, patients with early-stage melanoma (in situ or <1.0-mm thick, nonulcerated, lymph-node negative) have follow-up visits every 6 months for 2 years and then annually. Patients with thicker or ulcerated melanomas and those with positive lymph nodes generally return for follow-up visits more frequently—every 3 to 4 months up to 3 years, every 6 months during years 3 and 4, and annually thereafter. At each visit, the patient undergoes a physical examination, skin survey, chest radiography, and measurement of LDH. Exceptions to this "routine" clinic visit are made for patients with melanoma in situ, in whom chest radiography and measurement of LDH levels are not routinely performed, and patients with thin melanomas, in whom chest radiography and measurement of LDH levels are generally done annually. Abnormal findings may prompt further workup. Particular attention should be paid to signs or symptoms of central nervous system involvement. Extensive radiographic evaluation of asymptomatic patients with AJCC stage I, stage II, or stage III melanoma who are clinically free of disease rarely reveals metastases and thus is not routinely performed.

RECOMMENDED READING

Albertini JJ, Cruse CW, Rapaport D, et al. Intraoperative radio-lymph-scintigraphy improves sentinel lymph node identification for patients with melanoma. *Ann Surg* 1996;223: 217–224.

Aloia TA, Gershenwald JE. Management of early-stage cutaneous melanoma. *Curr Prob Surg* 2005;42:468–534.

American Joint Committee on Cancer (AJCC). Melanoma of the skin. In: Greene FL, Page DL, Fleming ID, et al., eds. *AJCC Cancer Staging Manual*. 6th ed. New York: Springer-Verlag; 2002:239–254.

Ang KK, Peters LJ, Weber RS, et al. Postoperative radiotherapy for cutaneous melanoma of the head and neck region. *Int J Radiat Oncol Biol Phys* 1994;30:795–798.

Bafaloukos D, Tsoutsos D, Kalofonos H, et al. Temozolomide and cisplatin versus temozolomide in patients with advanced melanoma: a randomized phase II study of the Hellenic Cooperative Oncology Group. *Ann Oncol* 2005;16:950–957.

Balch CM. The role of elective lymph node dissection in melanoma: rationale, results, and controversies. *J Clin Oncol* 1988;6:163–172.

Balch CM, Buzaid AC, Atkins MB, et al. A new American Joint Committee on Cancer staging system for cutaneous melanoma. *Cancer* 2000;88:1484–1491.

Balch CM, Buzaid AC, Soong SJ, et al. Final version of the American Joint Committee on Cancer staging system for cutaneous melanoma. *J Clin Oncol* 2001;19:3635–3648.

Balch CM, Soong S-J, Bartoluccci AA, et al. Efficacy of an elective regional lymph node dissection of 1 to 4 mm thick melanomas for patients 60 years of age and younger. *Ann Surg* 1996;224: 255–266.

Balch CM, Soong S-J, Gershenwald JE, et al. Prognostic factor analysis of 17,600 melanoma patients: validation of the American Joint Committee on Cancer melanoma staging system. *J Clin Oncol* 2001;19:3622–3634.

Balch CM, Soong S-J, Murad TM, et al. A multifactorial analysis of melanoma. II. Prognostic factors in patients with stage I (localized) melanoma. *Surgery* 1979;86: 343–351.

Balch CM, Soong S-J, Murad TM, et al. A multifactorial analysis of melanoma: III. Prognostic factors in melanoma patients with lymph node metastases (stage II). *Ann Surg* 1981;193:377–388.

Balch CM, Soong S-J, Ross MI, et al. Long-term results of a multi-institutional randomized trial comparing prognostic factors and surgical results for intermediate thickness melanomas (1.0 to 4.0 mm). Intergroup Melanoma Surgical Trial. *Ann Surg Oncol* 2000; 7:87–97.

Ballo MT, Ang KK. Radiotherapy for cutaneous malignant melanoma: rationale and indications. *Oncology (Huntingt)* 2004;18: 99–107, discussion 107–110, 113–114.

Ballo MT, Garden AS, Myers JN, et al. Melanoma metastatic to cervical lymph nodes: can radiotherapy replace formal dissection after local excision of nodal disease? *Head Neck* 2005; 27:718–721.

Ballo MT, Strom EA, Zagars GK, et al. Adjuvant irradiation for axillary metastases from malignant melanoma. *Int J Radiat Oncol Biol Phys* 2002;52:964–972.

Ballo MT, Zagars GK, Gershenwald JE, et al. A critical assessment of adjuvant radiotherapy for inguinal lymph node metastases from melanoma. *Ann Surg Oncol* 2004;11:1079–1084.

Bedrosian I, Faries MB, Guerry Dt, et al. Incidence of sentinel node metastasis in patients with thin primary melanoma (< or = 1 mm) with vertical growth phase. *Ann Surg Oncol* 2000;7:262–267.

Buzaid AC, Ross MI, Balch CM, et al. Critical analysis of the current American Joint Committee on Cancer staging system for cutaneous melanoma and proposal of a new staging system. *J Clin Oncol* 1997;15:1039–1051.

Cannon-Albright LA, Goldgar DE, Meyer LJ, et al. Assignment of a locus for familial melanoma, MLM, to chromosome 9p13-p22. *Science* 1992;258:1148–1152.

Cascinelli N, Morabito A, Santinami M, et al. Immediate or delayed dissection of regional nodes in patients with melanoma of the trunk: a randomised trial. *Lancet* 1998;351:793–796.

Cho E, Rosner BA, Feskanich D, et al. Risk factors and individual probabilities of melanoma for whites. *J Clin Oncol* 2005; 23:2669–2675.

Chung MH, Gupta RK, Hsueh E, et al. Humoral immune response to a therapeutic polyvalent cancer vaccine after complete resection of thick primary melanoma and sentinel lymphadenectomy. *J Clin Oncol* 2003;21:313–319.

Clary BM, Brady MS, Lewis JJ, et al. Sentinel lymph node biopsy in the management of patients with primary cutaneous melanoma: review of a large single-institutional experience with an emphasis on recurrence. *Ann Surg* 2001;233:250–258.

Cochran AJ, Wen DR, Huang RR, et al. Prediction of metastatic melanoma in nonsentinel nodes and clinical outcome based on the primary melanoma and the sentinel node. *Mod Pathol* 2004;17:747–755.

Cormier JN, Xing Y, Feng L, et al. Metastatic melanoma to lymph nodes in patients with unknown primary sites. *Cancer* 2006;106: 2012–2020.

Daponte A, Ascierto PA, Gravina A, et al. Temozolomide and cisplatin in advanced malignant melanoma. *Anticancer Res* 2005;25: 1441–1447.

Dudley ME, Wunderlich JR, Robbins PF, et al. Cancer regression and autoimmunity in patients after clonal repopulation with antitumor lymphocytes. *Science* 2002;298:850–854.

Dudley ME, Wunderlich JR, Yang JC, et al. Adoptive cell transfer therapy following non-myeloablative but lymphodepleting chemotherapy for the treatment of patients with refractory metastatic melanoma. *J Clin Oncol* 2005;23:2346–2357.

Elder DE, Guerry DT, VanHorn M, et al. The role of lymph node dissection for clinical stage I malignant melanoma of intermediate thickness (1.51–3.99 mm). *Cancer* 1985;56:413–418.

Essner R, Bostick PJ, Glass EC, et al. Standardized probe-directed sentinel node dissection in melanoma. *Surgery* 2000;127: 26–31.

Eton O, Buzaid AC, Bedikian AY, et al. A phase II study of "decrescendo" interleukin-2 plus interferon-alpha-2a in patients with progressive metastatic melanoma after chemotherapy. *Cancer* 2000;88:1703–1709.

Eton O, Legha SS, Bedikian AY, et al. Sequential biochemotherapy versus chemotherapy for metastatic melanoma: results from a phase III randomized trial. *J Clin Oncol* 2002;20: 2045–2052.

Evans GR, Friedman J, Shenaq J, et al. Plantar flap reconstruction for acral lentiginous melanoma. *Ann Surg Oncol* 1997;4:575–578.

Fraker DL, Alexander HR, Andrich M, et al. Palliation of regional symptoms of advanced extremity melanoma by isolated limb perfusion with melphalan and high-dose tumor necrosis factor. *Cancer J Sci Am* 1995;1:122.

Fraker DL, Alexander HR, Andrich M, et al. Treatment of patients with melanoma of the extremity using hyperthermic isolated limb perfusion with melphalan, tumor necrosis factor, and interferon gamma: results of a tumor necrosis factor dose-escalation study. *J Clin Oncol* 1996; 14:479–489.

Garbe C, Buttner P, Weiss J, et al. Risk factors for developing cutaneous melanoma and criteria for identifying persons at risk: multicenter case-control study of the Central Malignant Melanoma Registry of the German Dermatological Society. *J Invest Dermatol* 1994;102:695–699.

Gershenwald JE, Berman RS, Porter G, et al. Regional nodal basin control is not compromised by previous sentinel lymph node biopsy in patients with melanoma. *Ann Surg Oncol* 2000;7:226–231.

Gershenwald JE, Colome MI, Lee JE, et al. Patterns of recurrence following a negative sentinel lymph node biopsy in 243 patients with stage I or II melanoma. *J Clin Oncol* 1998;16:2253–2260.

Gershenwald JE, Mansfield PF, Lee JE, et al. Role for lymphatic mapping and sentinel lymph node biopsy in patients with thick (> or = 4 mm) primary melanoma. *Ann Surg Oncol* 2000;7:160–165.

Gershenwald JE, Prieto VG, Colome-Grimmer MI, et al. The prognostic significance of microscopic tumor burden in 945 melanoma patients undergoing sentinel lymph node biopsy. 36th Annual Meeting of the American Society of Clinical Oncology; 2003; New Orleans, La.

Gershenwald JE, Prieto VG, Johnson M. AJCC stage III (nodal) criteria accurately predict survival in sentinel node-positive melanoma patients. 3rd International Sentinel Node Congress; 2002; Yokohama, Japan.

Gershenwald JE, Thompson W, Mansfield PF, et al. Multi-institutional melanoma lymphatic mapping experience: the prognostic value of sentinel lymph node status in 612 stage I or II melanoma patients. *J Clin Oncol* 1999;17:976–983.

Gershenwald JE, Tseng CH, Thompson W, et al. Improved sentinel lymph node localization in patients with primary melanoma with the use of radiolabeled colloid. *Surgery* 1998;124:203–210.

Gill M, Celebi JT. B-RAF and melanocytic neoplasia. *J Am Acad Dermatol* 2005;53:108–114.

Gray-Schopfer VC, da Rocha Dias S, Marais R. The role of B-RAF in melanoma. *Cancer Metastasis Rev* 2005;24:165–183.

Hancock BW, Harris S, Wheatley K, et al. Adjuvant interferon-alpha in malignant melanoma: current status. *Cancer Treat Rev* 2000; 26:81–89.

Hawkins WG, Busam KJ, Ben-Porat L, et al. Desmoplastic melanoma: a pathologically and clinically distinct form of cutaneous melanoma. *Ann Surg Oncol* 2005;12:207–213.

Hayward N. New developments in melanoma genetics. *Curr Oncol Rep* 2000;2:300–306.

Heaton KM, Sussman JJ, Gershenwald JE, et al. Surgical margins and prognostic factors in patients with thick (>4 mm) primary melanoma. *Ann Surg Oncol* 1998;5:322–328.

Henderson RA, Mossman S, Nairn N, et al. Cancer vaccines and immunotherapies: emerging perspectives. *Vaccine* 2005;23: 2359–2362.

Holly EA, Aston DA, Cress RD, et al. Cutaneous melanoma in women. I. Exposure to sunlight, ability to tan, and other risk factors related to ultraviolet light. *Am J Epidemiol* 1995;141:923–933.

Holly EA, Cress RD, Ahn DK. Cutaneous melanoma in women. III. Reproductive factors and oral contraceptive use. *Am J Epidemiol* 1995;141:943–950.

Hsueh EC, Essner R, Foshag LJ, et al. Prolonged survival after complete resection of disseminated melanoma and active immunotherapy with a therapeutic cancer vaccine. *J Clin Oncol* 2002;20:4549–4554.

Jemal A, Devesa SS, Fears TR, et al. Cancer surveillance series: changing patterns of cutaneous malignant melanoma mortality rates among whites in the United States. *J Natl Cancer Inst* 2000;92:811–818.

Jemal A, Siegel R, Ward E, et al. Cancer statistics, 2006. *CA Cancer J Clin* 2006;56:106–130.

Kammula US, Ghossein R, Bhattacharya S, et al. Serial follow-up and the prognostic significance of reverse transcriptase-polymerase chain reaction—staged sentinel lymph nodes from melanoma patients. *J Clin Oncol* 2004;22: 3989–3996.

Kang JC, Wanek LA, Essner R, et al. Sentinel lymphadenectomy does not increase the incidence of in-transit metastases in primary melanoma. *J Clin Oncol* 2005;23:4764–4770.

Kirkwood JM, Ibrahim JG, Sondak VK, et al. High- and low-dose interferon alfa-2b in high-risk melanoma: first analysis of intergroup trial E1690/S9111/C9190. *J Clin Oncol* 2000;18:2444–2458.

Kirkwood JM, Ibrahim JG, Sosman JA, et al. High-dose interferon alfa-2b significantly prolongs relapse-free and overall survival compared with the GM2-KLH/QS-21 vaccine in patients with resected stage IIB–III melanoma: results of intergroup trial E1694/S9512/C509801. *J Clin Oncol* 2001;19:2370–2380.

Kirkwood JM, Manola J, Ibrahim J, et al. A pooled analysis of Eastern Cooperative Oncology Group and intergroup trials of adjuvant high-dose interferon for melanoma. *Clin Cancer Res* 2004;10:1670–1677.

Kirkwood JM, Strawderman MH, Ernstoff MS, et al. Interferon alfa-2b adjuvant therapy of high-risk resected cutaneous melanoma: the Eastern Cooperative Oncology Group Trial EST 1684. *J Clin Oncol* 1996;14:7–17.

Komenaka I, Hoerig H, Kaufman HL. Immunotherapy for melanoma. *Clin Dermatol* 2004;22:251–265.

Koops HS, Vaglini M, Suciu S, et al. Prophylactic isolated limb perfusion for localized, high-risk limb melanoma: results of a multicenter randomized phase III trial. European Organization for Research and Treatment of Cancer Malignant Melanoma Cooperative Group Protocol 18832, the World Health Organization Melanoma Program Trial 15, and the North American Perfusion Group Southwest Oncology Group-8593. *J Clin Oncol* 1998;16:2906–2912.

Krag DN, Meijer SJ, Weaver DL, et al. Minimal-access surgery for staging of malignant melanoma. *Arch Surg* 1995;130:654–658, discussion 659–660.

Li W, Stall A, Shivers SC, et al. Clinical relevance of molecular staging for melanoma: comparison of RT-PCR and immunohistochemistry staining in sentinel lymph nodes of patients with melanoma. *Ann Surg* 2000;231:795–803.

Lienard D, Ewalenko P, Delmotte JJ, et al. High-dose recombinant tumor necrosis factor alpha in combination with interferon gamma and melphalan in isolation perfusion of the limbs for melanoma and sarcoma. *J Clin Oncol* 1992;10:52–60.

Lindner P, Doubrovsky A, Kam PC, et al. Prognostic factors after isolated limb infusion with cytotoxic agents for melanoma. *Ann Surg Oncol* 2002;9:127–136.

Livingston PO, Wong GY, Adluri S, et al. Improved survival in stage III melanoma patients with GM2 antibodies: a randomized trial of adjuvant vaccination with GM2 ganglioside. *J Clin Oncol* 1994;12:1036–1044.

Mansfield PF, Lee JE, Balch CM. Cutaneous melanoma: current practice and surgical controversies. *Curr Probl Surg* 1994;31:253–374.

McCarthy WH, Shaw HM, Milton GW. Efficacy of elective lymph node dissection in 2,347 patients with clinical stage I malignant melanoma. *Surg Gynecol Obstet* 1985;161:575–580.

McMasters KM. The Sunbelt Melanoma Trial. *Ann Surg Oncol* 2001;8:41S–43S.

McMasters KM, Reintgen DS, Ross MI, et al. Sentinel lymph node biopsy for melanoma: how many radioactive nodes should be removed? *Ann Surg Oncol* 2001;8:192–197.

Milton GW, Shaw HM, McCarthy WH, et al. Prophylactic lymph node dissection in clinical stage I cutaneous malignant melanoma: results of surgical treatment in 1319 patients. *Br J Surg* 1982;69:108–111.

Morton DL. Immune response to postsurgical adjuvant active immunotherapy with Canvaxin polyvalent cancer vaccine: correlations with clinical course of patients with metastatic melanoma. *Dev Biol (Basel)* 2004;116:209–217, discussion 229–236.

Morton DL, Foshag LJ, Hoon DS, et al. Prolongation of survival in metastatic melanoma after active specific immunotherapy with a new polyvalent melanoma vaccine. *Ann Surg* 1992;216:463–482.

Morton DL, Wen DR, Wong JH, et al. Technical details of intraoperative lymphatic mapping for early stage melanoma. *Arch Surg* 1992;127:392–399.

Norman J, Cruse CW, Espinosa C, et al. Redefinition of cutaneous lymphatic drainage with the use of lymphoscintigraphy for malignant melanoma. *Am J Surg* 1991;162:432–437.

O'Meara AT, Cress R, Xing G, et al. Malignant melanoma in pregnancy. A population-based evaluation. *Cancer* 2005;103:1217–1226.

Parmiani G, Castelli C, Rivoltini L, et al. Immunotherapy of melanoma. *Semin Cancer Biol* 2003;13:391–400.

Pawlik TM, Gershenwald JE. Sentinel lymph node biopsy in managing melanoma. *Contemp Surg* 2005;61:175–182.

Pawlik TM, Ross MI, Gershenwald JE. Lymphatic mapping in the molecular era. *Ann Surg Oncol* 2004;11:362–374.

Pawlik TM, Ross MI, Johnson MM, et al. Predictors and natural history of in-transit melanoma after sentinel lymphadenectomy. *Ann Surg Oncol* 2005;12:587–596.

Pawlik TM, Ross MI, Prieto VG, et al. Assessment of the role of sentinel lymph node biopsy for primary cutaneous desmoplastic melanoma. 4th Annual International Sentinel Node Congress; 2004; Santa Monica, Calif.

Pawlik TM, Ross MI, Thompson JF, et al. The risk of in-transit melanoma metastasis depends on tumor biology and not the surgical approach to regional lymph nodes. *J Clin Oncol* 2005;23:4588–4590.

Pawlik TM, Sondak VK. Malignant melanoma: current state of primary and adjuvant treatment. *Crit Rev Oncol Hematol* 2003;45:245–264.

Pawlik TM, Zorzi D, Abdalla EK, et al. Hepatic resection for metastatic melanoma: distinct patterns of recurrence and prognosis for ocular versus cutaneous disease. The Society of

Surgical Oncology Annual Meeting; 2005; Atlanta, Ga.

Porter GA, Ross MI, Berman RS, et al. How many lymph nodes are enough during sentinel lymphadenectomy for primary melanoma? *Surgery* 2000; 128:306–311.

Porter GA, Ross MI, Berman RS, et al. Significance of multiple nodal basin drainage in truncal melanoma patients undergoing sentinel lymph node biopsy. *Ann Surg Oncol* 2000;7:256–261.

Ranieri JM, Wagner JD, Azuaje R, et al. Prognostic importance of lymph node tumor burden in melanoma patients staged by sentinel node biopsy. *Ann Surg Oncol* 2002;9:975–981.

Reintgen D, Balch CM, Kirkwood J, et al. Recent advances in the care of the patient with malignant melanoma. *Ann Surg* 1997; 225:1–14.

Reintgen D, Cruse CW, Wells K, et al. The orderly progression of melanoma nodal metastases. *Ann Surg* 1994;220:759–767.

Reintgen DS, Cox EB, McCarty KS, Jr, et al. Efficacy of elective lymph node dissection in patients with intermediate thickness primary melanoma. *Ann Surg* 1983; 198:379–385.

Rigel DS, Carucci JA. Malignant melanoma: prevention, early detection, and treatment in the 21st century. *CA Cancer J Clin* 2000;50:215–236, quiz 237–240.

Rosenberg SA, Yannelli JR, Yang JC, et al. Treatment of patients with metastatic melanoma with autologous tumor-infiltrating lymphocytes and interleukin 2. *J Natl Cancer Inst* 1994;86: 1159–1166.

Ross MI. Surgical management of stage I and II melanoma patients: approach to the regional lymph node basin. *Semin Surg Oncol* 1996;12:394–401.

Ross MI, Reintgen D, Balch CM. Selective lymphadenectomy: emerging role for lymphatic mapping and sentinel node biopsy in the management of early stage melanoma. *Semin Surg Oncol* 1993;9:219–223.

Rousseau DL, Jr, Gershenwald JE. The new staging system for cutaneous melanoma in the era of lymphatic mapping. *Semin Oncol* 2004;31:415–425.

Rousseau DL, Jr, Ross MI, Johnson MM, et al. Revised American Joint Committee on Cancer staging criteria accurately predict sentinel lymph node positivity in clinically node-negative melanoma patients. *Ann Surg Oncol* 2003;10:569–574.

Sharma A, Trivedi NR, Zimmerman MA, et al. Mutant V599EB-Raf regulates growth and vascular development of malignant melanoma tumors. *Cancer Res* 2005;65:2412–2421.

Shivers SC, Wang X, Li W, et al. Molecular staging of malignant melanoma: correlation with clinical outcome. *JAMA* 1998; 280:1410–1415.

Sim FH, Taylor WF, Pritchard DJ, et al. Lymphadenectomy in the management of stage I malignant melanoma: a prospective randomized study. *Mayo Clin Proc* 1986;61:697–705.

Smith MA, Fine JA, Barnhill RL, et al. Hormonal and reproductive influences and risk of melanoma in women. *Int J Epidemiol* 1998;27:751–757.

Sondak VK, Liu PY, Tuthill RJ, et al. Adjuvant immunotherapy of resected, intermediate-thickness, node-negative melanoma with an allogeneic tumor vaccine: overall results of a randomized trial of the Southwest Oncology Group. *J Clin Oncol* 2002;20:2058–2066.

Sosman JA, Unger JM, Liu PY, et al. Adjuvant immunotherapy of resected, intermediate-thickness, node-negative melanoma with an allogeneic tumor vaccine: impact of HLA class I antigen expression on outcome. *J Clin Oncol* 2002;20:2067–2075.

Sumner WE, III, Ross MI, Mansfield PF, et al. Implications of lymphatic drainage to unusual sentinel lymph node sites in patients with primary cutaneous melanoma. *Cancer* 2002; 95:354–360.

Sumner WE, III, Ross MI, Prieto VG. Patterns of failure in patients with thick (> or = 4 mm) melanoma undergoing sentinel node biopsy. Fifth World Conference on Melanoma; 2001; Venice, Italy.

Thompson JF, Kam PC. Isolated limb infusion for melanoma: a simple but effective alternative to isolated limb perfusion. *J Surg Oncol* 2004;88:1–3.

Thompson JF, Kam PC, Waugh RC, et al. Isolated limb infusion with cytotoxic agents: a simple alternative to isolated limb perfusion. *Semin Surg Oncol* 1998;14:238–247.

Thompson JF, McCarthy WH, Bosch CM, et al. Sentinel lymph node status as an indicator of the presence of metastatic melanoma in regional lymph nodes. *Melanoma Res* 1995;5:255–260.

Travis J. Closing in on melanoma susceptibility gene(s). *Science* 1992;258:1080–1081.

van Poll D, Thompson JF, Colman MH, et al. A sentinel node biopsy does not increase the incidence of in-transit metastasis in patients with primary cutaneous melanoma. *Ann Surg Oncol* 2005;12:597–608.

Veronesi U, Adamus J, Bandiera DC, et al. Delayed regional lymph node dissection in stage I melanoma of the skin of the lower extremities. *Cancer* 1982;49:2420–2430.

Veronesi U, Adamus J, Bandiera DC, et al. Inefficacy of immediate node dissection in stage 1 melanoma of the limbs. *N Engl J Med* 1977;297:627–630.

Veronesi U, Cascinelli N, Adamus J, et al. Thin stage I primary cutaneous malignant melanoma. Comparison of excision with margins of 1 or 3 cm. *N Engl J Med* 1988;318:1159–1162.

Wang X, Heller R, VanVoorhis N, et al. Detection of submicroscopic lymph node metastases with polymerase chain reaction in patients with malignant melanoma. *Ann Surg* 1994;220:768–774.

Wayne JD, Albo D, Hunt KK. Anaphylatic reaction to isosulfan blue dye during sentinel lymph node biopsy is more common in breast cancer than in melanoma. 37th Annual Meeting of the American Society of Clinical Oncology; 2001; San Francisco, Calif.

Wrightson WR, Wong SL, Edwards MJ, et al. Complications associated with sentinel lymph node biopsy for melanoma. *Ann Surg Oncol* 2003;10: 676–680.

Nonmelanoma Skin Cancer

Kelly Herne, Sharon R. Hymes, and
Jeffrey E. Gershenwald

EPIDEMIOLOGY AND ETIOLOGY

Most nonmelanoma skin cancers (NMSCs) are either basal cell carcinoma (BCC) or squamous cell carcinoma (SCC). Together, these cancers account for approximately 90% of all malignancies of the skin. BCC exceeds SCC in frequency by a factor of 4 or 5 to 1 in the United States, Australia, and the United Kingdom. However, in areas of decreasing latitude such as Africa, Japan, and Indonesia, SCC is more common. The male-to-female ratio of NMSC is 3:1, reflecting a greater tendency among men to expose skin to the sun. In addition, men are more likely than women to have these cancers on the lips, ears, and scalp, again reflecting patterns of solar exposure.

Many factors contribute to the development of NMSC, most notably ultraviolet (UV) radiation in the form of sunlight. UV radiation is accepted as the dominant risk factor for the development of both SCC and BCC, although the relationship between UV radiation and the development of BCC is less clear. Indeed, mutations of the p53 tumor suppressor gene induced by UV light are found in more than 90% of SCCs but only 50% of BCCs. Another important risk factor for both types of cancer is immunosuppression, especially in patients who have undergone organ transplantation. These patients tend to develop NMSC, especially SCC, more rapidly and with higher frequency than those in the general population, and it tends to follow a more aggressive course. Patients with AIDS also have an increased incidence of NMSC, although factors such as human papilloma virus (HPV) infection may act synergistically with UV exposure. HPV infection, especially HPV16 and 18, has also been implicated in the development of anogenital SCC. Arsenic exposure in well drinking water and hydrocarbon (tar) exposure have been linked to both SCC and BCC.

DIFFERENTIAL DIAGNOSIS

Several other epidermal tumors common to the skin can be either clinically confused with NMSC or are precursors to NMSC. Recognition of these tumors is important for both tumor surveillance and cancer prevention.

Seborrheic keratoses are benign proliferations of epidermis that appear on any part of the skin, except mucous membranes, and usually appear after age 30. They are not related to sun exposure but are common on the face, neck, and trunk, often in large numbers. They initially appear as flat brown macules, eventually becoming larger, “stuck on” brown plaques with dull, crumbly surfaces (Fig. 4.1A). Seborrheic keratoses can sometimes be

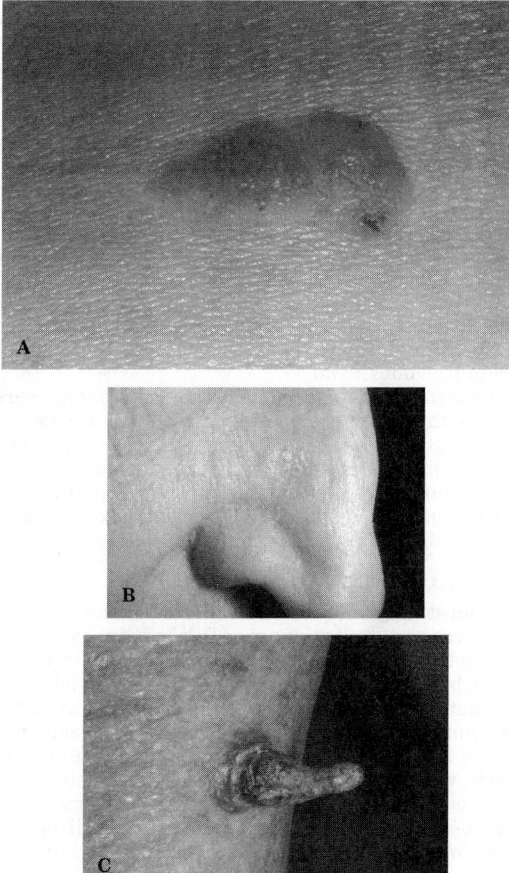

Figure 4.1. A: Seborrheic keratosis. B: Actinic keratosis. C: Cutaneous horn.

confused with melanoma. Biopsy of these lesions is prudent if sudden change in size or color occurs.

Actinic keratoses (AKs) are premalignant lesions with the potential to develop into SCC. They are found mainly on light-skinned individuals on sun-exposed areas. These lesions present as skin-colored, erythematous, or brown ill-defined patches with adherent scales (Fig. 4.1B). The mean size is approximately 3 to 4 mm. These lesions are extremely common on the face, scalp, ears, and lips and can often be better appreciated by palpation than by inspection with the naked eye.

Keratoacanthoma is a tumor that often occurs on older, sun-damaged skin, especially on the neck and face. They may rapidly grow as a red- or skin-colored dome-shaped nodules with a central crater. Maximum size may be attained by 6 to 8 weeks, with slow regression over a period of 2 to 12 months. Because these tumors can be confused both clinically and histologically with SCC, conservative excision is recommended.

Cutaneous horn is a clinical description for a growth that appears as a dense cone of epithelium resembling a horn (Fig. 4.1C). They range in size from several millimeters to over a centimeter, are generally white or yellowish in color, and appear on sun-exposed skin in older individuals. Histologically, cutaneous horns can develop from benign lesions such as warts or seborrheic keratoses and from premalignant or malignant lesions such as AK or SCC. Biopsy of these tumors is therefore always indicated to rule out the latter.

Nevus sebaceus is a benign tumor of the scalp that appears at or soon after birth as a yellowish-orange, well-demarcated plaque. Initially, the surface has a smooth or waxy appearance that gradually becomes more warty or verrucous during puberty. In adulthood, approximately 10% of these lesions develop into BCC. It is therefore recommended that these lesions be excised or closely monitored for the life of the patient.

BASAL CELL CARCINOMA

BCC is the most common cancer in humans and the most common type of skin cancer. The incidence of BCC continues to rise, with an annual estimated incidence of 200 per 100,000 in the United States. It is believed to arise from cells of the hair follicle and is therefore found almost exclusively on hair-bearing skin. Most lesions are found on sun-exposed areas such as the head and neck, but non–sun-exposed areas are also at risk. These tumors tend to grow slowly, with eventual invasion into local structures, including muscle, cartilage, and bone. Although the biological behavior of BCC is characterized by local and sometimes disfiguring invasiveness, metastasis is rare, occurring in less than 0.05% of cases.

In general, the histologic type of BCC is predictive of its behavior. Nodular BCC is the classic lesion of this type of NMSC. It appears as a pink translucent nodule, often described as "pearly." Overlying telangiectasias and ulceration are also common (Fig. 4.2). In dark-skinned individuals, these tumors are often pigmented and can resemble melanoma.

Superficial BCC is a variant that is more common on the limbs and trunk, as well as on areas with little or no sun exposure. It presents as a slow-growing, scaly pink plaque and can easily be confused with superficial SCC or squamous cell carcinoma in situ (Bowen's disease).

The sclerosing or morpheaform type represents the rarest form of BCC and often the most difficult to recognize. It presents as a poorly defined indurated or sclerotic plaque, often mistaken for a scar. In addition, this type of BCC frequently is found to be larger histopathalogically than clinically evident. Therefore, both diagnosis and treatment remain a challenge.

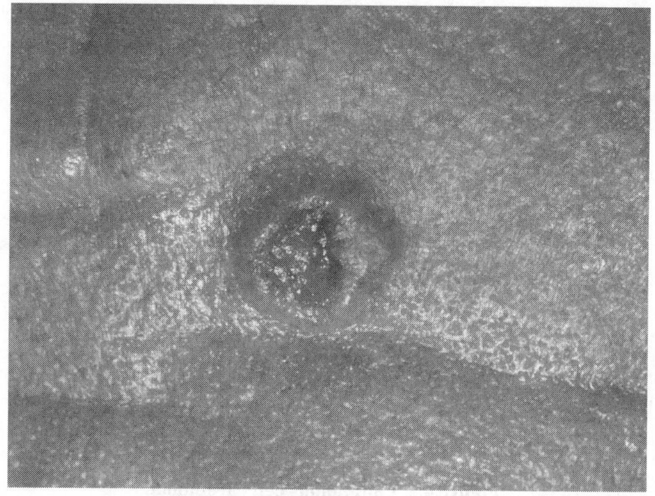

Figure 4.2. Nodular basal cell carcinoma.

SQUAMOUS CELL CARCINOMA

SCC is the second most common type of cutaneous cancer. In the United States, it occurs at a frequency one-fifth that of BCC. The development of SCC is principally related to two factors: solar damage and lighter skin types. SCC develops from the keratinocytes of the epidermis. SCC is also found in association with scars or areas of chronic inflammation such as non-healing ulcers. In addition, there are verrucous forms of SCC found on the mucous membranes of the oral cavity and genitals.

SCC has many clinical variants. As stated previously, it can arise from a precursor lesion such as an AK or can develop at the base of a cutaneous horn. Uncommonly, it presents de novo as a single lesion on otherwise normal-appearing skin. The most common lesion is found on a background of sun-damaged skin, especially on the head, neck, or arms. The lesions are usually red, poorly defined plaques or nodules with an ulcerated, friable surface (Fig. 4.3). Bowen's disease, or SCC in situ, is characterized by a well-demarcated pink plaque with a raised border and uniform scaling throughout.

SCC has a higher metastatic potential than does BCC, with an overall incidence of 2% to 3%. However, many factors affect the metastatic potential of any given tumor, such as histologic subtype based on nuclear pleomorphism and cytologic atypia (Broder classification I–IV); SCC types II and higher are more likely to metastasize. In addition, tumor size more than 2 cm and depth more than 4 mm (similar to Breslow thickness for melanoma) are risk factors for metastasis. Anatomic site also plays a role in the

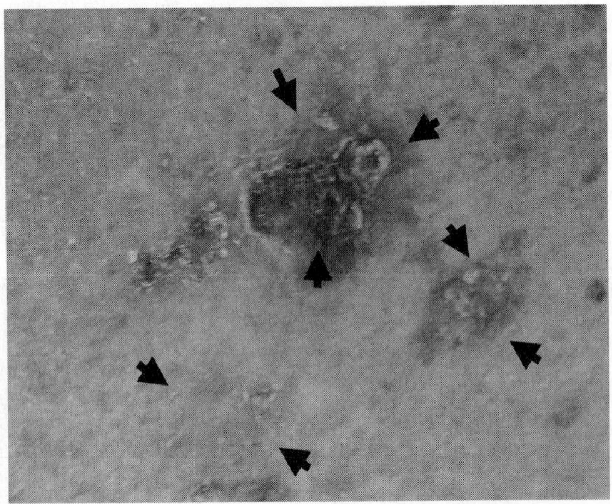

Figure 4.3. Squamous cell carcinoma.

tendency of SCC to metastasize. SCC of the lip has a metastatic rate up to 20%, and SCC of the ear, 11%. SCC arising in scars and other areas of chronic inflammation are also more likely to metastasize, with rates of 18% to 31% reported. Regional lymph nodes are the most common metastatic site, with distant sites such as bone, brain, and lungs occasionally reported. For tumors of the head and neck, the parotid gland is a common site for metastases.

SYNDROMES ASSOCIATED WITH NONMELANOMA SKIN CANCERS

Xeroderma pigmentosum is an autosomal recessive disease that occurs in approximately 1 in 250,000 individuals and is characterized by photophobia, severe sun sensitivity, and advanced sun damage. Affected individuals have defective DNA excision repair on exposure to UV radiation and develop malignancies of the skin and eyes, including melanoma, SCC, and BCC, at a rate 1,000 times that of the general population. Aggressive sun protection in the form of full-body sun suits and regular skin exams is important. Ideally, these patients should only go outside at night.

Nevoid basal cell syndrome is an autosomal dominant disorder characterized by the development of multiple BCCs. These patients are also exquisitely sensitive to radiation and should not undergo radiation therapy or excessive sun exposure. Often, these tumors are quite small, numbering in the hundreds on any given skin surface, and are thus difficult to monitor and treat. Again, regular follow-up and aggressive sun avoidance are important.

Albinism is an autosomal recessive disorder characterized by decreased or absent melanin in the skin and eyes. Patients may develop multiple SCCs, BCCs, and melanomas.

BIOPSY TECHNIQUES

Any cutaneous lesion suspicious for malignancy should be biopsied to assess pathology. Changes noted by patients may be quite subtle and include itching, tenderness, bleeding, or change in size, color, or texture. In addition, lesions that patients do not routinely observe themselves, such as those on the back, posterior legs, and buttocks, should be carefully examined.

Biopsy of pigmented lesions should be limited to punch or excisional biopsy techniques in which the full thickness of the dermis can be evaluated in the pathological specimen. A punch biopsy usually ranges in size from 2 to 8 mm and involves removing a round cylinder of tissue, ideally to the level of the subcutaneous fat. This site is then sutured or left to granulate. Often, entire lesions can be removed for pathological examination; if not, the most suspicious aspect of the tumor may be sampled.

Shave biopsy is an excellent technique for superficial lesions or nonpigmented lesions suspicious for BCC or SCC. It is also a good biopsy technique for cutaneous horns or keratoacanthomas, provided the base of the tumor is included in the specimen. A shave biopsy involves injecting local anesthesia into the epidermis and upper dermis to form a "plumped up" wheal below the lesion in question. A tangential sample is performed at the base of the wheal with either a sterile flexible razor blade or a no. 15 blade so that mid dermis is included in the biopsy specimen. If performed too superficially, invasion into the dermis cannot be evaluated, and rebiopsy may be indicated.

Excision involves removal of the entire lesion with a margin of clinically clear tissue and is generally used for classic lesions such as nodular or superficial BCC or superficial SCC. Margins can be evaluated in the specimen, and further treatment is often not necessary.

TREATMENT

The treatment of NMSC requires careful evaluation of tumor size, pathological characteristics, anatomical location, age and overall health of the patient, cost to the patient, and cosmesis. Treatment modalities can be divided into surgical and nonsurgical therapies.

Surgical excision is the mainstay of treatment of NMSC and is effective for all histologic types of tumors. Primary surgical excision with a margin of clinically normal tissue allows subsequent evaluation of the entire specimen for clear surgical margins. *Excisions with predetermined margins* are ideally performed along Langer's lines of cleavage to ensure a good cosmetic result. Elliptical excisions are usually performed on the scalp, forehead, cheeks, chin, trunk, and extremities. When dealing with lesions on the eyelids, alar rim of the nose, lips, and ears, however, wedge-shaped excisions may minimize distortion.

Mohs micrographic surgery is a useful modality for lesions of the head and neck, recurrent or large (i.e., >2 cm) lesions, or lesions of aggressive histologic type (e.g., sclerosing BCC or high-grade SCC). For NMSCs with metastatic potential, clinical evaluation of regional lymph nodes may be indicated.

Mohs micrographic surgery involves removal of the clinical margin of the tumor under local anesthesia, with immediate evaluation of the margins in frozen sections. Small incremental sections are removed until the margins are clear. This technique preserves normal tissue, thus allowing for the best cosmetic result. It also ensures that larger lesions with subclinical extension are entirely removed. Mohs micrographic surgery of primary NMSC of the head and neck has a cure rate (i.e., negative histologic margin) of 99%. The reconstructive choices after Mohs surgery are similar to those available after traditional excision. Although Mohs micrographic surgery is time-consuming, the benefits of superior cosmesis and excellent cure rates make it a treatment of choice for many patients.

Destructive techniques for superficial BCC and SCC include curettage, cryotherapy, and laser ablation. Curettage involves debulking the tumor under local anesthesia with a sharp curette until firm underlying dermis is reached. The base is hyphrecated and the process is repeated two or three times. This technique is reserved for small or superficial tumors.

Cryotherapy is a destructive method primarily reserved for the treatment of precancerous lesions such as AKs and occasionally for small superficial BCCs or SCCs. Liquid nitrogen is either sprayed with a cryogun or directly applied to the lesion with cotton-tipped applicators for a period of time such that the visible thawing of the lesions takes at least 15 seconds (30 seconds for superficial SCC or BCC).

Laser ablation with a carbon dioxide laser may be considered for pre-cancerous lesions. However, follicular involvement may be difficult to treat and lead to recurrence.

Nonsurgical therapies for the treatment of NMSC include radiation and several topical therapies. Radiation therapy is often reserved for patients unable or unwilling to undergo surgical treatment of primary lesions and for the adjuvant treatment of recurrent or histologically aggressive tumors (e.g., those exhibiting perineural invasion). In such patients, radiation therapy can be quite useful for tumors of the face, especially of the nose, lips, eyelids, and canthi. However, the number of treatment sessions depends on the size and location of the tumor. Although painless, radiation therapy may be associated with acute or chronic radiation-induced changes. For high-grade SCC with perineural involvement or invasion into bone, radiation therapy is generally recommended in conjunction with surgical excision or Mohs micrographic surgery.

Topical therapies for superficial NMSC and AKs include 5% fluorouracil (5-FU) and imiquimod creams. Treatment regimens for AKs vary widely; in general, 5-FU is applied to the entire affected area once or twice daily for a period ranging from 2 to 6 weeks. Significant erythema, stinging, oozing and crusting are often reported, especially with more aggressive treatment regimens. 5-FU can be applied to an entire region, such as the face, chest, arms, or hands. Retreatment several months later, either with cryotherapy or other modalities may be necessary.

For the treatment of superficial BCC, 5-FU can be applied daily to the tumor and to several millimeters of surrounding skin for a period of at least 4 weeks. After a several-week respite, the area is then evaluated clinically for residual tumor. Biopsy is often indicated to ensure adequate therapy.

Imiquimod therapy for AKs and superficial BCC has recently become popular. For AKs, the cream is applied 2 non-consecutive days a week for 16 weeks. In general, less irritation is reported with imiquimod, except on mucosal areas such as the lips. Imiquimod is also approved for the treatment of superficial BCC, although not for SCC. The cream should be applied 5 to 7 nights a week for at least 8 weeks. After a 2- to 3-month respite, the lesion is evaluated either clinically or histologically (rebiopsy) to confirm adequate therapy. This treatment regimen is often well tolerated and is particularly useful for multiple superficial BCCs in one area, such as the back or chest.

Photodynamic therapy is currently under investigation for the treatment of AKs and superficial BCC. A photosensitizer—most commonly, aminolevulinic acid—is applied to the skin and activated with a light source. The tumor cells retain the photosensitizer for longer periods of time than normal cells, resulting in preferential killing. Cure rates for AKs are reported to be as high as 90%, but no long-term data are available for rates for superficial BCC.

Chemoprevention with low-dose oral retinoids for chronically immunosuppressed patients who have undergone organ transplantation has shown some promise in the prevention of SCC. Ten years after organ transplantation, these patients have an 18-fold increased risk for the development of SCC. However, long term therapy is needed as beneficial effects are often lost when these drugs are discontinued.

SCREENING AND PREVENTION

Aggressive screening of patients at risk for skin cancer is essential to minimize the morbidity and mortality of NMSC. Patients at risk include those with light skin types, immunosuppression, and a family or personal history of skin cancer. Early exposure to UV should be limited in children, with regular use of sunscreen from an early age. Appropriate SPF level and application techniques should be emphasized for all patients, especially applications to the face and neck.

Regular examination of the skin by a dermatologist is recommended for all patients at risk for skin cancer, on at least a yearly basis. For patients with a history of AKs or NMSC, regular follow-up with a dermatologist is recommended. A complete skin exam includes examination of the entire skin surface, including the scalp, with particular attention to previous areas of skin cancer. In addition, patients with a history of SCC should undergo a thorough examination of all regional lymph node basins to evaluate for metastases.

RECOMMENDED READING

Bolognia JL, Jorizzo JL, Rapini RP. *Dermatology*. Philadelphia, Pa: Elsevier Limited; 2003.

Brodland AG, Zitelli JA. Surgical margins for excision of cutaneous SCC. *J Am Acad Dermatol* 1992;27(2pt): 241–248.

Chakrabarty A, Geisse JK. Medical therapies for non-melanoma skin cancer. *Clin Dermatol* 2004;22(3): 183–188.

Gupta AK, Cherman AM, Tyring SK. Viral and nonviral uses of imiquimod: a review. *J Cutan Med Surg* 2005; May 5. 8(5):338–352.

Harwood CA, Leedham-Green M, Leigh IM, Proby CM. Low-dose retinoids in the prevention of cutaneous squamous cell carcinomas in organ transplant recipients: a 16-year retrospective study. *Arch Dermatol* 2005;141(4): 456–464.

Miller SJ, Moresi JM. Actinic keratosis, basal cell carcinoma and squamous cell carcinomas. *Dermatology*. Philadelphia, PA: Elsevier Limited; 2003.

Pierson DM, Bandel C, Ehrig T, Cockerell CJ. Benign epithelial tumors and proliferations. *Dermatology*. Philadelphia, PA: Elsevier Limited; 2003.

Ponten F, Lundeberg J. Principles of tumor biology and pathogenesis of BCCs and SCCs. *Dermatology*. Philadelphia, PA: Elsevier Limited; 2003.

Smeets NW, Krekels GA, Ostertag JU, et al. Surgical excision vs Mohs' micrographic surgery for basal-cell carcinoma of the face: randomised controlled trial. *Lancet* 2004;364(9447):1766–1772.

Wolf DJ, Zitelli JA. Surgical margins for basal cell carcinoma. *Arch Dermatol* 1987;123(3):340–344.

5

Soft-tissue and Bone Sarcoma

Keith A. Delman and Janice N. Cormier

EPIDEMIOLOGY

In 2005, an estimated 9,400 new cases of soft-tissue sarcoma were diagnosed in the United States, with 3,400 patients expected to die of the disease. These rare tumors account for less than 1% of all newly diagnosed adult cancers and 7% of all newly diagnosed cancers in children. Several distinct groups of sarcomas have been recognized: soft-tissue sarcomas, bone sarcomas (osteosarcomas/chondrosarcomas), Ewing sarcomas, and peripheral primitive neuroectodermal tumors.

Encompassing more than 50 histologic types, soft-tissue sarcomas can occur anywhere in the body. The majority of primary lesions originate in an extremity (59%), with the next most frequent anatomical site of origin being the trunk (19%), followed by the retroperitoneum (13%) and the head/neck region (9%). The most common histologic types of soft-tissue sarcoma in adults (excluding Kaposi sarcoma) are malignant fibrous histiocytoma (24%), leiomyosarcoma (21%), liposarcoma (19%), synovial sarcoma (12%), and malignant peripheral nerve sheath tumors (6%). Rhabdomyosarcoma is the most common soft-tissue sarcoma of childhood and accounts for approximately 250 cases annually.

During the past 25 years, a multimodality treatment approach has been successfully applied to patients with extremity sarcomas, and this has led to improvements in both survival and quality of life. However, patients with abdominal sarcomas continue to have high rates of recurrence and poor overall survival. The overall 5-year survival rate for patients with all stages of soft-tissue sarcoma is 50% to 60%. Of the patients who die of sarcoma, most will succumb to metastatic disease, which 80% of the time occurs within 2 to 3 years of the initial diagnosis.

ETIOLOGY

Numerous factors have been associated with an increased risk of soft-tissue sarcoma. These factors are discussed in the following sections.

Trauma

Although patients with sarcoma frequently report a history of trauma in the tumor area, a causal relationship has not been established. More often, a minor injury calls attention to a pre-existing tumor that may be accentuated by edema or a hematoma.

Occupational Chemicals

Exposure to some herbicides such as phenoxyacetic acids and wood preservatives containing chlorophenols has been linked to an increased risk for soft-tissue sarcoma. Several chemical carcinogens, including Thorotrast (thorium oxide), vinyl chloride, and arsenic, have been associated with hepatic angiosarcoma. Exposure to asbestos has been associated with mesothelioma.

Previous Radiation Exposure

External radiation therapy is a rare but well-established cause of soft-tissue sarcoma. An 8- to 50-fold increase in the incidence of sarcomas has been noted for patients treated for cancers of the breast, cervix, ovary, testes, and lymphatic system. In addition, the risk for sarcomas after radiation therapy increases with higher dosage. The interval between irradiation and the development of sarcoma is usually at least 10 years. In a review of 160 patients with postirradiation sarcomas, the most common histologic types were osteogenic sarcoma, malignant fibrous histiocytoma, angiosarcoma, and lymphangiosarcoma. Postirradiation sarcomas are often diagnosed at a more advanced stage and are therefore associated with a poorer prognosis compared with other sarcomas.

Chronic Lymphedema

In 1948, Stewart and Treves were the first to describe the association of chronic lymphedema following axillary dissection with subsequent lymphangiosarcoma. Lymphangiosarcoma has also been observed in patients following filarial infections and in the lower extremities of patients with congenital primary lymphedema.

Genetic Predisposition

Specific inherited genetic alterations have been associated with an increased risk of bone and soft-tissue sarcomas. For example, patients with Gardner syndrome (familial polyposis) have a higher than normal incidence of desmoids, patients with germline mutations in the tumor suppressor gene *p53* (Li-Fraumeni syndrome) have a high incidence of sarcomas, and patients with von Recklinghausen disease who have abnormalities in the neurofibromatosis type 1 gene have an increased risk of neurofibrosarcomas. Soft-tissue sarcomas can also occur in patients with hereditary retinoblastoma as a second primary malignancy.

Oncogene Activation

Oncogenes are genes that are capable of inducing malignant transformation and tend to drive cells toward proliferation. Several oncogenes have been identified in association with soft-tissue sarcomas, including *MDM2*, *N-myc*, *c-erB2*, and members of the *ras* family. Amplification of these genes has been shown to correlate with an adverse outcome in patients with various soft-tissue sarcomas.

Cytogenetic analysis of soft-tissue tumors has led to the identification of distinct chromosomal translocations in oncogenes that are associated with certain histologic subtypes. These include the TLS-CHOP fusion, which is observed in myxoid liposarcoma, and the EWS-ATF1 fusion, which is observed in clear-cell sarcoma, among others. The gene rearrangements best characterized to date are those found in Ewing sarcoma, clear cell sarcoma, myxoid liposarcoma, alveolar rhabdomyosarcoma, desmoplastic small round cell tumors, and synovial sarcoma.

Tumor Suppressor Genes

Tumor suppressor genes play a critical role in suppressing tumor cell growth. However, these genes can be inactivated as a result of hereditary or sporadic mechanisms. Two genes that have shown the greatest relevance to soft-tissue tumors are the retinoblastoma (*Rb*) tumor suppressor gene and the *p53* tumor suppressor gene. Mutations or deletions in *Rb* can lead to the development of retinoblastoma, as well as sarcomas of soft tissue and bone. Mutations in the *p53* tumor suppressor gene are the most common mutations in human solid tumors and have been observed in 30% to 60% of cases of soft-tissue sarcomas.

PATHOLOGY

Sarcomas are a heterogeneous group of tumors that not only arise predominantly from the embryonic mesoderm, but can also arise from the ectoderm (e.g., peripheral nervous sheath tumors). Mesodermal cells give rise to the connective tissues distributed throughout the body, including pericardium, pleura, blood vessel endothelium, smooth and striated muscle, bone, cartilage, and synovium. These are the cells from which nearly all sarcomas originate. Consequently, sarcomas develop in a wide variety of anatomical sites.

Despite the various histologic subtypes, sarcomas have many common clinical and pathological features. The overall clinical behavior of most types of sarcoma is similar and determined by anatomical location (depth, specifically related to fascial boundaries), grade, and size. The dominant route of metastasis is hematogenous. Tumor grade has been firmly established to have prognostic significance and has therefore been incorporated into the staging of soft-tissue sarcomas. However, some experts have suggested that the pathological classification is far more important than grade when other pretreatment variables are taken into account. Table 5.1 shows a breakdown of the histologic types of tumors by their aggressiveness. Tumors with little or no metastatic potential include desmoids, atypical lipomatous tumors (also called well-differentiated liposarcoma), dermatofibrosarcoma protuberans, and hemangiopericytomas. Those subtypes with an intermediate risk of metastatic spread include myxoid liposarcoma, myxoid malignant fibrous histiocytoma, and extraskeletal chondrosarcoma. Highly aggressive tumors that have a substantial metastatic potential include angiosarcoma, clear cell sarcoma, pleomorphic and dedifferentiated liposarcoma, leiomyosarcoma, rhabdomyosarcoma, and synovial sarcoma. Approximately 15% of all soft-tissue sarcomas occur in the retroperitoneum. Approximately 80% are malignant, with liposarcoma, fibrosarcoma, leiomyosarcoma, and malignant fibrous histiocytoma accounting for the vast majority of the histologic types.

In as many as 25% to 40% of cases, expert sarcoma pathologists may disagree about specific histologic diagnoses or criteria for defining tumor grade. This low concordance rate may stem from the fact that few pathologists have the opportunity to study many of these rare tumors during their careers. It also emphasizes the need for more objective molecular and biochemical markers to improve the accuracy of conventional histologic assessment.

Table 5.1. Breakdown of sarcoma histologic type by tumor aggressiveness

Low metastatic potential
Desmoid tumor
Atypical lipomatous tumor
Dermatofibrosarcoma protuberans
Hemangiopericytoma
Intermediate metastatic potential
Myxoid liposarcoma
Myxoid malignant fibrous histiocytoma
Extraskeletal chondrosarcoma
High metastatic potential
Alveolar soft part sarcoma
Angiosarcoma
Clear cell sarcoma ("melanoma of soft parts")
Epithelioid sarcoma
Extraskeletal Ewing sarcoma
Extraskeletal osteosarcoma
Malignant fibrous histiocytoma
Liposarcoma (pleomorphic and dedifferentiated)
Leiomyosarcoma
Neurogenic sarcoma (malignant schwannoma)
Rhabdomyosarcoma
Synovial sarcoma

STAGING

The staging criteria for soft-tissue sarcomas in the current version of the American Joint Committee on Cancer (AJCC) staging guidelines consist of the histopathological grade (G), tumor size and depth (T), and the presence of metastases (distant [M] or nodal [N]) (Table 5.2). This system does not apply to visceral sarcomas, Kaposi sarcoma, dermatofibrosarcoma, or desmoid tumors.

Histopathological Grade

Histopathological grade remains the most important prognostic factor for determining disease-free and overall survival rate. In the 2002 AJCC staging system, grades 1 and 2 (well and moderately differentiated), N0, M0 lesions are classified as stage I lesions, regardless of tumor size and depth. To accurately determine tumor grade, an adequate tissue sample must be well fixed, well stained, and reviewed by an experienced sarcoma pathologist. The pathological features that define grade include cellularity, differentiation, pleomorphism, necrosis, and the number of mitoses.

Table 5.2. American Joint Committee on cancer staging criteria for soft-tissue sarcomas

Primary tumor (T)		
TX	Primary tumor cannot be assessed	
T0	No evidence of primary tumor	
T1	Tumor ≤5 cm in greatest dimension	
	T1a Tumor above superficial fascia	
	T1b Tumor invading or deep to superficial fascia	
T2	Tumor >5 cm in greatest dimension	
	T2a Tumor above superficial fascia	
	T2b Tumor invading or deep to superficial fascia	
Regional lymph nodes (N)		
NX	Regional lymph nodes cannot be assessed	
N0	No regional lymph node metastasis	
N1	Regional lymph node metastasis	
Distant metastasis (M)		
MX	Distant metastasis cannot be assessed	
M0	No distant metastasis	
M1	Distant metastasis	
Histopathological grade (G)		
GX	Grade cannot be assessed	
G1	Well differentiated	
G2	Moderately differentiated	
G3	Poorly differentiated	
G4	Undifferentiated	
Stage grouping		
Stage I		
A	G1–2, T1a–1b, N0, M0	(low grade, small, superficial, and deep)
B	G1–2, T2a, N0, M0	(low grade, large, and superficial)
Stage II		
A	G1–2, T2b, N0, M0	(low grade, large, and deep)
B	G3–4, T1a–1b, N0, M0	(high grade, small, superficial, and deep)
C	G3–4, T2a, N0, M0	(high grade, large, and superficial)
Stage III	G3–4, T2b, N0, M0	(high grade, large, and deep)
Stage IV	Any G, any T, N1, M0 Any G, any T, N0, M1	(any metastasis)

Adapted from Greene FL, Page DL, Fleming ID, et al., eds. *Cancer Staging Manual*. 6th ed. Philadelphia, Pa: Lippincott-Raven; 2002, with permission.

Tumor Size

Tumor size at presentation is also an important determinant of outcome. Sarcomas have classically been stratified into two groups based on size: T1 lesions (≤5 cm) and T2 lesions (>5 cm). The 2002 AJCC staging system continues to use depth (i.e., superficial or deep) to define prognosis. Extremity soft-tissue sarcomas that are superficial to the investing muscular fascia are designated *a* lesions in the T score (Ta), whereas tumors deep to the fascia and all retroperitoneal and visceral lesions are designated *b* (Tb).

Nodal Metastases

Lymph node metastases are rare, with less than 5% of soft-tissue sarcomas metastasizing to the nodes. Nodal metastases are associated with a poor prognosis and continue to be classified as stage IV disease. A few histologic subtypes, such as epithelioid sarcoma, rhabdomyosarcoma, clear cell sarcoma, angiosarcoma, and malignant fibrous histiocytoma, have been found to be associated with a higher incidence of nodal involvement (10%–20%).

Distant Metastasis

Distant metastases occur most frequently in the lung. Resection of the pulmonary lesions in selected patients with isolated lung metastases may offer up to a 30% 5-year survival rate. Other potential sites of metastasis include bone, brain, and liver. Visceral and retroperitoneal sarcomas have a propensity to metastasize to the liver and peritoneum.

EXTREMITY SOFT-TISSUE SARCOMAS

More than 50% of soft-tissue sarcomas originate in an extremity. The most common histologic subtypes that occur in the extremity include malignant fibrous histiocytoma, liposarcoma, synovial sarcoma, and fibrosarcoma, although various other histologic types are also seen in the extremities.

Clinical Presentation

Most extremity soft-tissue sarcomas present as an asymptomatic mass, but the size at presentation usually depends on the anatomical site of the tumor. For example, although a 2- to 3-cm tumor may become readily apparent on the back of the hand, a tumor in the thigh may grow to 10 to 15 cm in diameter before it becomes apparent. Frequently, trauma to the affected area will call attention to the pre-existing lesion. Small lesions that on the basis of the clinical history remain unchanged for several years may be closely observed without biopsy. However, all other tumors should be biopsied.

Biopsy

Accurate preoperative histologic diagnosis is a critical step in determining the primary treatment of a soft-tissue sarcoma. The biopsy should yield enough tissue so that a pathological diagnosis can be made without increasing the risk of complications.

Core-needle biopsy and fine-needle aspiration have been demonstrated to be reliable means of obtaining enough material for an accurate pathological diagnosis to be made, particularly when the pathological findings correlate closely with clinical and imaging findings. Biopsy performed under ultrasound or computed tomography (CT) guidance can improve the positive yield rate by helping pathologists more accurately locate the needle in the tumor, particularly in patients with deep extremity or retroperitoneal tumors.

Evaluation

The goals of pretreatment radiologic imaging are to accurately define the local extent of a tumor and to look for metastatic disease. Magnetic resonance imaging (MRI) has supplanted CT as the imaging technique of choice in the evaluation of soft-tissue sarcomas of the extremity, except in patients who do not have access to MRI or who have a contraindication to MRI, in whom CT remains the preferable technique. MRI accurately delineates muscle groups and distinguishes between bone, vascular structures, and tumor. In addition, sagittal and coronal views allow three-dimensional evaluation of anatomical compartments.

CT remains the imaging technique of choice for evaluating retroperitoneal sarcomas. The current generation of CT scanners can rapidly provide a detailed survey of the abdomen and pelvis and delineate adjacent organs and vascular structures. A CT scan of the abdomen and pelvis should be obtained when the histologic assessment of an extremity sarcoma reveals myxoid liposarcoma, because this histologic subtype is known to metastasize to the abdomen. Chest CT is used most often in patients with high-grade lesions. Searches for bone and brain metastases are rarely indicated, unless a patient has symptoms of metastases to these sites.

Management of Local Disease

The success of local tumor control depends on several tumor- and treatment-related prognostic factors. In multivariate analyses, high histologic grade, large tumor size (>5 cm), positive surgical margins, and intraoperative violation of the tumor capsule have been associated with a high rate of local recurrence. Histologic grade and tumor size are the most significant risk factors for distant metastasis and tumor-related mortality.

Surgery

The type of surgical resection performed in patients with extremity soft-tissue sarcomas is determined by a number of factors, including tumor location, tumor size, the depth of invasion, the involvement of nearby structures, the need for skin grafting or autogenous tissue reconstruction, and the patient's performance status. In the 1970s, 50% of patients with extremity sarcomas were treated with amputation for local control of their tumors. However, despite a local recurrence rate of less than 10% following radical surgery, large numbers of patients continued to die from metastatic disease. This realization led to the development and adoption of other methods of local therapy that combined conservative surgical excision with postoperative radiation therapy, with resultant local control rates of 78% to 91%.

Wide local excision is the primary treatment for patients with extremity sarcomas. It is important, when planning surgery and radiotherapy, to remember that there is generally a zone of compressed reactive tissue that forms a pseudocapsule around the tumors and that tumors may extend beyond this pseudocapsule. The inexperienced surgeon may mistakenly use this to guide resection. The goal of local therapy is to resect the tumor with a 2-cm margin of surrounding normal soft tissue. In some anatomical areas, however, these margins are not attainable because of the proximity of vital structures. When possible, the biopsy site or tract should also be included en bloc with the resected specimen.

Elective regional lymphadenectomy is rarely indicated in patients with soft-tissue sarcomas. However, in patients with rhabdomyosarcoma or epithelioid sarcoma with suspicious clinical or radiologic findings, fine-needle aspiration of the lymph nodes should be performed preoperatively. In these rare cases, a lymph node dissection may be indicated for regional control of the disease. A prospective trial is currently under way to evaluate the role of lymphatic mapping and sentinel lymph node biopsy in pediatric patients with extremity rhabdomyosarcomas.

There have been several studies that have shown favorable local control rates for patients with extremity tumors treated with conservative resection combined with radiation therapy. For example, in a small study from the National Cancer Institute, there was no difference in survival among patients treated with conservative surgery plus radiation therapy compared with patients treated with amputation. In 1985, on the basis of the limited data available, the National Institutes of Health developed a consensus statement recommending limb-sparing surgery for the majority of patients with high-grade extremity sarcomas. However, amputation remains the treatment of choice for patients whose tumor cannot be grossly resected with a limb-sparing procedure that preserves function (<5% of cases).

Radiation Therapy

The primary goal of radiation therapy is to optimize local tumor control. The evidence for adjunctive radiation therapy in patients eligible for conservative surgical resection comes from two randomized trials and a number of large single-institution reports. In one of these randomized trials, conducted by the National Cancer Institute, 91 patients with high-grade extremity tumors were treated with limb-sparing surgery followed by chemotherapy alone or radiation therapy plus adjuvant chemotherapy. A second group of 50 patients with low-grade tumors were treated with resection alone versus resection with radiation therapy. The 10-year local control rate for all patients receiving radiation therapy was 98% compared with 70% for those not receiving radiation therapy.

In the second randomized trial, which was performed at Memorial Sloan-Kettering Cancer Center, 164 patients were randomized to observation or brachytherapy following conservative surgery. The 5-year local control rate for patients with high-grade tumors was 66% in the observation group and 89% in the group treated with brachytherapy. There was no significant difference between the groups of patients with low-grade tumors.

Until recently, the policy at the M. D. Anderson Cancer Center was to administer radiation therapy as an adjunct to surgery for all patients with intermediate- and high-grade tumors of any size. However, because T1 tumors are less frequently associated with local recurrences, radiation therapy for these patients is currently considered on an individual basis because it may not confer a significant clinical benefit. In fact, two recent studies have failed to demonstrate an improvement in the 5-year recurrence or survival rates in patients with small sarcomas who received postoperative radiation therapy.

Preoperative Versus Postoperative External-beam Radiation Therapy

The optimal timing of external-beam radiation therapy for sarcomas located either in an extremity or in the retroperitoneum remains a focus of active investigation. Currently, the only randomized trial comparing preoperative and postoperative radiation therapy is a multicenter trial performed in Canada. In this trial, from October 1994 to December 1997, patients were randomized to receive either 50 Gy of external-beam radiation therapy preoperatively or 66 Gy of external-beam radiation therapy postoperatively. One hundred and ninety patients were entered into the study. With a median follow-up of 3.3 years, the recurrence and progressionfree survival rates were similar between the groups, with the only statistically significant difference being in the rates of wound complications. That is, the incidence of wound complications was 35% in the patients who received preoperative therapy, but only 17% in the patients who received postoperative radiation therapy.

At M. D. Anderson, despite the potential for increased wound problems, radiation therapy is preferentially given preoperatively for several reasons. First, this enables multidisciplinary planning with the radiation oncologist, medical oncologist, and surgeon to occur early in the course of therapy while the tumor is in place. Also, preoperative radiation therapy allows lower doses of radiation to be delivered to an undisturbed tissue bed that is potentially better oxygenated. In addition, the size of the preoperative radiation fields and the number of joints included in the fields is significantly smaller than those of postoperative radiation fields, which may result in an improved functional outcome.

Critics of preoperative radiation therapy cite the difficulty with the pathological assessment of margins and the increased incidence of wound complications as deterrents to preoperative radiation therapy. However, plastic surgery techniques that include advanced tissue transfer procedures are being used more frequently in patients with such high-risk wounds. The outcomes in patients treated in this fashion have been encouraging, with a high success rate (>90%) of healed wounds from a single-stage operation.

Brachytherapy

Brachytherapy, which involves the placement of multiple catheters in the tumor resection bed, has been reported to achieve local control rates comparable to those achieved with external-beam radiation therapy. Guidelines have been established that recommend placing the afterloading catheters at 1-cm intervals with a 2-cm margin around the surgical bed. Usually, after the fifth postoperative day, the catheters are then loaded with radioactive wires (iridium 192) that deliver 42 to 45 Gy to the tumor bed over 4 to 6 days. The frequency of wound complications associated with brachytherapy is similar to that seen for postoperative radiation therapy (approximately 10%).

The primary benefit of brachytherapy is the shorter overall treatment time of 4 to 6 days, compared with the 4 to 6 weeks generally consumed by preoperative or postoperative regimens. Brachytherapy also produces less radiation scatter in critical anatomical regions (e.g., gonads, joints), with improved function a potential clinical benefit. Cost-analysis comparisons of brachytherapy versus external-beam radiation therapy have further shown that the charges for adjuvant irradiation with brachytherapy are lower than those for external-beam radiation therapy.

Systemic Chemotherapy

Despite improvements in the local control rate, metastasis and death remain significant problems for patients with high-risk soft-tissue sarcomas. This includes patients presenting with metastatic disease and localized sarcomas that are in nonextremity sites, show an intermediate- or high-grade histology, or are large (T2). The treatment regimen for patients with high-risk localized disease, metastatic disease, or both, often includes chemotherapy.

As a group, sarcomas include histologic subtypes that are very responsive to cytotoxic chemotherapy as well as subtypes that are universally resistant to current agents. Only three drugs, doxorubicin, dacarbazine, and ifosfamide, have consistently achieved response rates of 20% as single-agent treatments in patients with advanced soft-tissue sarcomas. The majority of active chemotherapeutic trials have included doxorubicin as part of the treatment regimen. The response rate to ifosfamide has been found to vary from 20% to 60% in single-institution series in which higher-dose regimens have been used or in which it has been given in combination with doxorubicin.

Adjuvant (Postoperative) Chemotherapy

Individual randomized trials of adjuvant chemotherapy have failed to demonstrate an improvement in disease-free and overall survival in patients with soft-tissue sarcomas. However, there are several criticisms of these individual trials that may explain why they failed to demonstrate improvement in survival. First, the chemotherapy regimens used were suboptimal, in that single-agent drugs (most commonly doxorubicin) were studied and dosing schedules were less intensive. Second, the sample sizes in these trials were not large enough to allow the detection of clinically significant differences in survival. Third, the majority of patients who did not respond to the initial treatment regimen were started on other chemotherapeutic regimens that potentially affected disease-free and overall survival. Finally, most studies included patients at low risk for metastasis and death, that is, those with small (<5 cm) and low-grade tumors.

Hence, adjuvant chemotherapy for patients with soft-tissue sarcomas remains controversial. To help settle this issue, a formal meta-analysis called the Sarcoma Meta-Analysis Collaboration was conducted in 1997. This group analyzed the data on 1,568 patients from 14 trials of doxorubicin-based adjuvant chemotherapy to determine the effect of adjuvant chemotherapy on localized, resectable soft-tissue sarcomas. With a median follow-up of 9.4 years, doxorubicin-based chemotherapy was found to have significantly lengthened the time to local and distant recurrence and the overall recurrence-free survival. However, the absolute improvement in the overall survival rate for the entire group was only by 4%, which was not statistically significant. When subsets of patients were examined, there was a 7% increase in the survival rate in those patients with extremity tumors.

Neoadjuvant (Preoperative) Chemotherapy

The rationale for neoadjuvant/preoperative chemotherapy for soft-tissue sarcomas is that, given that only 30% to 50% of patients will respond to standard chemotherapeutic regimens, it enables the oncologist to identify those select patients in whom specific regimens are effective, as shown by measuring the primary tumor in situ. Patients whose tumors shrink after two or four courses subsequently undergo local treatment with surgery and/or radiation therapy, followed by postoperative chemotherapy with the same agents that were administered preoperatively. At the same time, patients who do not respond to short courses of preoperative chemotherapy are spared the toxic effects of prolonged postoperative chemotherapy with agents to which they are insensitive.

In an effort to better assess the role of chemotherapy, a cohort analysis of the combined databases from both M. D. Anderson and Memorial Sloan-Kettering was recently performed. The data on 674 patients with stage III extremity sarcoma who received either preoperative or postoperative doxorubicin-based chemotherapy were reviewed to determine their outcomes (5-year disease-specific survival, as well as 5-year local and distant recurrence rates) from systemic therapy. The 5-year disease-specific survival rate was 61%, and the probability of local and distant recurrences at 5 years was 83% and 56%, respectively. An important conclusion from this study was that the clinical benefits of doxorubicin-based chemotherapy in patients with high-risk extremity sarcomas were not sustained beyond 1 year after therapy. The investigators then went on to compare their study with the Sarcoma Meta-Analysis Collaboration and made the following observations. First, the patient population of the Sarcoma Meta-Analysis Collaboration was more heterogeneous than that of the cohort study, in that it included patients with both primary and recurrent extremity and nonextremity sarcomas. Second, there were also fewer uncontrolled variables in the cohort study. On the basis of these findings, the authors urged caution when reviewing studies of chemotherapeutic regimens with a short-term follow-up and concluded that there remains no consensus regarding the role of chemotherapy in patients with localized high-risk soft-tissue sarcomas.

Regional Chemotherapy/Isolated Limb Perfusion

Isolated limb perfusion (ILP) is an investigational approach for treating extremity sarcomas in the approximately 10% of patients with extremity sarcomas for whom amputation is the only option for local treatment. It has been used mainly as a limb-sparing alternative in these patients and consists of the regional administration of high-dose chemotherapy via ILP.

The technique of ILP involves isolation of the main artery and vein of the perfused limb from the systemic circulation. The specific tumor site determines the choice of the specific anatomical approach. External iliac vessels are used for thigh tumors, femoral or popliteal vessels for calf tumors, and axillary vessels for upper-extremity tumors. The vessels are dissected, and all collateral vessels are ligated. The vessels are then cannulated and connected to a pump oxygenator similar to that used in cardiopulmonary bypass. A tourniquet or Esmarch bandage is applied to the limb to achieve complete vascular isolation. The chemotherapeutic agents are then added to the perfusion circuit and recirculated for 90 minutes. The temperature of the perfused limb is maintained during the entire procedure by both external heating and warming of the perfusates. At the end of the procedure, the drugs are washed out of the limb, the cannulas are removed, and the blood vessels repaired.

There are several problems with trying to interpret the data from studies of ILP performed to date. These problems include the heterogeneous nature of the patients treated and the wide variety of chemotherapeutic agents used. Despite these problems, favorable response rates of 18% to 80% with overall 5-year survival rates of 50% to 70% have been reported.

Recently, interest has developed in a less invasive technique termed *isolated limb infusion*. This technique has also been termed *minimally invasive isolated limb perfusion*. Regardless of the nomenclature, the procedure involves the placement of infusion catheters by interventional radiologists, after which the patient is transferred to the operating room with the catheters in place. Under ischemic conditions, chemotherapy is administered via a nonoxygenated bypass circuit. The ischemic conditions are vital to this technique because this is believed to enhance the efficacy of the chemotherapeutic agents. Currently, isolated limb infusion is only available as an experimental protocol at certain centers.

Management of Local Recurrence

Disease can recur in up to 20% of patients with extremity sarcoma, but patients with microscopically positive surgical margins are the ones in whom the risk of local recurrence is greatest. It remains a matter of controversy, however, as to what the impact of local failures is on survival and distant disease-free survival. Many believe recurrence represents a harbinger of distant metastatic disease. Regardless, the adequacy of the surgical resection clearly plays a role in determining whether disease recurs locally.

An isolated local recurrence should be treated aggressively with margin-negative re-resection (possibly amputation) plus radiation therapy. Patients previously treated with external-beam radiation therapy may be considered for brachytherapy or intraoperative radiation therapy. Several small studies have shown that patients with isolated local recurrences may be successfully retreated, with local recurrence-free survival rates approaching 72%.

Management of Distant Disease

Distant metastases occur in 40% to 50% of patients with intermediate- and high-grade extremity sarcomas, compared with only 5% of patients with low-grade sarcomas. Most metastases to distant sites occur within 2 years of the initial diagnosis. The predominant site of distant metastases from primary extremity sarcomas is the lung (73% of cases).

Lung metastases should be resected if there are no extrapulmonary metastases, the patient is medically fit enough to withstand a thoracotomy, and the lesions are amenable to resection. Large series have revealed 3-year survival rates of 40% to 50% in patients with completely resected pulmonary metastases. A disease-free interval of more than 12 months, the ability to resect all metastatic disease, age younger than 50 years, and absence of preceding local recurrence were found to be independent prognostic factors in a multivariate analysis of patients who underwent resection of pulmonary metastases.

General Recommendations

General recommendations for the management of extremity soft-tissue sarcomas are as follows:

1. Soft-tissue tumors that are enlarging or greater than 3 cm in diameter should be evaluated with radiologic imaging (ultrasonography or CT), and a tissue diagnosis made on the basis of fine-needle aspiration or core-needle biopsy findings.
2. Evaluate for metastatic disease once a sarcoma diagnosis is established: chest radiography for low- or intermediate-grade lesions and T1 tumors, and chest CT for high-grade or T2 tumors.
3. A wide local excision with 2-cm margins is adequate therapy for low-grade lesions and T1 tumors.
4. Radiation therapy plays a critical role in the management of T2 tumors.
5. Patients with recurrent high-grade sarcomas or distant metastatic disease should be considered for preoperative (neoadjuvant) or postoperative (adjuvant) chemotherapy.
6. An aggressive surgical approach should be taken in the treatment of patients with an isolated local recurrence or resectable distant metastases.

RETROPERITONEAL SARCOMAS

Fifteen percent of soft-tissue sarcomas in adults occur in the retroperitoneum. Most retroperitoneal tumors are malignant, and approximately one-third are soft-tissue sarcomas. The differential diagnosis in a patient presenting with a retroperitoneal tumor includes lymphoma, germ cell tumors, and undifferentiated carcinomas. The most common sarcomas occurring in the retroperitoneum are liposarcomas, malignant fibrous histiocytomas, and leiomyosarcomas.

Although significant advances in our understanding of extremity soft-tissue sarcomas have resulted in improved treatments and outcomes, similar progress has not been achieved in our understanding and treatment of retroperitoneal soft-tissue sarcomas. For several reasons, patients with retroperitoneal soft-tissue sarcomas generally have a worse prognosis than those with extremity sarcomas. One reason is that retroperitoneal soft-tissue sarcomas commonly grow to large sizes before they become clinically apparent, by which time they often involve important vital structures, which precludes surgical resection. A second reason is that the surgical margins that can be obtained around these sarcomas are often inadequate because of anatomical constraints.

Clinical Presentation

Retroperitoneal sarcomas generally present as large masses; nearly 50% are larger than 20 cm at the time of diagnosis. They typically do not produce symptoms until they grow large enough to compress or invade contiguous structures. On occasion, patients may present with neurologic symptoms, resulting from the compression of lumbar or pelvic nerves, or obstructive gastrointestinal symptoms, resulting from the displacement or direct tumor involvement of an intestinal organ.

Evaluation

The workup in a patient with a retroperitoneal mass begins with an accurate history that should exclude signs and symptoms of lymphoma (e.g., fever, night sweats). A complete physical examination with particular attention to all nodal basins and a testicular examination in males are critically important. Laboratory assessment can be helpful; an increased lactate dehydrogenase concentration can be suggestive of lymphoma, whereas an increased β-human chorionic gonadotropin level, alpha-fetoprotein level, or both can indicate a germ cell tumor.

The radiologic assessment should include a CT scan of the abdomen and pelvis to define the extent of the tumor and its relationship to surrounding structures, particularly vascular structures. Imaging should include the liver in a search for metastases and discontinuous abdominal disease. The kidneys should also be evaluated to assess bilateral renal function. Thoracic CT is indicated to look for lung metastases. A CT-guided core-needle biopsy is appropriate for obtaining a tissue diagnosis in patients presenting with an equivocal history, an unusual-appearing mass, an unresectable tumor, or distant metastasis and in patients who are potentially eligible for a neoadjuvant protocol.

Management

Complete surgical resection is the most effective treatment for primary or recurrent retroperitoneal sarcomas, but it is frequently not possible. For example, in several retrospective assessments of patients with retroperitoneal sarcoma, complete surgical excision was achieved in only 40% to 60% of patients. The effects of an incomplete surgical resection on outcome are quite demonstrable. In an analysis of 500 patients with retroperitoneal soft-tissue sarcomas treated at Memorial Sloan-Kettering Cancer Center, the median survival duration of patients who underwent complete resection was 103 months versus 18 months for patients who underwent incomplete resection, which was no different than the survival seen in patients treated with observation without resection.

Surgical resection should not be offered to patients unless radiographic evidence indicates the potential for complete resection, although palliative surgical procedures may be performed to reduce the symptoms of intestinal obstruction or bleeding. In particular, patients with atypical lipomatous tumors, also termed *well-differentiated liposarcomas,* may benefit symptomatically from repeated tumor debulking.

Adjuvant Therapy

Chemotherapy has not been shown to be an effective treatment for retroperitoneal sarcomas. Several centers have ongoing protocols to determine the role of preoperative chemotherapy and radiation therapy for these tumors, but the findings from these studies have not yet been released. A trial sponsered by the American College of Surgeon's Oncology Group evaluating the benefit of preoperative radiation in patients with retro peritoneal sarcomas recently closed for failure to meet accrual targets.

Management of Recurrent Disease

Retroperitoneal sarcomas recur in two-thirds of patients. In addition to recurring locally in the tumor bed and metastasizing to the lungs, retroperitoneal leiomyosarcomas frequently spread to the liver. Retroperitoneal sarcomas can also recur diffusely throughout the peritoneal cavity (sarcomatosis). The approach to resectable recurrent disease after the treatment of a retroperitoneal sarcoma is similar to the approach taken after the recurrence of an extremity sarcoma. However, the ability to resect a recurrent retroperitoneal sarcoma declines precipitously with each recurrence. In a large series of patients treated at Memorial Sloan-Kettering Cancer Center, the authors were able to resect recurrent tumors in 57% of patients with a first recurrence, but in only 20% of patients after a second recurrence and 10% after a third recurrence. Isolated liver metastases, if stable over several months, may be amenable to resection, radiofrequency ablation, or chemoembolization.

In as many as 25% of patients, well-differentiated liposarcoma may recur in a poorly differentiated form or develop areas of dedifferentiation. Dedifferentiated retroperitoneal liposarcoma is more aggressive with a greater propensity for distant metastasis than its well-differentiated precursor.

Follow-up

The rationale behind follow-up strategies to detect the recurrence of any type of cancer is that the early recognition and treatment of recurrent, local, or distant disease can prolong survival. The ideal follow-up strategy should therefore be easy to implement, accurate, and cost-effective.

The development of metastases is the primary determinant of survival in patients with soft-tissue sarcoma. The site of recurrence is related to the anatomical site of the primary tumor. Extremity sarcomas generally recur in the form of distant pulmonary metastases, whereas retroperitoneal or intra-abdominal sarcomas tend to recur as frequently locally as they do in the lungs.

Whether the early detection of recurrence can improve overall survival depends on the availability of effective therapeutic interventions. A few reports involving small numbers of patients have shown that it is possible to salvage patients with recurrent local disease with radical re-excision with or without radiation therapy. Similarly, several groups have reported on patients who have experienced prolonged survival following the resection of pulmonary metastases. These limited data form the impetus for the aggressive surveillance strategies taken in patients with soft-tissue sarcomas.

The majority of soft-tissue sarcomas that recur do so within the first 2 years after the completion of therapy. Patients should therefore be evaluated with a complete history and physical examination every 3 months with a chest radiograph and tumor site imaging during this high-risk period. If the chest radiograph reveals a suspicious nodule, a CT scan of the chest should be obtained for further assessment. Most experts recommend that the tumor site be evaluated with either MRI for an extremity tumor or CT for intra-abdominal or retroperitoneal tumors. In some circumstances, ultrasonography can be used to look for the recurrence of an extremity tumor either locally or at a distant site. Follow-up intervals may be lengthened to every 6 months, with annual imaging during years 2 through 5 after the completion of therapy. After 5 years, patients should be assessed annually and a chest radiograph should be obtained.

GASTROINTESTINAL STROMAL TUMORS

Gastrointestinal stromal tumors (GISTs) constitute the majority of mesenchymal tumors involving the gastrointestinal tract. It is estimated that there are 2,500 to 6,000 cases per year in the United States. Although the clinical presentation of these tumors varies depending on the tumor size and anatomical location, most tumors are found incidentally at the time of endoscopy or radiologic imaging. GISTs arise most frequently in the stomach (60%–70%), followed by the small intestine (20%–25%), colon and rectum (5%), and esophagus (<5%). Most GISTs are sporadic and, in 95% of cases, solitary. Most patients with GISTs present in the fifth to the seventh decades of life, and these tumors are equally distributed between the genders. Symptoms of these lesions include pain and gastrointestinal bleeding, with abdominal mass a frequent finding.

Since the late-1990s, it has been recognized that GISTs have distinctive immunohistochemical and genetic features. GISTs originate from the intestinal pacemaker cells (the interstitial cells of Cajal), which express CD117, a transmembrane tyrosine kinase receptor that is the product of the c-KIT proto-oncogene. The expression of CD117 has emerged as an important defining feature of GISTs, being found in nearly 95% of cases. The pathogenesis of these tumors is related to mutations in the *c-KIT* gene. Exploitation of this genetic characteristic has led to significant inroads into the development of successful experimental therapy for these tumors.

Treatment

Surgical resection remains the treatment of choice for GISTs. However, despite complete surgical resection, the majority of patients (76% in one study from Memorial Sloan-Kettering Cancer Center) will suffer local recurrence. Salvage surgery for these recurrences is associated with a 15-month median survival.

Promising preclinical results have been the driving force for the rapid clinical development of imatinib mesylate (Gleevec, formerly known as STI571; Novartis), a selective tyrosine kinase inhibitor of *c-KIT*. This agent represents a novel intervention and has demonstrated the merits of specifically targeted molecular therapies in the management of oncologic diseases. In February 2002, imatinib mesylate was approved by the U.S. Food and Drug Administration for use in the treatment of GISTs on the basis of the results of trials conducted in patients with metastatic and locally advanced disease (Table 5.3). Initial results have shown that nearly 54% of patients with GISTs respond to imatinib and that there is no benefit to doses over 400 mg per day. Little is currently known about the optimal length of treatment, the duration of benefit, or the long-term toxicity of this drug. At M. D. Anderson, there are three ongoing clinical protocols involving the use of imatinib in different settings. The first protocol is part of the American College of Surgeons Oncology Group Z9001 phase III prospective randomized trial; in it, adjuvant imatinib treatment plus surgery is being compared with surgery alone in patients with GISTs who have undergone R0 or R1 resection. The second protocol (Z9000) is a phase II prospective randomized study in which combined preoperative and postoperative imatinib is being used for patients with primary, recurrent, or metastatic resectable GIST. The third protocol is a phase II trial that is investigating whether preoperative and postoperative imatinib will reduce the recurrence rate in patients with primary and recurrent operable GIST.

OTHER SOFT-TISSUE LESIONS

Sarcoma of the Breast

Sarcomas of the breast are rare tumors, accounting for less than 1% of all breast malignancies and less than 5% of all soft-tissue sarcomas. Various histologic subtypes have been reported to occur within the breast, including angiosarcoma, stromal sarcoma, fibrosarcoma, and malignant fibrous histiocytoma. Cystosarcoma phyllodes is generally considered to be a separate entity from other soft-tissue sarcomas because these tumors are believed to originate from hormonally responsive stromal cells of the breast and the majority are benign.

As with sarcomas at other anatomical sites, the histopathological grade and size of the tumor are important prognostic factors. Likewise, the likelihood of local recurrences increases as the tumor size increases; tumors smaller than 5 cm are associated with better overall survival. Local and distant recurrence are more common in patients with high-grade lesions. Complete excision with negative margins is the primary therapy. Simple mastectomy carries no additional benefit if complete excision can be accomplished by segmental mastectomy. Because of low rates

Table 5.3. Summary of clinical trials of imatinib mesylate in patients with advanced gastrointestinal stromal tumor

Study, Year	Phase	No. of Patients	Overall Response	CR	PR	2-y Overall Survival	Progression free Survival
Van Oosterom, 2001	I	36	53%	0%	53%	—	—
Demetri, 2002	II	147	54%	0%	54%	—	—
Verwiej, 2003	II	27	71%	4%	67%	—	73% (1 y)
Rankin, 2004	III	746					
– 400 mg daily			48%	3%	45%	78%	50% (2 y)
– 800 mg daily			48%	3%	45%	73%	53% (2 y)
Verwij, 2004	III	946					
– 400 mg daily			50%	5%	45%	69%	44% (2 y)
– 800 mg daily			54%	6%	48%	74%	55% (2 y)

CR, complete response; PR, partial response.

of regional lymphatic spread, axillary dissection is not routinely indicated. Neoadjuvant chemotherapy or radiation therapy may be considered for patients with large, high-risk tumors.

Desmoids

Desmoid tumors do not metastasize and are considered low-grade sarcomas. Approximately half of these tumors arise in the extremity, with the remaining lesions located on the trunk or in the retroperitoneum. Abdominal wall desmoids are associated with pregnancy and are believed to arise as the result of hormonal influences. Patients with Gardner syndrome may have retroperitoneal desmoids as an extracolonic manifestation of the disease. Surgical resection with wide local excision should be the primary therapy for desmoid tumors. Local recurrence may occur in up to one-third of patients. Adjuvant radiation therapy has been associated with a reduced incidence of local recurrence.

Dermatofibrosarcoma Protuberans

Dermatofibrosarcoma protuberans is a neoplasm arising in the dermis that may occur anywhere in the body. Approximately 40% arise on the trunk, with most of the remaining tumors distributed between the head and neck and extremities. The lesion presents as a nodular, cutaneous mass that shows slow and persistent growth. Satellite lesions may be found in patients with larger tumors. Wide local excision is recommended, although recurrence rates can be as high as 30% to 50%.

BONE SARCOMAS

Epidemiology

Malignant tumors of the musculoskeletal system constitute 10% of newly diagnosed cancers in the population younger than 30 years of age, with 1,000 cases diagnosed annually in the United States. However, malignant tumors arising from the skeletal systems represent only 0.2% of all primary cancers. Osteosarcoma and Ewing sarcoma are the two most common malignant conditions of bone. Osteosarcoma has a peak frequency during adolescent growth, whereas Ewing sarcoma occurs most frequently in the second decade of life.

Clinical Presentation

The most common presentation of bone sarcomas (Ewing sarcoma or osteosarcoma) is pain or swelling in a bone or joint. As with soft-tissue sarcomas in adults, often a traumatic event draws attention to the swelling and can throw off the correct diagnosis. Osteosarcoma most commonly involves the metaphysis of long bones, especially the distal femur, proximal tibia, or humerus. Ewing sarcoma may involve flat bones or the diaphysis of tubular bones such as the femur, pelvis, tibia, and fibula. Ewing sarcoma may also occur in soft tissues. Chondrosarcoma occurs most commonly in the pelvis, proximal femur, and shoulder girdle.

Up to 25% of patients presenting with osteosarcoma or Ewing sarcoma have metastatic disease at presentation. The most frequent metastatic sites for osteosarcoma include the lung (90% of cases) and the bone (10%), whereas Ewing sarcoma metastases occur in the lung (50%), bone (25%), and bone marrow (25%).

Staging

As with soft-tissue sarcomas, histopathological grade is a crucial component of the staging of bone sarcomas. The surgical staging system for musculoskeletal sarcoma is based on the system by Enneking and includes prognostic variables such as histopathological grade (G), the location of the tumor (T), and the presence or absence of metastases (M). The three stages are stage I, low grade (G1); stage II, high grade (G2); and stage III, G1 or G2 with the presence of metastases (M1). Each stage is then designated *a* if the lesion is anatomically confined within well-delineated surgical compartments (T1) and *b* if the lesion is located beyond such compartments in ill-defined fascial planes and spaces (T2).

Diagnosis

The evaluation of patients with a suspected bone tumor should include a thorough history and physical examination, plain radiographs, and MRI of the entire affected bone. Bone scanning and CT of the chest are also necessary.

On plain radiographs, malignant bone tumors show irregular borders, and there is often evidence of bone destruction and a periosteal reaction. Soft-tissue extension is also frequently seen.

Biopsy

A core-needle biopsy is the diagnostic procedure of choice in a patient suspected of harboring an osteosarcoma. A core-needle biopsy performed under radiographic guidance should yield diagnostic findings in almost all cases of osteosarcoma.

Treatment

Effective multimodality therapy for childhood musculoskeletal tumors has dramatically improved the 5-year survival rates from 10% to 20% in 1970 to the current 60% to 70%. Limb salvage is the standard treatment for most patients with osteosarcoma.

Surgery

Whenever feasible, limb salvage is the standard surgical approach to bone sarcomas. Successful limb-sparing surgery consists of three phases: tumor resection, bone reconstruction, and soft-tissue coverage. Complete surgical extirpation of the primary tumor and any metastases is essential in patients with osteosarcoma because this tumor is relatively resistant to radiation therapy.

It is also desirable to resect a Ewing sarcoma, if this can be done. If surgical removal with a wide surgical margin can be achieved, the prognosis is favorable (12-year relapsefree survival of 60%). However, Ewing sarcoma most typically involves the pelvis with an extensive soft-tissue mass that invades the pelvic cavity, which makes it difficult to carry out radical surgery.

Surgical resection is usually the only treatment indicated for the management of chondrosarcomas because this type of tumor is unresponsive to existing systemic therapies.

Chemotherapy

Chemotherapy has revolutionized the treatment of most bone sarcomas and is considered standard care for osteosarcoma and

Ewing sarcoma. The bleak 15% to 20% survival rate achieved with surgery alone during the 1960s has improved to 55% to 80% through the addition of chemotherapy to surgical resection. The timing of chemotherapy, the mode of delivery, and the drug combinations continue to be studied in multi-institutional trials, so further improvements in the clinical outcome are anticipated. Effective agents include doxorubicin, cisplatin, methotrexate, ifosfamide, and cyclophosphamide. Randomized clinical trials of patients with osteosarcoma have shown that the use of combination chemotherapy in addition to surgery results in cure rates of 58% to 76%. Preoperative chemotherapy is an attractive option because it can lead to the downstaging of tumors, which then enables the maximal application of limb-sparing surgery. In addition, tumor necrosis following preoperative chemotherapy has been shown to be the most important prognostic variable determining survival.

Multiagent chemotherapy has also been demonstrated to be essential in the treatment of Ewing sarcoma. Trials spanning more than 20 years performed by the Intergroup Study of Ewing's Sarcoma have established the efficacy of multidrug regimens (i.e., regimens that involve combinations of vincristine, doxorubicin, cyclophosphamide, ifosfamide, and etoposide) in increasing the 5-year relapsefree survival rates to up to 70% in patients with nonmetastatic disease. Agents currently being investigated as treatments for osteosarcoma include trastuzumab, inhaled granulocyte-macrophage colony-stimulating factor, and imatinib mesylate, among others.

Radiation Therapy

Because osteosarcomas are generally radiation resistant, radiation therapy is predominantly used for the palliation of large, unresectable tumors. In contrast, radiation therapy is the primary mode of treatment for most localized Ewing sarcomas. Preoperative irradiation may also be considered to reduce tumor volume before surgical resection is attempted.

Recurrent Disease

Bone tumors disseminate through the bloodstream and commonly metastasize to the lungs and bony skeleton. In the past, only 10% to 30% of patients presenting with detectable metastatic osteosarcoma became long-term disease-free survivors. More recent studies have shown that combined modality approaches consisting of surgical resection of the primary tumor and metastatic deposits in conjunction with multiagent chemotherapy can improve 5-year disease-free survival rates to up to 47%.

Ewing sarcoma may recur in the form of distant disease as long as 15 years after the initial diagnosis. In a retrospective analysis of 241 patients with Ewing sarcoma of the pelvis, tumor volume, responsiveness to chemotherapy, and adequate surgical margins were found to be the major factors that influenced prognosis.

Patients with suspected tumor recurrence should undergo a complete evaluation to determine the extent of the disease. The resection of pulmonary metastases has become the mainstay of treatment for patients with osteosarcoma. Prognosis can generally be determined by the response to previous therapy, duration of remission, and extent of metastases. Multimodality therapy, including chemotherapeutic agents not previously used, is the general recommendation for treatment.

Sacrococcygeal Chordoma

The notochordal remnant is the site of origin of this rare tumor. Chordomas are locally aggressive tumors that have a high propensity to recur. Because symptoms can be vague, diagnosis can be delayed. Surgical resection should involve a multidisciplinary team that includes the surgical oncologist, neurosurgeon, and reconstructive plastic surgeon. A two-stage procedure is used at M. D. Anderson. At the first stage, the blood supply to the tumor arising from the iliac vessels is controlled through an anterior approach. Several days later, the tumor is resected via a posterior approach. Radiation therapy should be considered because of high rates of local recurrence.

RECOMMENDED READING

American Joint Committee on Cancer. *AJCC cancer staging manual*. 6th ed. Philadelphia: Lippincott-Raven, 2002.

Arndt CA, Crist WM. Common musculoskeletal tumors of childhood and adolescence. *N Engl J Med* 1999;341:342.

Ayala AG, Ro JY, Fanning CV, et al. Core needle biopsy and fine-needle aspiration in the diagnosis of bone and soft tissue lesions. *Hematol Oncol Clin North Am* 1995;9:633.

Baldini EH, Goldberg J, Jenner C, et al. Long-term outcomes after function-sparing surgery without radiotherapy for soft tissue sarcoma of the extremities and trunk. *J Clin Oncol* 1999;17:3252.

Barkley HT, Martin RG, Romsdahl MM, et al. Treatment of soft tissue sarcomas by preoperative irradiation and conservative surgical resection. *Int J Radiat Oncol Biol Phys* 1988;14:693.

Billingsley KG, Burt ME, Jara E, et al. Pulmonary metastases from soft tissue sarcoma: analysis of patterns of disease and postmetastasis survival. *Ann Surg* 1999;229:602.

Billingsley KG, Lewis JJ, Leung DH, et al. Multifactorial analysis of the survival of patients with distant metastasis arising from primary extremity sarcoma. *Cancer* 1999;85:389.

Brady MS, Gaynor JJ, Brennan MF. Radiation-associated sarcoma of bone and soft tissue. *Arch Surg* 1992;127:1379.

Brennan MF, Casper ES, Harrison LB, et al. The role of multimodality therapy in soft tissue sarcoma. *Ann Surg* 1991;214:328.

Casson AG, Putnam JB, Natarajan G, et al. Five year survival after pulmonary metastasectomy for adult soft tissue sarcoma. *Cancer* 1992;69:662.

Chang AE, Kinsella T, Glatstein E, et al. Adjuvant chemotherapy for patients with high-grade soft tissue sarcomas of the extremity. *J Clin Oncol* 1988;6:1491.

Chang AE, Matory YL, Dwyer AJ, et al. Magnetic resonance imaging versus computed tomography in the evaluation of soft tissue tumors of the extremities. *Ann Surg* 1997;205:340.

Cormier JN, Huang X, Xing Y, et al. Cohort analysis of patients with localized, high-risk, extremity sarcoma treated at two cancer centers: chemotherapy-associated outcomes. *J Clin Oncol* 2004;22:4567.

Davis AM, Bell RS, Goodwin PJ. Prognostic factors in osteosarcoma: a critical review. *J Clin Oncol* 1994;12:423.

Demetri GD, von Mehren M, Blanke CD, et al. Efficacy and Safety of imatinib mesulate in advanced gastrointestinal stromal tumors. *N Engl J Med* 2002;472–80.

Eggermont AM, Schrafford T, Koops H, et al. Isolated limb perfusion with tumor necrosis factor and melphalan for limb salvage in 186 patients with locally advanced soft tissue extremity sarcoma. The cumulative multicenter European experience. *Ann Surg* 1996;224:756.

Eilber FR, Eckardt J. Surgical management of soft tissue sarcomas. *Semin Oncol* 1997;24:526.

Fong Y, Coit DG, Woodruff JM, Brennan MF. Lymph node metastasis from soft tissue sarcoma in adults. Analysis of data from a prospective database of 1772 sarcoma patients. *Ann Surg* 1993;217:72.

Geer RJ, Woodruff J, Casper ES, et al. Management of small soft tissue sarcomas of the extremity in adults. *Arch Surg* 1992;127:1285.

Glenn J, Sindelar WF, Kinsella T, et al. Results of multimodality therapy of resectable soft tissue sarcomas of the retroperitoneum. *Surgery* 1985;97:316.

Gutman H, Pollock RE, Benjamin RS, et al. Sarcoma of the breast: implications for extent of therapy. The M. D. Anderson experience. *Surgery* 1994;116:505.

Heslin MJ, Smith JK. Imaging of soft tissue sarcomas. *Surg Oncol Clin North Am* 1999;8:91.

Hoffmann C, Ahrens S, Dunst J, et al. Pelvic Ewing sarcoma: a retrospective analysis of 241 cases. *Cancer* 1999;85:869.

Huth JF, Eilber FR. Patterns of metastatic spread following resection of extremity soft tissue sarcomas and strategies for treatment. *Semin Surg Oncol* 1988;4:20.

Jaques DP, Coit DG, Hajdu SI, et al. Management of primary and recurrent soft tissue sarcoma of the retroperitoneum. *Ann Surg* 1990;212:51.

Karakousis CP, Proimakis C, Rao U, et al. Local recurrence and survival in soft tissue sarcomas. *Ann Surg Oncol* 1996;3:255.

Lawrence W Jr., Donegan WL, Natarajan N, et al. Adult soft tissue sarcomas. A pattern of care survey of the American College of Surgeons. *Ann Surg* 1987;205:349.

Levine EA. Prognostic factors in soft tissue sarcoma. *Semin Surg Oncol* 1999;17:23.

Lewis JJ, Leung D, Woodruff JM, Brennan MF. Retroperitoneal soft tissue sarcoma: analysis of 500 patients treated and followed at a single institution. *Ann Surg* 1998;228:355.

Lienard D, Ewalenko P, Delmotte JJ, et al. High-dose recombinant tumor necrosis factor alpha in combination with interferon gamma and melphalan in isolation perfusion of the limbs for melanoma and sarcoma. *J Clin Oncol* 1992;10:52.

Lindberg RD, Martin RG, Romsdahl MM, et al. Conservative surgery and postoperative radiotherapy in 300 adults with soft tissue sarcomas. *Cancer* 1981;47:2391.

Localio AS, Eng K, Ranson JHC. Abdominosacral approach for retrorectal tumors. *Am Surg* 1980;179:555.

Mazanet R, Antman KH. Adjuvant therapy for sarcomas. *Semin Oncol* 1991;18:603.

Midis GP, Pollock RE, Chen NP, et al. Locally recurrent soft tissue sarcoma of the extremities. *Surgery* 1998;123:666.

National Institutes of Health consensus development panel on limb-sparing treatment of adult soft tissue sarcoma and osteosarcomas 1985;3:1.

Patel SR, Benjamin RS. New chemotherapeutic strategies for soft tissue sarcomas. *Semin Surg Oncol* 1999;17:47.

Pezzi CM, Pollock RE, Evans HL, et al. Preoperative chemotherapy for soft tissue sarcoma of the extremities. *Ann Surg* 1990;211:476.

Pisters PW, Harrison LB, Leung DH, et al. Long-term results of a prospective randomized trial of adjuvant brachytherapy in soft tissue sarcoma. *J Clin Oncol* 1996;14:859.

Pisters PWT, Harrison LB, Woodruff JM, et al. A prospective randomized trial of adjuvant brachytherapy in the management of low grade soft tissue sarcomas of the extremity and superficial trunk. *J Clin Oncol* 1994;12:1150.

Pisters PW, Leung DH, Woodruff J, et al. Analysis of prognostic factors in 1,041 patients with localized soft tissue sarcomas of the extremities. *J Clin Oncol* 1996;14:1679.

Pollock RE, Karnell LH, Menck HR, et al. The National Cancer Data Base report on soft tissue sarcoma. *Cancer* 1996;78:2247.

Potter DA, Kinsella T, Glatstein E, et al. High-grade soft tissue sarcomas of the extremities. *Cancer* 1986;58:190.

Ramanathan RC, A'Hern R, Fisher C, et al. Modified staging system for extremity soft tissue sarcomas. *Ann Surg Oncol* 1999;5:57.

Rankin C, von Mehren M, Blanke C, et al. Continued prolongation of survival by imatinib in patients with metastatic GIST. Update of results from North American Intergroup phase III study S0033. *Proc Am Soc Clin Oncol* 2004: Abstr 9005.

Razek A, Perez C, Tefft M, et al. Intergroup Ewing's sarcoma study: local control related to radiation dose, volume and site of primary lesion in Ewing's sarcoma. *Cancer* 1980;46:516.

Rosenberg SA, Tepper J, Glatstein E, et al. The treatment of soft tissue sarcomas of the extremities: prospective randomized evaluations of (1) limb-sparing surgery plus radiation therapy compared with amputation and (2) the role of adjuvant chemotherapy. *Ann Surg* 1982;196:305.

Sarcoma Meta-analysis Collaboration. Adjuvant chemotherapy for localized resectable soft tissue sarcoma of adults: meta-analysis of individual data. *Lancet* 1997;350:1647.

Singer S. New diagnostic modalities in soft tissue sarcoma. *Semin Surg Oncol* 1999;17:11.

Singer S, Corson JM, Demetri GD, et al. Prognostic factors predictive of survival for truncal and retroperitoneal soft tissue sarcoma. *Ann Surg* 1995;221: 185.

Storm FK, Mahvi DM. Diagnosis and management of retroperitoneal soft tissue sarcoma. *Ann Surg* 1991;214:2.

Suit HD, Mankin HJ, Wood WC, et al. Treatment of the patient with stage M0 soft tissue sarcoma. *J Clin Oncol* 1988;6:854.

Tanabe KK, Pollock RE, Ellis LM, et al. Influence of surgical margins on outcome in patients with preoperatively irradiated extremity soft tissue sarcomas. *Cancer* 1994;73:1652.

Van Geel AN, Pastorino U, Jauch KW, et al. Surgical treatment of lung metastases: the European Organization for Research and Treatment of Cancer-soft tissue and bone sarcoma group study of 255 patients. *Cancer* 1996;77:675.

Van Oosterom AT, Judson IR, Verweij J, et al. Safety and efficacy of imatinib (STI571) in metastatic gastrointestinal stromal tumours: a phase I study. *Lancet* 2001;1421–1423.

Varma DG. Optimal radiologic imaging of soft tissue sarcomas. *Semin Surg Oncol* 1999;17:2.

Verweij J, Casali PG, Zalcberg J, et al. Progression-free survival in gastrointestinal stromal tumours with high-dose imatinib: radnomised trail. *Lancet* 2004: 1127–34.

Verweij J, van Oosterom A, Blay JY, et al. Imatinib mesylate (STI-571 Glivec, Gleevec) is an active agent for gastrointestinal stromal tumours, but does not yield response in other soft-tissue sarcomas that are unselected for a molecular target. Results from an EORTC Soft Tissue and Bone Sarcoma Group phase II study. *Eur J Cancer.* 2003:2006–11.

Verweij J, van Oosterom A, Somers R, et al. Chemotherapy in the multidisciplinary approach to soft tissue sarcomas: EORTC soft tissue and bone sarcoma group studies in perspective. *Ann Oncol* 1992;3 [suppl 2]:75.

Whooley BP, Mooney MM, Gibbs JF, et al. Effective follow-up strategies in soft tissue sarcoma. *Semin Surg Oncol* 1999;17:83.

Yang JC, Chang AE, Baker AR, et al. Randomized prospective study of the benefit of adjuvant radiation therapy in the treatment of soft tissue sarcomas of the extremity. *J Clin Oncol* 1998;16:197.

Zahm SH, Fraumeni JR Jr. The epidemiology of soft tissue sarcoma. *Semin Oncol* 1997;24: 504.

Cancers of the Head and Neck

Kenneth A. Newkirk and
F. Christopher Holsinger

EPIDEMIOLOGY AND PATHOGENESIS

Cancers of the head and neck represent a relatively small, albeit significant, group of cancers. The treatment of these malignancies is associated with significant functional and aesthetic morbidities that have a dramatic impact on patients' quality of life. Although the majority of cancers of the head and neck arise in the upper aerodigestive tract and salivary glands, cancers of the skin, thyroid gland, and parathyroid glands deserve special consideration and are addressed in Chapters 3, 4, and 16.

Cancers of the head and neck represent approximately 3% of all cancers in the United States (and approximately 6% worldwide in 2002), with approximately 45,000 head and neck cancers diagnosed in 2004. The majority of head and neck cancers are diagnosed in the sixth to eighth decades, with males having a 4:1 ratio. Tobacco exposure represents the most significant risk factor for cancers of the head and neck, with alcohol consumption being both a synergistic and an independent risk factor. The risk of tobacco-related head and neck cancers increases proportionately with the degree of exposure. In addition, for some patients, genetic instability (e.g., hypopharyngeal cancers associated with Plummer-Vinson syndrome), viral infections (e.g., Ebstein-Barr virus [EBV] associated with nasopharyngeal cancer, human papilloma virus associated with tonsillar cancers), and occupational (e.g., saw dust exposures and sinonasal adenocarcinomas) and environmental exposures (e.g., ultraviolet [UV] exposure and lower lip cancers, betel nut use and buccal cancers, reverse cigarette smoking and palatal cancers) have been implicated in some head and neck cancers. A small group of patients (particularly young patients with oral tongue cancers) have no identifiable risk factors and have a particularly aggressive course. Some studies suggest that the disease course may be more aggressive in African Americans than in whites, with death rates for African American males being twice that for white males with the same disease (larynx and oral cavity cancers).

PATHOLOGY

Squamous cell carcinoma (SCC) represents the most common histologic type, accounting for more than 90% of tumors. Tumors may have either an ulcerative or an exophytic growth pattern. Histologically, the tumors may be in situ or invasive. Histologic differentiation (well, moderate, and poorly differentiated) has been reported to have prognostic implications, but this has not been universally confirmed. Basaloid, spindle-shaped SCCs and verrucous carcinoma are believed to be variants of SCC, and distinguishing among the variants may have prognostic implications.

Premalignant lesions, such as leukoplakia and erythroplakia, are associated with a high risk of cancer development.

CLINICAL PRESENTATION, EVALUATION, AND PROGNOSIS

The clinical signs and symptoms of cancer of the upper aerodigestive tract is site specific. The most common presenting symptom for head and neck cancers is pain. Other symptoms that are suggestive of cancer of the upper aerodigestive tract are the presence of a nonhealing ulcer, bleeding, hoarseness, dysphagia, odynophagia, otalgia (referred pain), facial pain, neck mass, or new lesion intraorally. Symptoms can occur secondary to local destruction or involvement of adjacent structures (neural, soft-tissue, or bony involvement). The clinician should be alerted to the fact that an adult, with any of these signs and symptoms that do not resolve within 2 weeks, should be referred to an experienced clinician for evaluation.

Clinical examination of the head and neck includes visual inspection and palpation (bimanual evaluation) of the scalp, external ears, ear canals, mucous membranes of the eyes, nasal passages, oral cavity, nasopharynx, oropharynx, hypopharynx, and larynx. Examination of the larynx and pharyngeal regions are performed by either mirror examination or flexible endoscopy. Care must be taken to examine the major salivary glands visually and manually. A detailed cranial nerve examination is important for documenting pretreatment function because locally aggressive cancers may cause functional deficits pretreatment and because various treatment modalities may be associated with posttreatment dysfunction. Examination of the neck for spread to cervical lymph nodes of the upper jugulodigastric chain is important prognostically. The grouping of cervical nodes of the jugulodigastric chain (Fig. 6.1) provides a uniform system for communicating between clinicians. Metastasis to specific nodal groups or echelons can be predictive of the location of the primary site when patients present with a cervical metastasis from an unknown primary.

Biopsies of suspicious lesions can be performed in either the clinic or the operating room. Biopsies are performed with either a scalpel or punch biopsy forceps of the primary lesion or fine-needle aspiration (FNA) of suspicious lymph nodes. FNA of neck masses is as accurate as open biopsy in experienced cytopathologists' hands and is preferred over open biopsy to reduce the risk of tumor spillage and seeding of the neck. Intraoperative panendoscopy (direct laryngoscopy, esophagoscopy, nasal endoscopy, and bronchoscopy) is performed to provide adequate tissue for diagnosis from areas inaccessible in the clinic, to allow for better hemostasis, and to detail the extent of the disease for treatment planning. Improvements in fiber-optic technology (e.g., transnasal esophagoscopy) are expanding the scope of what can be evaluated and successfully biopsied in the clinical setting.

Radiographic imaging includes plain x-rays, computed tomography (CT) scans, magnetic resonance imaging (MRI) scans, ultrasound, and positron emission tomography (PET) scanning. Chest x-rays help determine the presence of distant metastasis

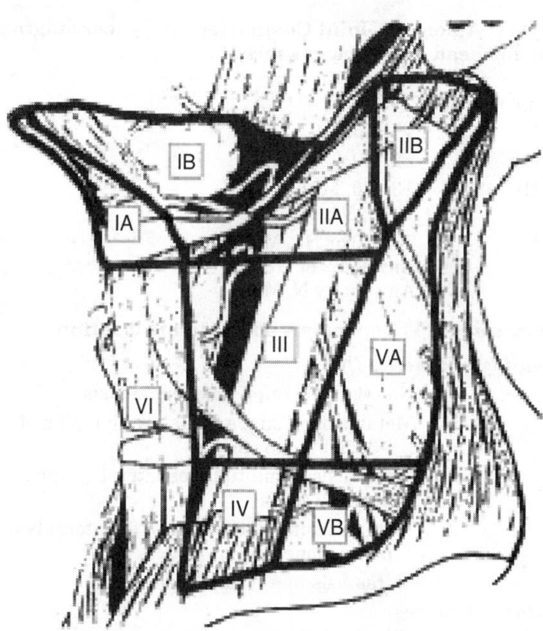

Figure 6.1. Lymph node groups. Level IA, submental, and level 1B, submandibular lymph node groups; levels IIA and IIB, upper jugular group; level III, middle jugular groups; level IV, lower jugular group; levels VA and VB, posterior triangle group; level VI, anterior compartment group.

(approximately 15% of patients) or second primaries (5%–10%). Panorex films help determine whether mandible involvement is present. CT scans from the skull base to the clavicles provide detailed information on the extent of local soft-tissue and bony involvement of upper aerodigestive tract tumors, and the presence of regionally metastatic disease to the upper cervical jugulodigastric chain.

In general, prognosis for upper aerodigestive tract cancers is determined by the size of the primary, as well as the presence of regional (cervical) nodal metastasis and distant metastasis, with bulkier disease being associated with a worse prognosis. The presence of nodal metastasis decreases survival by 50% and is associated with an increased risk of distant metastasis. Staging for head and neck cancer is based on the American Joint Committee on Cancer classification and is outlined in Table 6.1. The T stage defines the size and extent of the primary; the N stage defines the size, number, and location of nodal spread; and the M stage refers to the presence or absence of distant metastasis. Approximately 15% of head and neck cancer patients will develop distant metastasis.

Table 6.1. American Joint Committee on Cancer staging system for head and neck cancers

Stage grouping	
Stage I	T1, N0, M0
Stage II	T2, N0, M0
Stage III	T3, N0, M0 T1–3, N1, M0
Stage IV	T4, N0 or N1, M0 Any T, N2 or N3, M0 Any T, any N, M1
Primary tumor (T) dependent on anatomic location	
Regional lymph nodes (N)	
N0	No regional lymph node metastasis
N2a	Metastasis in single ipsilateral lymph node >3 cm but <6 cm
N2b	Metastasis in multiple ipsilateral lymph nodes, none >6 cm
N2c	Metastasis in bilateral or contralateral lymph nodes, none >6 cm
N3	Metastasis in a lymph node >6 cm
Metastatic disease	
M0	No evidence of distant metastasis
M1	Evidence of distant metastasis

Adapted from Greene FL, Page DL, Fleming ID, et al., eds. *AJCC Cancer Staging Manual.* 6th ed. New York, NY: Springer-Verlag; 2002, with permission.

In addition to the traditional prognostic markers, depth of invasion, perineural invasion and perivascular invasion at the primary tumor site, and lymph node extracapsular spread are associated with worse prognosis. Survival for early-stage disease (stages I and II) across sites falls in the 80% to 90% range, but drops to 3% to 40% for stage III and IV disease. Much research is currently being done to identify more selective biological and molecular predictive and prognostic markers, such as the expression of mutated p53, and epidermal growth factor receptor expression.

The mainstay for treatment of early-stage head and neck cancer is single modality therapy, either surgery or radiation therapy. More advanced disease is more appropriately treated with multimodality therapy. Chemotherapy has played an increasing role in the primary treatment of advanced head and neck cancer, in addition to maintaining its traditional role in treating recurrent or unresectable disease.

For most sites (oral cavity, sinonasal, salivary glands), surgery is the treatment of choice for early-stage disease and provides the best chance for cure if an adequate margin of resection is obtained. Limiting factors may be the potential functional deficit or cosmetic deformity to an organ system, or the accessibility of the tumor to complete surgical extirpation. Advances in surgical reconstructive techniques and prosthetics have expanded the envelope of what is appropriate surgical removal.

For early-stage disease at some sites (larynx, pharynx), radiation therapy is as effective a treatment modality as surgery, with the benefit of preserving anatomical structures. For more advanced disease, radiation is an important adjunct preoperatively and postoperatively in controlling local and regional disease and in sterilizing microscopic disease. Indications for postoperative radiation therapy are positive surgical resection margins, perineural or perivascular invasion, extracapsular spread, locally aggressive poorly differentiated tumors, tumor spillage during resection, and advanced-stage disease. Although it provides the benefit of potential "organ preservation," radiation is not without significant functional deficits. Mucositis may be severe with an acute onset. It may also be very painful, leading to dysphagia. Xerostomia (dry mouth) and dysphagia are often underappreciated but debilitating long-term sequelae. In addition to salivary gland dysfunction, thyroid dysfunction and fibrosis and scarring of soft tissues are potential long-term sequelae of radiation therapy. Multimodality therapy is the mainstay of therapy for advanced (stage II and IV) disease.

An important part of treatment is preservation of function posttreatment. Organ-specific system rehabilitation is particularly important in maintaining adequate voice and swallowing function.

Follow-up for cancers of the head and neck is important because most recurrences will occur within 2 years of treatment. At The University of Texas M. D. Anderson Cancer Center, follow-up of patients occurs every 3 months for the first 2 years postoperatively, every 6 months for the next 3 years, and yearly thereafter until 5 years. A chest x-ray and liver function studies are performed yearly.

NECK DISSECTION

Nodal metastases are associated with a 50% decrease in survival. Disease of the neck can be treated effectively with surgery and/or radiation. Limited disease (single node) with no extracapsular spread may be treated with single modality therapy, while more advanced disease may require combination therapy.

Traditionally, surgery of the neck consists of one of the following types of neck dissections: *radical neck dissection* (RND), *modified radical neck dissection* (MRND), and *selective neck dissection*. The RND consists of removal of all cervical lymph nodes in levels I to V, the sternocleidomastoid muscle, the internal jugular vein, and the spinal accessory nerve. The limits of the dissection are the inferior border of the mandible superiorly, the clavicle inferiorly, the trapezius posteriorly, the lateral border of the sternohyoid muscle anteriorly, and the deep cervical fascia overlying the levator scapulae and the scalene muscles deeply. In an attempt to decrease postoperative morbidity, the MRND was designed. It is similar to the RND but involves preservation of the spinal accessory nerve, internal jugular vein, and/or the sternocleidomastoid muscle.

A selective neck dissection involves removal of limited cervical lymph node groups (levels I–III [a *supraomohyoid neck dissection*], levels II–IV [a *lateral neck dissection*], levels II–V, VII, and postoccipital and retroauricular nodes [a *posterolateral neck dissection*]), along with preservation of the spinal accessory nerve, internal jugular vein, and sternocleidomastoid muscle. The type of selective neck dissection performed depends on the site and histology of the primary tumor and the most common routes of lymphatic spread. A supraomohyoid neck dissection is performed for clinically limited (nonpalpable) spread from oral cavity cancers, a lateral neck dissection for clinically limited (nonpalpable) spread from larynx cancers, and a posterolateral neck dissection for skin cancers (e.g., melanoma, SCC) of the scalp. Of note, a level VI or *anterior compartment neck dissection* is used in the management of thyroid cancer, along with a lateral neck dissection. More extensive disease encountered at surgery may warrant a more involved neck dissection. All patients undergoing dissection of the spinal accessory nerve will have some form of neuropraxia and should undergo postsurgical physical therapy rehabilitation.

In patients treated with surgery of the primary and neck dissection preradiation at M. D. Anderson, a selective neck dissection (e.g., supraomohyoid neck dissection for oral cavity cancers, lateral neck dissection for laryngeal cancers) is the procedure most commonly used for clinically occult disease. Clinical nodal disease is treated by a MRND. For postradiation patients, a selective neck dissection (levels II and III) is the procedure of choice for persistent adenopathy, and is associated with good local-regional control and functional outcomes.

CARCINOMA OF THE ORAL CAVITY

The oral cavity is the portion of the aerodigestive tract from the vermillion border of the lips to the junction of the hard and soft palate and the circumvallate papillae of the tongue. This region anatomically includes the lips, buccal mucosa, gingiva, floor of mouth, anterior floor of mouth, anterior two-thirds of the tongue, hard palate, and retromolar trigone region. Oral cavity cancer accounts for approximately 3% of cancers in the United States, is the sixth most common cancer worldwide, and comprises 30% of all head and neck cancers. In 2005, in the United States alone, an estimated 20,000 cancers occurred in the oral cavity, and approximately 5,000 deaths were attributable to oral cavity cancers. Men are more commonly affected than women (3–4:1), and the mean age of occurrence is in the sixth to seventh decades.

Staging of the primary is based on the TNM stage, with size of the primary tumor determining the T stage. T1 lesions measure less than 2 cm, T2 measure from 2 to 4 cm, T3 measure 4 cm, and T4 measure greater than 4 cm or involve extension to local tissues (Table 6.2).

Surgical excision is the mainstay of therapy for oral cavity cancers. An adequate margin of normal tissue (at least 1–1.5 cm) is taken to ensure proper resection. Surgical defects can be left to heal by secondary intention or are repaired by primary closure, split-thickness skin grafting, local rotational or advancement flap reconstruction, or free flap reconstruction for large defects. Neck dissections are done for clinically evident nodal disease and

Table 6.2. Staging system for oral cavity tumors

Tis	Carcinoma in situ
T1	Tumor ≥2 cm at greatest dimension
T2	Tumor >2 cm but not 4 cm at greatest dimension
T3	Tumor >4 cm at greatest dimension
T4	Tumor invades adjacent structures (e.g., cortical bone, deep extrinsic muscle of tongue, maxillary sinus, or skin)

Adapted from Greene FL, Page DL, Fleming ID, et al., eds. *AJCC Cancer Staging Manual.* 6th ed. New York, NY: Springer-Verlag; 2002, with permission.

electively for large primary tumors or tumors with a depth of invasion greater than 4 mm or other poor prognostic factors as listed previously. The traditional neck dissection for oral cavity lesions is a supraomohyoid neck dissection (levels I–III), although some data exist for including level IV lymph nodes due to the possibility of skip metastasis. Primary tumors close to the midline may require bilateral neck dissections because the risk of spread to the contralateral neck may be greater than 20%.

Radiation therapy is given in the form of external-beam therapy or brachytherapy implants (primary interstitial brachytherapy implants are used for small lesions of the anterior commisure of the lip, oral tongue, and floor of mouth [T1 lesions]). Radiation therapy is only rarely used as the primary therapy and is reserved for postoperative treatment of patients at high risk for local-regional recurrence (i.e., large primary tumors [T3 or T4], primary tumors with close or positive margins, evidence of perineural or lymphovascular invasion, tumors with a depth of invasion greater than 4 mm, nodal metastasis with evidence of extracapsular spread, or multiple positive nodes).

The prognosis for early lesions (T1 and T2) of the oral cavity is good, with a 5-year survival of 80% to 90%. Survival for advanced lesions (T3 and T4) can range from 30% to 60%, depending on the factors that affect prognosis as outlined previously.

LIP

Cancer of the lip accounts for approximately 25% to 30% of oral cavity cancers, with greater than 90% being SCC and greater than 90% occurring on the lower lip. Smoking and sun exposure are major risk factors. Surgery is the treatment of choice for small lesions, with the exception of commissure lesions, which may be better treated with radiation. Cure rates approaching 90% are achievable for early lesions, with more advanced lesions having a 5-year survival of less than 50%. Nodal metastases are associated with large primary tumors; tumors of the upper lip and commissure, as well as perineural spread along the mental nerve, portends a poorer prognosis.

BUCCAL MUCOSA

Buccal mucosa cancers represent 5% of oral cavity cancers. Tobacco smoking, alcohol use, smokeless tobacco use, and betel nut use have been associated with buccal cancers. The region near the lower third molar is a common site for buccal cancers, and patients may present with trismus due to involvement of the pterygoid muscles. Cervical metastases may be common (50%) and are associated with a poor prognosis. Wide local excision is the treatment of choice, and a possible marginal mandibulectomy may be necessary to obtain clear margins. Early-stage disease may be associated with cure rates in the 60% to 70% range, while advanced tumors have survival of approximately 40%. Local-regional recurrence is a significant problem. Survival may be improved with postoperative radiation. The surgical defect may be reconstructed with local advancement flaps (e.g., tongue) or may require free flap reconstruction.

FLOOR OF MOUTH

Approximately 10% to 15% of oral cavity cancers occur in the floor of the mouth. Approximately 50% of patients will present with cervical metastasis, which, as with other oral cavity sites, is a predictor of poor prognosis. Deep tongue muscle and mandible involvement is frequently seen, requiring partial glossectomy and marginal or segmental mandibulectomy with free flap reconstruction to obtain clean margins. Bilateral cervical metastasis is not uncommon. Overall 5-year survival rates range from 30% to 70%, with stages I and II approaching 70% to 80% and stage IV disease being less than 50%.

ORAL TONGUE

Oral tongue (anterior two-thirds of the tongue) carcinoma accounts for approximately 37% of estimated new oral cavity cancers in 2005. Partial glossectomy with healing by secondary intention, primary closure, skin grafting, or free flap reconstruction is the accepted treatment. In addition to the size of the primary and histologic grade, tumor thickness also has prognostic significance for local-regional recurrence, with lesions greater than 4 mm having a 40% to 50% incidence of nodal metastasis. For tumors of 4 mm or greater thickness, an ipsilateral supraomohyoid neck dissection (levels I–III) is recommended for management of the neck. There are some data that suggest that a level IV dissection may be warranted due to the presence of skip metastasis; however, this is usually done for patients' metastasis in levels I to III. Early-stage tumors have a good prognosis (70%–80% 3-year survival for stages I and II and 40%–50% for stage III and IV disease), while advanced lesions require combined modality treatment. A small subset of oral tongue cancers occurs in patients younger than 40 years of age with no known risk factors; these cancers appear to be more aggressive and therefore warrant more aggressive therapy. Speech and swallowing rehabilitation are essential for good postoperative function. SCC of the base of the tongue behaves differently and is reviewed in the Cancer of the Oropharynx, Nasopharynx, and Hypopharynx section later in this chapter.

HARD PALATE

Hard palate SCCs represent approximately 0.5% of all oral cavity cancers in the United States. Cancers of the hard palate and gingiva are treated with wide local excision. Tumors within close proximity to or involving bone and large tumors may require partial palatectomy or maxillectomy to obtain clear margins. Bony defects are best reconstructed with a palatal prosthesis or obturator. Five-year cure rates approach 40% to 70% in patients without nodal disease.

CANCER OF THE LARYNX

In the United States, larynx cancers will have an estimated incidence of 10,000 new cases in 2005. Cancers occur in the sixth to eighth decades with a male-to-female ratio of 4:1. Tobacco and alcohol abuse are the most common risk factors associated with development of laryngeal cancer. The larynx is divided into three subsites—the *supraglottis, glottis,* and *subglottis*—that have implications for behavior, treatment, and prognosis.

The *supraglottis* is the portion of the larynx above the laryngeal ventricle and below the laryngeal surface of the epiglottis. The supraglottis contains the epiglottis, arytenoids, aryepiglottic folds, false cords, and ventricles. The lymphatic drainage is into the upper and mid-jugulodigastric chain via the pyriform sinuses and is bilateral, which makes addressing both sides of the neck for a supraglottic cancer a necessity. Sensation is via the internal branch of the superior laryngeal nerve. Cancers of the supraglottis account for 35% of laryngeal cancers. The *glottis* is the portion of the larynx that comprises the true vocal folds. The lymphatic drainage is minimal due to the close adherence of the mucosa to the underlying vocal ligament. Sensation is via the superior laryngeal nerve. Glottic cancers comprise 65% of laryngeal cancers. The *subglottis* extends from the inferior portion of the true vocal folds to the inferior border of the cricoid cartilage. Lymphatic drainage is via efferents that enter into the deep cervical jugulodigastric nodes and the paratracheal and pretracheal lymph nodes bilaterally. Subglottic cancers comprise less than 5% of laryngeal cancers. Subsite division is important for diagnosis and treatment of early tumors; however, in advanced stages, laryngeal cancers may have extensive *paraglottic* (submucosal spread around the laryngeal framework) and *transglottic* (extension across subsites) spread. Staging for laryngeal cancers varies and is listed in Table 6.3.

Presenting symptoms for laryngeal cancers include hoarseness, pain, dysphagia, and respiratory distress. Evaluation of the larynx is essential for staging of laryngeal cancers. Impaired vocal fold mobility and subsite extension portend a more advanced cancer and poorer prognosis. Cancers that affect the true vocal fold usually present early due to the impairment in function (voice and respiration). Supraglottic cancers usually present late, with submucosal and local spread, and symptoms are due to invasion of local tissues causing hoarseness, dysphagia, odynophagia, otalgia (referred pain), and respiratory distress. Imaging of the larynx (CT scanning) is important in determining local extension of the primary disease, laryngeal cartilage destruction, and the presence of clinically occult disease.

Treatment

Because glottic cancers are the most common laryngeal cancers seen, these are discussed in detail. The goal of treatment of

Table 6.3. Staging system for cancers of the larynx

Supraglottis	
T1	Tumor confined to site of origin
T2	Tumor involving adjacent supraglottic sites, without glottic fixation
T3	Tumor limited to the larynx, with fixation and/or extension to the postericoid medial wall of the pyriform sinus or pre-epiglottic space
T4	Massive tumor extending beyond the larynx to involve the oropharynx, soft tissues of the neck, or destruction of thyroid cartilage
Glottis	
T1	Tumor confined to vocal folds, with normal vocal cord mobility
T1a	Limited to one vocal fold
T1b	Involves both vocal folds
T2	Tumor extension to supraglottis and/or subglottis with normal or impaired vocal cord mobility
T3	Tumor confined to larynx, with fixation of the vocal cords
T4	Massive tumor, with thyroid cartilage destruction and/or extension beyond the confines of the larynx

Adapted from Greene FL, Page DL, Fleming ID, et al., eds. *AJCC Cancer Staging Manual*. 6th ed. New York, NY: Springer-Verlag; 2002, with permission.

laryngeal cancer is eradication of the disease, as well as preservation of function and anatomy when possible. Both surgery and radiation provide excellent control rates for T1 and T2 glottic lesions. Estimated 5-year survival for all cancers of the larynx is 65%. Local control rates in the literature for both treatment modalities range from 70% to 100%, which improves with salvage laryngectomy. T3 and T4 tumors have control rates in the 80% to 85% and 60% to 70% range, respectively. Five-year survival for T1 and T2 lesions is 80% to 90%, and for T3 and T4 disease, 50% to 60%. More advanced laryngeal cancers require combined modality therapy with total laryngectomy (or a modification thereof) and postoperative radiation therapy.

Surgery

Early-stage glottic disease may be treated effectively with surgery or radiation therapy. Surgical options for early glottic disease include vocal cord stripping, transoral laser microsurgery, hemilaryngectomy, subtotal laryngectomy (supracricoid partial laryngectomy [SCPL]), and total laryngectomy. The advantages of surgery are complete extirpation of the disease and reservation of other treatments (e.g., radiation) for future recurrences. Both vocal cord stripping and laser microsurgery may leave the cord with scarring that can make it difficult to evaluate for recurrence. A *vertical partial laryngectomy* (*VPL* or *hemilaryngectomy)* involves removal of half of the larynx vertically, as well as preservation of half of the larynx vertically, to maintain voice and function. Patients with small volume disease after radiation are good candidates for this procedure. For early-stage supraglottic cancers (T1 and T2), a *supraglottic or horizontal laryngectomy* may be performed. The cricoid and at least one arytenoid is preserved and sutured onto the base of the tongue, again in an attempt to preserve adequate respiration, voice, and swallowing function. Candidates for this procedure require adequate pulmonary reserve and cardiac function to prevent aspiration pneumonia.

The SCPL is an extended horizontal partial laryngectomy technique that preserves the patient's native voice and permits near-total laryngectomy without permanent tracheostoma. SCPL can include removal of the false and true vocal cords, the entire thyroid cartilage including the entire paraglottic spaces, and a portion or all of the supraglottis and pre-epiglottic space. In selected cases, one arytenoid may be resected. Phonatory function and deglutition is maintained by the movement of the spared arytenoid(s) against the tongue base. It represents a dramatic advance because it uses the patient's laryngeal framework to preserve the patient's native voice, while providing a true en bloc tumor resection.

Total laryngectomy is reserved for more advanced disease (T3 and T4) or patients who have failed previous therapy and who are likely to have poor functional outcomes (voice and swallowing) with voice-sparing surgical procedures. A bilateral lateral neck dissection can be performed at the same time for more extensive disease (a wide-field laryngectomy), and hemi- or total thyroidectomy is performed for disease that destroys cartilage or involves the pyriform sinuses, subglottis, or paratracheal nodes. In cases with significant hypopharyngeal or cervical esophageal extension, a laryngopharyngectomy can be performed and repaired with a free tissue transfer microvascular reconstruction. Postoperative radiation is typically given in advanced disease. Speech pathology consultation is essential preoperatively for adequate voice and swallowing rehabilitation postoperatively. Voice rehabilitation with an electrolarynx, tracheoesophageal puncture, or esophageal speech can lead to good voice quality. In addition to being monitored for recurrence, patients also need to be followed for potential hypothyroidism (either from surgery or radiation).

Radiation Therapy

Given the good rates of local-regional control, radiation therapy has been advocated as the treatment of choice for early-stage disease. The advantages of radiation are sparing of the anatomy with preservation of voice. The disadvantages are postradiation sequelae (e.g., xerostomia, potential radionecrosis of the laryngeal framework) and the inability to use radiation again in the event of a recurrence. Postoperative radiation therapy is typically given to patients with extensive primary disease (submucosal spread, subsite extension [i.e., supra- or subglottic, extralaryngeal extension]), disease with positive margins, multiple positive lymph nodes, or lymph nodes with extracapsular spread, and patients requiring prelaryngectomy tracheotomy (who have a higher risk of stomal recurrence).

Typical doses of primary radiation for early laryngeal disease are in the 65 to 70 Gy range. For glottic cancers, the radiation can be focused on the primary site due to the low incidence of nodal metastasis. For supraglottic cancers with a higher propensity of cervical metastasis at the time of diagnosis, fields should encompass the primary nodal drainage basins (levels II–V), with doses in the 50 to 60 Gy ranges.

CANCER OF THE OROPHARYNX, NASOPHARYNX, AND HYPOPHARYNX

The pharynx is a tubular structure that contains the larynx. The pharynx can be divided into three anatomical subsites: the nasopharynx, the oropharynx, and the hypopharynx. The anatomical boundaries of the oropharynx are the anterior tonsillar pillar, uvula and base of tongue, and the vallecular surface of the epiglottis inferiorly. Included in this subsite are the pharyngeal tonsils and the base of tongue. The nasopharynx is separated from the oropharynx by the soft palate. The boundaries of the hypopharynx are the laryngeal surface of the epiglottis, the pyriform sinuses, the posterior pharyngeal wall, and the postcricoid area above the cricopharyngeus muscle. Lymphatic drainage for the nasopharynx is the retropharyngeal lymph node basin, the parapharyngeal lymph nodes, and the upper and posterior jugulodigastric nodes. Lymphatics for the oropharynx are in the deep, upper jugulodigastric chain, while the hypopharynx drains into the mid- and lower deep jugulodigastric chain. Bilateral cervical metastases are not uncommon. The parapharyngeal space is a potential space located outside the pharynx proper. It is pyramidal shape and extends from the skull base to the hyoid bone. Most tumors of this region are benign; the most common tumors arise from the deep lobe of the parotid gland and include unusual histologic variants such as pleomorphic adenomas, paragangliomas, and neurogenic tumors (schwannomas and neurofibromas), rather than the common squamous tumors of the upper aerodigestive tract.

The most common presenting symptoms are pain, dysphagia, referred otalgia, and a neck mass. In an attempt to cure disease with decreased morbidity and to preserve function (swallowing), external-beam radiation (tonsil, hypopharynx, base of tongue) has become the treatment of choice for oropharyngeal and hypopharyngeal cancers. Survival rates have been in the 70% to 80% range for stage I and II disease and 50% for stage II disease. Surgery is reserved for small lesions and recurrent disease, due to the increased morbidity associated with surgery. Brachytherapy is also used in some centers for base of tongue tumors.

Nasopharyngeal cancers are malignancies that arise from or near the fossa of Rosenmüller in the nasopharynx. These cancers are most commonly seen in regions of China and Africa, where there is a strong association with EBV. Indeed, EBV viral capsid IgA antigen (VC) and early antigen IgA (EA) titers serve as a tumor marker for recurrence. The average age at presentation is in the fifth and sixth decades. Most patients present with a painless neck mass, nasal obstruction, unilateral serous otitis media, or epistaxis. Cranial neuropathy (particularly involving cranial nerves II, IV, V, and VI) may occur as a result of skull base invasion, which may be seen in as many as 25% of patients. An irregular mass is seen on nasopharyngoscopy. Tumors are classified according to the World Health Organization classification (type I being well-differentiated keratinizing SCC, type II being nonkeratinizing carcinoma, and type III being poorly differentiated [undifferentiated] carcinoma, which includes lymphoepitheliomas and anaplastic carcinomas).

The mainstay of therapy is cisplatin-based chemotherapy and radiation therapy to the nasopharyngeal bed and primary draining lymph node echelons. Tumors are staged based on extent of disease with stage I tumors limited to the nasopharynx; stage II disease involving extension into the oropharynx, nasal fossa, and parapharyngeal space; stage III disease involving extension into the skull base fossa and paranasal sinuses; and stage IV disease involving the infratemporal fossa, orbit, and hypopharynx, or with intracranial extension and/or cervical adenopathy. Five-year survival for nasopharyngeal carcinoma is less than 20% for type I tumors and approaches 50% for type II and III tumors. Surgery may be used for limited, early-stage disease, but is associated with significant morbidity. Neck dissections are performed for residual disease post chemoradiotherapy.

Cancers of the hypopharynx usually present at advanced stages (greater than 60% are stage III and IV) and are associated with poor local control and survival. The majority of cancers occur in the pyriform sinus (70%–80%), and nodal disease at the time of presentation is common (70%–80%). Chemoradiation is the mainstay of therapy, although total laryngectomy or laryngopharyngectomy may be suitable for some patients. Five-year survival for hypopharyngeal cancers is dismal, ranging from 20% to 40%.

CANCER OF THE NASAL CAVITY AND PARANASAL SINUSES

The nasal cavity extends from the external nasal dorsum and pyriform aperture to the choana and the nasopharynx, and from the nasal floor (which is comprised of the maxilla anteriorly and the palatine bone posteriorly) to the nasal roof (which houses the olfactory bulbs and cranial nerve I). The nasal septum, which is composed of cartilage anteriorly and the vomer and perpendicular plate of the ethmoid bones posteriorly, separates the nose into halves. The lateral nasal walls house the ostia for the paranasal sinuses; the nasofrontal duct; and the inferior, middle, and superior turbinates. The nasal cavity and paranasal sinuses are lined by respiratory epithelium (pseudostratified ciliated columnar epithelium), except at the nasal vestibule, which is lined by keratinizing squamous epithelium. The sensory innervation to the nasal and paranasal mucosa is from branches of the trigeminal nerve (V1 and V2). The blood supply is from the external carotid (superior labial, angular, and internal maxillary arteries) and internal carotid (anterior and posterior ethmoidal arteries) arteries.

There are four paired paranasal sinuses: the maxillary, frontal, ethmoid, and sphenoid sinuses. The sinuses communicate with the nasal cavity through their ostia. The ostium of the maxillary sinus drains underneath the middle turbinate at the osteomeatal complex, as do the ostia of the anterior and middle ethmoid sinuses. The frontal sinus drains through the nasofrontal duct located at the anterior aspect of the nose. The ostia of the sphenoid sinuses are located above and medial to the superior turbinate on the face of the sinus. Lymphatic drainage of the paranasal sinuses occurs via the retropharyngeal, parapharyngeal, and deep upper jugulodigastric lymph nodes.

The most common presenting symptoms for sinonasal tumors are unilateral nasal obstruction, facial pain, facial numbness, and epistaxis. Patients may also present with unilateral serous otitis media (due to obstruction of the eustachian tube orifice), epiphora, or excessive tearing (due to obstruction of the nasolacrimal duct, which drains underneath the inferior turbinate). Nodal metastases are uncommon in sinonasal malignancies. Occupational exposures are associated with certain sinonasal malignancies (e.g., wood dust with adenocarcinomas, smoking nickel and heavy metal exposures with SCCs).

Evaluation of the nose and paranasal sinuses includes external and endoscopic inspection. Biopsies of nasal and paranasal tumors should be done cautiously because of the risk of bleeding and cerebrospinal fluid leak due to intracranial extension, and may warrant imaging prior to biopsy. Imaging (both CT scan and MRI scan) is important in determining the extent of the disease (i.e., extension beyond the nose and paranasal sinuses into the brain, orbit, skull base, and infratemporal fossa). Contrast CT scan is used to determine the presence of bony destruction and the vascularity of the lesion. MRI scanning is helpful in delineating the extent of soft-tissue destruction (intracranial and intraorbital involvement) and distinguishing tumor from inspissated fluid on T2-weighted images.

Benign tumors of the nasal cavity include nasal papillomas and angiofibromas. Nasal papillomas are divided into squamous and Schneiderian papillomas (the most common). Schneiderian papillomas usually present with unilateral nasal obstruction, epistaxis, and rhinorrhea. There are three subtypes of Schneiderian papillomas: cylindrical, septal, and inverting, the latter two being the most common. Septal papillomas account for 50% of Schneiderian papillomas. They arise from the nasal septum, are exophytic in nature, and occur most commonly in males in the third to sixth decades of life. Inverting papillomas most commonly arise from the lateral nasal wall, are polypoid in nature, occur most commonly in males (fifth to eighth decades), and, as the name implies, push the stroma inward (hence, the term inverting papilloma). Up to 15% of tumors may harbor SCC, and there is a risk (10%) of squamous degeneration. Surgical excision is the treatment of choice; this involves a medial maxillectomy, or an open or endoscopic resection of the lateral nasal wall.

Angiofibromas are benign locally destructive vascular tumors. They are seen most commonly in young males (second to fourth decades) who present with a history of unilateral nasal obstruction and recurrent, refractory epistaxis. It is a smooth lobulated mass arising in the posterior lateral nose near the sphenopalatine foramen (derives its blood supply from the sphenopalatine artery). Contrast CT scan or MRI is diagnostic (anterior bowing of the posterior maxillary sinus wall [Holman-Miller sign]). Office biopsy should not be performed due to the risk of bleeding.

Surgery following embolization (within 48 hours) is the treatment of choice.

Sinonasal malignancies are rare, accounting for less than 5% of head and neck malignancies. The differential for sinonasal malignancies include mucosal melanomas, sarcomas, SCCs, sinonasal undifferentiated carcinomas (SNUCs), lymphomas (angiocentric T-cell lymphoma), esthesioneuroblastomas (also called olfactory neuroblastomas), extramedullary plasmacytomas, adenocarcinomas, and adenoid cystic carcinomas. Hematoxylin and eosin staining may only reveal small blue cells, making the diagnosis difficult. Immunohistochemical analysis is important in establishing the diagnosis.

The most common type of sinonasal tumor is SCC, occurring predominantly in males in the sixth to eighth decades. Histologically, they are similar to SCCs elsewhere in the head and neck. Mucosal melanomas are rare (1%–2% of all melanomas), with a fairly equal male-to-female ratio. Up to one-third may be amelanotic, and immunohistochemical staining is important in establishing the diagnosis. Survival is poor, with less than 30% of patients alive at 5 years. Esthesioneuroblastoma is a rare tumor arising from the olfactory neuroepithelium with intranasal extension. Epistaxis, anosmia, pain, and nasal obstruction are common presenting symptoms. Combined nasal and intracranial surgery (craniofacial resection) followed by radiation is the preferred treatment. Five-year survival approaches 70% for resectable disease, although there is a high incidence of local recurrence. Angiocentric T-cell lymphoma is a non-Hodgkin lymphoma that may present with nasal obstruction, epistaxis, and local tissue destruction of the midline midface (septum). The tissues are friable and necrotic on endoscopy. Multiple biopsies may be needed to confirm the diagnosis. Radiation is the treatment of choice. Sinonasal sarcomas are rare and associated with a poor prognosis. Treatment usually involves some combination of surgery and radiation. Chemotherapy may be used, based on the histologic subtype. SNUC is also rare and associated with a poor prognosis. Local extension is common (intracranial and intraorbital). Craniofacial resection with postoperative radiation is the treatment of choice. Extramedullary plasmacytoma is the most common type of localized plasma cell neoplasm in the head and neck; yet, it accounts for less than 1% of all head and neck neoplasms. Males are more commonly affected than females (3:1), and up to 70% occur in the head and neck. Nasal obstruction and epistaxis are common. CT and MRI are nondiagnostic, and biopsy is important in establishing the diagnosis. Staining for lambda and kappa light chains confirms the diagnosis. Systemic workup for multiple myeloma is important because these tumors may progress to multiple myeloma in up to 30% of cases. Radiation is the treatment of choice with local control rates of 70% to 80% and 5-year survival of 60% to 70%. Adenocarcinomas and adenoid cystic carcinomas are commonly seen in sinus malignancies, and are associated with local extension and perineural spread.

Surgery followed by radiation has been the accepted treatment for these disorders. Small tumors are amenable to surgical extirpation via open or endoscopic approaches. Small squamous cell tumors of the nasal vestibule respond well to brachytherapy.

However, due to the late presentation of many sinonasal tumors and local extension to the skull base and orbit, surgery may be associated with high morbidity (e.g., neurologic sequelae and sacrifice of the orbit). Surgery may entail a partial or total rhinectomy, partial or total maxillectomy and adjacent sinuses (ethmoid and frontal), orbital exenteration, and combined approaches with neurosurgery for intracranial extension (craniofacial resection). Neck dissection is reserved for clinically gross disease. There are some data that suggest that preoperative chemotherapy may be beneficial in minimizing the extent of surgery, but this remains investigational. Prognosis for sinonasal malignancies is poor, with overall 5-year survival rates of 20% to 30%. Survival for early-stage disease (60%–70% for T1) is better than for latter stages (10%–20% for T4).

UNKNOWN PRIMARY WITH CERVICAL METASTASIS

Approximately 2% to 9% of patients who present with SCC metastatic to the neck will have an undiagnosed or unknown primary at the time of presentation. However, after careful evaluation and workup, approximately 90% of these patients will have a primary diagnosis. Thus, only approximately 10% of patients have an unknown primary tumor. Although persistent adenopathy can be associated with numerous inflammatory or infectious conditions (e.g., cat scratch disease, atypical mycobacterium), malignant cervical adenopathy should be suspected in patients with adenopathy that persists for more than 2 weeks after appropriate medical (antibiotic) therapy. The most common pathology seen is ACC, although lymphoma, melanoma metastasis from the skin, and metastatic thyroid, lung, and breast cancer may rarely present with persistent adenopathy in the head and neck.

A thorough history and physical, which should include endoscopy to rule out the primary, should be performed on all patients. Random biopsies of potential sites are not recommended. However, goal-directed biopsies of suspicious areas and bilateral tonsillectomy are indicated, depending on the site of the nodal metastasis, because as many as 25% of tonsils may harbor an occult primary. The site of nodal metastasis may indicate the site of the primary. For example, cystic or level II adenopathy may suggest an oropharyngeal primary (base of tongue or tonsil), while level V adenopathy may be suggestive of a nasopharyngeal or thyroid primary and a supraclavicular node may suggest a lung or gastrointestinal primary. Common occult upper aerodigestive tract sites for primary disease are the tonsil, base of tongue, pyriform sinus, and nasopharynx. If FNA suggests a primary other than SCC, then an appropriate, systemic metastatic workup needs to be performed. Directed diagnostic imaging of the head and neck, such as CT or MRI scanning, is important. The role of PET scans has not been established in head and neck cancers, but data are promising in the setting of known and unknown primary disease, depending on the volume of disease present.

Treatment for true unknown cervical primaries is surgery (neck dissection), radiation, or surgery followed by postoperative radiation, either to the nodal basin alone or with elective irradiation of the most common mucosal sites (i.e., the nasopharynx, oropharynx, hypopharynx, and supraglottis). Data suggest that there may be a decrease in the occurrence of an occult primary with the latter approach. Some authors view this as controversial and recommend reserving radiation to the elective sites until a primary develops to reduce the morbidity associated with radiation.

Surgery for squamous cell primaries usually entails a selective or MRND. If there is single nodal disease with no poor prognostic criteria (e.g., extracapsular spread, multiple nodes, less than 3 cm), then surgery alone or radiation alone may result in a good outcome. For bulkier, more aggressive disease, surgery (e.g., MRND, RND) and radiation (usually postoperative, but sometimes preoperative) is the treatment of choice. Surgery is also indicated for the diagnosis of metastatic well-differentiated thyroid cancer, which would entail a total thyroidectomy and neck dissection (lateral and anterior compartment).

Surgery for tumors of infraclavicular origin (e.g., breast or gastrointestinal) must be carefully considered in light of the high risk of systemic metastasis elsewhere in the body. If the tumor is limited to the neck with no other distant metastasis, then surgery and postoperative radiation may improve local control. For poorly differentiated tumors suggestive of nasopharyngeal origin, the preferred treatment is radiation.

Five-year survival for treatment of unknown squamous cervical metastases approaches 40% to 60% in many studies, whether using surgery alone or surgery and radiation. Close follow-up is important because the primary will declare itself in as many as 20% of patients. Prognosis for metastatic disease from an infraclavicular primary is poor, being less than 10% in most studies.

CANCERS OF THE EAR AND TEMPORAL BONES

The ear is composed of the external ear (pinna, auricle, and external canal), the middle ear, and the inner ear. The epithelium over the external ear is squamous with adjacent adnexal and glandular (sebaceous) structures, while ciliated epithelium and glands line the middle ear. The framework of the auricle and outer third of the external canal is comprised of elastic cartilage, while the inner third of the external canal and middle ear is made up of the temporal bone.

Cancers of the ear and temporal bones are rare and account for less than 1% of all head and neck cancers. Although cutaneous malignancies of the pinna and auricle are common, cancers of the temporal bone are rare. The majority of tumors of the ear involve the auricle (>80%), followed by the ear canal and middle ear and mastoid. Males are more commonly affected, and sun exposure is a major risk factor. SCC is the most common histologic cancer of the outer ear, followed by basal cell carcinomas. Rhabdomysarcomas and adenocarcinomas can occur in the middle ear. Pain, aural fullness, conductive hearing loss, ulceration, and chronic otorrhea are common presenting symptoms. Extension toward the middle ear may be associated with cranial neuropathies such as facial paralysis and sensorineural hearing loss in up to one-third of patients.

Surgery is often the preferred therapy for SCC and basal cell carcinomas, although radiation therapy may play a role in highly selected cases. Small lesions of the outer ear are treated effectively by partial or total auriculectomy. Early external canal lesions can be effectively treated by sleeve resection. Lateral temporal bone resection is reserved for large tumors with medial extension, which may include parotidectomy for parotid nodal metastasis.

Survival for cancers of the outer ear approaches 90% for cancers confined to the auricle, with decreasing prognosis for those with medial extension and middle ear extension to less than 30%. Temporal bone malignancies have a survival rate of 20% to 30% at 5 years.

NEOPLASMS OF THE SALIVARY GLAND

Salivary gland tissue in the upper aerodigestive tract consists of three pairs of major salivary glands—parotid glands, submandibular or submaxillary glands, and sublingual glands—and thousands of minor salivary glands that exist in the mucosa of the lips, buccal mucosa, hard and soft palate, and oropharynx. The parotid glands lie lateral and posterior to the mandible, and can be divided into a superficial and a deep lobe by the course of the facial nerve. The deep lobe of the parotid gland abuts the prestyloid, parapharyngeal space, and deep lobe parotid tumors (e.g., pleomorphic adenomas) are the most common tumors in this region. The duct of the parotid gland (Stenson duct) drains intraorally near the second maxillary molar. Lymph nodes are present in the substance of the gland, and the nodal basin for the parotid gland is the preauricular and upper jugulodigastric nodes. Of note, the parotid gland and associated lymph nodes are a primary nodal drainage basin for scalp and auricular malignancies, and a parotidectomy should be included in any comprehensive treatment of these malignancies. The submandibular glands are located beneath the mandible and their ducts (Wharton ducts), and drain near the frenulum of the tongue in the floor of the mouth. The marginal mandibular branch of the facial nerve overlies the gland superficially, the facial vessels (and associated lymph nodes) are intimately associated with gland, and the lingual and hypoglossal nerves are closely associated with the deep surface of the gland. The sublingual glands are located deep to the mucosa of the floor of the mouth on top of the mylohyoid muscle.

Tumors of the salivary glands can occur in both major and minor salivary glands, with the majority occurring in the major salivary glands. The majority of tumors occur in the parotid glands (90%), and the majority of these are benign (80%). As the size of the gland decreases, the risk of malignancy increases, with 50% of submandibular gland tumors being malignant and 80% of sublingual gland tumors being malignant. Some tumors are associated with previous radiation exposure or smoking (e.g., Warthin tumors). However, the majority of salivary gland tumors have no identifiable risk factors.

Most salivary gland tumors present as a painless mass, although rapid growth and pain may be seen but are not always suggestive of more ominous or aggressive disease because inflammatory or infectious diseases can present with similar symptoms (e.g., parotitis or collagen vascular diseases such as Sjögren syndrome or Wegner granulomatosis). Facial paralysis, nodal metastasis, and local tissue invasion may be indicative of a more aggressive disease. Of note, Bell palsy (idiopathic facial nerve paralysis) is a diagnosis of exclusion, and the patient with a sudden facial nerve paralysis should have a parotid malignancy (either primary or metastatic from a skin primary) ruled out.

FNA is helpful in establishing the diagnosis but is highly dependent on the skill of the cytopathologist (accuracy ranges from 60%–90%). If an FNA cannot establish the diagnosis, then an open, excisional biopsy should be performed. In the case of the parotid gland, an excisional biopsy would entail performing a *superficial parotidectomy* to identify and preserve the facial nerve. Incisional biopsy should be avoided to prevent tumor violation, tumor spillage, and, in the case of the parotid gland, facial nerve injury. CT and MRI scans are helpful in detailing the extent of disease (e.g., parapharyngeal space extension of deep lobe parotid tumors or skull base involvement).

The majority of tumors in the salivary glands are benign, with pleomorphic adenomas being the most common. Other benign tumors include Warthin tumors (which are associated with smoking and are bilateral in 10% of cases), monomorphic adenomas, and oncocytomas. Malignant tumors include mucoepidermoid carcinomas, adenoid cystic carcinomas, adenocarcinomas, and SCCs.

Treatment

Surgery is the mainstay of therapy for all parotid tumors. For benign tumors, superficial parotidectomy and submandibular gland excision are both diagnostic and curative. Because of the intimate relationship of the parotid gland and submandibular glands to the facial nerve and its branches, as well as the morbidity associated with facial nerve paralysis, only gross involvement of the nerve by tumor is an indication for sacrifice. Pleomorphic adenomas are the most common benign tumors of the salivary glands. Care must be taken to remove a rim of normal tissue around the tumor, as well as to avoid rupture of the pseudocapsule and tumor spillage, to reduce the risk of recurrence.

Malignant tumors of the salivary glands typically require surgery and radiation. The exceptions are low-grade neoplasms (e.g., low-grade mucoepidermoid carcinomas and polymorphous low-grade adenocarcinomas), which may be treated with surgery alone. Superficial parotidectomy is indicated for small lesions. For parotid tumors with deep lobe extension, total parotidectomy with facial nerve preservation is the treatment of choice. Gross involvement of the facial nerve by tumor is an indication for sacrifice of the nerve. In such cases, the nerve should be traced proximally (as far back as the brainstem, if necessary) until tumor is cleared. This is especially true of adenoid cystic carcinomas, which are neurotropic tumors. Sacrifice of the facial nerve should be repaired immediately either by interpositional nerve grafting (using the sural nerve from the leg or medial antebrachial cutaneous nerve from the arm) or a cranial nerve XII to VII grafting. Parotid tumors with local extension (skin or external canal involvement) may require a mastoidectomy (to trace the nerve proximally) and removal of the lateral part of the temporal bone. Excision of the submandibular gland and adjacent facial lymph nodes is the treatment for submandibular tumors. As with the parotid, only gross involvement with tumor is an indication for nerve sacrifice (e.g., lingual and hypoglossal nerves), and local extension to surrounding tissues (e.g., floor of mouth musculature, tongue) necessitates more radical surgery. Neck dissection (selective) is reserved for clinically apparent neck disease.

Radiation is reserved for primary treatment of malignant tumors in patients who are poor surgical candidates or who do not want to undergo surgery, as well as for the postoperative treatment of high-grade or recurrent disease. Adenoid cystic carcinomas, high-grade mucoepidermoid carcinomas, high-grade adenocarcinomas, SCCs, and metastatic disease to the neck are typically irradiated. In addition, patients with pleomorphic adenomas that are recurrent or involve gross tumor spillage may be candidates for postoperative radiation. Doses to the primary tumor bed are in the range of 50 to 70 Gy.

Five-year survival for benign tumors approaches 100%, with the greatest risk of recurrence occurring in patients who have had inadequate initial operations. For malignant tumors, 5-year survival is 70% to 90% for low-grade tumors and 20% to 30% for high-grade malignancies. Regional and distant recurrences range from 15% to 20% and are common in tumors with perineural invasion (e.g., adenoid cystic carcinomas). Adenoid cystic carcinomas have a propensity to spread along nerves and metastasize to the lung; therefore, surveillance should entail imaging (i.e., MRI scans and chest x-rays) to exclude recurrence.

RECOMMENDED READING

Al-Sarraf M, LeBlanc M, Giri PG, et al. Chemoradiotherapy versus radiotherapy in patients with advanced nasopharyngeal cancer: phase III randomized intergroup study 0099. *J Clin Oncol* 1998;16(4):1310–1317.

Ang KK, Jiang GL, Frankenthaler RA, et al. Carcinoma of the nasal cavity. *Radiother Oncol* 1992;24:163–168.

Benner SE, Pajak TF, Lippman SM, Earley C, Hong WK. Prevention of second primary tumors with isotretinoin in patients with squamous cell carcinoma of the head and neck: long-term follow-up. *J Natl Cancer Inst* 1994;84:140–141.

Byers RM, Clayman GL, McGill D, et al. Selective neck dissections for squamous carcinoma of the upper aerodigestive tract: patterns of regional failure. *Head Neck* 1999;21:499–505.

Byers RM, Wolf PF, Ballantyne AJ. Rationale for elective modified neck dissection. *Head Neck Surg* 1988;10:160–167.

Carrau RL, Segas J, Nuss DW, et al. Squamous cell carcinoma of the sinonasal tract invading the orbit. *Laryngoscope* 1999;109:230–235.

Clayman GL, Johnson CJ II, Morrison W, Ginsberg L, Lippman SM. The role of neck dissection after chemoradiotherapy for oropharyngeal cancer with advanced nodal disease. *Arch Otolaryngol Head Neck Surg* 2001;172(2):135–139.

Colletier PJ, Garden AS, Morrison WH, Goepfert H, Geara F, Ang KK. Postoperative radiation for squamous cell carcinoma metastatic to cervical lymph nodes from an unknown primary site: outcomes and patterns of failure. *Head Neck* 1998;20(8):674–681.

Diaz EM, Jr, Holsinger FC, Zuniga ER, Roberts DB, Sorensen DM. Squamous cell carcinoma of the buccal mucosa: one institution's experience with 119 previously untreated patients. *Head Neck* 2003;25(4):267–273.

Disa JJ, Hu QY, Hidalgo DA. Retrospective review of 400 consecutive free flap reconstructions for oncologic surgical defects. *Ann Surg Oncol* 1997;4(8):663–669.

Eden BV, Debo RF, Larner JM, et al. Esthesioneuroblastoma. Long-term outcome and patterns of failure—the University of Virginia experience. *Cancer* 1994;73:2556–2562.

Fagan JJ, Collins B, Barnes L, D'Amico F, Myers EN, Johnson JT. Perineural invasion in squamous cell carcinoma of the head and neck. *Arch Otolaryngol Head Neck Surg* 1998;124:637–640.

Fee WE, Roberson JB, Goffinet DR. Long-term survival after surgical resection for recurrent nasopharyngeal cancer after radiotherapy failure. *Arch Otolaryngol Head Neck Surg* 1991;117(11):1233–1236.

Forastiere A, Koch W, Trotti A, Sidransky D. Head and neck cancer [review]. *N Engl J Med* 2001;345(26):1890–1900.

Fordice J, Kershaw C, El Naggar A, Goepfert H. Adenoid cystic carcinoma of the head and neck: predictors of morbidity and mortality. *Arch Otolaryngol Head Neck Surg* 1999;125:149–152.

Frankenthaler RA, Byers RM, Luna MA, Callender DL, Wolf P, Goepfert H. Predicting occult lymph node metastasis in parotid cancer. *Arch Otolaryngol Head Neck Surg* 1993;119:517–520.

Frankenthaler RA, Luna MA, Lee SS, et al. Prognostic variables in parotid gland cancer. *Arch Otolaryngol Head Neck Surg* 1991;117:1251–1256.

Garden AS, Morrison WH, Clayman GL, Ang KK, Peters LJ. Early squamous cell carcinoma of the hypopharynx: outcomes of treatment with radiation alone to the primary disease. *Head Neck* 1996;18:317–322.

Garden AS, Weber RS, Ang KK, Morrison WH, Matre J, Peters LJ. Postoperative radiation therapy for malignant tumors of minor salivary glands. *Cancer* 1994;73(10):2563–2569.

Greenberg JS, Fowler R, Gomez J, et al. Extent of extracapsular spread: a critical prognosticator in oral tongue cancer. *Cancer* 2003;97(6):1464–1470.

Gwozdz JT, Morrison WH, Garden AS, Weber RS, Peters LJ, Ang KK. Concomitant boost radiotherapy for squamous carcinoma of the tonsillar fossa. *Int J Radiat Oncol* 1997;39(1):127–135.

Harrison LB, Zelefsky MJ, Sessions RB, et al. Base of tongue cancer treated with external beam irradiation plus brachytherapy: oncologic and functional outcome. *Radiology* 1992;184:267–270.

Hong WK, Endicott J, Itri LM, et al. 13-cis Retinoic acid in the treatment of oral leukoplakia. *N Engl J Med* 1986;315: 1501–1505.

Induction chemotherapy plus radiation compared with surgery plus radiation in patients with advanced laryngeal cancer. The Department of Veterans Affairs Laryngeal Cancer Study Group. *N Engl J Med* 1991;324(24): 1685–1690.

Johnson JT, Myers EN, Hao SP, Wagner RL. Outcome of open surgical therapy for glottic carcinoma. *Ann Otol Rhinol Laryngol* 1993;102:752–755.

Jungehulsing M, Scheidhauer K, Damm M, et al. 2[F]-Fluoro-2-deoxy-D-glucose positron emission tomography is a sensitive tool for the detection of occult primary cancer (carcinoma of unknown primary syndrome) with head and neck lymph node manifestation. *Otolaryngol Head Neck Surg* 2000;123:294–301.

Khuri FR, Lippman SM, Spitz MR, et al. Molecular epidemiology and retinoid chemoprevention of head and neck cancer. *J Natl Cancer Inst* 1997;89:199.

Kirchner JA, Cornog JL, Holmes RE. Transglottic cancer. *Arch Otolaryngol* 1974;99:247–251.

Kraus DH, Dubner S, Harrison LB, et al. Prognostic factors for recurrence and survival in head and neck soft tissue sarcomas. *Cancer* 1994;74:697–702

Kraus DH, Zelefsky MJ, Brock HA, Huo J, Harrison LB, Shah JP. Combined surgery and radiation therapy for squamous cell carcinoma of the hypopharynx. *Otolaryngol Head Neck Surg* 1997;116:637–641.

Laccourreye H, Laccourreye O, Weinstein G, Menard M, Brasnu D. Supracricoid laryngectomy with cricohyoidoepiglottopexy: a partial laryngeal procedure for glottic carcinoma. *Ann Otol Rhinol Laryngol* 1990;99(6 pt 1): 421–426.

Laccourreye H, Laccourreye O, Weinstein G, Menard M, Brasnu D. Supracricoid laryngectomy with cricohyoidopexy: a partial laryngeal procedure for selected supraglottic and transglottic carcinomas. *Laryngoscope* 1990;100(7):735–741.

Machtay M, Rosenthal DI, Hershock D, et al. Organ preservation therapy using induction plus concurrent chemoradiation for advanced resectable oropharyngeal carcinoma: a University of Pennsylvania phase II trial. *J Clin Oncol* 2002;20(19):3964–3971.

Mendenhall WM, Parsons JT, Stringer SP, Cassisi NJ. Management of Tis, T1, and T2 squamous cell carcinoma of the glottic larynx. *Am J Otolaryngol* 1994;15(4):250–257.

Myers EN, Alvi A. Management of carcinoma of the supraglottic larynx: evolution, current concepts and future trends. *Laryngoscope* 1996;106:559–567.

Myers EN, Suen JC, eds. *Cancer of the Head and Neck*. Philadelphia, Pa: WB Saunders; 1996.

Papadimitrakopoulou VA, Clayman GL, Shin DM, et al. Biochemoprevention for dysplastic lesions of the upper aerodigestive tract. *Arch Otolaryngol Head Neck Surg* 1999;125:1083–1089.

Spiro RH. Salivary neoplasms: overview of a 35 year experience with 2807 patients. *Head Neck Surg* 1986;8:177–184.

Spiro RH, DeRose G, Strong EW. Cervical node metastasis of occult origin. *Am J Surg* 1983;146:441–446

Spiro RH, Huvos AG, Wong GY, Spiro JD, Gnecco CA, Strong EW. Predictive value of tumor thickness in squamous carcinoma confined to the tongue and floor of the mouth. *Am J Surg* 1986;152:345–350.

Steiner W. Results of curative laser microsurgery of laryngeal carcinomas. *Am J Otolaryngol* 1993;14:116–121.

Stern SJ, Goepfert H, Clayman G, Byers R, Wolf P. Orbital preservation in maxillectomy. *Otolaryngol Head Neck Surg* 1993;109:111–115.

Stern SJ, Goepfert H, Clayman G, et al. Squamous cell carcinoma of the maxillary sinus. *Arch Otolaryngol Head Neck Surg* 1993;119(9):964–969.

Sturgis EM, Potter BO. Sarcomas of the head and neck region. *Curr Opin Oncol* 2003;15(3):239–252.

Urken ML, Weinberg H, Buchbinder D, et al. Microvascular free flaps in head and neck reconstruction. *Arch Otolaryngol Head Neck Surg* 1994;120:633–640.

Wanebo HJ, Koness RJ, MacFarlane JK, et al. Head and neck sarcoma: report of the Head and Neck Sarcoma Registry. Society of Head and Neck Surgeons Committee on Research. *Head Neck* 1992;14:1–7.

Weber RS, Benjamin RS, Peters LJ, Ro JY, Achon O, Goepfert H. Soft tissue sarcomas of the head and neck in adolescents and adults. *Am J Surg* 1986;152(4):386–392.

Weber RS, Berkey BA, Forastiere A, et al. Outcome of salvage total laryngectomy following organ preservation therapy: the Radiation Therapy Oncology Group trial 91-11. *Arch Otolaryngol Head Neck Surg* 2003;129(1):44–49.

Thoracic Malignancies

Shanda H. Blackmon and Ara A. Vaporciyan

PRIMARY NEOPLASMS OF THE LUNG

In 2005, lung cancer accounted for an estimated 163,510 deaths and 172,570 new cases of cancer in the United States. Although less publicized than breast or prostate cancer, lung cancer is the most common cause of cancer-related death in both men and women. Approximately 30% of all cancer deaths are attributable to lung cancer. However, as seen in Figure 7.1, the overall age-adjusted death rates for lung cancer have begun to level off. This leveling off is attributable to an overall decrease in the number of males who smoke and no further increase in the number of women who smoke. Unfortunately, this good news is countered by a disturbing increase in smoking among certain minority and adolescent age groups. The overall 5-year survival rate for lung cancer is only 15%, primarily because the disease is usually advanced at presentation. If found at an early stage, the 5-year survival rate approaches 60% to 70%.

Epidemiology

Smoking is the primary etiology in more than 80% of lung cancers, and secondhand smoke increases the risk of lung cancer by 30%. Despite the strong association of lung cancer with smoking, such cancers develop in only 15% of heavy smokers. Giant bullous emphysema and airway obstructive disease can act synergistically with smoking to induce lung cancer, perhaps because of poor clearance and trapping of carcinogens. Industrial and environmental carcinogens have been implicated, including residential radon gas, asbestos, uranium, cadmium, arsenic, and terpenes.

Pathology

Lung cancer can be broadly separated into two groups: non–small-cell lung cancers (NSCLCs) and small-cell lung cancers (SCLCs). This is a popular division because, for the most part, NSCLC is often managed with surgery when the tumor is localized, whereas SCLC is almost always managed nonsurgically with chemotherapy and radiation therapy. The three major types of NSCLC are adenocarcinoma, squamous cell carcinoma, and large-cell carcinoma (Table 7.1).

Non–small-cell Lung Carcinoma

Adenocarcinoma is the most common type of NSCLC and accounts for more than 40% of cases. It is the most common lung cancer found in nonsmokers and women. The lesions tend to be located in the periphery and develop systemic metastases, even in the face of small primary tumors.

Bronchoalveolar cell carcinoma is a subset of adenocarcinoma, whose incidence appears to be increasing. This tumor is more frequent in women and nonsmokers, and can present as a single

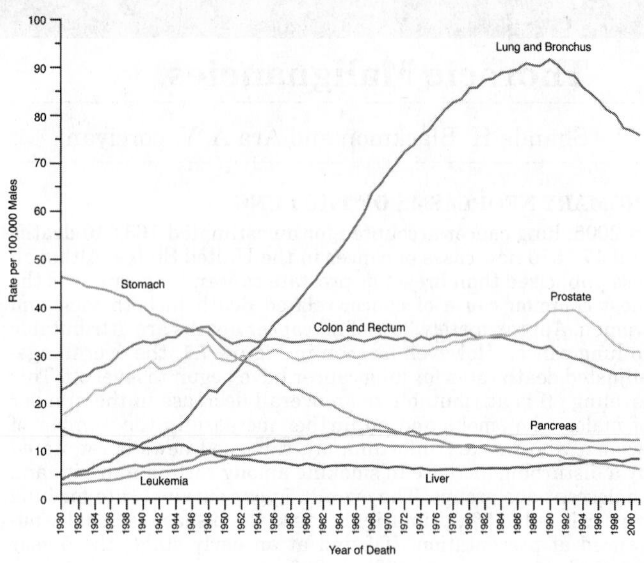

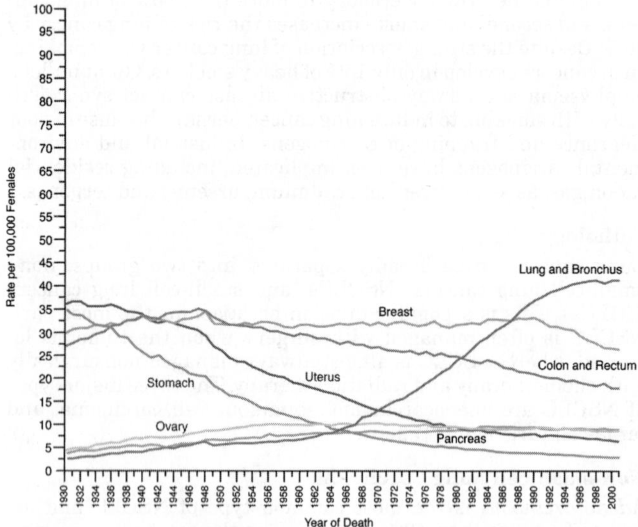

Figure 7.1. Annual age-adjusted cancer death rates for selected cancer types in males *(top)* and females *(bottom)*, United States, 1930 to 2001.

Table 7.1. Frequency of histologic subtypes of primary lung cancer

Cell Type	Estimated Frequency (%)
Non-small-cell lung cancer	
Adenocarcinoma	40
Bronchoalveolar	2
Squamous cell carcinoma	25
Large-cell carcinoma	7
Small-cell lung cancer	
Small-cell carcinoma	20
Neuroendocrine, well differentiated	1
Carcinoids	5

mass, multiple nodules, or an infiltrate. The clinical course can vary from indolent progression to rapid diffuse dissemination.

Squamous cell carcinoma accounts for approximately 25% of all lung cancers. Most (66%) present as central lesions. Cavitation is found in 7% to 10% of cases. Unlike adenocarcinoma, the tumor often remains localized, tending to spread initially to regional lymph nodes rather than systemically.

Large-cell carcinoma accounts for approximately 7% to 10% of all lung cancers. Clinically, large-cell carcinomas behave aggressively, with early metastases to the regional nodes in the mediastinum and distant sites such as the brain.

Small-cell Lung Carcinoma

Small-cell carcinoma is associated with neuroendocrine carcinoma because of ultrastructural and immunohistochemical similarities. Some pathologists think small-cell carcinomas represent a spectrum of disease beginning with the well-differentiated, benign carcinoid tumor (Kulchitsky I), including the less differentiated atypical carcinoids (Kulchitsky II) or neuroendocrine carcinomas, and ending with the undifferentiated small-cell carcinomas (Kulchitsky III). Small-cell carcinomas tend to present with metastatic and regional spread, and are usually treated with chemotherapy with or without radiation therapy. Surgery is only used to remove the occasional localized peripheral nodule.

Carcinoids tend to arise from major bronchi and are central tumors. Metastasis is rare. Immunohistochemically, carcinoids express neuron-specific enolase, chromogranin, and synaptophysin virtually without exception.

Neuroendocrine carcinomas or *atypical carcinoids* occur more peripherally than carcinoids and have a more aggressive course, although surgery should still be considered according to clinical stage. Without appropriate immunostaining, they may inadvertently be classified as large-cell carcinomas.

Diagnosis

Signs and symptoms occur in 90% to 95% of patients at the time of diagnosis. Intraparenchymal tumors cause cough, hemoptysis, dyspnea, wheezing, and fever (often due to infection from proximal bronchial tumor obstruction). Regional spread of the tumor within the thorax can lead to pleural effusions or chest wall pain. Less common symptoms are superior vena cava syndrome, Pancoast syndrome (shoulder and arm pain, Horner syndrome, and weakness and atrophy of the hand muscles), and involvement of the recurrent laryngeal nerve, the phrenic nerve, the vagus nerve, or the esophagus. Paraneoplastic syndromes are found in 10% of patients with lung cancer, most commonly those with SCLC. These syndromes are numerous and can affect endocrine, neurologic, skeletal, hematologic, and cutaneous systems.

A standard chest radiograph (CXR) is the initial diagnostic study for the evaluation of suspected lung cancer, followed routinely by computed tomography (CT). CT should include imaging of the liver and adrenal glands to rule out two common sites for intra-abdominal metastases. CT helps assess local extension to other thoracic structures and the presence of mediastinal adenopathy. At present, magnetic resonance imaging (MRI) adds little to the information gained by CT imaging. Positron emission tomography (PET), especially integrated PET-CT, has become a frequent method of distinguishing benign from malignant pulmonary nodules. Although the accuracy of PET scanning in evaluating a pulmonary nodule can exceed 90% in some studies, clinicians should be aware that false-negative PET scans occur in patients with neoplasms having low metabolic activity (carcinoid and bronchioalveolar neoplasms). Even with advances in imaging, histologic confirmation will frequently be required to distinguish benign from malignant disease and to determine the histologic type of cancer. For a solitary lesion with a high index of suspicion, histologic confirmation can be obtained at the time of surgery (thoracotomy or video-assisted thoracic surgery [VATS]) using frozen sectioning of a wedge resection or a needle biopsy. If immediate surgery is not appropriate, then tissue can be obtained by sputum cytology and bronchoscopy (central lesions) or by fluoroscopic fine-needle aspiration (FNA), or CT-guided biopsy (peripheral lesions). Patients with benign lesions should be followed for interval growth over a period of at least 2 years.

Staging

The primary goal of pretreatment staging is to determine the extent of disease so prognosis and treatment can be determined. In SCLC, most patients present with metastatic or advanced locoregional disease. A simple two-stage system classifies the SCLC as limited or extensive disease. Limited disease is confined to one hemithorax, ipsilateral or contralateral hilar or mediastinal nodes, and ipsilateral supraclavicular lymph nodes. Extensive disease has spread to the contralateral supraclavicular nodes or distant sites such as the contralateral lung, liver, brain, or bone marrow. Staging for SCLC requires a bone scan;

bone marrow biopsy; and CT scans of the abdomen, brain, and chest.

Staging of NSCLC has most recently involved a system proposed in 1985: the International Lung Cancer Staging System or International Staging System (ISS). This system is based on TNM classifications as shown in Table 7.2. Survival rates for patients with NSCLC by stage of disease are shown in Figure 7.2. Because of heterogeneity within groups, further modifications to the ISS have been proposed that involve splitting stage I into IA (T1N0) and IB (T2N0) and stage II into IIA (T1N0) and IIB (T2N0) and moving the good-prognosis T3N0 patients (chest wall involvement without nodal spread) into IIB. Staging of NSCLC involves a thorough history and physical examination, CXR, and CT scans of the chest and upper abdomen, with the adjunctive use of PET scanning when available. Unfortunately, CT cannot definitively predict mediastinal nodal involvement because not all malignant lymph nodes are enlarged, and many enlarged nodes are simply larger because of proximal infection. Lymph nodes larger than 1 cm have a 30% chance of being benign, whereas lymph nodes smaller than 1 cm still have a 15% chance of containing tumor. PET-CT has a higher negative predictive value in the evaluation of mediastinal N2 disease, although false positives can occur in patients with infectious granulomas, inflammatory processes, and rheumatoid nodules. Most investigators agree that tissue confirmation of PET localized mediastinal disease and metastases is required. Because of the low yield in asymptomatic early-stage patients (T1N0), a bone scan, CT, or MRI of the brain should only be obtained when suspected by history.

Treatment

Pretreatment Assessment

Once a patient has been staged clinically with noninvasive tests, a physiological assessment should be performed to determine the patient's ability to tolerate different therapeutic modalities. In addition to a general evaluation of the patient's overall medical status, specific attention should be paid to the cardiovascular and respiratory systems. Cardiovascular screening should include a history and physical examination, as well as a CXR and electrocardiography. Patients with signs and symptoms of significant cardiac disease should undergo further noninvasive testing, including either exercise testing, echocardiography, or nuclear perfusion scans. Significant reversible cardiac problems should be addressed before therapy (i.e., chemotherapy, radiation therapy, or surgery).

The pulmonary reserve of patients with lung cancer is commonly diminished as a result of tobacco abuse. Simple spirometry is an excellent initial screening test to quantify a patient's pulmonary reserve and ability to tolerate surgical resection. A predicted postoperative forced expiratory volume in 1 second (FEV_1) of less than 0.8 L or less than 35% of predicted postoperative FEV_1 is associated with an increased risk of perioperative complications, respiratory insufficiency, and death. The predicted postoperative FEV_1 is estimated by subtracting the contribution of the lung to be resected from the preoperative FEV_1. In certain

Table 7.2. TNM descriptors

Primary tumor (T)	
Tx	Primary tumor cannot be assessed or tumor proven by the presence of malignant cells in sputum or bronchial washings but not visualized by imaging or bronchoscopy
T0	No evidence of primary tumor
Tis	Carcinoma in situ
T1	Tumor $\leq$3 cm in greatest dimension, surrounded by lung or visceral pleura, without bronchoscopic evidence of invasion more proximal than the lobar bronchus[a] (i.e., not in the main bronchus)
T2	Tumor with any of the following features of size or extent: >3 cm in greatest dimension Involving main bronchus, $\geq$2 cm distal to the carina Invading the visceral pleura Associated with atelectasis or obstructive pneumonitis that extends to the hilar region but does not involve the entire lung
T3	Tumor of any size that directly invades any of the following: chest wall (including superior sulcus tumors), diaphragm, mediastinal pleura, parietal pericardium; or tumor in the main bronchus <2 cm distal to the carina but without involvement of the carina; or associated atelectasis or obstructive pneumonitis of the entire lung
T4	Tumor of any size that invades any of the following—mediastinum, heart, great vessels, trachea, esophagus, vertebral body, carina—or tumor with a malignant pleural or pericardial effusion,[b] or with satellite tumor nodule(s) within the ipsilateral primary tumor lobe of the lung
Regional lymph nodes (N)	
Nx	Regional lymph nodes cannot be assessed
N0	No regional lymph node metastasis
N1	Metastasis to ipsilateral peribronchial and/or ipsilateral hilar lymph nodes, and intrapulmonary nodes involved by direct extension of the primary tumor
N2	Metastasis to ipsilateral mediastinal and/or subcarinal lymph nodes(s)
N3	Metastasis to contralateral mediastinal, contralateral hilar, ipsilateral or contralateral scalene, or supraclavicular lymph node(s)
Distant metastasis (M)	
Mx	Presence of distant metastasis cannot be assessed
M0	No distant metastasis
M1	Distant metastasis present[c]

[a]The uncommon superficial tumor of any size with its invasive component limited to the bronchial wall, which may extend proximally to the main bronchus, is also classified T1.

[b]Most pleural effusions associated with lung cancer are due to tumor. However, there are a few patients in whom multiple cytopathological examinations of pleural fluid show no tumor. In these cases, the fluid is nonbloody and is not an exudate. When these elements and clinical judgment dictate that the effusion is not related to the tumor, the effusion should be excluded as a staging element, and the patient's disease should be staged T1, T2, or T3. Pericardial effusion is classified according to the same rules.

[c]Separate metastatic tumor nodule(s) in the ipsilateral nonprimary tumor lobe(s) of the lung are also classified M1.

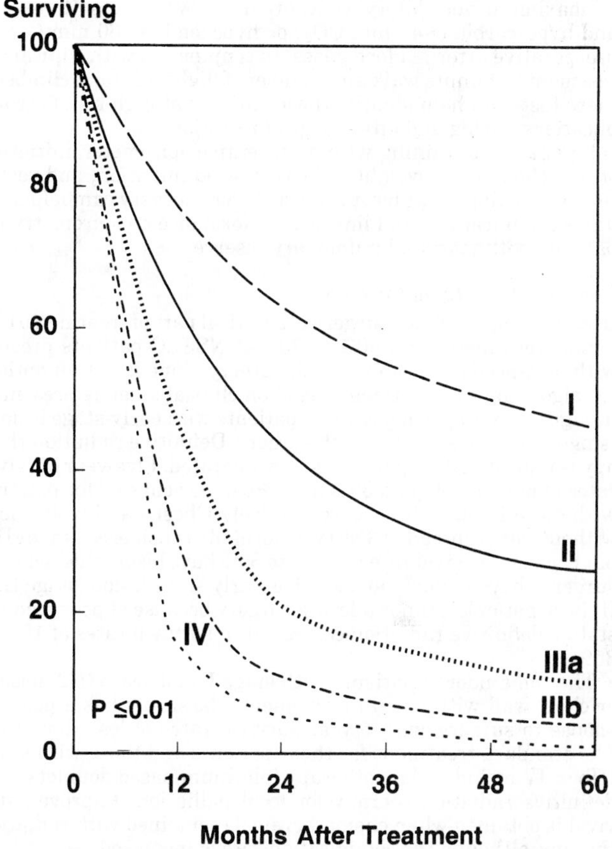

Figure 7.2. Cumulative survival according to clinical stage of non–small-cell lung cancer.

instances, the lung to be resected does not contribute much to the preoperative FEV_1 because of tumor, atelectasis, or pneumonitis. Thus, more accurate determination of predicted postoperative FEV_1 can be obtained by performing a ventilation-perfusion scan and subtracting the exact contribution of the lung to be resected. In good performance patients with borderline spirometry criteria, oxygen consumption studies can be obtained that measure both respiratory and cardiac capacity. A maximum oxygen consumption (VO_2 max) of greater than 15 mL min^{-1} kg^{-1} indicates low risk, whereas a VO_2 max of less than 10 mL min^{-1} kg^{-1} is associated with high risk (a mortality rate of more than 30% in some series). Additional risk factors for lung resection include a predicted postoperative diffusing capacity (DLCO) or maximum ventilatory ventilation (MVV) of less than 40% and hypercarbia (>45 mm CO_2) or hypoxemia (<60 mm O_2) on preoperative arterial blood gases. In conjunction with clinical assessment (6-minute walk and number of flights of stairs climbed), these tests can help identify those patients at high risk for complications during and after surgical resection.

Preoperative training with an incentive spirometer, initiation of bronchodilators, weight reduction, good nutrition, and cessation of smoking for at least 2 weeks before surgery can help minimize complications and improve performance on spirometry for patients with marginal pulmonary reserve.

Non–small-cell Lung Carcinoma

In early-stage NSCLC, surgery is a critical part of treatment. Unfortunately, more than 50% to 70% of NSCLC patients present with advanced disease for which surgery alone is not an option. An algorithm for treatment based on clinical stage is presented in Figure 7.3. Physiologically fit patients with early-stage lesions (stage I or II) are treated with surgery. Definitive radiation therapy is indicated if surgery cannot be tolerated. Five-year survival rates of 60% to 70% and 39% to 43% can be achieved for patients with stage I and II disease, respectively. Chest wall involvement without nodal spread (T3N0) was formally considered stage IIIa, but because survival rates of 33% to 60% have been achieved with surgery, they are now considered as early-stage lesion (stage IIa). If these patients cannot tolerate surgery because of poor medical status, definitive radiation can result in survival rates of 15% to 35%.

The remainder of patients with stage IIIa disease (N2 disease or chest wall with nodal involvement) classically has a poor response to surgery, with 5-year survival rates of less than 15%. The standard treatment for these patients and those with stage IIIb or IV includes chemotherapy (platinum-based doublets) and definitive radiation therapy for local palliation. Improved survival is obtained when chemotherapy is combined with radiation therapy, although the complication rate is increased.

A small subset of stage IIIb tumors can be approached surgically. These tumors are considered stage IIIb because of local extension (T4N0) into adjacent structures rather than systemic spread (nodes, hematogenous metastases) and may benefit from aggressive surgical resection of the atrium, carina, or vertebrae. Survival rates of up to 30% have been reported. Metastatic disease is only treated surgically in the unusual circumstance of an isolated brain metastasis with a node-negative lung primary. Several reports have documented better local control (in the brain and lung) with surgery and a subset of long-term survivors. The presence of mediastinal nodes, however, contraindicates surgical resection and mandates radiation therapy for the lung primary.

SURGERY

PNEUMONECTOMY. The removal of the whole lung was previously the most commonly performed operation for NSCLC; it now accounts for only 20% of all resections. Although a more

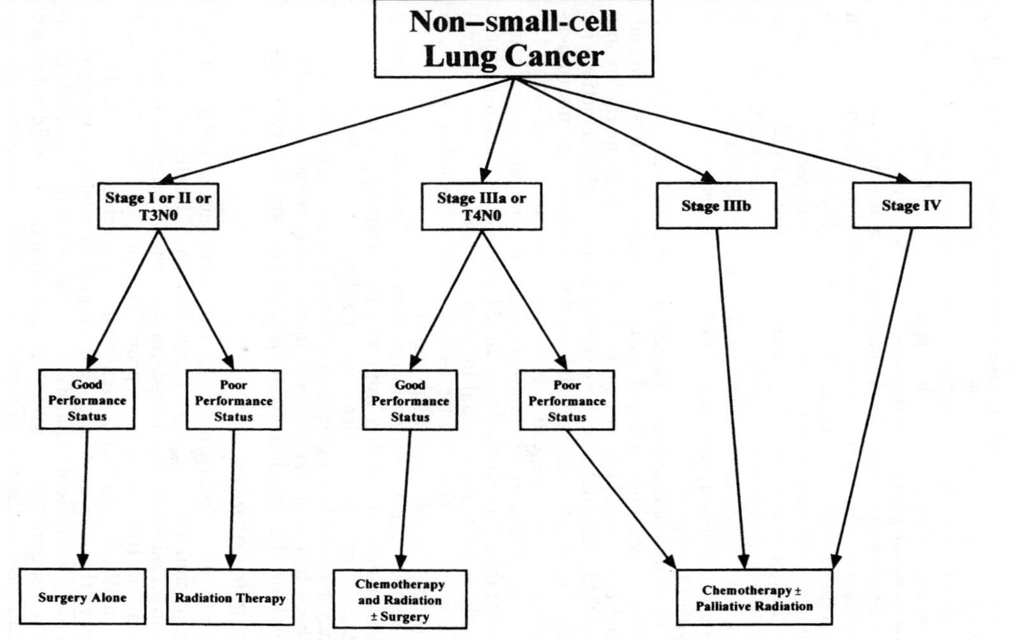

Figure 7.3. Algorithm for treatment of non–small-cell lung cancer.

complete resection is accomplished using pneumonectomy versus parenchyma-conserving techniques (lobectomy), it comes at the cost of higher mortality (4%–10%) and morbidity without clear survival benefits.

LOBECTOMY. The similar survival of patients treated by lobectomy versus pneumonectomy, along with the lower morbidity and mortality (1%–3%) associated with lobectomy, make lobectomy the preferred method of resection. Sleeve lobectomies and bronchoplasty procedures in which portions of the main bronchus are removed without loss of the distal lung have further decreased the need for pneumonectomies.

LESSER RESECTIONS. Segmentectomies and nonanatomical resections (wedge resection and lumpectomy) are associated with increased local recurrence when compared with lobectomy. The general consensus remains that these procedures should be performed only in high-risk patients with minimal pulmonary reserve who could not tolerate a lobectomy. The advent of CT screening for lung cancer has identified more subcentimeter cancers. The use of lesser resections will need to be reassessed for these types of cancers.

EXTENDED OPERATIONS. Recent improvements in surgery and critical care have allowed certain tumors, previously considered unresectable, to be removed with acceptable morbidity and mortality. Carinal sleeve resections and extended resections for superior sulcus tumors with hemivertebrectomy and instrumentation of the spine can now be performed in a small subset of patients whose tumors were previously considered surgically unresectable. These procedures should only be performed in patients without mediastinal nodal involvement because 5-year survival rates are less than 5% for patients with extended resections in the presence of nodal involvement.

MEDIASTINAL LYMPH NODE DISSECTION. Complete mediastinal lymph node dissection improves the accuracy of lung cancer staging, improves indications for subsequent adjuvant therapy, may decrease locoregional recurrence, and may improve survival. There has been no increase in morbidity associated with the addition of a complete nodal dissection in experienced hands.

CHEMOTHERAPY

Almost 50% of patients present with extrathoracic spread, and an additional 15% are unresectable because of locally advanced tumor. In addition, the long-term survival for resectable stage II and IIIa tumors remains poor. Therefore, the use of adjuvant chemotherapy to treat patients with unresectable tumors and improve the results of surgery is an area of intense investigation. A meta-analysis of these studies demonstrated a survival advantage using platinum-based therapy, although this did not reach statistical significance. These data spawned numerous large adjuvant trials in Europe and America. The European study was the International Adjuvant Lung Cancer Trial and enrolled nearly 1,900 completely resected stage I, II, and IIIA patients. The group that received cisplatinum-based doublet therapy had a 4.1% improvement in overall survival ($p < 0.03$). Since this publication, two additional positive trials (NCIC BR10 and CALGB 9633) have been presented. Although the inclusion criteria were slightly different, both studies demonstrated a more than 30% improvement in survival. These studies have required a significant shift in the postoperative management of completely resected early-stage lung cancers. Although the risk associated with adjuvant chemotherapy is small, it must be considered before initiating therapy. Therefore, we now have all patients with completely resected IB or higher stage cancers evaluated by an oncologist for possible adjuvant chemotherapy.

Studies examining the role of neoadjuvant chemotherapy, common in the late 1990s, have been difficult to complete due to the data regarding adjuvant treatment. Although multimodality therapy has achieved a strong foothold, the optimum timing of chemotherapy, adjuvant versus neoadjuvant, remains to be determined.

Small-cell Lung Carcinoma

Unlike NSCLC, SCLC tends to be disseminated at presentation and is therefore not amenable to cure with surgery or thoracic radiation therapy alone. Without treatment, the disease is rapidly fatal, with few patients surviving more than 6 months. Fortunately, SCLC is very sensitive to chemotherapy, and more than two-thirds of patients achieve a partial response after systemic therapy with multidrug regimens. Treatment of SCLC therefore revolves around systemic chemotherapy. An algorithm based on the extent of disease is presented in Figure 7.4. Complete response is seen in as many as 20% to 50% of patients with limited disease, but these responses are not durable, and the 5-year survival rate is still less than 10%.

Chemotherapeutic regimens for SCLC most commonly include combinations of cyclophosphamide, cisplatin, etoposide, doxorubicin, and vincristine. Thoracic radiation therapy has been shown to improve local control of the primary tumor and is often included as part of the treatment for limited SCLC. In addition, because brain metastases are noted in 80% of patients with SCLC during the course of their disease, patients who show no evidence of brain metastases on CT scans and who achieve a good response from therapy are usually treated with prophylactic brain irradiation to minimize the chances of developing this morbid site of treatment failure.

A small role for surgical resection of SCLC does exist. Solitary peripheral pulmonary nodules with no evidence of metastatic disease after evaluation with bone scan, PET-CT, and CT of the abdomen, brain, and chest can be treated with lobectomy and postoperative chemotherapy if mediastinoscopy is negative. In these select patients, a 5-year survival rate of 50% has been achieved for T1N0, T2N0, and completely resected N1 disease. Surgery for more central lesions, however, has not been demonstrated to improve survival over that achieved with chemotherapy and radiation therapy alone.

Surveillance

The few treatment options for tumor recurrence in NSLC have limited the cost-effectiveness of aggressive radiologic surveillance

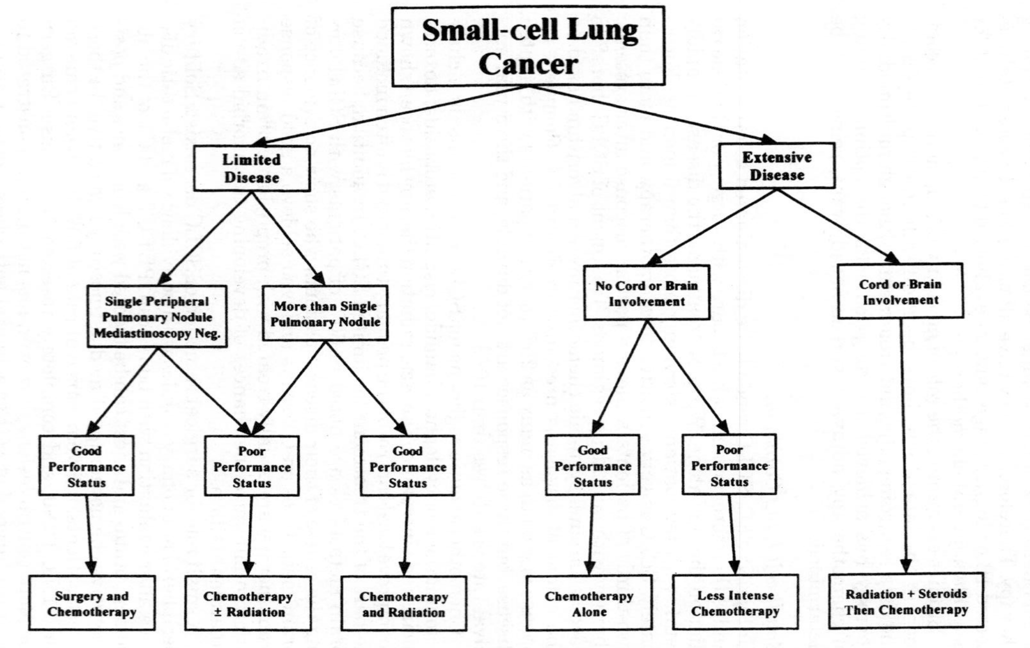

Figure 7.4. Algorithm for treatment of small-cell lung cancer.

following surgical resection. Nevertheless, there is an increased incidence of second primary lung cancers (2% per year), and annual or semiannual CXR may help detect these lesions. Any patient who experiences symptoms in the interim should also be evaluated aggressively for recurrence or a new primary. The advent of low-dose helical CT scanning may change this standard, and its role in the surveillance of resected lung cancer patients is being evaluated. The lung and liver are the most common sites of metastases. Patients with isolated lung metastases can achieve survival rates of 25% to 40% if complete surgical resection is obtained. Because metastases can recur, resection involves nonanatomical wedge or laser resections to preserve the lung parenchyma.

METASTATIC NEOPLASMS TO THE LUNG

Pathology

The biology of the underlying primary malignancy determines the behavior of its metastases. Metastases may occur via hematogenous, lymphatic, direct, or aerogenous routes.

Diagnosis

Because of their predominantly peripheral localization, most pulmonary metastases remain asymptomatic, with fewer than 5% showing symptoms at presentation. Diagnosis is commonly made during radiographic follow-up after treatment of the primary malignancy.

Routine CXR during surveillance after cancer treatment is an effective means of screening patients for pulmonary metastases. Indeed, several studies have demonstrated the increased sensitivity of CT over standard CXR. However, the cost-effectiveness of CT for screening remains low, and no data as yet suggest that early detection with CT leads to improved survival. Planning of surgical interventions, however, should be based on CT findings, even though CT scanning still misses approximately 30% to 50% of the nodules found at surgery.

When multiple pulmonary nodules are present in patients with a known previous malignancy, the likelihood of metastatic disease approaches 100%. New solitary lesions, however, can represent primary lung cancers because many of the risk factors are similar.

Staging

No valid staging system exists for pulmonary metastases. The International Registry of Lung Metastases has identified three parameters of prognostic significance: resectability, disease-free interval, and number of metastases. The present criteria for resectability include resectable pulmonary nodules, control of the primary tumor, adequate predicted postoperative pulmonary reserve, and no extrathoracic metastases. Patients who meet these criteria should be offered metastasectomy. Favorable histologies for long-term survival following resection include sarcoma, breast, colon, and genitourinary metastases. Unfavorable histologies include melanomas, esophageal, pancreatic, and gastric cancers.

Treatment

Surgery

Preoperative evaluation for resection of pulmonary metastases is similar to that of any other pulmonary resection. Because of the increased risk of recurrent metastases and need for future thoracotomies, parenchyma-conserving procedures are performed whenever possible (wedge resection, laser, or cautery excision). The various surgical approaches include the following.

Median sternotomy allows bilateral exploration with one incision. Lesions located near the hilum can be difficult to reach, and exposure of the left lower lobe—especially in patients with obesity, cardiomegaly, or an elevated left hemidiaphragm—is poor.

Bilateral anterothoracosternotomy (clamshell procedure) allows excellent exposure of both hemithoraces, including the left lower lobe, although some surgeons think the incision increases postoperative pain.

Posterolateral thoracotomy is a more common incision for access to the lung. The limitation to one hemithorax, however, necessitates a second staged operation for removing bilateral metastases.

Thoracoscopic resection allows visualization of both hemithoraces during the same anesthetic. Pleural-based lesions are therefore easily visualized and excised. Unfortunately, the ability to carefully evaluate the parenchyma for deeper or smaller nonvisualized lesions is poor, and some reports suggest an increased risk of local recurrence with thoracoscopy.

At surgery, wedge resections with a 1-cm margin are preferred. If multiple nodules within one segment, lobe, or lung preclude resection of multiple wedges, then laser resections can be performed.

Adjuvant Therapy

The role of radiation therapy in the treatment of pulmonary metastases is limited to the palliation of symptoms of advanced lesions with extensive pleural, bony, or neural involvement. The value of chemotherapy preoperatively or postoperatively remains controversial. There are many isolated reports of the benefit of chemotherapy, especially when the primary tumor is sensitive (e.g., osteosarcoma, teratoma, other germ cell tumors). However, improvements in survival are more difficult to achieve when the primary is of other types.

Surveillance

The frequency and intensity of follow-up after resection are determined by the primary tumor but usually involve annual or biannual CT scans.

NEOPLASMS OF THE MEDIASTINUM

The mediastinal compartment can harbor numerous lesions of congenital, infectious, developmental, traumatic, or neoplastic origin. Earlier recommendations advocated a direct surgical approach to all mediastinal tumors, with biopsy or debulking of unresectable lesions. However, recent advances in imaging and noninvasive diagnostic techniques, as well as improvements in

Table 7.3. Overall incidence of mediastinal tumors

Thymic	19 (3)[a]
Neurogenic	23 (39)[a]
Lymphoma	12
Germ cell	12
Cysts	18
Mesenchymal	8
Miscellaneous	8

[a]Numbers in parentheses represent incidence in children.

chemotherapy and radiation therapy, have led to a more conservative approach, with management decisions based on better preoperative evaluation.

Pathology

A recent study combining nine previous series was performed to better approximate the true incidence of mediastinal lesions (Table 7.3). In adults, neurogenic and thymic tumors contribute 23% and 19%, respectively, to the overall incidence, whereas in children they contribute 39% and 3%, respectively. This section does not attempt to describe the myriad cystic and other rare miscellaneous lesions but instead concentrates on the more common diagnoses.

Neurogenic tumors include schwannoma, neurofibroma, ganglioneuroblastoma, neuroblastoma, pheochromocytoma, and paraganglioma. They are the most common tumors arising in the posterior compartment.

Thymoma arises from thymic epithelium, although its microscopic appearance is a mixture of lymphocytes and epithelial cells. Thymomas are classified as lymphocytic (30% of cases), epithelial (16%), mixed (30%), and spindle cell (24%). Histologic evidence of malignancy is difficult to obtain because benign and malignant lesions can have similar histologic and cytologic features. Surgical evidence of invasion at the time of resection is the most reliable method of differentiating between malignant and benign thymomas.

Lymphomas comprise approximately 50% of childhood and 20% of adult anterior mediastinal malignancies. They are treated nonsurgically but may require surgery to secure a diagnosis.

Germ cell tumors are comprised of teratomas, seminomas, and nonseminomatous germ cell tumors. Teratomas are the most common and are mostly benign. Malignant teratomas are very rare and often widely metastatic at the time of diagnosis. Seminomas progress in a locally aggressive fashion. Nonseminomatous malignant tumors include embryonal carcinoma and choriocarcinoma, both of which carry a poor prognosis, and the more favorable endodermal sinus tumor.

Miscellaneous cysts and mesenchymal tumors include thyroid goiters, thyroid malignancies, mediastinal parathyroid adenomas, bronchogenic cysts, pericardial cysts, duplications, diverticula, and aneurysms.

Diagnosis

Mediastinal lesions are most commonly asymptomatic. When symptoms do occur, they result from compression of adjacent structures or systemic endocrine or autoimmune effects of the tumors. Children, with their smaller chest cavities, tend to have symptoms at presentation (two-thirds of children vs. only one-third of adults) and more commonly have malignant lesions (greater than 50%). Symptoms can include cough, stridor, and dyspnea (more common in children), as well as symptoms of local invasion such as chest pain, pleural effusion, hoarseness, Homer syndrome, upper-extremity and back pain, paraplegia, and diaphragmatic paralysis.

Chest radiography remains a mainstay of diagnosis. Fifty percent of lesions are diagnosed by CXR. The position of the tumor within the mediastinum on lateral projection can help tailor the differential diagnosis (Fig. 7.5, Table 7.4). The standard for further assessment of the lesion is CT, specifically with contrast enhancement. Certain tumors and benign conditions can be

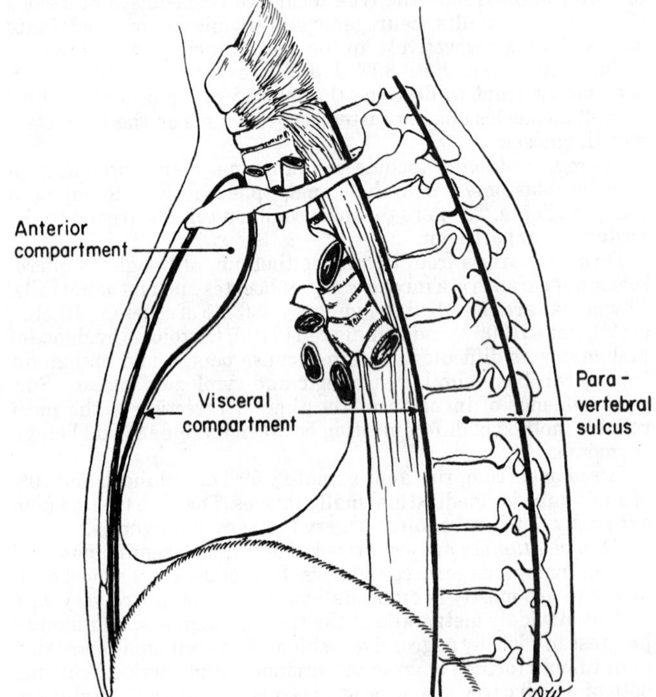

Figure 7.5. Anatomical boundaries of mediastinal masses according to one commonly used classification.

Table 7.4. Usual location of common primary tumors and cysts of mediastinum

Anterior Compartment	Visceral Compartment	Paravertebral Sulci
Thymoma	Enterogenous cyst	Neurilemoma (schwannoma)
Germ cell tumors	Lymphoma	Neurofibroma
Lymphoma	Pleuropericardial cyst	Malignant schwannoma
Lymphangioma	Mediastinal granuloma	Ganglioneuroma
Hemangioma	Lymphoid hamartoma	Ganglioneuroblastoma
Lipoma	Mesothelial cyst	Neuroblastoma
Fibroma	Neuroenteric cyst	Paraganglioma
Fibrosarcoma	Paraganglioma	Pheochromocytoma
Thymic cyst	Pheochromocytoma	Fibrosarcoma
Parathyroid adenoma	Thoracic duct cyst	Lymphoma
Aberrant thyroid		

diagnosed or strongly suggested by their appearance on CT scans. Angiography or MRI may be required if a major resective procedure is planned and vascular involvement suspected. Nuclear imaging such as thyroid and parathyroid scanning, gallium scanning for lymphoma, and metaiodobenzylguanidine scanning for pheochromocytomas may also be indicated.

The use of serum markers can be of some assistance in the diagnosis of some germ cell and neuroendocrine tumors. In addition, the association of myasthenia gravis with thymoma can also assist in the diagnosis.

Because many mediastinal tumors are treated without surgery, a determined effort should be made to achieve a tissue diagnosis noninvasively. FNA, with its reasonable sensitivity, is an excellent starting point, but the diagnosis of lymphoma can be difficult because only a limited number of cells are retrieved. Bronchoscopy and esophagoscopy can also be useful if symptoms or imaging studies suggest tumor involvement.

If these procedures cannot facilitate a diagnosis, then a mediastinoscopy to access paratracheal lesions can be performed. Although the risk of vascular or tracheobronchial injury is present, the incidence of complications is very low in experienced hands. If more invasive procedures are required to make the diagnosis, an anterior or parasternal mediastinotomy (Chamberlain procedure) or thoracoscopy can be performed. Rarely, a sternotomy or thoracotomy will be required to obtain a tissue diagnosis.

Staging

Staging is determined by the specific histologic characteristics and its extent at the time of diagnosis.

Table 7.5. Frequency and treatment of malignant chest wall tumors

Cell Type	Estimated Frequency (%)	Standard Therapy
Chondrosarcoma	35	Surgical resection
Plasmacytoma	25	Radiation + chemotherapy
Ewing sarcoma	15	Surgery + chemotherapy
Osteosarcoma	15	Surgery + chemotherapy
Lymphoma	10	Chemotherapy ± radiation

Treatment

Therapy, like staging, is determined by the type of tumor and its histologic characteristics (Table 7.5). The primary determination to be made is whether the lesion will require resection as part of its treatment or whether chemotherapy or radiation therapy is sufficient. Thymomas should all be resected, with the possibility of postoperative radiation therapy. Benign neurogenic tumors are sometimes observed in older debilitated patients; however, if the patient is otherwise healthy or if malignant potential is suspected, then resection should be pursued. Germ cell tumors should be treated on the basis of their histologic characteristics. In particular, benign teratomas should be resected, seminomas should be treated with radiation therapy, and nonseminomatous tumors should be treated initially with chemotherapy. In the subset of nonseminomatous tumors that have a residual mass but negative markers, surgical resection should be performed to rule out residual tumor. Lymphomas should not be resected and should be treated with radiation therapy or chemotherapy on the basis of their stage and histologic appearance (i.e., Hodgkin vs. non-Hodgkin).

Surveillance

The frequency and intensity of follow-up after resection are determined by the primary tumor. CXR remains the mainstay of surveillance, with CT scanning reserved for evaluation subsequent to abnormal CXR findings.

NEOPLASMS OF THE CHEST WALL

Primary chest wall malignancies account for less than 1% of all tumors, and include a wide variety of bone and soft-tissue lesions. The absence of large series makes the prospective evaluation of treatment options difficult. As more patients with these tumors are treated at large referral institutions, the initiation of multi-institutional trials will help settle some of the more controversial aspects of therapy.

Pathology

Primary chest wall tumors include chondrosarcoma (20%), Ewing sarcoma (8%–22%), osteosarcoma (10%), plasmacytoma

(10%–30%), and, infrequently, soft-tissue sarcoma. Chondrosarcomas arise from the ribs in 80% of cases and from the sternum in the remaining 20%. They are related to prior chest wall trauma in 12.5% of cases and are very resistant to radiation and chemotherapeutic agents. Ewing sarcoma is part of a spectrum of disease having primitive neuroectodermal tumors at one end and Ewing sarcoma at the other. Multimodality therapy, including both radiation therapy and chemotherapy, has been shown to be beneficial for this tumor. Osteosarcomas are best treated with neoadjuvant therapy, with prognosis being predicted by the tumor's response to chemotherapy. Plasmacytoma confined to the chest must be confirmed by evaluating the remaining skeletal system. Surgery can then be used to confirm the diagnosis. If radiation therapy is unable to achieve local control, then resection may be indicated. Soft-tissue sarcomas are rare and are primarily resected. Adjuvant therapy is based on tumor histologic findings.

Diagnosis

Chest wall tumors are asymptomatic in 20% of patients, whereas the remaining 80% have an enlarging mass. Fifty percent to 60% of these patients will have associated pain. Radiographic assessment usually includes CXR and CT; however, MRI is being used instead with increasing frequency because of its ability to image in multiple planes with superior anatomical distinction, which can better reveal the extent of disease than CT or plain radiography. Pathological diagnosis is made with FNA (64% accuracy) or core cutting biopsy (96% accuracy). Incisional biopsies should be avoided if possible because they may interfere with subsequent surgical treatment and reconstruction.

Staging

Chest wall lesions are staged according to the primary tumor identified. Most progress to pulmonary or hepatic metastases without lymphatic involvement.

Treatment

As outlined previously, the treatment of chest wall lesions is determined by the diagnosis. Most, with few exceptions, require resection as part of the treatment. Posterior lesions reaching deep to the scapula or that require resection of less than two ribs do not require reconstruction of the chest wall. However, all other lesions require some form of stable reconstructive technique. A simple mesh closure using Marlex or Proline mesh is acceptable as long as the material is secured in position under tension. Some surgeons believe there is a loss of tensile strength over time. A more rigid prosthesis is methyl methacrylate sandwiched between two layers of Marlex mesh. Long-term seroma formation plagues all types of repair, particularly this latter repair technique.

If the chest wall lesion involves the overlying muscle or the skin, a large defect may be present after resection. This may require a muscle flap for final reconstruction, especially if postoperative radiation therapy is considered. Although description of the techniques available is beyond the scope of this manual, a combination of muscle flap with primary skin closure, muscle flap with skin grafting, or myocutaneous flap coverage can be used.

Surveillance

Once treated and in remission, chest wall tumors tend to recur locally or with pulmonary or hepatic metastases. Regular follow-up with careful examination and CT scanning should suffice to detect all significant sites of recurrence.

NEOPLASMS OF THE PLEURA

There are two main types of pleural neoplasms. The first, malignant pleural mesothelioma, remains an uncommon and highly lethal tumor with no adequate method of treatment. It behaves primarily as a locally aggressive tumor with locally invasive failure after therapy and only metastasizes late in its course. Its relationship with asbestos exposure was suggested in the 1940s and 1950s, and clearly established in 1960. The second, a more localized pleural tumor known as localized fibrous tumor of the pleura, can also occur; when malignant, it is frequently classified as a localized mesothelioma.

Pathology

Localized mesotheliomas and malignant localized fibrous tumors of the pleura are very rare. There is some controversy as to whether these lesions are even mesothelial at all because no epithelial component may be identifiable. More commonly, a benign localized fibrous tumor of the pleura is found. However, diffuse pleural mesothelioma is always a malignant process. There is a 20-year latency for development of this disease after exposure to asbestos. A recent surge in the incidence of this disease reflects the widespread use of asbestos in the 1940s and 1950s, and this surge should continue because mechanisms for limiting occupational asbestos exposure were not instituted until the 1970s. Mesothelioma commonly presents as an epithelial histology and less commonly as a sarcomatoid or mixed histology. It can be hard to differentiate this lesion from metastatic adenocarcinoma. Immunohistochemistry and electron microscopy, however, have aided in establishing the diagnosis.

Diagnosis

The presentation of mesothelioma is often vague and nonspecific, with dyspnea and pain common in 90% of patients. Radiographic diagnosis in the early stage is often difficult, with the findings limited to a pleural effusion in many cases. Even CT may fail to identify any other abnormalities at this stage. The classic finding of a thick, restrictive pleural rind is a late finding. Thoracentesis is diagnostic in 50% of patients, and pleural biopsy is positive in 33%. If the diagnosis remains elusive, thoracoscopy is diagnostic in 80% of patients.

Staging

A staging system for mesothelioma has been proposed by Rusch and the International Mesothelioma Interest Group (IMIG) and is shown in Table 7.6.

Table 7.6. Staging of mesothelioma

T	
T1	TIa tumor limited to the ipsilateral parietal, including mediastinal and diaphragmatic pleura No involvement of the visceral pleura Tib tumor involving the ipsilateral parietal, including mediastinal and diaphragmatic pleura Scattered foci of tumor also involving the visceral pleura
T2	Tumor involving each of the ipsilateral pleural surfaces (parietal, mediastinal, diaphragmatic, and visceral pleura), with at least one of the following features: • Involvement of diaphragmatic muscle • Confluent visceral pleural tumor (including the fissures), or extension of tumor from visceral pleura into the underlying pulmonary parenchyma
T3	Describes locally advanced but potentially resectable tumor Tumor involving all ipsilateral pleural surfaces (parietal, mediastinal, diaphragmatic, and visceral pleura), with at least one of the following features: • Involvement of the endothoracic fascia • Extension into the mediastinal fat • Solitary, completely resectable focus of tumor extending into the soft tissues of the chest wall • Nontransmural involvement of the pericardium
T4	Describes locally advanced technically unresectable tumor Tumor involving all ipsilateral pleural surfaces (parietal, mediastinal, diaphragmatic, and visceral), with at least one of the following features: • Diffuse extension or multifocal masses of tumor in the chest wall, with or without associated rib destruction • Direct transdiaphragmatic extension of tumor to the peritoneum • Direct extension of tumor to the contralateral pleura • Direct extension of tumor to one or more mediastinal organs • Direct extension of tumor into the spine • Tumor extending through to the internal surface of the pericardium with or without a pericardial effusion, or tumor involving the myocardium
N	Lymph nodes
NX	Regional lymph nodes cannot be assessed
N0	No regional lymph node metastases
N1	Metastases in the ipsilateral bronchopulmonary or hilar lymph nodes

(continued)

Table 7.6. (***Continued***)

N2	Metastases in the subcarinal or the ipsilateral mediastinal lymph nodes, including the ipsilateral internal mammary nodes
N3	Metastases in the contralateral mediastinal, contralateral internal mammary, ipsilateral, or contralateral supraclavicular lymph nodes
M	Metastases
MX	Presence of distant metastases cannot be assessed
M0	No distant metastasis
M1	Distant metastasis present
Stage	
Stage I	I_a T_{Ia} N_0 M_0 I_b T_{Ib} N_0 M_0
Stage II	T_2 N_0 M_0
Stage III	Any T_3 M_0 Any N_1 M_0 Any N_2 M_0
Stage IV	Any T_4 Any N_3 Any M_1

Treatment

The treatment of mesothelioma is still evolving. Attempts at radical resections, such as extrapleural pneumonectomy, have led to some improvements in local control, but only limited impact on survival at the cost of a significantly increased operative risk. The addition of adjuvant radiotherapy can increase local control and the removal of the entire lung can facilitate its delivery. Unfortunately, better local control has led to an increase in the number of patients who succumb to systemic disease. The effectiveness of chemotherapy is limited, although new agents may be on the horizon (i.e., Pemextred). By themselves, chemotherapy and radiation therapy have had only limited effects, with less impact on palliation.

Surveillance

Mesotheliomas tend to recur locally. CT scans are required to detect recurrences or follow residual disease. Unfortunately, treatment options are limited, but they do include radiation therapy and chemotherapy.

RECOMMENDED READING

PET Scanning

Detterbeck FC, Vansteenkiste JF, Morris DE, Dooms CA, Khandani AH, Socinski MA. Seeking a home for a PET, part 3: emerging applications of positron emission tomography imaging in the management of patients with lung cancer. *Chest* 2004;126(5): 1656–1666.

Erasmus JJ, Connolly JE, McAdams HP, Roggli VL. Solitary pulmonary nodules: part I.

Morphologic evaluation for differentiation of benign and malignant lesions. *Radiographics* 2000;20(1):43–58.

Erasmus JJ, McAdams HP, Connolly JE. Solitary pulmonary nodules: part II. Evaluation of the indeterminate nodule. *Radiographics* 2000;20(1):59–66.

Gonzalez-Stawinski GV, Lemaire A, Merchant F, et al. A comparative analysis of positron emission tomography and mediastinoscopy in staging non-small cell lung cancer. *J Thorac Cardiovasc Surg* 2003;126(6):1900–1905.

Reed CE, Harpole DH, Posther KE, et al. American College of Surgeons Oncology Group Z0050 trial. Results of the American College of Surgeons Oncology Group Z0050 trial: the utility of positron emission tomography in staging potentially operable non-small cell lung cancer. *J Thorac Cardiovasc Surg* 2003;126(6):1943–1951.

Adjuvant Chemotherapy for Early-stage Lung Cancer

The International Adjuvant Lung Cancer Trial Collaborative Group. Cisplatin-based adjuvant chemotherapy in patients with completely resected NSCLC. *N Engl J Med* 2004;350: 351–360.

Strauss GM, Herndon J, Maddaus MA, et al. Randomized clinical trial of adjuvant chemotherapy with paclitaxel and carboplatin following resection in stage IB non-small cell lung cancer (NSCLC): report of Cancer and Leukemia Group B (CALGB) Protocol 9633 [abstract 7019]. *Proc Am Clin Oncol* 2004;23:17b.

Winton TL, Livingston R, Johnson D, et al. A prospective randomized trial of adjuvant vinorelbine (VIN) and cisplatin (CIS) in completely resected stage Ib and II non-small cell lung cancer (NSCLC) Intergroup JBR. 10 [abstract 7018]. *Proc Am Clin Oncol* 2004;23.

Additional References

Anderson BO, Burt ME. Chest wall neoplasms and their management. *Ann Thorac Surg* 1994;58:1774.

Dartevelle PG. Extended operations for the treatment of lung cancer. *Ann Thorac Surg* 1997;63:12.

Ginsberg RJ, Rubinstein LV. Randomized trial of lobectomy versus limited resection for T1 N0 non–small cell lung cancer: lung cancer study group. *Ann Thorac Surg* 1995;60:615.

Jemal A, Murray T, Ward E, et al. Cancer statistics, 2005. *CA Cancer J Clin* 2005;55(1):10–30.

Mountain CF. Revisions in the international system for staging lung cancer. *Chest* 1997;111: 1710.

Nesbitt JC, Putnam JB, Walsh GL, et al. Survival in early-stage non–small cell lung cancer. *Ann Thorac Surg* 1995;60:466.

Pastorino U, Buyse M, Friedel G, et al. Long-term results of lung metastasectomy: prognostic analyses based on 5206 cases. *J Thorac Cardiovasc Surg* 1997;113:37.

Rusch VW. The international mesothelioma interest group: a proposed new international TNM staging system for malignant pleural mesothelioma. *Chest* 1995;108:1122–1128.

Roth JA, Fossella F, Komaki R, et al. A randomized trial comparing perioperative chemotherapy and surgery with surgery alone in resectable stage III non–small cell lung cancer. *J Natl Cancer Inst* 1994;86:673.

Shields TW. Primary mediastinal tumors and cysts and their diagnostic investigation In: Shields TW, ed. *Mediastinal Surgery*. Philadelphia, Pa: Lea & Febiger; 1991.

Sugarbaker DJ, Jaklitsch MT, Liptay MJ. Mesothelioma and radical multimodality therapy: who benefits? *Chest* 1995;107:3455.

Walsh GL, Morice RC, Putnam JB, et al. Resection of lung cancer is justified in high-risk patients selected by exercise oxygen consumption. *Ann Thorac Surg* 1994;58:704.

Walsh GL, O'Connor M, Willis KM, et al. Is follow-up of lung cancer patients after resection medically indicated and cost effective? *Ann Thorac Surg* 1995;60:1563.

8

Esophageal Carcinoma

Alexander A. Parikh, Ara A. Vaporciyan, and Wayne L. Hofstetter

Cancer of the esophagus is uncommon, believed to represent approximately 1.5% of newly diagnosed invasive malignancies in the United States; it is the ninth most common malignancy worldwide. It is highly virulent, however, and causes 2% of all cancer-related deaths. Surgical resection is the mainstay of therapy, although most cases are diagnosed at a late stage. Since the mid-1970s, the overall 5-year survival rate has improved from 3% to only 15%. Recent treatment strategies have included multimodality approaches that combine surgery, radiation therapy, and chemotherapy. These approaches have resulted in 5-year survival rates of 40% to 75% in the subset of patients who have a complete histologic response after preoperative therapy.

EPIDEMIOLOGY

Carcinoma of the esophagus accounts for approximately 15,000 new cases and 13,000 deaths in the United States each year. In the past, squamous cell carcinomas (SCC) accounted for more than 95% of cases, but in recent years, adenocarcinoma arising in the background of Barrett esophagus has become increasingly common, and it now accounts for more than 50% of the esophageal cancers at many major centers. Esophageal carcinoma, particularly SCC, has substantial geographic variation, from 1.5 to 7 cases per 100,000 people in most parts of the world, including the United States, to 100 to 500 per 100,000 people in its endemic areas such as northern China, South Africa, Iran, Russia, and India. Males have a two to three times higher risk than females, and a seven to ten times higher risk for the development of adenocarcinoma. Furthermore, in the United States, SCC is approximately five times more common among African Americans than it is among whites, whereas adenocarcinoma occurs approximately three to four times more often in whites, particularly in men. The typical patient with esophageal adenocarcinoma is a middle-class, overweight male in his sixties or seventies. Both major histologic types are rare in patients younger than 40 years, but the incidence increases thereafter.

ETIOLOGY AND RISK FACTORS

Several different environmental and genetic risk factors have been identified as potential causes of esophageal cancers, particularly SCC. In geographic areas where esophageal cancer is endemic, such as in China, diets are deficient in vitamins A, C, riboflavin, and protein, and have excessive nitrates and nitrosamines. Fungal contamination of foodstuffs and the associated aflatoxin production may be another important risk factor.

The combination of smoking and alcohol consumption has a synergistic effect on the development of esophageal SCC, increasing the risk by as much as 44 times. Other causes and risk factors include SCC of the head and neck (presumably because of the risk associated with alcohol and smoking), achalasia (as high as 30 times increased risk), strictures resulting from ingestion of caustic agents such as lye, Zenker diverticulae, esophageal webs in Plummer-Vinson syndrome, prior radiation, and familial connective tissue diseases such as tylosis (50% have cancer by age 45 years). For adenocarcinoma, the primary etiologic factor is Barrett esophagus, with an estimated annual incidence of malignant transformation of 0.5% to 1%, representing a 125 times greater risk than that in the general population. Similar to colon cancers, esophageal adenocarcinomas are known to progress through a metaplasia–dysplasia–cancer sequence. Gastroesophageal reflux disease results in the overexposure of the esophageal mucosa to acid and bile. Specifically, the conjugated bile salts (secondary bile acids) are believed to synergistically damage the mucosa, leading to increased DNA methylation (as well as other genetic and molecular changes) and the formation of specialized intestinal metaplasia (Barrett mucosa) or cardiac metaplasia. Both are recognized as precursor lesions to esophageal/gastroesophageal junction cancers. Obesity, tobacco use, and the eradication of *Helicobacter pylori* are also linked to the increased incidence of esophageal adenocarcinoma in the United States.

PATHOLOGY

Esophageal cancer is seen in two main histologic types: SCC and adenocarcinoma. In the United States, approximately 20% of cases of SCC involve the upper third of the esophagus, 50% involve the middle third, and the remaining 30% extend from the distal part of the esophagus to the gastroesophageal junction. SCC rarely invades the stomach, and there is usually a discrete segment of normal mucosa between the cancer and the gastric cardia. In contrast, nearly 97% of adenocarcinomas develop in the middle and distal esophagus, and many extend into the stomach if they are located near the gastroesophageal junction. Cancers arising in Barrett esophagus are believed to comprise upward of 70% of all adenocarcinomas involving the distal esophagus and gastroesophageal junction. They can vary in length and range in contour from flat, infiltrative lesions to fungating polypoid masses. Ulceration is often present and may even be deep enough to cause perforation. The typical esophageal carcinoma is a circumferential, exophytic, fungating mass that is nearly or completely transmural. Access to the submucosal lymphatics allows tumors to spread freely along a submucosal plane and present with very long tumors or multiple mucosal lesions. Similarly, early metastases to lymph nodes or distant sites are common. Microscopically, adenocarcinomas can resemble cells in the gastric cardia or colon, and most are well or moderately differentiated. Signet ring differentiation on histology may signify a gastric cardia origin, but this is not an absolute rule.

Other less common primary malignant neoplasms of the esophagus include neuroendocrine tumors, gastrointestinal stromal tumors, variants of SCC or adenocarcinomas (e.g., adenosquamous), melanomas, sarcomas, and lymphomas.

CLINICAL FEATURES

Clinical presentation is generally insidious, and typical symptoms occur late in the course of the disease, usually precluding early intervention. Most patients experience symptoms for 2 to 6 months before they seek medical attention. The most common symptom is progressive dysphagia, which occurs in as many as 80% to 90% of patients. This is usually a late sign because 50% to 75% of the esophageal lumen must be reduced before patients experience this symptom. Typically, malignant dysphagia will begin when the esophageal functional diameter approaches 12 to 13 mm, about the size of a normal adult endoscope. Weight loss is also common, with an estimated mean weight loss of 10 kg from the onset of symptoms and weight loss of greater than 10% of normal body weight has been associated with decreased long-term survival in many publications. Other symptoms include varying degrees of odynophagia (in approximately 50%), as well as emesis, cough, regurgitation, anemia, hematemesis, and aspiration pneumonia. Hoarseness is usually due to invasion of the recurrent laryngeal nerve, and Horner syndrome indicates invasion of the sympathetic trunk. Hematemesis and melena usually indicate friability of the tumor or its invasion into major vessels. Erosion into the aorta resulting in exsanguinating hemorrhage has been reported. Bleeding from the tumor mass can occur in 4% to 7% of patients.

DIAGNOSTIC EVALUATION

Results of the physical examination depend in large part on the degree of weight loss and cachexia. Enlarged cervical or supraclavicular lymph nodes can be biopsied with fine-needle aspiration (FNA), and bone pain should be evaluated with a bone scan to exclude distant metastases. All neurologic symptoms (e.g., headaches, visual disturbances) should also be assessed with computed tomography (CT) or magnetic resonance imaging (MRI) of the brain.

Plain posteroanterior and lateral chest radiographs provide assessment of the status of the pulmonary parenchyma (i.e., metastasis, coexisting bronchogenic carcinoma, and pneumonia). A double-contrast barium esophagogram provides information about the location, length, and anatomical configuration of the lesion, as well as an evaluation of the stomach for evidence of disease or abnormalities that would preclude its use as a conduit. The esophagogram is also useful in showing the degree of luminal compromise or stricture and the presence of a tumor-related tracheoesophageal fistula. CT scans of the chest and abdomen should also be obtained to rule out the presence of local invasion of mediastinal structures, adenopathy, and distant metastasis.

Positron emission tomography (PET) is being used with increasing frequency in the diagnostic staging algorithm. When combined with CT, it has been shown to alter the treatment course in approximately 15% of patients studied, which in itself has rendered it cost efficient. This modality is helpful in determining the significance of regional adenopathy or distant lesions and may carry prognostic information in terms of the level of initial nucleotide uptake and midterm response to preoperative treatment.

Upper endoscopy is currently the most widely used technique for the diagnosis of esophageal cancer. Flexible endoscopy allows magnified visual observation and histologic sampling of the esophagus, as well as observation of the stomach, pylorus, and duodenum in search of coexisting disease. Biopsy and brush cytology can produce diagnostic accuracy of nearly 100% with adequate sampling, and endoscopic dilation of tight strictures can be performed to allow passage of the endoscope beyond the tumor. The addition of endoscopic ultrasound (EUS) can be used to predict the TNM stage of the lesion with reliable accuracy. EUS is most accurate in predicting the depth of invasion of the primary lesion, and this can lead to very good insight to the potential of surrounding organ involvement or lymph node involvement. Thoracic, paraesophageal, paragastric, portohepatic, and celiac lymph nodes are routinely identified and can be biopsied via aspiration (FNA) for diagnosis. Tumors that involve the upper or middle third of the esophagus should be evaluated by flexible and/or rigid bronchoscopy to rule out tracheobronchial involvement.

STAGING

The staging system of the American Joint Committee on Cancer uses the TNM classification and is the most commonly used system in the United States (Table 8.1). Although CT scanning is probably the most widely used noninvasive staging modality, its accuracy is quite limited. Overall accuracy in determining resectability and T stage have been estimated at 60% to 70%, whereas accuracy in determining N stage is generally less than 60%. Accuracy in detection of metastatic disease is somewhat better, estimated at 70% to 90% for lesions larger than 1 cm. The use of combined imaging with PET-CT has improved the accuracy of both tests. The ability to combine anatomical irregularity to areas of abnormal Flouro-Deoxy Glucose (FDG) uptake on a superimposed image increases the predictive value of PET alone or CT alone. Recent studies with this technique have reported overall accuracy levels of nearly 60% and 90% in the ability to detect both locoregional nodal metastases and distant disease, respectively.

EUS is probably the most accurate means currently available for T and N staging. Reported overall accuracy for T staging is 76% to 90%; overall accuracy in predicting resectability is approximately 90% to 100% for adenocarcinoma, but decreases to 75% to 80% for SCC. Studies comparing EUS and CT scanning generally agree that EUS is superior in overall T staging and assessment of regional lymph nodes (70%–86% accuracy). The precise differentiation between benign and malignant nodes occasionally remains problematic, however, due to micrometastases that are undetectable by EUS and enlarged inflammatory lymph nodes that are incorrectly classified as metastatic. FNA can be helpful in making this diagnosis. Minimally invasive techniques such as thoracoscopy and laparoscopy are increasingly important in the staging of esophageal cancer. Thoracoscopy allows visualization of the entire thoracic esophagus and the periesophageal nodes (N1), when performed through the right hemithorax, or the aortopulmonary and periesophageal nodes and the lower esophagus, when performed through the left chest. Lymph nodes can be

Table 8.1. TNM staging for esophageal cancer

Primary tumor (T)	
Tx	Primary tumor cannot be assessed
T0	No evidence of primary tumor
Tis	Carcinoma in situ
T1	Tumor invades lamina propria or submucosa
T2	Tumor invades muscularis propria
T3	Tumor invades adventitia
T4	Tumor invades adjacent structures
Regional lymph nodes (N)	
Nx	Regional nodes cannot be assessed
N0	No regional node metastasis
N1	Regional node metastasis
Distant metastasis (M)	
Mx	Presence of distant metastasis cannot be assessed
M0	No distant metastases
M1	Distant metastasis
	Tumors of the lower thoracic esophagus
	M1a Metastasis in celiac lymph nodes
	M1b Other distant metastasis
	Tumors of the midthoracic esophagus
	M1a Not applicable
	M1b Nonregional lymph nodes or other distant metastasis
	Tumors of the upper thoracic esophagus
	M1a Metastasis in cervical nodes
	M1b Other distant metastasis

Stage grouping			
Stage 0	Tis	N0	M0
Stage I	T1	N0	M0
Stage IIA	T2	N0	M0
	T3	N0	M0
Stage IIB	T1	N1	M0
	T2	N1	M0
Stage III	T3	N1	M0
	T4	Any N	M0
Stage IV	Any T	Any N	M1
Stage IVA	Any T	Any N	M1a
Stage IVB	Any T	Any N	M1b

Adapted from Fleming ID, Cooper JS, Henson DE, et al., eds. *AJCC Manual for Staging of Cancer.* 5th ed. Philadelphia, Pa: Lippincott-Raven; 1997, with permission.

sampled for histologic evaluation, the pleura can be examined, and adjacent organ invasion (T4) can be confirmed. The overall accuracy for detecting lymph node involvement has been reported to be as high as 81% to 95%. Laparoscopy and laparoscopic ultrasonography (LUS) are useful in evaluating the peritoneum, liver, gastrohepatic ligament, gastric wall, diaphragm, and the perigastric and celiac lymph nodes. Biopsies and peritoneal washings can be performed to confirm N1 and M1 disease. These modalities are especially useful in patients with gastroesophageal junction or proximal gastric tumors. In addition, a feeding jejunostomy can be placed for nutritional support before treatment begins. Studies have suggested that the overall accuracy of laparoscopy in staging and determination of resectability in esophageal cancer is as high as 90% to 100%, and that invasive staging procedures may prevent unnecessary surgical resection in as many as 20% of patients. Prospective comparisons with CT and EUS have suggested that laparoscopy and LUS have superior overall accuracy in staging, particularly for lymph nodes and metastatic disease. Mediastinoscopy can also prove helpful to assess regional lymph nodes (N1) at the right and left paratracheal lymph node stations, along the mainstem bronchi, in the aortopulmonary window, or in the subcarinal area.

TREATMENT

Patients should be approached with the intent of performing a surgical resection as it affords the best chance for long-term survival (Fig. 8.1). Because accurate clinical staging is so difficult, all patients who can physiologically tolerate resection and have no clinically evident distant metastases should generally undergo exploration. If distant metastases or unresectable advanced locoregional disease is found at exploration, nonoperative palliation should be undertaken because of the high perioperative mortality rate (approximately 20%) associated with palliative surgical bypass.

Distal esophageal tumors located at the gastroesophageal junction can be managed by subtotal esophagectomy, esophagogastrectomy, or segmental esophagectomy with bowel interposition. The extent of gastric and esophageal involvement, as well as the stage of the primary tumor, should guide the surgeon to an appropriate approach. A subtotal esophagectomy through a right thoracotomy and laparotomy (Ivor Lewis or Tanner-Lewis esophagectomy) allows for generous resection of the stomach because the esophageal reconstruction takes place in the chest at the level of the azygous vein. Locally advanced tumors with involvement of the distal esophagus and proximal stomach lend themselves to this approach because a lymphadenectomy is easily performed in two fields and negative margins can be obtained in the stomach with less worry of gastric necrosis. However, tumors with extensive involvement of the stomach and esophagus may require an esophagogastrectomy, with interposition of small or large bowel for reconstruction. Early distal tumors or short segment Barrett esophagus with high-grade dysplasia can be treated with segmental esophagectomy and small bowel interposition (Merendino procedure) or vagal-sparing esophagectomy with gastric or bowel interposition.

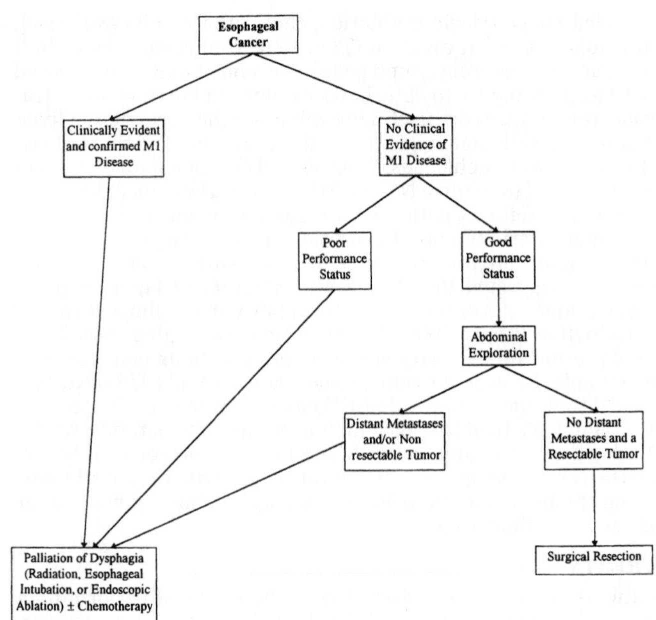

Figure 8.1. Algorithm for treatment of esophageal cancer.

Proximally located (e.g., upper and midesophageal) tumors often require a total esophagectomy because it is difficult to achieve negative margins with segmental or subtotal resections (e.g., Ivor Lewis esophagectomy). Given the propensity for esophageal cancers to spread in the submucosal lymphatic system, it is recommended that a minimum of a 5-cm margin, and preferably a 10-cm margin, should be taken on the esophagus. This is a critical decision-making factor when formulating a treatment algorithm for an individual patient. The two most popular methods to achieve a total or near-total esophagectomy differ according to whether thoracotomy is used for esophageal mobilization. The esophagus can be mobilized using a right thoracotomy with the conduit brought either through the posterior mediastinum (preferred) or substernally to the neck for anastomosis (McKowen approach). Alternatively, a transhiatal esophagectomy can be performed with mobilization of the intrathoracic esophagus from the esophageal hiatus to the thoracic inlet without the need for thoracotomy. The advantage of the transhiatal technique is that it avoids thoracotomy while achieving a complete removal of the esophagus. The potential disadvantages of this technique include a limited periesophageal and mediastinal lymphadenectomy, the risk of causing tracheobronchial or vascular injury during blunt dissection of the esophagus, and potentially higher locoregional recurrence rates. In addition, the use of a cervical anastomosis is associated with a higher rate of anastomotic leakage than an intrathoracic anastomosis (12% vs. 5%, respectively), although the morbidity is much less with a cervical leak than it is with a thoracic leak. Other potential downsides to a cervical anastomosis include pharyngeal reflux, nocturnal aspiration, prolonged swallowing dysfunction after surgery, and an increased incidence of recurrent laryngeal nerve palsy. Intrathoracic anastomoses are hampered by reflux and a striking incidence of recurrent esophageal metaplasia, which has been reported to occur in 80% of long-term survivors.

Patients that present with cervical esophageal carcinomas have several treatment options. Advances in chemoradiotherapy have relegated resection of most localized cervical lesions to salvage procedures. Patients that have persistent locoregional, limited disease after definitive medical therapy are candidates for segmental resections with immediate or delayed reconstruction. Small bowel, neck, or musculocutaneous free flaps are well suited to esophageal reconstructions in the cervical area, with or without pharyngolaryngectomy. An alternative option for patients with early-stage disease is immediate resection and reconstruction. At the other end of the spectrum, lengthy lesions with involvement into the thoracic esophagus may require a complete esophagectomy via a three-field approach.

Although it is generally agreed that surgical resection is the primary form of therapy for local and locoregional disease, great controversy remains over the extent of the resection necessary and over the value and extent of lymphadenectomy. There is one group of thought that lymph node metastases are markers for systemic disease and that removal of involved nodes in most cases offers no survival benefit. However, many well-respected and experienced surgeons believe that some patients with affected lymph nodes can be successfully cured with an aggressive surgical approach that focuses on wide peritumoral excision and extended lymphadenectomy using a transthoracic/thoracoabdominal and cervical approach (en bloc esophagectomy). There is currently no definitive evidence to support either philosophy; however, many reports that have focused on specific subsets of patients in stages IIb to III have shown that patients who have undergone complete lymphadenectomy and have less than 10% of their resected nodes involved with metastatic disease can still look forward to prolonged survival and excellent locoregional control. The downside to this approach is that we are currently unable to predict which patients with locally advanced disease would benefit from immediate resection and extensive lymphadenectomy versus neoadjuvant chemoradiotherapy followed by resection. Proponents of radical resection have reported increased survival rates with more extensive surgical procedures and excellent locoregional control, but most of these comparisons have been retrospective. Furthermore, it is unclear whether more extensive dissection actually leads to improved survival or whether these superior results are a function of more accurate staging (stage migration effect). Recent prospective randomized studies in the United States and Western Europe have failed to show any significant difference in morbidity, mortality, or recurrence rates, or in the overall survival rate when comparing transhiatal esophagectomy with transthoracic or total thoracic esophagectomy or when comparing the number of lymph nodes resected. Either technique is acceptable, and it is unlikely that a prospective randomized trial will ever be performed that could conclusively prove an advantage in overall survival rate with a particular type of surgery. The choice among surgical resection techniques should be left to the preference of the surgeon and individualized to the particular characteristics of the patient. The salient points that emerge from historical comparisons of these procedures is that a transhiatal resection has a tendency toward higher locoregional recurrence, but a lower incidence of ICU care, and does not require thoracotomy to complete.

Minimally invasive esophagectomy is gaining popularity in some high-volume centers. Patients with appropriate lesions have the option of undergoing esophageal resection with combined thoracoscopic and laparoscopic resection followed by a small neck incision with an esophagogastric anastomosis performed in the neck. Complete laparoscopic (transhiatal) resections can also be accomplished, but again, this approach makes extensive en bloc resection of mediastinal lymph nodes difficult. Early results on several hundred patients resected in this manner show no difference in survival, and a formal phase I/II trial is currently underway. Disadvantages of this modality include a fairly steep learning curve, especially for surgeons with limited laparoscopic esophageal experience, and prolonged anesthetic times (although very experienced surgeons can effectively resect the esophagus in a similar amount of time as open procedures).

Reconstruction After Resection

The stomach, colon, and jejunum have all been successfully used as replacement conduits after esophagectomy. The stomach is used far more frequently because of the ease of mobilization, a hearty and redundant blood supply, limited perioperative morbidity, and the need to perform only one anastomosis.

The colon is a commonly used alternative replacement conduit. However, some surgeons prefer this conduit over the stomach in younger patients who are expected to have a prolonged survival because it provides a barrier between the stomach remnant and the residual esophagus, and this may prevent significant pharyngeal reflux and future esophageal metaplasia or dysplasia within the esophageal remnant. Either the right colon or the left colon can be used, but the segment of left and transverse colon that is supplied by the ascending branch of the left colic artery, arc of Riolan, and the marginal artery is generally a better size match to the esophagus and has more reliable arterial arcades. The colonic arterial anatomy should be evaluated preoperatively by arteriography in any patient who is expected to have extensive limiting atherosclerosis or is suspected to have had a previous bowel resection. Otherwise, in patients with a naïve abdomen, evaluation of the vasculature can take place in the operating theater. Another alternative is CT or MR angiography. Colonoscopy is necessary to rule out pathological conditions, such as telangiectasia, polyposis, synchronous neoplasm, or extensive diverticulosis, that would preclude use of the colon.

Jejunal reconstruction can be performed for lesions anywhere in the esophagus. Segmental jejunal free flaps transferred to the neck have been used successfully after resection of hypopharyngeal or upper cervical esophageal tumors. In this case, the mesenteric vessels are usually anastomosed to the external carotid artery and the internal jugular vein. Pedicled grafts are being used when segmental distal esophageal resection is performed for benign lesions requiring resection or confirmed (no evidence of cancer in the specimen) short segment Barrett esophagus with high-grade dysplasia. Pedicled jejunal flaps with proximal microvascular augmentation will allow for total esophageal replacement with the small bowel.

Finally, musculocutaneous flaps are also frequently used for segmental cervical reconstruction and can be harvested from any of multiple areas with minimal physiological or aesthetic effect.

Few prospective studies have been performed to evaluate the use of different replacement conduits, but evidence from several nonrandomized and small randomized trials supports that overall survival is unchanged regardless of the technique used. Review performed by Urschel et al. was unable to reach definitive results that would cause one technique to be favored over another. The basic principles are that the stomach has the most reliable blood supply, is a hearty conduit, and is associated with the lowest immediate postoperative morbidity. Cervical leaks from a colon interposition tend to be well tolerated and stricture rarely occurs. If strictures do occur, they are more easily dilated than those in esophagogastric anastomoses. Graft loss can occur with any conduit in any position. Pyloroplasty or pyloromyotomy is required to avoid gastric stasis secondary to the division of the vagus nerves during esophagectomy. No difference has been seen in the leak rate or in the development of strictures between stapled and hand-sewn anastomoses.

Results of Surgical Therapy

Mortality rates for transhiatal or transthoracic esophagectomies are now less than 5%, and realistic morbidity rates range from 35% to 65%. Overall survival rates after surgical resection correspond to the stage of the disease and vary from 5% to 50%. The 5-year survival rates have been reported to be 60% to 90% for stage I, 30% to 60% for stage II, 5% to 30% for stage III, and 0% to 20% for stage IV (Fig. 8.2). Unfortunately, the vast majority (70%) of patients already has stage III or IV disease at diagnosis.

When examining the pattern of failure after surgical resection, one finds that most patients experience either distant metastasis or both locoregional and distant recurrence, and a small percentage experience solely a recurrence of localized disease. Novel treatment modalities focusing on the patterns of failure need to be explored to improve on the relatively poor prognosis afforded by surgery alone in most patients with esophageal carcinoma.

Adjuvant Therapy

Results of several randomized prospective trials on the use of adjuvant radiation therapy (45–56 Gy) after resection have been published. Some studies have shown the potential benefit of adjuvant radiotherapy in specific subsets of patients. Both those undergoing unplanned yet noncurative (palliative) esophagectomy

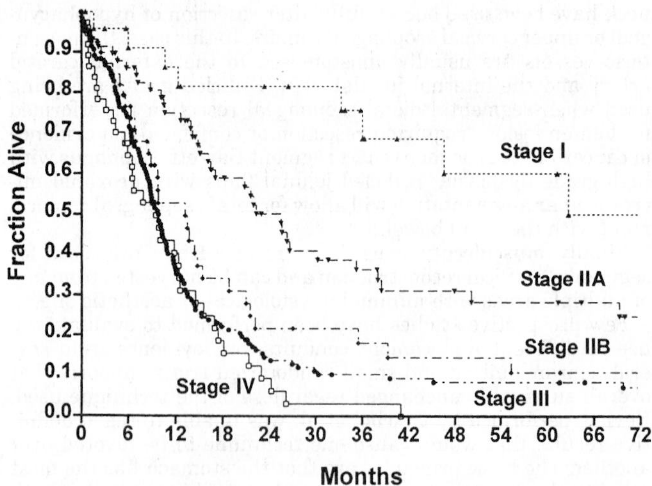

Figure 8.2. Survival curves for patients with esophageal cancer.

and those who are found to have stage III or higher disease may benefit. Most would give consideration for radiation therapy in patients with positive margins or R2 resection as well, although there is no scientific proof of benefit. Treatment-related toxicity can be severe. Overall, although reductions in local recurrences have been noted and specific subsets may benefit, no significant survival advantage has been found using adjuvant radiotherapy for esophageal carcinoma.

According to the results of prospective randomized trials, postoperative combination chemotherapy with various agents, including 5-fluorouracil (5-FU), cisplatin, mitomycin C, vindesine, and paclitaxel, also has no proven role in the treatment of completely resected lesions. Furthermore, adjuvant chemotherapy is generally poorly tolerated, and many patients fail to complete their treatment regimen. This treatment modality, therefore, is not recommended outside clinical trial settings.

Adjuvant chemoradiotherapy may benefit patients with esophageal carcinoma. This modality has the advantage of better patient selection because the pathological stage will guide the decision to proceed to therapy. Patients with a high risk of recurrence (stage IIb and above) would be chosen to selectively undergo treatment. This may increase overall survival because the resection rate remains high (a frequent criticism for neoadjuvant therapy is that overall resection rates drop secondary to treatment toxicity), and patients that are found to be earlier stage can avoid the potential toxicity. In theory, chemoradiotherapy may increase survival by decreasing both distant and local disease. To date, there is some phase II evidence that has shown promising results, but compliance with treatment has not been ideal and formal prospective, randomized phase III trials are needed before final recommendations can be made regarding its efficacy.

Neoadjuvant Therapy

Largely because of the difficulty administering adjuvant therapy to postesophagectomy patients and the disappointing results of trials with adjuvant chemotherapy or radiation monotherapy, researchers have turned their attention toward the use of preoperative or neoadjuvant therapy. Preoperative radiation therapy has been investigated in several prospective randomized trials, and the results have been subjected to meta-analysis. Despite some initial response, the results of these trials have shown marginal overall benefit in terms of survival rate. Preoperative radiation therapy alone is therefore not generally recommended, even in the face of clinical trials.

Although results of phase II studies of induction chemotherapy had been promising, most of the subsequent prospective randomized trials using multiple different agents and combinations have failed to show any advantage in recurrence or survival. Evidence that neoadjuvant chemotherapy was capable of significant tumor response and even complete responses was reported by multiple authors. Complete responders were also found to have better survival rates than partial or nonresponders, and the R0 resection rate seemed to improve overall. However, the net gain in survival was not significantly different from controls (surgery alone). Conjecture on the reasons for this are that nonresponders frequently fare worse than controls; the overall resection rate was lower in patients undergoing neoadjuvant therapy, thereby abolishing any overall benefit; or there was a study design flaw, possibly representing a β-error. Unfortunately, benefits seen in phase II trials were mainly believed to be secondary to selection bias. In contrast, the largest trial on induction chemotherapy involving more than 800 patients with esophageal carcinoma (squamous and adeno) performed in Europe (MRC trial, 2002) did show a significant survival advantage over surgery alone. The fact that the largest U.S. intergroup trial, however, failed to find any advantage in survival rate with the same agents in more than 400 patients leaves the issue open for debate. At this point, interest in chemotherapy as monotherapy neoadjuvant treatment has been mostly diverted to combined chemoradiotherapy.

Neoadjuvant chemoradiation therapy for esophageal carcinoma has been shown to be feasible and effective. Phase II trials have reported excellent overall response rates (complete responses in 25%–35%) and relatively decent compliance with therapy. Survival and local control compare favorable to historical controls. However, despite the fact that there have been eight prospective randomized studies, only one to date has shown a benefit to this therapy over surgery alone. This study has been widely criticized, and the results have not been repeated in any other randomized trial. This trial, conducted at the University of Dublin with 113 patients with adenocarcinoma, evaluated neoadjuvant cisplatin plus 5-FU and 40 Gy of radiation with surgery alone. The investigators reported a 25% complete pathological response, as well as a significant increase in median survival (16 vs. 11 months) and 3-year survival rate (32% vs. 6%) for the patients receiving the neoadjuvant treatment. Much of the debate over this study has focused on the poor survival in the surgery-only arm of 6% at 3 years, erratic preoperative clinical staging, and questions of miscalculations within the statistics. The seven other randomized trials that have been performed around the world as multi-institutional and single institutional trials have not shown a significant survival advantage. The significant contributions of these works, however, have improved our understanding of esophageal cancer biology. Locoregional recurrence is reported to be low after neoadjuvant chemoradiotherapy, and patients that have had a complete response fare very well. Patients who are significantly downstaged (to N0 status) perform equal to pathologically similarly staged patients who have undergone surgery alone. Radiation to 50.4 Gy is equivalent to higher doses of radiation and is well tolerated without significantly increasing perioperative mortality (in experienced centers).

Three large meta-analyses have been conducted on the use of neoadjuvant chemoradiotherapy in esophageal cancer. The trend toward survival advantage in most of the smaller trials translated to a significant survival advantage in the three published meta-analyses for treated patients. It is probable that there is an overall benefit to chemoradiotherapy; however, a trial that would adequately define this would require approximately 2,000 patients and a decade or more to complete. Furthermore, many clinicians have questioned whether including a surgery-only arm is scientifically ethical for a trial this large and, therefore, there is doubt that this trial will ever be performed.

Definitive Radiation Therapy and Chemoradiation Therapy

Although surgical resection remains the preferred therapy for esophageal cancer, definitive radiation therapy and chemoradiation therapy have been used in patients who are not candidates for surgical resection. Local control rates ranged between 40% and 75%, and median and 2-year survival rates ranged from 9 to 24 months and from 18% to 38%, respectively. Several prospective randomized trials have shown that definitive chemoradiation therapy is superior to radiation therapy alone in the treatment of esophageal cancer. Although direct comparisons against surgical therapy (with or without neoadjuvant therapy) have been attempted in the United States and Europe, both trials have failed to recruit patients, largely because of physicians' reluctance to accept a nonsurgical approach in patients who are operative candidates. One trial out of Europe that sought to evaluate the additional benefit of surgery after neoadjuvant chemoradiotherapy showed significantly improved locoregional control in the surgery arm compared with chemoradiotherapy alone. At this time, therefore, definitive chemoradiation therapy should be reserved for those patients who are poor surgical candidates.

Other Therapeutic Modalities

In certain parts of the world, particularly in areas where esophageal cancer is endemic, mass screening and advances in diagnostic techniques have led to the detection of increased numbers of superficial esophageal cancers. Studies from Japan and the United States have suggested that for lesions confined to the epithelium and lamina propria, lymphatic spread is rare. In some of these patients, endoscopic mucosal resection is a feasible option, although experience with this technique is still limited. Ablation therapy with Nd-YAG laser or argon-beam coagulation are primarily used for palliation, but in patients who are not candidates for surgery with superficial cancers and carcinoma in situ, these methods can also be useful. Although experience with these techniques is limited, investigators have reported tumor-free survival for several months after therapy, although recurrence rates after about 1 year can be significant. Similarly, photodynamic therapy has been used in nonsurgical candidates, and results of preliminary studies in patients with early-stage tumors have suggested that tumor-free survival can last several months and that complete remission is possible in some patients (at 2-year follow-up). However, long-term studies are still needed.

Palliation for Unresectable Tumors

Common indications for palliation in patients with advanced disease include dysphagia, presence of esophagorespiratory fistula, recurrent bleeding, and prolongation of survival. Tumor debulking surgery has been performed, and although survival duration seems somewhat improved relative to that in patients who did not undergo resection, few randomized trials have been performed, and morbidity can be significant. Other options for palliation include (a) dilation, which is a safe and effective method to relieve dysphagia, although it usually requires multiple procedures; (b) stents, both rigid and expandable, which have become very popular in recent years for relieving dysphagia and for treating fistulas and bleeding; (c) laser therapy, which has been effective in relieving dysphagia from shorter strictures and those with intraluminal rather than infiltrative growth; (d) photodynamic therapy, which results in fewer perforations than do dilations or laser therapy and is tolerated better but requires more frequent sessions; (e) bipolar electrocautery and coagulation with tumor probes that use heat to destroy tumor cells and cause circumferential injury; and (f) brachytherapy, which delivers radioactive seeds intraluminally.

All of these techniques have advantages and disadvantages, and short-term success rates of 80% to 100% have been reported. If these treatment options fail, an endoscopic prosthesis can often be placed with good results. These techniques are not without complications, however, and ulceration, obstruction, dislocation, and aspiration have all been reported. Recently, improvements in definitive radiation therapy and chemotherapy have also provided excellent means for short-term palliation. With nonoperative treatment, however, long-term local control is still poor (40% locoregional failure). Which method to use therefore depends on the experience of the physician and the particular needs and condition of the patient.

Surveillance

A barium swallow study should be obtained in the first preoperative month as a baseline study. Asymptomatic patients can be assessed with yearly physical examinations and chest radiography. Any symptoms (e.g., pain, dysphagia, weight loss) should be evaluated aggressively with CT scanning, barium studies, or endoscopy. Benign strictures at the anastomosis should be treated with dilation. Unfortunately, treatment options are limited for locoregional or distant recurrences. If radiation therapy was not given preoperatively or postoperatively, it can be used along with the previously mentioned nonoperative methods of palliation (i.e., dilation, stenting, laser, photodynamic, or thermal resection).

RECOMMENDED READING

Ajani JA. Current status of new drugs and multidisciplinary approaches in patients with carcinoma of the esophagus. *Chest* 1998;113(suppl 1):112S.

Akiyama H, Tsurumaru M, Udagawa H, et al. Esophageal cancer. *Curr Probl Surg* 1997;34:767.

Bosset JF, Gignoux M, Triboulet JP, et al. Chemoradiotherapy followed by surgery compared with surgery alone in squamous-cell cancer of the esophagus. *N Engl J Med* 1997;337:161.

Goldminc M, Maddern G, LePrise E, et al. Oesophagectomy by transhiatal approach or thoracotomy: a prospective randomized controlled trial. *Br J Surg* 1993;80:367.

Gore RM. Esophageal cancer: clinical and pathologic features. *Radiol Clin North Am* 1997;35:243.

Herskovic A, Martz K, Al-Sarraf M, et al. Combined chemotherapy and radiotherapy compared with radiotherapy alone in patients with cancer of the esophagus. *N Engl J Med* 1992;326:1593.

Kelsen DP, Ginsberg R, Pajak TF, et al. Chemotherapy followed by surgery compared with surgery alone for localized esophageal cancer. *N Engl J Med* 1998;339:1979.

Kolh P, Honore P, Degauque C, et al. Early stage results after oesophageal resection for malignancy-colon interposition versus gastric pull-up. *Eur J Cardiothorac Surg* 2000;18:293–300.

Knyrim K, Wagner HJ, Bethge N, et al. A controlled trial of an expansile metal stent for palliation of esophageal obstruction due to inoperable cancer. *N Engl J Med* 1993; 329:1302.

Orringer MB, Marshall B, Iannettoni MD. Transhiatal esophagectomy: clinical experience and refinements. *Ann Surg* 1999;230:392.

Roth JA, Pass HI, Flanagan MM, et al. Randomized clinical trial of preoperative and postoperative adjuvant chemotherapy with cisplatin, vindesine and bleomycin for carcinoma of the esophagus. *J Thorac Cardiovasc Surg* 1988;96:242.

Swisher SG, Holmes EC, Hunt KK, et al. The role of neoadjuvant therapy in surgically resectable esophageal cancer. *Arch Surg* 1996;131:819.

Swisher SG, Hunt KK, Holmes EC, et al. Changes in the surgical management of esophageal cancer from 1970 to 1993. *Am J Surg* 1995;169:609.

Urba SG, Orringer MB, Turrisi A, et al. Randomized trial of preoperative chemoradiation versus surgery alone in patients with locoregional esophageal carcinoma. *J Clin Oncol* 2001;19:305.

Urschel JD. Does the interponat affect outcome after esophagectomy for cancer? *Dis Esophagus* 2001;14(2):124–130.

Walsh TN, Noonan N, Hollywood D, et al. A comparison of multimodal therapy and surgery for esophageal adenocarcinoma. *N Engl J Med* 1996;335:462.

Gastric Cancer

Waddah B. Al-Refaie, Eddie K. Abdalla, Syed A. Ahmad, and Paul F. Mansfield

INTRODUCTION

Because 95% of gastric cancers are adenocarcinomas, they are the primary focus of this chapter on gastric cancer. As with other cancers, evolution in the evaluation and treatment of gastric adenocarcinoma since the mid-1990s has led to a shift in the management of this disease. Now, laparoscopy is an essential component of pretreatment staging for resectable gastric adenocarcinoma. The American Joint Committee on Cancer (AJCC) staging system has been altered to consider the number rather than the location of nodes involved by metastatic tumor, which has been shown to yield a more accurate prognosis in patients with this disease. Finally, evidence that the combination of chemoradiation therapy and potentially curative surgical resection increases disease-free and overall survival duration has led many investigators to recommend multimodality treatment in patients with advanced resectable gastric adenocarcinomas. This chapter covers the epidemiology, preoperative evaluation, and surgical and adjuvant treatment of gastric cancer, as well as management of advanced disease. Less common tumors such as gastric lymphoma, gastric carcinoids, and gastrointestinal stromal tumors (GISTs) of the stomach are also briefly discussed.

EPIDEMIOLOGY

In the United States in 2005, 21,860 new cases of adenocarcinoma of the stomach and 11,550 deaths due to this disease were expected, which would make gastric cancer the 14th most common cancer and the 8th leading cause of cancer death in the United States. There has been a decline in its incidence since the 1930s, when gastric adenocarcinoma was the most common malignancy in the country. Although the reasons for the decreasing incidence are suspected, they are not completely clear. Nonetheless, even though the incidence of distal gastric cancer is decreasing in the United States, the incidence of proximal gastric tumors continues to increase. Cancers of the gastric cardia currently account for nearly 50% of all cases of gastric adenocarcinoma. There are also wide variations in the incidence worldwide: The approximate incidence of gastric carcinoma in the United States is 10 cases per 100,000 people, whereas the incidence in Japan is upward of 78 cases per 100,000 people, although the incidence is dropping in Japan as well. Nonetheless, rates remain high in Korea and Costa Rica.

Gender- and ethnic group-related differences influence the presentation and outcome of gastric adenocarcinoma patients. In particular, gastric cardia tumors are five times more common, and noncardia gastric tumors are twice as common in men as in women. In addition, whites are affected twice as frequently as blacks. However, the incidence is also higher in low socioeconomic populations, and the populations of developing countries.

Survival rates in patients with gastric cancer remain poor, with virtually no change in the overall 5-year survival rates ranging from 53% in Japan to 10% in Eastern Europe. A recent analysis of the National Cancer Data Base in the United States revealed a 6% to 12% better 5-year survival rate for women than for men, for patients with distal as opposed to proximal tumors, and for Japanese or Japanese Americans compared with members of other ethnic groups.

RISK FACTORS

Many factors have been associated with an increased risk for intestinal-type gastric adenocarcinoma, with diet believed to play a major role. For example, the incidence of gastric carcinoma tends to be high in geographic regions where people consume diets high in salt and smoked foods. Indeed, animal studies have shown that polycyclic hydrocarbons and dimethylnitrosamines, substances produced after prolonged smoking of fish and meat, can induce malignant gastric tumors. In contrast, diets high in raw vegetables, fresh fruits, vitamin C, and antioxidants may be protective.

In the United States, male gender, black race, and low socioeconomic class are associated with a higher risk of gastric carcinoma. Obesity is associated with proximal gastric cancers. A specific occupational hazard may exist for metal workers, miners, and rubber workers, as well as for workers exposed to wood or asbestos dust. Cigarette smoking poses a clear risk, possibly as a result of the associated decreased vitamin C levels, but alcohol consumption has not been as consistently correlated with the development of gastric carcinoma. An association between gastric carcinoma and blood group A was first described in 1953, but the relative risk is only 1.2. Familial clustering of gastric adenocarcinoma, although rare, has been reported and is discussed more later in this chapter.

Helicobacter pylori, a gram-negative microaerophilic bacterium living within the mucous layer in the gastric pits, has been implicated in the genesis of gastric carcinoma. In keeping with this, the incidence of *H. pylori* infection is increased in areas where there is a high rate of gastric cancer and is increased among patients with gastric cancer in the United States. *H. pylori* is common in patients with distal cancer but not in patients with proximal cancer. It also appears that there is a marked geographic association with *H. pylori* infection, in that it is more prevalent in the populations of developing nations than in industrialized nations. Furthermore, nearly 90% of patients with intestinal-type gastric cancer have *H. pylori* detected in adjacent, histologically normal mucosa, whereas only 32% of patients with diffuse-type gastric cancer have this finding. Likewise, *H. pylori* is essential for the development of mucosa-associated lymphoid tissue (MALT) and gastric lymphoma. (Intestinal- and diffuse-type gastric cancers are discussed in the Pathology section.) Finally, the risk of adenocarcinoma appears to be increased in patients with serologic evidence of immunoglobulin G antibody to *H. pylori* bacterial proteins and with infection of greater than 10 years' duration. By strongly impairing the bioavailability of vitamin C, *H. pylori* infection appears to heighten the risk for gastric cancer by causing decreased levels of circulating vitamin C.

Gastric polyps are unusual and rarely precursors of gastric cancer. Hyperplastic polyps, the polyps most commonly found in the stomach, are benign lesions. The finding of villous adenomas does, however, indicate an increased risk of malignancy, not only within the polyp itself, but also elsewhere in the stomach. However, villous adenomas represent only 2% of all gastric polyps.

Pernicious anemia is associated with a 10% incidence of gastric cancer, a risk that is about three to five times that seen in the normal population. Even though the risk of carcinoma developing in a chronic gastric ulcer is small, of concern is the fact that up to 10% of patients with gastric carcinoma are misdiagnosed as having a benign gastric ulcer when evaluated by only a double-contrast study of the upper gastrointestinal tract. Also, initial endoscopic biopsies may miss the cancer, thus requiring the endoscopy to be repeated to ensure the ulcer has resolved. Operations for benign peptic ulcers also appear to be associated with an increased risk of stomach cancer. Typically appearing 25 or more years after gastrectomy for the treatment of gastric ulcers, gastric stump cancer has been variously reported to occur from zero to five times more often in patients who have had gastrectomy than in individuals without previous gastric resection. Chronic atrophic gastritis and the intestinal metaplasia that often result from these procedures are also risk factors for gastric carcinoma but may not be direct precursor conditions. To date, no association has been demonstrated between long-term H_2 blockade and gastric cancer incidence.

Mutations in the *CDH1* gene that encodes *E-cadherin,* an epithelial cell adhesion molecule, may be found in intestinal cancers but are more common in diffuse-type gastric cancers. Furthermore, defects in E-cadherin–mediated cell adhesion are characteristic of diffuse-type gastric tumors. It also appears that a *CDH1* gene mutation occurs in a cluster of patients with hereditary diffuse gastric cancer. Therefore, prophylactic gastrectomy is offered to carriers of these mutations. Virtually all carriers of this mutation so far have been found to harbor an early malignancy in the resected specimen, despite negative initial endoscopy findings, pointing to the advisability of the gastrectomy.

Vascular endothelial growth factor C (VEGF-C) is a glycoprotein that belongs to the VEGF family. VEGFs are cytokines that play an important role in angiogenesis and, as shown in recent studies, in lymphangiogenesis as well. Several in vivo and in vitro studies have also demonstrated that VEGF-C and VEGF-D promote the formation of new lymphatic channels in solid tumors. In gastric adenocarcinomas, expression of VEGF-C mRNA is associated with lymphatic invasion, lymph node metastasis, and possibly a less favorable outcome.

Most recently, several genetic alterations have been found to be associated with gastric cancer. A study of *p53* expression in 418 patients with gastric cancer revealed *p53* expression in more than 55% of tumors; however, there was no correlation between *p53* expression and depth of invasion, lymph node involvement, or survival. Other reported risk factors include prior radiation therapy and Epstein-Barr virus infection.

PATHOLOGY

Ninety-five percent of gastric cancers are adenocarcinomas that arise almost exclusively from the mucous-producing rather than the acid-producing cells of the gastric mucosa. Lymphoma, carcinoid, leiomyosarcoma, GISTs of the stomach, and adenosquamous and squamous cell carcinoma comprise the remaining 5% of gastric cancers. In the United States, gastric cancer is divided into ulcerative (75%), polypoid (10%), scirrhous (10%), and superficial (5%) subtypes on the basis of macroscopic findings. Adenocarcinoma of the stomach is an aggressive tumor, often metastasizing early by both lymphatic and hematogenous routes and directly extending into adjacent structures. Extension through the serosal surface can lead to peritoneal tumor spread.

According to the Lauren classification, there are two histologic types of gastric adenocarcinoma: intestinal and diffuse. Each type has distinct clinical and pathological features. The intestinal type is found in geographic regions where there is a high incidence of gastric cancer and is characterized pathologically by the tendency of malignant cells to form glands. These tumors are usually well to moderately differentiated and associated with metaplasia or chronic gastritis. They occur more commonly in older patients and tend to spread hematologically to distant organs. The diffuse type typically lacks organized gland formation, is usually poorly differentiated, and has many signet ring cells. If more than 50% of the tumor contains intracytoplasmic mucin, then it is designated signet ring type. Diffuse-type tumors are more common in younger patients with no history of gastritis and spread transmurally and by lymphatic invasion. Diffuse-type tumors appear to be associated with obesity. Although the incidence of these tumors varies little from country to country, their overall incidence appears to be increasing worldwide. Although Lauren classification separates gastric tumors into two types, the World Health Organization classifies them according to their histomorphologic appearance, which includes tubular, mucinous, papillary, and signet ring cell types.

In the past, most gastric carcinomas (60%–70%) were found in the antrum. However, between 1980 and 1990, the proportion of gastric carcinomas arising in the antrum decreased, and the proportion arising in the cardia increased. Nine percent of patients have tumor that involves the entire stomach; this is known as linitis plastica or "leather bottle" stomach, and the prognosis for these patients is dismal. In general, gastric tumors are more common on the lesser curve of the stomach than on the greater curve. In the United States, the incidence of synchronous lesions is 2.2%, compared with an incidence of up to 10% in Japanese patients with pernicious anemia.

CLINICAL PRESENTATION

Gastric adenocarcinoma is usually not associated with specific symptoms early in the course of the disease. Patients often ignore the vague epigastric discomfort and indigestion that portend the cancer and may be treated presumptively for benign disease for 6 to 12 months before diagnostic studies are performed. Rapid weight loss, anorexia, and vomiting are usually a sign of advanced disease. These presenting features are simply due to the presence of a partially obstructing (either mechanical or physiological) lesion. The most frequent presenting symptoms of 1,121 patients at Memorial Sloan-Kettering Cancer Center were weight loss, pain, vomiting, and anorexia. The epigastric pain is usually similar to the pain caused by benign ulcers and is often relieved by eating food; however, it can mimic angina. Dysphagia is usually associated with tumors of the cardia or gastroesophageal junction. Antral tumors may cause symptoms of gastric outlet obstruction. Although very rare, large tumors that directly invade the transverse colon may present with colonic obstruction. Physical examination will reveal a palpable mass in up to 30% of patients.

Approximately 10% of patients present with one or more signs of metastatic disease. The most common indications of distant metastasis are a palpable supraclavicular lymph node (Virchow node), a mass palpable on rectal examination (Blumer shelf), a palpable periumbilical mass (Sister Mary Joseph node), ascites, jaundice, or a liver mass. The most common site of hematogenous spread is the liver; tumor also frequently spreads directly to the lining of the peritoneal cavity.

Gastric tumors may be associated with chronic blood loss, but massive upper gastrointestinal bleeding is rare. In Japan, the high incidence of gastric cancer has led to routine endoscopic screening; as a result, in that country, more than 50% of gastric cancers are diagnosed at an early stage.

PREOPERATIVE EVALUATION

National Comprehensive Cancer Network Guidelines for Initial Evaluation

The National Comprehensive Cancer Network has developed consensus guidelines for the clinical evaluation and staging of patients suspected of having gastric adenocarcinoma. The recommended initial evaluation includes a complete history and physical examination, laboratory studies (e.g., complete blood cell and platelet counts; measurement of electrolytes, creatinine, and liver function), chest radiography, and computed tomography (CT) of the abdomen and pelvis. For proximal gastric tumors, CT of the chest is also performed. Upper gastrointestinal contrast-enhanced studies are not mandatory. Esophagogastroduodenoscopy is necessary, and provides both tissue for a pathological diagnosis and anatomically localizes the primary tumor in more than 90% of patients. Four to six biopsy specimens and cytologic brushings are usually sufficient for establishing an accurate diagnosis. This initial workup enables the stratification of patients into two clinical stage groups: those with locoregional disease (AJCC stages I–III) and those with systemic disease (AJCC stage IV) (Table 9.1). Palliative therapy is considered in patients with systemic disease, depending on their symptoms and functional status, because several randomized studies have shown a quality of life benefit from treatment in patients with stage IV disease. Patients with locoregional disease are further stratified on the basis of their functional status and comorbid

Table 9.1. TNM classification of carcinoma of the stomach

Category	Criteria		
Primary tumor (T)			
Tx	Primary tumor cannot be assessed		
T0	No evidence of primary tumor		
Tis	Carcinoma in situ		
T1	Tumor invades lamina propria or submucosa		
T2	Tumor invades muscularis propria or subserosa		
T2a	Tumor invades muscularis propria		
T2b	Tumor invades subserosa		
T3	Tumor penetrates serosa (visceral peritoneum) without invasion of adjacent structures		
T4	Tumor invades adjacent structures		
Regional lymph nodes (N)			
Nx	Regional lymph nodes cannot be assessed		
N0	No regional lymph node metastasis		
N1	Metastases in 1–6 lymph nodes		
N2	Metastases in 7–15 lymph nodes		
N3	Metastases in >15 lymph nodes		
Distant metastasis (M)			
Mx	Distant metastasis cannot be assessed		
M0	No distant metastasis		
M1	Distant metastasis		
Stage grouping			
Stage 0	Tis	N0	M0
Stage IA	T1	N0	M0
Stage IB	T1	N1	M0
	T2a/b	N0	M0
Stage II	T1	N2	M0
	T2a/b	N1	M0
	T3	N0	M0
Stage IIIA	T2a/b	N2	M0
	T3	N1	M0
	T4	N0	M0
Stage IIIB	T3	N2	M0
Stage IV	T4	N1–3	M0
	T1–3	N3	M0
	Any T	Any N	M1

Adapted from Stomach. In: Greene FL, Page DL, Fleming ID, et al., eds. *AJCC Cancer Staging Manual.* 6th ed. New York, NY: Springer-Verlag; 2002:99–103, with permission.

conditions. Additional studies in patients with localized disease include laparoscopy and endoscopic ultrasonography (EUS). Pulmonary function tests may also be necessary in select patients. Patients with locoregional disease who are considered candidates for surgery receive definitive (frequently multimodality) therapy, including laparotomy and resection. Patients with occult M1 disease found at laparoscopy are considered for palliative therapy.

Upper Gastrointestinal Endoscopy and Endoscopic Ultrasonography

Upper gastrointestinal endoscopy with biopsy is essential for the diagnosis of gastric tumors and enables anatomical assessment of the proximal extent of the tumor, tumor size, and, often, provided that luminal obstruction does not prevent passage of the gastroscope beyond the tumor, the distal extent of the tumor. Tumor location can guide surgical or palliative treatment planning. In selected patients with advanced disease, esophagogastroduodenoscopy enables palliative treatment consisting of laser ablation, dilatation, or tumor stenting to be performed.

Depth of tumor invasion is a major determinant of stage and directly correlates with prognosis. Gastric mural EUS can achieve spatial resolution of 0.1 mm, which allows for a reasonably accurate assessment of the degree of tumor penetration through the layers of the gastric wall. However, because EUS cannot reliably distinguish between tumor and fibrosis (either treatment related or secondary to peptic ulceration), EUS has some limitation and is thus used primarily for initial staging rather than for assessing response to neoadjuvant therapy.

Pathological confirmation of preoperative EUS findings has shown the overall staging accuracy of EUS to be 75%. However, EUS correctly identifies T2 lesions only 38.5% of the time; it is better at identifying T1 (80%) and T3 (90%) lesions. Technical improvements and experience have improved the accuracy of EUS in the nodal evaluation of N1 disease to approximately 65%. The information yielded by EUS-guided fine-needle aspiration may further improve the accuracy of nodal staging, but this technique is technically more challenging. Given the operator dependence of EUS, it is largely performed at regional referral centers.

Computed Tomography

Abdominal and pelvic CT is performed early in the overall staging of patients with newly diagnosed gastric cancer. This allows unnecessary laparotomy to be avoided in many patients with visceral metastatic disease or malignant ascites. CT of the chest may be required for the complete staging of proximal gastric tumors.

The major limitations of CT as a staging tool are in the evaluation of early gastric tumors and small (<5 mm) metastases on peritoneal surfaces or in the liver. Even with the use of helical CT scan, the overall accuracy in determining tumor stage is approximately 66% to 77%. CT can be used to accurately determine nodal stage in 25% to 86% of patients.

Laparoscopy and Laparoscopic Ultrasonography

The value of further staging with laparoscopy is apparent on recognition of the low sensitivity of CT—even high-quality helical

CT performed with gastric-specific protocols for the detection of small (<5 mm) metastases on the peritoneal surface. Laparoscopy is done either separately or immediately before surgical resection. A full technical description of diagnostic laparoscopy is beyond the scope of this chapter. In brief, a laparoscopic inspection is usually performed in a systematic manner and includes a search for metastases on the peritoneal surfaces and the liver. Biopsy of the nodal basin for staging purposes is not routinely performed, but it can be done in selected cases. When it is done, the lesser sac should be evaluated via the gastrocolic omentum. The identification of advanced disease afforded by laparoscopy allows many patients to be spared an ultimately nontherapeutic laparotomy. Patients with small-volume metastatic disease in the peritoneum or liver identified at laparotomy have a life expectancy of only 3 to 9 months; thus, despite some reports that palliative gastrectomy may confer a survival advantage, such patients rarely benefit from expectant palliative resection. An argument for performing a second-look laparoscopy can be made in the case of patients who receive neoadjuvant chemotherapy for unresectable disease and appear to have a good clinical response.

Researchers at Memorial Sloan-Kettering Cancer Center and M. D. Anderson Cancer Center have evaluated the feasibility, yield, and clinical benefit of laparoscopic staging after high-quality abdominal CT staging and found that laparoscopy identified CT-occult metastatic disease in 23% to 37% of patients. Moreover, less than 2% of the patients in whom CT-occult metastases were identified by laparoscopy required subsequent laparotomy for palliation. On the basis of the available data, the National Comprehensive Cancer Network has integrated laparoscopy into the recommended routine staging algorithm for patients with locoregional gastric cancers and select patients with advanced gastric cancer.

Laparoscopic ultrasonography (LUS) has been proposed as a means to overcome some of the limitations of laparoscopy and to improve the diagnostic yield. However, the majority of studies of LUS in the staging of gastric cancer are difficult to interpret because the use of state-of-the-art prelaparoscopy staging (particularly CT) has varied, and results have been reported in a manner that makes it difficult to determine the specific added benefit of LUS over high-quality CT plus laparoscopy alone. Given the limitations of the available data, the high cost of LUS equipment, and the operator-dependent nature of the technique, it is best to regard LUS as requiring further investigation to define its role.

Peritoneal Cytology

Cytologic analysis of peritoneal fluid or fluid obtained by peritoneal lavage may identify occult carcinomatosis. For this reason, many institutions have included the cytologic assessment of peritoneal fluid in the preoperative staging of patients. The fluid is usually obtained by percutaneous or laparoscopic aspiration (with or without peritoneal lavage) performed at the time of staging laparoscopy. Peritoneal cytologic analysis can be relatively simple and fast and is therefore also feasible intraoperatively, although one must be on the watch for false-positive readings.

In most series, patients with positive peritoneal cytology findings have a prognosis similar to that of patients with macroscopic visceral or peritoneal disease (3- to 9-month median survival). Some researchers have investigated the impact of peritoneal cytology findings on outcome and noted that the median survival in those with positive cytology findings was 122 days; others have used it as an indication for neoadjuvant treatment rather than an absolute contraindication to resection. The primary concerns regarding the use of peritoneal cytology are the possibility of false-positive results and the fact that some reports do not confirm the uniformly poor prognosis in patients with positive findings. Given that cytologic analysis is very much an operator-dependent visual interpretation, efforts are ongoing to develop more sensitive and specific techniques for identifying peritoneal dissemination, including immunostaining and reverse transcriptase-polymerase chain reaction testing for carcinoembryonic antigen (CEA) mRNA. Although some success has been seen using these techniques because they take more time than peritoneal cytology, they may not be practical for use in the operating room.

Lymphatic Mapping

Given the essential role of nodal status in gastric cancer staging and the controversy that surrounds the extent of lymphadenectomy, there has been interest in evaluating the feasibility of sentinel lymph node mapping in gastric cancer. However, unlike breast cancer and melanoma, lymphatic drainage of the stomach is complex and thus there is a risk of a "skip" metastasis in up to 15% of cases. Although lymphatic mapping of stomach tumors has been most commonly performed via an open laparotomy, it has also been done using a laparoscopic approach. Mapping agents such as radiocolloid with or without vital dye and activated carbon particles have been used. The identification rate varies from 90% to 100%, and the sensitivity of the findings ranges from 61% to 100%. However, lymphatic mapping has several drawbacks. First, the number of patients with gastric cancer in which it has been studied is small in comparison with melanoma or breast cancer. Second, it is associated with a false-negative rate as high as 39%. Third, the number of sentinel lymph nodes per patient is quite varied (two to seven sentinel nodes per patient). Fourth, the findings are significantly different in the typically obese Western patients from those in Asian patients, in whom most of the studies of lymphatic mapping have been done. Therefore, for these reasons, sentinel lymph node mapping for stomach cancer remains investigational.

Other Studies

Positron emission tomography (PET), which estimates tumor metabolism on the basis of the uptake of a radiotracer—most commonly, fluorodeoxyglucose—is currently being evaluated as a staging tool for gastric cancer. This technique may reveal CT-occult metastases (particularly extra-abdominal disease) and may be used to assess response to neoadjuvant therapy. Current drawbacks to PET are its high cost and its limited availability.

Also, the additional yield of PET over standard staging studies in the evaluation of gastric cancer has thus far not been shown.

Increased levels of (CEA) Chorioembryonic Antigen are seen in only 30% of patients with gastric carcinoma. Because the CEA level is usually normal in early gastric cancer, CEA is not a useful screening marker. Serial determinations of the CEA level may be helpful, however, in detecting tumor recurrence or in monitoring response to treatment in patients who present with an increased CEA level.

STAGING SYSTEMS

Many staging systems for gastric adenocarcinoma have been proposed. The pathological staging system currently in use worldwide is the Union Internationale Contrele Cancer (UICC)/American Joint Committee on Cancer (AJCC) TNM staging system, with the addition of the term *R status* to denote residual disease remaining after resection. Several other largely abandoned systems have been developed in an attempt to describe both the extent of *disease* and the resultant extent of *resection* or *lymphadenectomy* necessary in a given patient. The various staging systems in use are explained as follows.

American Joint Committee on Cancer Staging System

The staging of gastric adenocarcinoma has changed significantly since the mid-1990s. In 1997, the AJCC released a revised TNM staging system in which patients are stratified on the basis of the number rather than the location of any involved lymph nodes. In 2002, this TNM staging system underwent minimal revision in the most current AJCC staging system (Table 9.1). Survival is closely linked to the AJCC pathological stage, particularly the nodal stage.

The validity of the newer TNM staging system is now well established. Because it is a pathological rather than a clinical staging system, however, a patient's TNM status is only fully known following resection. Three important clinicopathological factors have been shown to reliably stratify patients into distinct groups with different risks of tumor-related death: the depth of penetration of the primary tumor through the gastric wall (T), the absence or presence and extent of lymph node involvement (N), and the absence or presence of distant metastases (M). To adequately assess N status, no fewer than 15 lymph nodes should be retrieved. If metastasis is found in more than 15 lymph nodes (N3), this is considered stage IV disease. Some investigators (e.g., Roder et al., 1998) argued that survival is also independently predicted by tumor location (i.e., cardia as opposed to distal tumors) and suggested that future AJCC staging systems should reflect the poorer prognosis for patients with proximal tumors seen in their analyses.

Residual Disease: R Status

The *R status,* which was first described by Hermanek and Wittekind in 1994, is commonly used to describe the tumor status in a patient following resection and is designated following pathological evaluation of the resection margins (Table 9.2). R0 indicates that microscopic margins are free of tumor and that no gross or

Table 9.2. Current description of completeness of resection based on presence or absence of residual disease following resection and pathological evaluation of resection margins

Description	Gross or Pathological Extent of Residual Disease
R0	No residual gross disease and negative microscopic margins
R1	Microscopic residual disease only
R2	Gross residual disease

microscopic disease remains. R1 indicates that all gross disease has been extirpated but that microscopic margins are positive for tumor. R2 indicates that gross residual disease remains. Long-term survival can be expected only in patients who undergo an R0 resection for gastric adenocarcinoma, and significant effort is therefore made to avoid R1 or R2 resections.

Japanese R System

The R status described in the previous section should not be confused with an older Japanese classification of gastric resection that also included an R status. This R status has now been replaced with a D status and is mentioned here for informational purposes only because it has not been used after 1992.

Japanese Classification: Extent of Resection

The extent of pathological lymph node involvement relative to the scope of the lymphadenectomy performed is the distinguishing characteristic of the Japanese classification scheme, which is based on the assumption that extended lymph node clearance beyond the level of pathological involvement may prolong survival. In yet another Japanese system (Table 9.3), the completeness of nodal dissection is designated D1 (removal of all nodal tissue within 3 cm of the primary tumor), D2 (D1 plus clearance of hepatic, splenic, celiac, and left gastric nodes), or D3 (total gastrectomy, omentectomy, splenectomy, distal pancreatectomy, and celiac and portal lymphadenectomy). Although these classifications are not part of the AJCC staging system, the D terminology

Table 9.3. "D" Nomenclature: extent of surgical resection and lymphadenectomy

Description	Regions Included in Resection
D1	Removal of all nodal tissue within 3 cm of the primary tumor
D2	D1 plus clearance of hepatic, splenic, celiac, and left gastric lymph nodes
D3	D2 plus omentectomy, splenectomy, distal pancreatomy, and clearance of porta hepatis lymph nodes and para-aortic lymph nodes

is important in comparing the results of surgical therapy, as is discussed later in the chapter.

SURGICAL TREATMENT

As long as there is no documented metastatic disease, the surgical resection of gastric tumors is the mainstay of treatment. We recommend a wide macroscopically negative margin of 5 to 6 cm, along with the en bloc resection of lymph nodes and adherent surrounding organs. D2 lymphadenectomy, sparing the spleen and distal pancreas, is employed if it can be done with low morbidity and mortality. The appropriate surgical procedure for a given patient must take into account the location of the lesion and the known pattern of spread.

Proximal Tumors

Proximal tumors account for about 50% of all gastric carcinomas. These tumors are usually advanced at presentation and are associated with a poorer long-term prognosis than are distal cancers. There are three types of gastroesophageal junction tumors according to the Siewert classification: Type I are associated with Barrett esophagus or true esophageal cancer growing into the gastroesophageal junction, type II cancers are true junctional tumors that lie within 2 cm of the squamocolumnar junction, and type III cancers are present within the subcardial region of the stomach. The optimal surgical management of type II and III cancers is controversial. The options include total gastrectomy and proximal subtotal gastrectomy. Because of the advanced stage of most tumors of the cardia at diagnosis, some authors argue that any operation is realistically only a palliative procedure and that, therefore, one should always perform the simpler proximal subtotal gastrectomy, especially because total gastrectomy does not improve prognosis for patients with stage III and IV disease. However, some studies have shown a poorer quality of life in patients who undergo a proximal subtotal gastrectomy than in patients who undergo a total gastrectomy.

At M. D. Anderson, we usually perform a total gastrectomy with a Roux-en-Y reconstruction and regional lymphadenectomy for proximal gastric lesions. This procedure has the advantage of avoiding the alkaline reflux esophagitis often associated with proximal subtotal gastrectomy. Furthermore, lymph nodes along the lesser curvature, a common site of spread, are easily removed during a total gastrectomy. There is also no greater mortality or morbidity in patients who undergo total gastrectomy compared with those who undergo a proximal subtotal gastrectomy.

Midbody Tumors

Midstomach tumors account for 15% to 30% of all gastric cancers. For the same reasons as those given for our approach to the treatment of proximal tumors, we recommend total gastrectomy with regional lymphadenectomy if the node dissection can be done with low morbidity.

Distal Tumors

Distal tumors account for approximately 35% of all gastric cancers. The standard operation for these lesions is a distal subtotal gastrectomy with appropriate lymphadenectomy. Subtotal gastrectomy entails resection of approximately three-fourths of the stomach, including the majority of the lesser curvature. This procedure is performed for two reasons. First, randomized prospective trials demonstrated no survival benefit to total gastrectomy over subtotal gastrectomy. Second, the quality of life is better in those who have subtotal gastrectomy than in those who have total gastrectomy.

Because studies have shown that microscopic invasion beyond 6 cm from the gross tumor is rare, we therefore recommend a 5- to 6-cm luminal resection margin when possible. Even if this distance is achieved, however, the surgical margins should be evaluated by frozen-section preparations.

Splenectomy

Splenectomy is not performed unless the tumor adheres to or invades the spleen or its vascular supply. Routine splenectomy does not improve survival but does increase the morbidity and mortality associated with gastrectomy in western patients. If a splenectomy is anticipated preoperatively because of tumor adherence shown by CT, we give pneumococcal polysaccharide, meningococcal, and *Haemophilus* influenza vaccines before surgery. There is a large ongoing trial in Japan that is specifically examining the role of splenectomy in the treatment of patients with gastric adenocarcinomas.

Lymphadenectomy

Despite prospective randomized trials, controversy still exists about the role of extended lymphadenectomy in the treatment of gastric cancer. Radical lymphadenectomy was adopted based on an initial report published in 1981 by Kodama et al. that described a survival benefit for patients with serosal or regional lymph node involvement who underwent a D2 or D3 lymphadenectomy (R2 or R3 in the old Japanese nomenclature). Specifically, the 5-year survival rate in patients who underwent a radical lymphadenectomy was 39% as opposed to only 18% in patients who underwent D1 lymphadenectomy. Many other nonrandomized studies from Japan have shown a similarly significant survival benefit in patients undergoing radical lymphadenectomy. Unfortunately, Western studies have not been able to reproduce the Japanese results.

The reported differences in survival seen in Japanese and Western studies may have multiple reasons. One potential reason is that most Japanese patients present with early-stage disease, which makes overall survival appear better. However, stage for stage, the differences are not quite so dramatic. Furthermore, the Japanese approach to nodal dissection and pathological analysis is much more meticulous than the approach used in the West, and there is likely to be an element of stage migration. It is not very common for nodes distant from the stomach to be evaluated in the United States. Also, proximal tumors, which behave more aggressively, are less common in Japan than in the West. Finally, the more aggressive surgery performed in Japan may confer a small increase in survival rates.

In 1996, Wanebo et al. reviewed the outcomes in 18,346 patients with gastric cancer whose records had been gathered in a database that included information from 200 tumor registries in the United States. Compared with patients undergoing D1 dissection, patients undergoing D2 nodal dissection (including lymph nodes ≥3 cm from the primary tumor) (Table 9.3) had no increase in the median survival time (D2, 19.7 months; D1, 24.8 months) or in the 5-year survival rate (D2, 26.3%; D1, 30%). In 1987, Shiu et al. retrospectively reviewed 210 patients with gastric cancer treated at Memorial Sloan-Kettering Cancer Center and found that a lymphadenectomy that did not include lymph nodes at least one echelon beyond the histologically involved nodes was predictive of a poor prognosis. This study also showed that there was not a significant difference in the morbidity associated with D1 and D2 lymphadenectomies.

Thus far, five randomized trials evaluating the extent of lymphadenectomy for gastric cancer have been conducted. Three trials compared D1 versus D2 lymphadenectomy. Two trials compared D3 versus D2 or D1 lymphadenectomy.

To compare the morbidity and outcome in patients who underwent D1 and D2 lymphadenectomy, Dent et al., from South Africa, randomized 43 patients into each arm. Those who underwent D2 dissection had a higher morbidity rate (D1, 15%; D2, 30%; $P = 0.06$), longer hospital stay (D1, 4.2 days; D2, 9.2 days; $P < 0.008$), and longer operative time (D1, 1.8 hours; D2, 2.5 hours; $P < 0.001$). However, the 5-year survival rate was similar in both groups (D1, 69%; D2, 67%). In 2004, Bonenkamp et al. reported on a study conducted in the Netherlands in which 711 patients were prospectively randomized to undergo D1 or D2 lymphadenectomy. Patients undergoing the more extended lymphadenectomy (D2) had a significantly higher operative morbidity rate (D2, 43%; D1, 25%; $P < 0.001$) and significantly higher mortality rate (D2, 10%; D1, 4%; $P = 0.004$). The 5-year relapse rates (D1, 43%; D2, 37%) and 5-year survival rates (D1, 45%; D2, 47%) were similar, however. Similar results were obtained in the Medical Research Council trial reported in the United Kingdom by Cuschieri et al. in 1999. In this study, 400 patients with gastric adenocarcinoma were prospectively randomized, as in the Dutch trial, to undergo D1 or D2 lymphadenectomy. Similarly, there was no difference in the overall 5-year survival rate between the two groups (D1, 35%; D2, 33%). In this study, as in the Dutch trial, pancreaticosplenectomy performed as part of the D2 resection resulted in increased postoperative morbidity and mortality. These data therefore do not support the routine performance of D2 lymphadenectomy in patients with gastric adenocarcinoma, particularly if pancreaticosplenectomy is necessary to effect the dissection.

In a comparison of D1 and D3 lymphadenectomy, Robertson et al., from Hong Kong, randomized 54 patients to undergo either D1 lymphadenectomy with subtotal gastrectomy or D3 lymphadenectomy with total gastrectomy. In addition to poorer survival in the D3 group, the hospital stay and blood loss were greater in the patients in the D3 group than in the D1 group.

In 2004, the Japanese Cooperative Oncology Group (JCOG 9501) reported the findings from a prospective randomized trial evaluating R0 gastrectomy with D2 lymphadenectomy versus

D2 plus para-aortic lymphadenectomy. In this multicenter trial, surgeons experienced in performing extended lymphadenectomy operated on more than 500 patients. In addition to the preoperative staging, age younger than 75 years and negative peritoneal lavage cytology findings were some of the inclusion criteria. There were two deaths in each arm, accounting for a remarkably low hospital mortality of 0.8%. Although the morbidity rate in patients who underwent the D2 plus para-aortic lymphadenectomy (28.1%) was higher than that in the patients who underwent the D2 lymphadenectomy (20.9%), the difference did not reach statistical significance. Patients who underwent the D2 plus para-aortic lymphadenectomy also had longer operations ($P < 0.001$) with increased blood loss ($P < 0.001$), and hence higher blood transfusion requirements ($P < 0.001$), than did those who had only a D2 lymphadenectomy. The survival results of this trial are expected in 2006.

At M. D. Anderson, spleen-sparing D2 lymphadenectomy is standard. Analysis of patients who underwent curative resection after neoadjuvant therapy at M. D. Anderson between 1991 and 1998 showed a perioperative mortality rate of 2%. Current standard recommendations include a D1 dissection (perigastric lymphadenectomy), although major centers continue to study the potential benefit and morbidity associated with more extended nodal dissections in the setting of low operative mortality.

SURGICAL TECHNIQUE

Total Gastrectomy

For a total gastrectomy, the dissection is begun by separating the omentum from the mesocolon. The right gastroepiploic vessels are ligated at their origin, and the subpyloric nodes are resected with the specimen. The first portion of the duodenum is mobilized and divided 2 cm distal to the pylorus. The gastrohepatic ligament is opened, and the left gastric artery is ligated at its origin. It is important to remember that an aberrant or accessory left hepatic artery may originate from the left gastric artery and reside in the gastrohepatic ligament. If an extended lymphadenectomy is done, the celiac, hepatic artery, and splenic artery nodes are cleared of nodal tissue and removed along with the specimen. The short gastric vessels are ligated sequentially up to the gastroesophageal junction. Dissection around the gastroesophageal junction can free up 7 to 8 cm of distal esophagus, which facilitates transection of the esophagus with an adequate proximal margin. Stay sutures of 2-0 silk are placed, and after the esophagus is divided, the resection margins are evaluated by frozen-section examination. If the tumor adheres to the spleen, pancreas, liver, diaphragm, colon, or mesocolon, the involved organ or organs are removed en bloc.

There are many types of reconstructions, but the one most frequently used is a Roux-en-Y anastomosis. If a significant portion of the distal esophagus is resected, a left thoracoabdominal or right thoracotomy (Ivor-Lewis approach) may be used. Although some studies have shown that reconstruction with pouches and loops to act as reservoirs are beneficial, the data are far from conclusive. The one more advanced reconstruction, which makes physiological sense and has data supporting the benefit of the procedure, is jejunal interposition between the esophagus and the duodenum. In this reconstruction, care is taken to ensure the interposition limb is at least 45 cm long. A feeding jejunostomy tube is placed for postoperative nutritional support.

Subtotal Gastrectomy

The mobilization for subtotal gastrectomy is identical to that for total gastrectomy described in the preceding section, except that only approximately 80% of the distal stomach is resected. The dissection of the distal short gastric vessels is performed first to ensure splenic preservation. The small remnant of stomach that is left is supplied by the remaining short gastric vessels and the posterior gastric artery arising from the splenic artery. We often use Roux-en-Y reconstruction after subtotal gastrectomy, although a loop gastrojejunostomy (Billroth II) is also acceptable. Other recommendations include a Billroth I.

Figure 9.1 shows the M. D. Anderson treatment algorithm for potentially resectable gastric carcinoma.

COMPLICATIONS OF SURGERY

Complications of gastric resection and their relative incidences are given in Table 9.4. The most devastating complication is an anastomotic leak, which occurs in 3% to 21% of patients. Because leaks can occur late, an intact anastomosis early in the postoperative period is not a guarantee of an uncomplicated course. Oral feeding is begun 5 to 7 days postoperatively if the patient is asymptomatic. Upper gastrointestinal tract contrast studies are performed on the basis of clinical indications only (e.g., fever, tachycardia, tachypnea). Because the food reservoir is gone, many patients must initially change their eating habits such that they consume six small meals per day, otherwise called a "postgastrectomy diet." Alternatively, they may eat regular meals plus snacks. Supplemental jejunostomy feedings are started the same day or the day after surgery and continued until oral intake is adequate. Within several months, most patients are able to increase their intestinal capacity and eat larger meals less frequently (three or four meals per day).

Less than 10% of patients will develop clinically significant dumping syndrome. Early dumping typically occurs 15 to 30 minutes after a meal and includes diaphoresis, abdominal cramps, palpitations, and watery diarrhea. Late dumping is usually associated with hypoglycemia and hyperinsulinemia. The medical management for dumping symptoms should include dietary modification (fiber diet and avoidance of hyperosmolar liquids) and, if refractory, a somatostatin analog.

Figure 9.1. The University of Texas M. D. Anderson Cancer Center algorithm for the evaluation and treatment of potentially resectable gastric adenocarcinoma. *Occasionally, metastatic disease is found at the time of open surgical exploration for tumors believed to be resectable on the basis of radiologic and laparoscopic staging. In this situation, the decision to perform palliative resection is made on an individualized basis. Patients with metastatic disease have a dismal prognosis (see text).

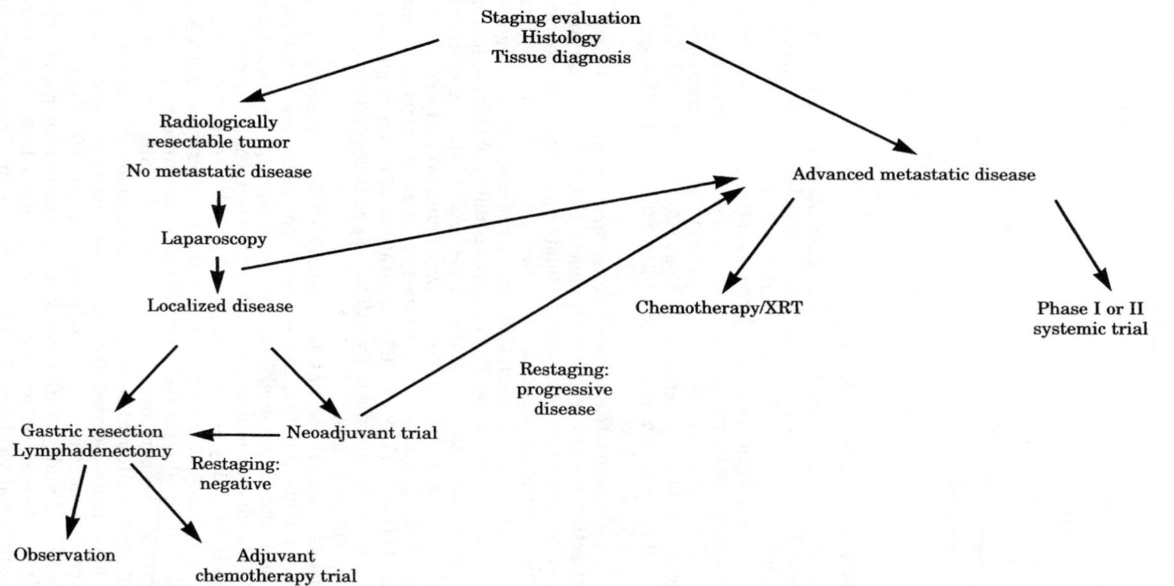
Staging evaluation
Histology
Tissue diagnosis
Radiologically
resectable tumor
No metastatic disease
Laparoscopy
Localized disease
Gastric resection
Lymphadenectomy
Neoadjuvant trial
Restaging:
negative
Observation
Adjuvant
chemotherapy trial
Restaging:
progressive
disease
Advanced metastatic disease
Chemotherapy/XRT
Phase I or II
systemic trial

Table 9.4. Complications of gastric resection

Complication	Percentage of Patients Affected
Pulmonary	3–55
Infectious	3–22
Anastomotic	3–21
Cardiac	1–10
Renal	1–8
Bleeding	0.3–5
Pulmonary embolus	1–4

OUTCOMES OF SURGERY

The overall 5-year survival rate in patients with gastric cancer in most Western series is 10% to 21%, which is a consequence of the high proportion of tumors that are at an advanced stage at presentation. Patients who undergo potentially curative resection have a slightly better prognosis (5-year survival rate of 24%–57%). The 5-year survival rate in patients who undergo curative resection in Japan is reported to be at least 50%. Overall 5-year survival rates in Japan and the United States by TNM stage are listed in Table 9.5.

To determine gastric cancer disease-specific survival following R0 resection, researchers from Memorial Sloan-Kettering Cancer Center developed an internally validated prognostic nomogram. In this nomogram, variables included age, gender, tumor location, Lauren classification, size, number of positive and negative lymph nodes, and depth. The predictive ability of this nomogram was compared with that of the current AJCC staging system in 1,039 patients, and the nomogram was found to be superior in predicting both 5- and 9-year disease-specific survival (concordance index 0.80 vs. 0.77; $P < 0.001$). Limitations of this nomogram are that it needs to be externally validated and it depends on several postoperative factors.

Disease recurrence has been analyzed in autopsy, reoperative, and clinical series. Some component of disease recurrence can be found in up to 80% of patients following gastrectomy. In 1982, Gunderson and Sosin analyzed patterns of recurrence in a prospective study of 109 patients who underwent gastric resection and subsequent reoperation at the University of Minnesota. Of the 107 evaluable patients, 86 (80%) had recurrent disease. Locoregional recurrence alone arose in 22 (25.6%) of these 86 patients, but peritoneal seeding was a component of recurrence in 54% of patients. Isolated distant metastases were uncommon but occurred as some component of recurrence in 29% of patients.

In 1990, Landry et al. from Massachusetts General Hospital analyzed disease recurrence in 130 patients treated by resection with curative intent. The overall locoregional recurrence rate was 38% (49/130); 21 patients (16%) had locoregional recurrence alone, 28 patients (22%) had locoregional recurrence and distant metastasis, and 39 patients (30%) had distant metastasis

Table 9.5. Five-year survival rates after gastrectomy with complete resection and >15 lymph nodes examined

	5-Year Survival Rate (%)			
	United States[a]			
AJCC Stage	All ($n = 32{,}532$)	Japanese Americans ($n = 697$)	Japan[b] ($n = 587$)	Germany[c] ($n = 1{,}017$)
IA	78	95	95	86
IB	58	75	86	72
II	34	46	71	47
IIIA	20	48	59	34
IIIB	8	18	35	25
IV	7	5	17	16
Overall	28	42	NR	NR

AJCC, American Joint Committee on Cancer; *n*, number of patients; NR, not reported.

[a]Data from Hundahl SA, Phillips JL, Menck HR. The National Cancer Data Base Report on poor survival of U.S. gastric carcinoma patients treated with gastrectomy: fifth edition American Joint Committee on Cancer staging, proximal disease, and the "different disease" hypothesis. *Cancer* 2000;88:921–932.

[b]Data from Ichikura T, Tomimatsu S, Uefuji K, et al. Evaluation of the New American Joint Committee on Cancer/International Union against cancer classification of lymph node metastasis from gastric carcinoma in comparison with the Japanese classification. *Cancer* 1999;86:553–558.

[c]Data from Roder JO, Bottcher K, Busch R, et al. Classification of regional lymph node metastasis from gastric carcinoma. German Gastric Cancer Study Group. *Cancer* 1998;82:621–631.

alone. However, when viewed only in terms of the patients in whom treatment failed, locoregional recurrence developed in 57% (49/88). The risk of locoregional recurrence increased with the degree of tumor penetration through the gastric wall. The most frequent sites of locoregional recurrence were the gastric remnant at the anastomosis, the gastric bed, and the regional nodes. The overall incidence of distant metastasis was 52% (67 patients), and the incidence of distant metastasis increased with advancing stage of disease. The overall recurrence rate was 68% (88 patients).

In 2004, D'Angelica reported the patterns of recurrence in 1,172 patients who underwent R0 resection at Memorial Sloan-Kettering Cancer Center. At a median follow-up of 22 months, various types of tumor recurrence had developed in 42.3% of the 1,172 patients. In this analysis, disease recurred in 79% of patients with recurrence within the first 2 years of treatment. Locoregional recurrence was the most frequent (54%), followed by distant (51%) and peritoneal (29%) recurrence. On multivariate analysis, factors predictive of locoregional recurrence were male gender and proximal lesions. The median time to death from the time of recurrence was 6 months. Interestingly, the nodal status and the extent of lymphadenectomy were not associated with locoregional recurrence. Although this analysis identified the recurrence pattern and predictors of recurrence, this retrospective study had some limitations. First, 26% of patients with recurrence did not have a recurrence pattern documented. Second, postoperative follow-up and adjuvant treatments were not consistent. The effect of adjuvant therapy on recurrence was also not evaluated.

EARLY GASTRIC CANCER

In the early 1960s, the Japanese defined early gastric cancer as carcinoma limited to the mucosa and submucosa, regardless of whether there were lymph node metastasis. This pathological classification was based on the high cure rate in this group of patients. In the United States, the proportion of patients with early gastric cancer at diagnosis has increased since the mid-1980s to approximately 10% to 15%. In Japan, aggressive screening has resulted in early gastric cancer being diagnosed in greater than 50% of Japanese patients with gastric cancer. Not surprisingly, therefore, the mean age of patients at diagnosis is 63 years in Western studies, whereas it is 55 years in Japanese studies. Most patients with early gastric cancer present with gastrointestinal symptoms similar to those of peptic ulcer disease, including epigastric pain and dyspepsia or even no symptoms.

Endoscopy is critical for the diagnosis of early gastric cancer. For example, in collected Western series, although only 22% of early gastric cancers were diagnosed with an upper gastrointestinal tract barium study, 80% were diagnosed with endoscopy. The Japanese have classified early gastric cancer pathologically on the basis of gross endoscopic appearance into three basic morphologic types: type I, protruded or polypoid; type II, superficial (IIa, elevated; Iib, flat; IIc, depressed); and type III, excavated or ulcerated. Early gastric cancers include all TNM T1 tumors.

Despite a high potential cure rate, up to 10% to 15% of early gastric tumors may be associated with positive lymph nodes. Therefore, although gastrectomy with D1 or D2 lymphadenectomy generally remains the treatment of choice in Japan, specific criteria have been developed for identifying patients who require only endoscopic mucosal resection. Recognition that tumor size (mucosal area), differentiation, lymphovascular invasion, and submucosal invasion are significant predictors of nodal metastases in patients with T1 tumors has also provided the means of identifying select patients with early tumors who require less aggressive treatment. In 1994, Takekoshi reported the findings from an analysis of cases of early gastric cancer from 104 centers in Japan. In particular, analysis of the endoscopic appearance (previously described) of early tumors in patients who underwent mucosal resection enabled the formulation of specific criteria for the mucosal resection of early gastric cancers without submucosal invasion. Subsequent analyses have led to refinements in the criteria that must be met to ensure the safe endoscopic mucosal resection of AJCC T1 gastric cancers. These criteria include only the following: (a) well- or moderately differentiated endoscopic type I or Iia tumor that is less than 2 cm in area, or (b) well- or moderately differentiated endoscopic type Iic tumor, without an ulcer scar, that is less than 1 cm in area. The incidence of nodal metastases in patients identified by these criteria was 0.01%. Although close endoscopic follow-up is necessary in patients who undergo this localized treatment, the cure rate has exceeded 90%. Conventional gastrectomy with at least a D1 lymphadenectomy is mandated if submucosal invasion is found on permanent serial sectioning in a patient after an endoscopic mucosal resection.

ADJUVANT THERAPY

Some form of recurrence develops in most patients who undergo a potentially curative resection for gastric cancer. However, although adjuvant therapy is needed in these patients, results have generally been inconsistent. Only recently has a survival benefit of adjuvant therapy been convincingly demonstrated. Unfortunately, poor tolerance of postoperative treatment is an obstacle that can frequently hamper the effectiveness of the treatment.

Postoperative Chemotherapy

Randomized trials investigating the effects of adjuvant chemotherapy alone on survival after complete resection of gastric adenocarcinoma have produced inconsistent results. Meta-analyses performed to resolve this issue have also yielded inconsistent findings regarding the impact of postoperative chemotherapy in gastric cancer. For example, in 2002, Janunger conducted a meta-analysis of 21 randomized studies of adjuvant systemic chemotherapy and found survival duration was significantly better in those who received postoperative chemotherapy than in controls (odds ratio [OR] 0.84, 95% confidence interval [CI] 0.74–0.96). However, when the data from Asian and Western studies were analyzed separately, no survival benefits were seen for the Western patients treated with chemotherapy (OR 0.96; 95% CI 0.83–1.12). Given the flaws in the conduct of some of the randomized trials, the authors noted that the results of their meta-analysis should be interpreted with caution when it came to recommending postoperative chemotherapy in patients with gastric cancer. Likewise, Mari et al. noted in their 2000 meta-analysis of 20 randomized trials that adjuvant chemotherapy was associated with a survival benefit (hazard ratio 0.82, 95% CI 0.75–0.89, $P < 0.001$). However, these authors were also reluctant to recommend adjuvant chemotherapy in patients with gastric cancer because of the inconsistencies in the findings from meta-analyses.

Postoperative External-beam Radiation Therapy

Most studies of radiation therapy for gastric cancer have examined radiation therapy as an adjuvant to surgery or combined with sensitizing chemotherapy (usually 5-fluorouracil [5-FU]).

Studies from the Mayo Clinic in the 1960s of low-dose bolus 5-FU with 40 Gy external-beam radiation therapy versus radiation therapy alone showed that combination therapy improved survival. The improvement in survival was attributed to a radiation-sensitizing effect of the chemotherapy because the 5-FU dose was relatively low.

Two randomized studies have examined patients assigned to receive no additional therapy or radiation therapy with concurrent 5-FU after complete tumor resection. In their 1979 study of 142 patients, Dent et al. found no benefit from this combined regimen, although the findings may have been influenced by the fact that some patients may have had an incomplete resection and the radiation therapy dose was only 20 Gy. In a second study in 1984, Moertel et al. found a benefit to chemotherapy plus radiation therapy, but the study results may have been skewed because ten patients who were randomized to the experimental arm refused treatment. Nonetheless, interest was generated by this study because the 5-year survival rate was slightly higher and the local recurrence rate was lower in the adjuvant therapy group than in the surgery-only group.

Many investigators believe that the standard of care for patients with resectable gastric cancer has changed in the past 5 years on the basis of the national intergroup trial (INT-0116) initiated by the Southwest Oncology Group that evaluated two cycles of 5-FU and leucovorin followed by radiation therapy with concurrent chemotherapy following R0 resection of gastric adenocarcinoma (MacDonald et al., 2001). More than 600 patients were randomized; of these, 556 were evaluable and were randomly assigned to curative resection (n = 275 patients) or curative resection with chemoradiation therapy (n = 281 patients) consisting of 45 Gy external-beam radiation therapy delivered concurrently with 5-FU and leucovorin. The first cycle used the Mayo Clinic regimen (425 mg/m^2 5-FU and 20 mg/m^2 leucovorin) for 4 consecutive days, followed by concurrent chemoradiation therapy, with chemotherapy doses decreased at this point and near the end of radiation therapy. One month after the completion of radiation therapy, two additional cycles of 5-FU and leucovorin were given. Three deaths were attributed to the adjuvant therapy (1%), and morbidity was acceptable; however, only 65% of the patients were able to complete the adjuvant treatment. Nonetheless, adjuvant therapy produced a significant improvement in the disease-free and overall 3-year survival rates. The median survival in the surgery-only group was 27 months, compared with 36 months in the chemoradiation therapy group; the 3-year survival rates were 41% and 52%, respectively. Concerns have been voiced regarding the surgery performed and the high percentage of D0 lymphadenectomies, with some investigators arguing that the principal benefit of this regimen is that it makes up for suboptimal surgery. Although 54% of patients had what was described as less than a D1 lymphadenectomy, this trial did not demonstrate any difference in overall or relapse-free survival among the three node dissection groups ($P = 0.80$).

Intraoperative Radiation Therapy

Most of the data available on intraoperative radiation therapy (IORT) for gastric cancer comes from the 1981 report of Abe and Takahashi from Japan. In a prospective nonrandomized trial, these authors compared 110 patients treated with surgery alone with 84 patients treated with surgery plus IORT. The 5-year survival rates were similar in patients with stage I disease; however, a suggestion of a survival benefit from IORT was seen in patients with stage II, III, or IV disease. In contrast, a small (<40 patients) randomized study of IORT done at the National Cancer Institute showed neither a disease-free nor an overall survival benefit from IORT, despite a marked decrease in the frequency of locoregional recurrence. Other studies of IORT have generally examined it in combination with other therapies (see the next section).

Neoadjuvant Therapy

The use of neoadjuvant chemotherapy in the treatment of gastric cancer evolved from preoperative treatment strategies used for esophageal and rectal cancers. Wilke et al. also sparked interest in this treatment as a result of their findings in patients with locally advanced gastric cancer (deemed unresectable either clinically or intraoperatively) who underwent R0 resection after receiving systemic preoperative chemotherapy. There are several potential advantages of neoadjuvant chemotherapy for gastric cancer (Ajani, 1998; Minsky, 1996). These include theoretical biological advantages (decreased tumor seeding at surgery), and the potential opportunity to assess tumor sensitivity to a chemotherapeutic regimen. That is, if the tumor responds to the neoadjuvant therapy, the same treatment can be continued postoperatively. Another theoretical advantage is an improved R0 resection rate. An advantage to preoperative radiation therapy is smaller treatment volume and displacement of contiguous structures by the intact tumor leading to reduced radiation therapy toxicity. Finally, the interval required for neoadjuvant therapy provides a time in which to evaluate for progression of disease, thus improving patient selection for resection. A potential disadvantage of neoadjuvant treatment is that there is a risk of overtreating patients with early-stage disease, although improved pretreatment staging with EUS minimizes this risk.

The combination of etoposide, cisplatin, and either 5-FU (ECF) or doxorubicin as neoadjuvant treatment has been evaluated in several trials. Clinical response rates have ranged from 21% to 31%, and complete pathological response rates have ranged from 0% to 15%. Multivariate analysis of the three phase II trials of neoadjuvant therapy at M. D. Anderson (Lowy et al., 1999) revealed that the response to neoadjuvant chemotherapy was the single most important predictor of overall survival after such treatment for gastric cancer.

Several important lessons have been learned from phase II trials regarding the role of neoadjuvant chemotherapy; the most important one has been that the treatment-related toxicities are acceptable. Furthermore, as previously mentioned, the outcome in those who respond to preoperative treatment is better than that in nonresponders.

In 2005, survival results of the UK Medical Research Council Adjuvant Gastric Infusion Chemotherapy (MAGIC) trial were presented at the American Society of Clinical Oncology annual meeting. In this multi-institutional, prospective randomized trial, 503 patients with stage II or higher gastric cancer were randomized to receive preoperative chemotherapy followed by surgery or to undergo surgery alone. Those randomized to the preoperative treatment arm received three cycles of ECF, followed by surgery and then three cycles of ECF. Only 42% of patients completed their postoperative regimen. Both progression-free survival and overall survival were improved in the treatment arm ($P < 0.001$ and $P = 0.009$ respectively). The 5-year survival rate was 36% in the treatment plus surgery group and 23% in the surgery-only group. Despite these promising results, the MAGIC trial is not without some criticism. First, the trial included patients with distal esophageal cancers, which may affect the results of the trial. Second, the staging in this trial may have been suboptimal due to lack of EUS or staging laparoscopy.

The approach to adjuvant therapy for gastric adenocarcinoma at M. D. Anderson has been largely to deliver the therapy preoperatively. Multimodality neoadjuvant therapy combining chemotherapy with external-beam radiation therapy is continuing to be studied. These studies are best exemplified by a pilot study of preoperative chemoradiation therapy with IORT for resectable gastric cancer done at M. D. Anderson (Lowy et al., 2001) in which 24 patients were treated with 45 Gy external-beam radiation therapy and concurrent infusional 5-FU (300 mg/m^2). Patients were restaged 4 to 6 weeks after completing treatment and, if free of disease, underwent resection and IORT (10 Gy). Several findings were of significant interest. Twenty-three (96%) of the 24 patients completed chemoradiation therapy, a rate significantly higher than that in trials of postoperative adjuvant therapy. Four patients had progression of disease and did not undergo resection; the remaining 19 patients underwent resection with D2 lymphadenectomy and IORT. The morbidity and mortality rates were acceptable (32% and one death; respectively). Of the patients who underwent resection, two (11%) had complete pathological responses, and 12 (63%) had significant pathological evidence of a treatment effect.

In 2004, Ajani et al. demonstrated that a pathological complete response (30%) can be achieved through a three-step approach in patients with localized gastric adenocarcinoma. In this trial, 28 of 34 patients received induction chemotherapy (5-FU [200 mg/m^2/d], leucovorin [20 mg/m^2], and cisplatin [20 mg/m^2/d]), followed by chemoradiation therapy (45 Gy plus concurrent 5-FU) and gastrectomy. R0 resection was achieved in 70% of patients, and a complete pathological response was noted in 30%. At a median follow-up of 50 months, the median survival was 33.7 months, and 2-year survival rate was 54%. There were two treatment-related deaths. This multi-institutional trial thus also demonstrated that a pathological response to treatment is associated with a significant survival benefit.

To discern whether it is the pathological response to preoperative chemotherapy, and not pretreatment parameters, that determine a patient's outcome, in 2005, Ajani et al. reported a prospective nonrandomized study of preoperative paclitaxel-based chemoradiation therapy. In this analysis, 43 patients received two cycles of 5-FU, cisplatin, and paclitaxel for 28 days, followed by chemoradiation therapy. The radiation regimen included 25 fractions of 1.8 Gy up to a total dose of 45 Gy. Then, patients underwent gastrectomy with spleen-preserving D2 lymphadenectomy after radiographic and endoscopic restaging. At the time of analysis, 78% of patients had undergone an R0 resection, 20% had had a complete pathological response, and 15% had had a partial pathological response. In this study, R0 resection ($P < 0.001$), pathological complete response ($P = 0.02$), pathological partial response ($P = 0.006$), and postsurgical T and N status ($P = 0.01$ and $P < 0.001$, respectively) were factors associated with overall survival. Although the authors acknowledged the importance of pretreatment parameters in the staging of gastric cancer, pathological response was a major determinant of outcome.

In summary, current trials of neoadjuvant chemoradiation therapy are yielding promising results; however, these results need to be validated in the setting of large, prospective randomized trials.

MANAGEMENT OF ADVANCED DISEASE

Many patients (20%–30%) present with stage IV disease, and an additional 28% to 37% initially believed to have localized disease are found to have metastatic disease after complete staging. The 5-year survival rate for patients with stage IV disease approaches zero—hence, a large percentage of newly diagnosed gastric cancer patients are incurable. Because of this overall low cure rate for gastric cancer and the advanced disease stage at presentation in many patients, palliation is an essential component of gastric cancer management. An appropriate understanding and use of palliative techniques is therefore essential.

Optimal palliation relieves or abates symptoms, while causing minimal morbidity and improving the patient's quality of life. Prolonged survival is generally not a goal of palliative treatment, but palliation may relieve debilitating and potentially life-threatening problems, such as gastrointestinal bleeding or gastric outlet obstruction, which may diminish survival.

Palliative Surgery

Surgical palliation of advanced gastric cancer may include resection or bypass alone or in combination with other interventions. Complete staging is required for determination of the best palliative approach.

Palliation by endoscopic means may be appropriate for patients with peritoneal disease, hepatic metastases, extensive nodal metastases, or ascites and for patients with problems that include bleeding or proximal or distal gastric obstruction. Both morbidity and mortality are relatively high in these patients with a short life expectancy. Laser recanalization or simple dilatation with or without stent placement can be used to treat obstruction. Repeat endoscopy may be required at periodic intervals. Patients who undergo stent placement for gastric outlet obstruction are frequently able to eat solid or semisolid food and may not require any further intervention before death.

The selection of patients for palliative resection is complex. In patients with an excellent performance status, experienced surgeons can perform palliative distal gastrectomy with minimal morbidity and acceptable mortality rates. Palliative total gastrectomy and esophagogastrectomy, however, should be approached with greater caution because the morbidity from these procedures is higher. Surgery achieves good palliation less than 50% of the time. In 2004, Minor retrospectively reviewed patients who underwent R1 or R2 resections and divided them into palliative (R1/R2) resections and nonpalliative resections (R1/R2). They reported a perioperative mortality rate of 7% associated with palliative resections versus 4% associated with nonpalliative resections; the median survival was 8.3 and 13.5 months, respectively ($P < 0.001$).

Specific indications for palliative resection, surgical bypass (open or laparoscopic), and endoscopic palliation remain undefined. However, assessment of morbidity, mortality, and quality of life has revealed that carefully selected patients (particularly those without macroscopic metastatic disease) may benefit from palliative resection. Advanced endoscopic techniques, including laser or argon-beam tumor ablation and endoscopic placement of coated metallic stents, provide better palliation of dysphagia than surgical bypass with lower morbidity. Multimodality therapy consisting of radiotherapy, surgery, and endoscopy is likely to lead to improvements in quality of life and lower morbidity with palliative therapy. However, earlier diagnosis and advances in curative therapy are ultimately the only way in which the high incidence and morbidity associated with advanced disease in patients with gastric adenocarcinoma will be definitively reduced.

Palliative Chemotherapy

Given the minimal survival benefit from combination chemotherapy in patients with advanced gastric cancer, investigators have debated its role versus that of best supportive care. As a result, four randomized trials have been conducted to assess the impact of combination chemotherapy on survival and quality of life. The combination regimens included FAMTX (5-FU, doxorubicin, and high-dose methotrexate), FEMTX (5-FU, epirubicin, and high-dose methotrexate), and ELF (etoposide, leucovorin, and 5-FU). Patients who received combination chemotherapy had both better survival (3–9 months) and quality of life than did patients given best supportive care. Despite this, the outcome from advanced gastric cancer remains poor.

Palliative Radiation Therapy

There are several isolated case reports describing the benefit of radiation therapy for the palliative treatment of advanced gastric carcinoma. However, no large prospective trial has demonstrated a long-term benefit from radiation therapy alone in patients with advanced disease. This modality is most likely best used in combination with chemotherapy, as described previously in this chapter.

Intraperitoneal Hyperthermic Perfusion

Intraperitoneal hyperthermic perfusion has been examined in several trials as a treatment for advanced gastric cancer. For example, in 1988, Koga et al. reviewed their experience with a combination of hyperthermia and mitomycin C as adjuvant treatment for patients with peritoneal recurrence of gastric cancer. These researchers reported that this procedure was technically feasible and safe. In 1990, Fujimoto et al. evaluated 59 patients with advanced gastric cancer who underwent gastrectomy and were then randomly assigned to receive either no further therapy or intraperitoneal hyperthermic perfusion. The patients treated with perfusion survived longer than did the controls (1-year survival rate of 80% vs. 34%). A significant survival benefit was also seen in patients with peritoneal seeding who underwent perfusion with hyperthermic mitomycin C. Similarly, in 1996, Yonemura et al. reported that adjuvant hyperthermic intraperitoneal chemotherapy with mitomycin C, etoposide, and cisplatin after gastric resection in patients with peritoneal seeding resulted in complete response in 8 (19%) of 43 patients and partial responses in 9 (21%) of 43 patients. A randomized trial conducted by Yu in patients who were treated at the time of complete resection of tumors that penetrated the gastric serosa but had no evidence of peritoneal metastases showed that hyperthermic intraperitoneal chemotherapy with mitomycin C led to a reduced incidence of peritoneal recurrence and a small survival advantage at 3 years. In 2005, Yonemura et al. prospectively reviewed 107 patients with peritoneal dissemination from gastric adenocarcinomas. Over a 10-year period, 65 patients underwent cytoreductive surgery in combination with intraperitoneal hyperthermic perfusion before 1995, and 42 patients underwent cytoreductive surgery in combination with intraperitoneal hyperthermic perfusion with peritonectomy after 1995. The perfusion regimen included mitomycin C, cisplatin, and etoposide. Complete cytoreductive surgery was achieved in 43% of 107 patients. There was a 21% postoperative complication rate, and there were three postoperative deaths (all in the peritonectomy group), accounting for 7% of the patients in this group. At a median follow-up of 46 months, the 5-year survival rates in those who had complete and incomplete cytoreductive surgery were 13% and 2%, respectively ($P < 0.001$), with a median survival of 19 and 7.8 months, respectively. Furthermore, the 5-year survival rate for patients who underwent cytoreductive surgery by peritonectomy was 27% ($P < 0.001$). Multivariate analysis showed that complete cytoreductive surgery ($P = 0.010$) and peritonectomy ($P = 0.012$) were associated with a more favorable outcome. However, peritonectomy was also associated with higher postoperative morbidity (43%) and mortality (7%) rates. Other centers, however, have not found such encouraging results. This technique is currently under investigation in a few centers around the world.

In summary, there is no standard treatment for patients with peritoneal carcinomatosis stemming from gastric adenocarcinoma other than systemic chemotherapy in selected cases. Prospective randomized studies are required to clarify the role of intraperitoneal therapy in this setting.

Immunotherapy and Hormonal Therapy

Numerous investigators have examined the use of immunologic agents alone and in combination with chemotherapy as adjuvant treatment in patients with advanced gastric adenocarcinoma, but the findings have been conflicting. In 1994, Maehara et al. reported that the rates of peritoneal recurrence were significantly lower and survival times significantly longer in patients randomly assigned to receive standard chemotherapy plus intraperitoneal injections of the streptococcal preparation OK-432 than in patients who received chemotherapy alone. Similarly, data from Japan and Korea suggested that immunochemotherapy consisting of *Microbacterium*-derived polysaccharides provides a survival benefit in patients following potentially curative resection. However, more recent trials have not demonstrated any difference in survival. For example, in 2004, Sato et al. conducted a prospective randomized trial in patients with gastric adenocarcinoma who underwent either R0 resection followed by adjuvant OK-432 and 5'-deoxy-5 fluorouridine treatment ($n = 144$) or R0 resection only ($n = 143$). The 5-year survival rate in both groups was virtually the same: 63.8% and 62.9%, respectively ($P = 0.7996$). The outcome from adjuvant hormonal therapy with tamoxifen in patients with advanced gastric cancer has also been disappointing. Nevertheless, studies of immunotherapy and hormonal therapy are ongoing. The role of immunomodulators in gastric cancer remains to be defined.

SURVEILLANCE

We typically see patients every 3 months for the first 2 years following curative resection of gastric adenocarcinoma. At each follow-up, a careful history and physical examination are performed, along with laboratory studies (complete blood cell count and liver function tests). Chest radiographs are obtained every 6 months, and abdominal and pelvic CT is performed 6 months after surgery and then yearly thereafter. Endoscopy should be considered at the end of the first year in patients who have undergone subtotal gastrectomy and can then be done yearly for 4 to 5 years. Patients who receive protocol-based therapy often have more frequent staging studies, but this has never been proven to impact patient survival. Perhaps the most important reasons to follow patients closely are to enable any postgastrectomy sequelae to be dealt with and to acquire accurate recurrence and survival data on patients in clinical trials.

GASTRIC LYMPHOMA

In contrast to the decreasing incidence of gastric adenocarcinoma, the incidence of gastric lymphoma is steadily increasing, with non-Hodgkin lymphomas now the second most common malignancy of the stomach after adenocarcinoma. *H. pylori* appears to be a causative agent in the development of both gastric lymphoma and MALT lymphoma. The stomach is the most common site of lymphoma in the gastrointestinal tract, accounting for two-thirds of gastrointestinal lymphomas. The average age of patients with gastric lymphoma is 60 years. The most frequent symptoms at the time of presentation are pain (68%), weight loss (28%), bleeding (28%), and fatigue (16%). Obstruction, perforation, and massive bleeding are uncommon.

Before the advent of endoscopy, the diagnosis of gastric lymphoma was usually made at operation. Endoscopy now permits a correct tissue diagnosis to be made in approximately 80% of cases. Most lesions are located in the distal stomach and spread locally by submucosal infiltration. Once the diagnosis has been made, a careful workup—including a physical examination (with special attention to adenopathy); routine laboratory tests, along with lactate dehydrogenase and β2-microglobulin determinations; a bone marrow biopsy; chest radiograph; and CT scan of the chest, abdomen, and pelvis—should be done to fully determine the extent of disease. Pathological examination shows most cases to be B-cell non-Hodgkin lymphoma, and the diffuse histiocytic subtype is predominant. The disease is staged using the modified

Ann Arbor staging system (see Chapter 17). Histologic grade and pathological stage are two variables that independently predict survival. However, one should be familiar with the international index when caring for these patients.

Treatment for MALT lymphoma typically includes acid suppression therapy (proton pump inhibitors or H_2 blockers), metronidazole, and other antibiotics. Patients need close endoscopic surveillance to both document regression and detect relapse, as well as to determine when anti-*H. pylori* treatment should be repeated. External-beam radiation (30 Gy) and/or chemotherapy is offered to (a) those who do not respond to an antibiotic eradication regimen and (b) high-risk patients (i.e., those with lymph node involvement or t[11;18] chromosomal translocation). At present, gastric resection is rarely performed for patients with MALT lymphomas.

The treatment of gastric lymphoma varies among institutions, with some centers advocating surgery alone, although the numbers of such institutions are decreasing, and others advocating chemotherapy and radiation therapy alone. Surgery is necessary in some cases to confirm the diagnosis. Surgical resection is curative in patients with localized disease, although half of resected patients require chemotherapy. Although more accurate staging is obtained at surgery, this is not a sufficient reason to perform resection. If surgery is performed, an attempt should be made to resect the area grossly involved with lymphoma but leave grossly normal stomach intact. Negative margins are not necessary for cure. In a 1990 nonrandomized study of patients with stage I and II gastrointestinal lymphomas, Talamonti et al. noted that surgery alone produced a 5-year survival rate of 82%, whereas radiation therapy produced a 5-year survival rate of only 50%.

Many patients with gastric lymphoma who undergo initial resection also receive chemotherapy. However, some authors have found no survival benefit associated with adjuvant chemotherapy. Still other authors believe that patients can benefit from a combination of radiation therapy and chemotherapy without any need for surgery. In fact, 10-year survival rates of 80% have been seen in patients with Ann Arbor stage IE and IIE gastric lymphoma treated with chemotherapy alone.

At M. D. Anderson, patients with gastric lymphoma are initially treated with a chemotherapeutic regimen based on doxorubicin and cyclophosphamide, with a complete response documented in more than 80% of patients treated with this protocol. Patients with a high international index (indicative of aggressive disease) may be candidates for bone marrow transplant. Radiation therapy and surgery are reserved for patients who do not have a complete response to chemotherapy or who have recurrent disease.

GASTRIC CARCINOIDS

Carcinoids of the stomach, first reported in 1923, are a rare entity and distinct from other carcinoid tumors. Despite earlier reports in which gastric carcinoids were reported to constitute only 2% of carcinoid tumors, evidence from the Surveillance, Epidemiology, and End Results database is now suggesting that gastric carcinoids constitute up to 5% of all carcinoids. Contemporary data from case series are also suggesting a rising incidence of these tumors.

Gastric carcinoids arise from enterochromaffin-like cells of the fundus of the stomach. Owing to the reported relationship between proton pump inhibitors and carcinoids seen in rats, gastric carcinoids have gained wider recognition. The presenting features of gastric carcinoids are variable; however, they are commonly discovered as an incidental finding during the workup for other symptoms, when a yellow nodule is found in the fundus of the stomach.

Gastric carcinoids are classified into three types: Type I carcinoids are associated with type A chronic atrophic gastritis, type II carcinoids are associated with Zollinger-Ellison syndrome with multiple endocrine neoplasia-I (MEN-I) syndrome, and type III are sporadic gastric carcinoids. Type I carcinoids are the most common type of gastric carcinoid (65%–83%) and are found predominantly in women. These patients typically have elevated plasma gastrin levels and low gastric acid production. On macroscopic examination, the lesions are multicentric, small (<1 cm), and located in the fundus. Overall, they grow slowly and rarely metastasize to other organs. Type II gastric carcinoids are the least common type, accounting for 8% of cases with an equal gender distribution. Although type II gastric carcinoids are associated with Zollinger-Ellison syndrome in conjunction with MEN-1 syndrome, they share features with type I carcinoids, such as location in the fundus, multicentricity, elevated plasma gastrin level, and small size (<1 cm). Type III gastric carcinoids, which are sporadic carcinoids, represent 23% of cases and are found predominantly in men (80%); the mean age of patients at diagnosis is 49 years. Patients may complain of histamine-producing symptoms, such as cutaneous flushing, bronchospasm, itching, and lacrimation. Unlike the other two types of gastric carcinoids, sporadic tumors are single, solitary, often large (2–5 cm), and located in the antrum or fundus of the stomach. Furthermore, the natural course of type III gastric carcinoids is more aggressive, with hepatic metastasis found at diagnosis in up to 50% of cases.

Gastric carcinoids are diagnosed by both biochemical and histologic means. Upper gastrointestinal endoscopy, including EUS, is also essential to evaluate the number, size, extent, and location of lesions. In addition, the endoscopist should carefully look for duodenal carcinoids, especially in patients with type II gastric carcinoids associated with Zollinger-Ellison–MEN-I syndrome. Extensive gastric biopsy should be performed in those with suspected gastric carcinoids, checking for histologic chromogranin, features of dysplasia, mucosal atrophy, and the degree of mucosal invasion. It appears that the rate of diagnosis correlates with the number of biopsies performed. Furthermore, CT of the abdomen is essential to exclude metastasis to the liver and nodal involvement.

The type of gastric carcinoid dictates the nature of treatment. For patients with either type I or II carcinoids, and with tumors less than 1 cm or with fewer than three to five lesions, treatment typically consists of an endoscopic polypectomy or endoscopic mucosal resection, with endoscopic surveillance every 6 months. Endoscopic mucosal resection should be approached with caution, however, given the reports of positive margins in tumors removed by this means. Antrectomy or local excision may be performed in a young patient with an elevated gastrin level who has recurrent or multifocal disease. This treatment will decrease gastrin levels and frequently leads to the regression of other tumors. Older patients with many lesions may be followed if the lesions are small. For diffuse or recurrent disease, a completion gastrectomy may be recommended, depending on the patient's age and course of disease. In contrast, those with type III disease should be considered for en bloc resection with lymphadenectomy, depending on the tumor size, although the high incidence of hepatic metastasis should temper this decision.

The prognosis for patients with gastric carcinoids is variable and depends mainly on the type. Several studies have suggested that the 5-year survival rates for all types of gastric carcinoids are between 48% and 52%; these studies did not categorize the carcinoids according to their types, so differences in the survival rates between the types were not shown. It appears that the 5-year survival rates for patients with type I or II gastric carcinoids are between 60% and 75%, although lymph node involvement is more common in type II disease, which would likely translate into a lower rate. In contrast, the 5-year survival rate in patients with type III gastric carcinoids is less than 50%.

Follow-up in patients with gastric carcinoids primarily consists of plasma chromogranin determinations. Plasma gastrin and urinary 5-hydroxyindoleacetic acid (5-HIAA) levels may also be evaluated, although urinary 5-HIAA levels are less sensitive.

GASTRIC INTESTINAL STROMAL TUMORS OF THE STOMACH

GISTs are the most common mesenchymal tumors of the stomach, with the stomach being the most common location of these tumors in the gastrointestinal tract (40%), followed by the small intestine (32%). GISTs of the stomach are predominantly found in males, with a median age at diagnosis of 63 years. The presenting features in these patients are varied and include bleeding (38%), abdominal pain (11.8%), and rupture (1%); 12% of patients have no symptoms. The median size of GISTs of the stomach is 6 cm.

Regardless of the location of these tumors in the stomach, R0 resection remains the treatment of choice, conferring a 5-year survival of 55%. Several studies have shown that the features recommended in the NIH guidelines, tumor size (>5 cm) and mitotic index (>5/50 hpf), are associated with a less favorable outcome. In the largest retrospective analysis of GISTs of the stomach performed by Miettiten et al. in 2005, tumor location in the gastroesophageal junction or fundus, ulceration, coagulative necrosis, and mucosal invasion were found to be associated with a poor outcome ($P < 0.001$). Antral tumors, however, were found to be associated with a more favorable outcome ($P < 0.001$).

Those patients with unresectable or metastatic disease are offered treatment with Imatinib (Gleevec, an oral tyrosine kinase inhibitor). They may then be re-evaluated for potential resection if they demonstrate response to treatment. Further specific details regarding GISTs are discussed in Chapter 5.

CONCLUSION

Strides are being made in the treatment of gastric cancer. However, although several diagnostic modalities are available for staging gastric cancer and ongoing trials of neoadjuvant treatment are yielding promising results, better systemic agents and better-designed trials are still needed. Despite the current progress, the outcome in patients with gastric cancer generally remains poor. As we enter the era of targeted therapy, it is imperative that such therapy also be developed for gastric cancer and that molecular predictors are identified to help in selecting appropriate treatment for patients.

RECOMMENDED READING

Ajani JA, Baker J, Pisters PW, et al. Irinotecan plus cisplatin in advanced gastric or gastroesophageal junction carcinoma. *Oncology (Huntingt)* 2001;15:52–54.

Ajani JA, Mansfield PF, Crane CH. Paclitaxel-based chemoradiotherapy in localized gastric carcinoma: degree of pathologic response and not clinical parameters dictated patient outcome. *J Clin Oncol* 2005;23:1237–1244.

Ajani JA, Mansfield PF, Janjan J, et al. Multi-institutional trials of preoperative chemoradiotherapy in patients with potentially resectable gastric carcinoma. *J Clin Oncol* 2004;22:2274–2280.

Ajani JA, Mansfield PF, Lynch PM, et al. Enhanced staging and all chemotherapy preoperatively in patients with potentially resectable gastric carcinoma. *J Clin Oncol* 1999;17:2403–2411.

Ajani JA, Ota DM, Jessup JM, et al. Resectable gastric carcinoma. An evaluation of preoperative and postoperative chemotherapy. *Cancer* 1991;68:1501–1506.

Alexander HR, Grem JL, Pass HI, et al. Neoadjuvant chemotherapy for locally advanced gastric adenocarcinoma. *Oncology (Huntingt)* 1993;7:37–42.

Behrns KE, Dalton RR, van Heerden JA, Sarr MG. Extended lymph node dissection for gastric cancer. Is it of value? *Surg Clin North Am* 1992;72:433–443.

Bonenkamp JJ, Hermans J, Sasako M, et al. Extended lymph-node dissection for gastric cancer. Dutch Gastric Cancer Group. *N Engl J Med* 1999;340:908–914.

Bonenkamp JJ, Songun I, Hermans J, et al. Randomised comparison of morbidity after D1 and D2 dissection for gastric cancer in 996 Dutch patients. *Lancet* 1995; 345:745–748.

Bozzetti F, Bonfanti G, Bufalino R, et al. Adequacy of margins of resection in gastrectomy for cancer. *Ann Surg* 1982;196:685–690.

Bozetti F, Marubini E, Bonfanti G, et al. Total versus subtotal gastrectomy: surgical morbidity and mortality rates in multicenter Italian randomized trial. The Italian Gastrointestinal Tumor Study Group. *Ann Surg* 1997;226:613.

Brady MS, Rogatko A, Dent LL, et al. Effect of splenectomy on morbidity and survival following curative gastrectomy for carcinoma. *Arch Surg* 1991; 126:359–364.

Burke EC, Karpeh MS, Conlon KC, et al. Laparoscopy in the management of gastric adenocarcinoma. *Ann Surg* 1997;225:262–267.

Burke EC, Karpeh MS, Conlon KC, et al. Peritoneal lavage cytology in gastric cancer: an independent predictor of outcome. *Ann Surg Oncol* 1998;5:411–415.

Cady B, Rossi RL, Silverman ML, Piccione W, Heck TA. Gastric adenocarcinoma. A disease in transition. *Arch Surg* 1989;124:303–308.

Conlon KC, Karpeh MS. Laparoscopy and laparoscopic ultrasound in the staging of gastric cancer. *Semin Oncol* 1996;23:347–351.

Correa P, Shiao YH. Phenotypic and genotypic events in gastric carcinogenesis. *Cancer Res* 1994;54:1941s–1943s.

Crew KD, Neugut AI. Epidemiology of upper gastrointestinal malignancies. *Semin Oncol* 2004;31:450–464.

Cuschieri A, Weeden S, Fielding J, et al. Patient survival after D1 and D2 resections for gastric cancer: long-term results of the MRC randomized surgical trial. Surgical Cooperative Group. *Br J Cancer* 1999;79:1522–1530.

D'Angelica M, Gonen M, Brennan M, Turnbull A, Bains M, Karpeh MS. Pattern of initial recurrence in completely resected gastric adenocarcinoma. *Ann Surg* 2004;240:808–816.

D'Ugo DM, Pende V, Persiani R, et al. Laparoscopic staging of gastric cancer: an overview. *J Am Coll Surg* 2003;196(6):965–974.

Davies J, Chalmers AG, Sue-Ling HM, et al. Spiral computed tomography and operative staging of gastric carcinoma: a comparison with histopathological staging. *Gut* 1997;41:314–319.

Dent DM, Werner ID, Novis B, et al. Prospective randomized trial of combined oncological therapy for gastric carcinoma. *Cancer* 1979;44:385–391.

Duff SE, Li C, Jeziorska M, et al. Vascular endothelial growth factors C and D lymphangiogenesis in gastrointestinal tract malignancies. *Br J Cancer* 2003;89:426–430.

Dupont JB, Lee JR, Burton GR, et al. Adenocarcinoma of the stomach: review of 1,497 cases. *Cancer* 1978;41(3):941–947.

Earle CC, Maroun JA. Adjuvant chemotherapy after curative resection for gastric cancer in non-Asian patients: revisiting a meta-analysis of randomised trials. *Eur J Cancer* 1999;35:1059–1064.

Ell C, May A. Self-expanding metal stents for palliation of stenosing tumors of the esophagus and cardia: a critical review. *Endoscopy* 1997;29: 392–398.

Estape J, Grau JJ, Alcobendas F, et al. Mitomycin C as an adjuvant treatment to resected gastric cancer. A 10-year follow-up. *Ann Surg* 1991;213:219–221.

Fujii K, Isozaki H, Okajima K, et al. Clinical evaluation of lymph node metastasis in gastric cancer defined by the fifth edition of the TNM classification in comparison with the Japanese system. *Br J Surg* 1999;86:685–689.

Fujimoto S, Shrestha RD, Kokubun M, et al. Positive results of combined therapy of surgery and intraperitoneal hyperthermic perfusion for far-advanced gastric cancer. *Ann Surg* 1990;212: 592–596.

Gastrointestinal Tumor Study Group. A comparison of combination chemotherapy and combined modality therapy for locally advanced gastric carcinoma. *Cancer* 1982;49: 1771–1777.

Geoghegan JG, Keane TE, Rosenberg IL, et al. Gastric cancer: the case for a more selective policy in surgical management. *J R Coll Surg Edinb* 1993;38(4):208–212.

Goh PM, So JB. Role of laparoscopy in the management of stomach cancer. *Semin Surg Oncol* 1999;16:321–326.

Greenlee RT, Murray T, Bolden S, et al. Cancer statistics, 2000. *CA Cancer J Clin* 2000;50:7–33.

Gunderson LL, Sosin H. Adenocarcinoma of the stomach: areas of failure in a re-operation series (second or symptomatic look): clinicopathologic correlation and implications for adjuvant therapy. *Int J Radiat Oncol Biol Phys* 1982;8:1–11.

Hartgronk HH, van de Velde CJ, Putter H, et al. Extended lymph node dissection for gastric cancer: who may benefit? Final results of the randomized Dutch gastric cancer group trial. *J Clin Oncol* 2004;22:2069–2077.

Hamazoe R, Maeta M, Kaibara N. Intraperitoneal thermochemotherapy for prevention of peritoneal recurrence of gastric cancer. Final results of a randomized controlled study. *Cancer* 1994;73:2048–2052.

Hermanek P, Wittekind C. Residual tumor (R) classification and prognosis. *Semin Surg Oncol* 1994;10:12–20.

Hermans J, Bonenkamp JJ, Boon MC, et al. Adjuvant therapy after curative resection for gastric cancer: meta-analysis of randomized trials. *J Clin Oncol* 1993;11:1441–1447.

Hermans J, Bonenkamp JJ. Meta-analysis of adjuvant chemotherapy in gastric cancer: a critical reappraisal [letter]. *J Clin Oncol* 1994;12: 877–880.

Hundahl SA, Phillips JL, Menck HR. The National Cancer Data Base Report on poor survival of U.S. gastric carcinoma patients treated with gastrectomy: fifth edition American Joint Committee on Cancer staging, proximal disease, and the "different disease" hypothesis. *Cancer* 2000;88:921–932.

Ichikura T, Tomimatsu S, Uefuji K, et al. Evaluation of the New American Joint Committee on Cancer/International Union against cancer classification of lymph node metastasis from gastric carcinoma in comparison with the Japanese classification. *Cancer* 1999;86:553–558.

Jatzko GR, Lisborg PH, Dent H, et al. A 10-year experience with Japanese-type radical lymph node dissection for gastric cancer outside of Japan. *Cancer* 1995;76:1302–1312.

Jentschura D, Winkler M, Strohmeier N, et al. Quality-of-life after curative surgery for gastric cancer: a comparison between total gastrectomy and subtotal gastric resection. *Hepatogastroenterology* 1997;44:1137–1142.

Kattan MW, Karpeh MS, Mazumdar M, et al. Postoperative nomogram for disease-specific survival after an R0 resection for gastric carcinoma. *J Clin Oncol* 2003;19:3647–3650.

Kajitani T. The general rules for gastric cancer study in surgery and pathology. Part I. Clinical classification. *Jpn J Surg* 1981; 11:127–139.

Karpeh MS, Kelsen DP, Tepper JE. Cancer of the stomach. In: DeVita VT, Hellman S, Rosenberg SA, eds. *Cancer: Principles and Practice of Oncology*, 6th ed. Philadelphia, Pa: Lippincott Williams & Wilkins; 2001: 1092–1126.

Kodama Y, Sugimachi K, Soejima K, et al. Evaluation of extensive lymph node dissection for carcinoma of the stomach. *World J Surg* 1981;5: 241–248.

Koga S, Hamazoe R, Maeta M, et al. Prophylactic therapy for peritoneal recurrence of gastric cancer by continuous hyperthermic peritoneal perfusion with mitomycin C. *Cancer* 1988;61:232–237.

Kuntz C, Herfarth C. Imaging diagnosis for staging of gastric cancer. *Semin Surg Oncol* 1999;17:96–102.

Landry J, Tepper JE, Wood WC, et al. Patterns of failure following curative resection of gastric carcinoma. *Int J Radiat Oncol Biol Phys* 1990;19:1357–1362.

Lightdale CJ. Endoscopic ultrasonography in the diagnosis, staging and follow-up of esophageal and gastric cancer. *Endoscopy* 1992;24(suppl 1): 297–303.

Lordick F, Stein HJ, Peschel C, et al. Neoadjuvant therapy for esophagogastric cancer. *Br J Surg* 2004;91:540–551.

Lowy AM, Feig BW, Janjan N, et al. A pilot study of preoperative chemoradiotherapy for resectable gastric cancer. *Ann Surg Oncol* 2001;8:519–524.

Lowy AM, Mansfield PF, Leach SD, Ajani J. Laparoscopic staging for gastric cancer. *Surgery* 1996;119:611–614.

Lowy AM, Mansfield PF, Leach SD, et al. Response to neoadjuvant chemotherapy best predicts survival after curative resection of gastric cancer. *Ann Surg* 1999;229:303–308.

MacDonald JS. Gastric cancer: chemotherapy of advanced disease. *Hematol Oncol* 1992;10:3–42.

MacDonald JS, Smalley S, Benedetti J, et al. Chemoradiotherapy after surgery compared with surgery alone for adenocarcinoma of the stomach or gastroesophageal junction. *N Engl J Med* 2001;345:725–730.

Maehara Y, Okuyama T, Kakeji Y, et al. Postoperative immunochemotherapy including streptococcal lysate OK-432 is effective for patients with gastric cancer and serosal invasion. *Am J Surg* 1994;168:36–40.

Makuuchi H, Kise Y, Shimada H, et al. Endoscopic mucosal resection for early gastric cancer. *Semin Surg Oncol* 1999;17: 108–116.

Mansfield PF. Lymphadenectomy for gastric cancer. *J Clin Oncol* 2004;22:2759–2760.

Minsky BD. The role of radiation therapy in gastric cancer. *Semin Oncol* 1996;23:390–396.

Moertel CG, Childs DS, O'Fallon JR, et al. Combined 5-fluorouracil and radiation therapy as a surgical adjuvant for poor prognosis gastric carcinoma. *J Clin Oncol* 1984;2:1249–1254.

Monson JR, Donohue JH, McIlrath DC, et al. Total gastrectomy for advanced cancer. A worthwhile palliative procedure. *Cancer* 1991;68:1863–1868.

National Comprehensive Cancer Network. NCCN practice guidelines for upper gastrointestinal carcinomas. *Oncology (Huntingt)* 1998;12: 179–223.

Noguchi Y, Imada T, Matsumoto A, et al. Radical surgery for gastric cancer. A review of the Japanese experience. *Cancer* 1989;64: 2053–2062.

Nomura A, Stemmermann GN, Chyou PH, et al. *Helicobacter pylori* infection and gastric carcinoma among Japanese Americans in Hawaii. *N Engl J Med* 1991;325:1132–1136.

Oiwa H, Maehara Y, Ohno S, et al. Growth pattern and *p53* overexpression in patients with early gastric cancer. *Cancer* 1995;75(suppl):1454–1459.

Ono H, Kondo H, Gotoda T, et al. Endoscopic mucosal resection for treatment of early gastric cancer. *Gut* 2001;48:225–229.

Parsonnet J, Vandersteen D, Goates J, et al. *Helicobacter pylori* infection in intestinal- and diffuse-type gastric adenocarcinomas. *J Natl Cancer Inst* 1991;83:640–643.

Roder JD, Bottcher K, Busch R, et al. Classification of regional lymph node metastasis from gastric carcinoma. German Gastric Cancer Study Group. *Cancer* 1998;82:621–631.

Rugge M, Cassaro M, Leandro G, et al. *Helicobacter pylori* in promotion of gastric carcinogenesis. *Dig Dis Sci* 1996;41:950–955.

Sano T, Sasako M, Yamamoto S. Gastric cancer surgery: results of mortality and morbidity of prospective randomized controlled trials (JCOG 9501) comparing D2 and extended para-aortic lymphadenectomy. *J Clin Oncol* 2004;22:2767–2773.

Sarbia M, Becker KF, Hofler H. Pathology of upper gastrointestinal malignancies. *Semin Oncol* 2004;31:465–475.

Sawyers JL. Gastric carcinoma. *Curr Probl Surg* 1995;32:101–178.

Shiu MH, Moore E, Sanders M, et al. Influence of the extent of resection on survival after curative treatment of gastric carcinoma. A retrospective multivariate analysis. *Arch Surg* 1987;122:1347–1351.

Shiu MH, Perrotti M, Brennan MF. Adenocarcinoma of the stomach: a multivariate analysis of clinical, pathologic and treatment factors. *Hepatogastroenterology* 1989;36:7–12.

Skoropad VY, Berdov BA, Mardynski YS, et al. A prospective, randomized trial of preoperative and intraoperative radiotherapy versus surgery alone in resectable gastric cancer. *Eur J Surg Oncol* 2000;26:773–779.

Smith JW, Brennan MF. Surgical treatment of gastric cancer. Proximal, mid, and distal stomach. *Surg Clin North Am* 1992;72:381–399.

Smith JW, Shiu MH, Kelsey L, et al. Morbidity of radical lymphadenectomy in the curative resection of gastric carcinoma. *Arch Surg* 1991;126:1469–1473.

Songun I, Keizer HJ, Hermans J, et al. Chemotherapy for operable gastric cancer: results of the Dutch randomised FAMTX trial.

The Dutch Gastric Cancer Group (DGCG). *Eur J Cancer* 1999; 35:558–562.

Stomach. In: Greene FL, Page DL, Fleming ID, et al., eds. *AJCC Cancer Staging Manual*. 6th ed. New York, NY: Springer; 2002: 99–102.

Sugarbaker PH, Yonemura Y. Clinical pathway for the management of resectable gastric cancer with peritoneal seeding: best palliation with a ray of hope for cure. *Oncology* 2000;58: 96–107.

Svedlund J, Sullivan M, Liedman B, et al. Quality of life after gastrectomy for gastric carcinoma: controlled study of reconstructive procedures. *World J Surg* 1997;21:422–433.

Tada M, Tanaka Y, Matsuo N, et al. Mucosectomy for gastric cancer: current status in Japan. *J Gastroenterol Hepatol* 2000; 15 [suppl]:D98–D102.

Takekoshi T. [General view of gastric cancer with depth invasion into muscle layer (M cancer) from a survey of reports of the Japanese Research Society for Gastric Cancer]. *J Gastroenterol Mass Survey* 1994;32:93–132.

Talamonti MS, Dawes LG, Joehl RJ, et al. Gastrointestinal lymphoma. A case for primary surgical resection. *Arch Surg* 1990;125:972–976.

Wanebo HJ, Kennedy BJ, Chmiel J, et al. Cancer of the stomach. A patient care study by the American College of Surgeons. *Ann Surg* 1993;218:583–592.

Wanebo HJ, Kennedy BJ, Winchester DP, et al. Gastric carcinoma: does lymph node dissection alter survival? *J Am Coll Surg* 1996;183: 616–624.

Weese JL, Harbison SP, Stiller GD, et al. Neoadjuvant chemotherapy, radical resection with intraoperative radiation therapy (IORT): improved treatment for gastric adenocarcinoma. *Surgery* 2000;128:564–571.

Yim HB, Jacobson BC, Saltzman JR, et al. Clinical outcome of the use of enteral stents for palliation of patients with malignant upper GI obstruction. *Gastrointest Endosc* 2001;53: 329–332.

Yonemura Y, Kawamura T, Bandou E, et al. Treatment of peritoneal dissemination from gastric cancer by peritonectomy and chemohyperthermic peritoneal perfusion. *Br J Surg* 2005;92:370–375.

10

Small Bowel Malignancies and Carcinoid Tumors

Keith D. Amos and Rosa F. Hwang

EPIDEMIOLOGY

Malignancies of the small intestine are rare, with an estimated 5,400 new cases diagnosed in the United States in 2006. The small intestine represents 75% of the length and 90% of the surface area of the alimentary tract, accounting for only 1% of gastrointestinal (GI) neoplasms. Adenocarcinoma, carcinoid, lymphoma, and sarcoma account for the majority of small bowel malignancies. The incidence of this rare malignancy is 0.7 to 1.6 per 100,000 persons, with a slight male predominance. Mean age at presentation is 57 years. Associated conditions include familial polyposis, Gardner syndrome, Peutz-Jeghers syndrome, adult (nontropical) celiac sprue, von Recklinghausen neurofibromatosis, and Crohn disease. In addition, immunosuppressed patients such as those with immunoglobulin A (IgA) deficiency are believed to be at increased risk of small bowel malignancies. As many as 25% of affected patients have synchronous malignancies, including neoplasms of the colon, endometrium, breast, and prostate gland.

The peak incidence of carcinoid tumors is in the sixth and seventh decades of life, although these tumors have been reported in patients as young as 10 years. The sites of origin of carcinoid tumors are shown in Table 10.1. Approximately 85% of carcinoid tumors are found in the GI tract, with the appendix being the most common site. Nonintestinal sites include the lungs, pancreas, biliary tract, thymus, and ovary. Ileal carcinoids are the most likely to metastasize, even when small, in contrast to appendiceal carcinoids, which rarely metastasize.

RISK FACTORS

Several distinctive characteristics of the small intestine may explain its relative sparing from malignancy. Benzopyrene hydroxylase, an enzyme that converts benzopyrene to a less carcinogenic compound, is found in large amounts in the mucosa of the small intestine. In contrast, anaerobic bacteria, which convert bile salts into potential carcinogens, are generally lacking in the small intestine. Unlike the stomach or colon, the small intestine is protected from the tumorigenic effects of an acidic environment and from the irritating effects of solid GI contents. In addition, the rapid transit of liquid succus entericus through the small bowel is believed to reduce its tumorigenicity by minimizing the contact time between potential enteric carcinogens and the mucosa. Secretory IgA, also found in large quantities in the small intestine, safeguards against oncogenic viruses.

GI dysfunction may predispose the small intestine mucosa to tumorigenesis. Stasis secondary to partial obstruction or blind

Table 10.1. Sites of origin of carcinoid tumors

Tumor Site	Percentage of Cases
Stomach	2.8
Duodenum	2.9
Jejunoileum	25.5
Appendix	36.2
Colon	6.0
Rectum	16.4
Bronchus	9.9
Ovary	0.5
Miscellaneous	0.2
Unknown primary	3.3

loop syndrome leads to bacterial overgrowth and has been implicated in the development of small intestine malignancies.

CLINICAL PRESENTATION

Small Bowel Malignancy

GI symptoms develop in 75% of patients with malignant lesions of the small bowel, compared with only 50% of patients with benign tumors. Sixty-five percent will present with intermittent abdominal pain that is dull and crampy and radiates to the back, 50% with anorexia and weight loss, and 25% with signs and symptoms of bowel obstruction. Only 10% of patients with small bowel malignancies will develop bowel perforation, most commonly those with lymphomas or sarcomas. A palpable abdominal mass is present in 25% of patients. Jaundice may be present in patients with common bile duct obstruction from ampullary cancer. Episodic jaundice associated with guaiac-positive stool suggests an ampullary malignancy.

The nonspecificity of symptoms, when present, frequently results in a 6- to 8-month delay in diagnosis. The correct diagnosis is established preoperatively in only 50% of cases. Late detection and inaccurate diagnosis contribute not only to the advanced stage of disease at the time of surgery, but also to a 50% rate of metastasis at presentation and thus to the overall poor prognosis for patients with malignant tumors of the small intestine.

Carcinoid Tumors

The presentation of carcinoids varies, depending not only on their physical characteristics and site of origin, but also on whether they are producing substances that are hormonally active. In general, most carcinoids are small, indolent tumors that are categorized pathologically either by microscopic features or according to their embryologic site of origin. The embryologic classification of carcinoids is more commonly used and is outlined in Table 10.2.

Table 10.2. Characteristics of carcinoid tumors by embryologic site of origin

Characteristics	Foregut	Midgut	Hindgut
Location	Bronchus Stomach Pancreas	Jejunum Ileum Appendix	Colon Rectum
Histology	Trabecular	Nodular, solid nest of cells	Trabecular
Secretion			
Tumor 5-HT	Low	High	None
Urinary 5-HIAA	High	High	Normal
Carcinoid syndrome	Yes	Yes	No
Other endocrine secretions	Frequent	Frequent	No

5-HIAA, 5-hydroxyindoleacetic acid; 5-HT, 5-hydroxytryptamin or serotonin.

This classification system subdivides carcinoids into those of the foregut (stomach, pancreas, and lungs), midgut (small bowel and appendix), or hindgut (colon and rectum).

Foregut carcinoids are more commonly associated with an atypical presentation due to secretion of peptide hormone products other than serotonin, such as gastrin, adrenocorticotropic hormone, or growth hormone. Pulmonary carcinoids are usually perihilar, and patients present with recurrent pneumonia, cough, hemoptysis, or chest pain. Ectopic secretion of corticotropin or growth hormone-releasing factor from these tumors can produce Cushing syndrome or acromegaly, respectively. Gastric carcinoids are associated with chronic atrophic gastritis type A (CAG-A) in 75% of cases, predominantly women, of which half have pernicious anemia. These tumors are usually identified on endoscopic evaluation for anemia or abdominal pain and are located in the body or fundus of the stomach. Another 5% to 10% of gastric carcinoids are associated with Zollinger-Ellison syndrome in patients with multiple endocrine neoplasia type I. The remaining 15% to 25% of gastric carcinoids are sporadic and more frequently appear in men. Sporadic foregut carcinoids are associated with an atypical carcinoid syndrome, which is believed to be histamine mediated and exhibited mainly as intense erythematous flushing, itching, conjunctival suffusion, facial edema, and occasional urticaria.

Midgut carcinoids produce symptoms of hormone excess only when bulky or metastatic. Because 75% of the tumors are located in the distal one-third of the appendix, less than 10% cause symptoms, and the vast majority of appendiceal carcinoids are found incidentally. Patients with small bowel carcinoids usually present with symptoms similar to those described for other small bowel tumors. Not uncommonly, as a small bowel carcinoid progresses, it induces fibrosis of the mesentery, which may by itself cause intestinal obstruction and lead to varying degrees of mesenteric ischemia. Most patients with small bowel carcinoids present with metastases to lymph nodes or to the liver.

Hindgut carcinoids tend to be clinically silent tumors until they are advanced. Two-thirds are found in the right colon with the average tumor diameter at presentation being 5 cm. They rarely produce serotonin, even in the presence of metastatic disease. Patients with hindgut tumors most commonly present with bleeding and occasionally experience abdominal pain.

The hormonal manifestations of carcinoid tumors (carcinoid syndrome) are seen in only 10% of patients and occur when the secretory products of these tumors gain direct access to the systemic circulation and avoid metabolism in the liver. This clinical syndrome occurs in the following situations: (a) when hepatic metastases are present; (b) when retroperitoneal disease is extensive, with venous drainage directly into the paravertebral veins; and (c) when the primary carcinoid tumor is outside the GI tract, as with bronchial, ovarian, or testicular tumors. Ninety percent of cases of carcinoid syndrome are seen in patients with midgut tumors.

The main symptoms of carcinoid syndrome are watery diarrhea, flushing, sweating, wheezing, dyspnea, abdominal pain, hypotension, or right heart failure due to tricuspid regurgitation or pulmonic stenosis caused by endocardial fibrosis. The flush is often dramatic and is an intense purplish color on the upper body and arms. Facial edema is often present. Repeated attacks can lead to the development of telangiectasias and permanent skin discoloration. The flush can be precipitated by consuming alcohol, blue cheese, chocolate, or red wine, and by exercise. The mediators of these symptoms are shown in Table 10.3.

A life-threatening form of carcinoid syndrome called *carcinoid crisis* is usually precipitated by a specific event such as anesthesia, surgery, or chemotherapy. The manifestations include an

Table 10.3. Clinical symptoms of carcinoid syndrome and tumor products suspected of causing them

Symptom	Tumor Product
Flushing	Bradykinin Hydroxytryptophan Prostaglandins
Telangiectasia	Vasoactive intestinal polypeptide Serotonin Prostaglandins Bradykinin
Bronchospasm	Bradykinin Histamine Prostaglandins
Endocardial fibrosis	Serotonin
Glucose intolerance	Serotonin
Arthropathy	Serotonin
Hypotension	Serotonin

intense flush, diarrhea, tachycardia, hypertension or hypotension, bronchospasm, and alteration of mental status. The symptoms are usually refractory to fluid resuscitation and administration of vasopressors.

DIAGNOSTIC WORKUP

Small Bowel Malignancies

A high index of suspicion is essential to the early diagnosis and treatment of small intestine malignancies. The patient presenting with nonspecific abdominal symptoms should undergo a complete history, physical examination, and screening for occult fecal blood. Laboratory workup should include a complete blood cell count, measurement of serum electrolyte levels, and liver function tests. Further laboratory testing, including measurement of urinary 5-hydroxyindoleacetic acid (5-HIAA), should be directed by clinical suspicion.

Retrospective reviews report that 50% to 60% of small intestine neoplasms are detected by using conventional radiographic techniques, including upper GI series with small bowel followthrough (UGI/SBFT) and enteroclysis. Hypotonic duodenography, using anticholinergic agents or glucagon to reduce duodenal peristalsis, may enhance diagnostic yield to as high as 86% for more proximally located duodenal malignancies. Traditionally, computed tomography (CT) was not believed to be helpful in diagnosing small bowel neoplasms. However, several recent reviews have shown that CT was able to detect abnormalities in 97% of patients with small bowel tumors. Angiography demonstrates a tumor blush in specific subtypes of small bowel malignancies, most notably, carcinoid and leiomyosarcoma, but is rarely indicated in the initial diagnostic workup.

Enteroscopy should be considered when all previous diagnostic studies are negative. In 1991, Lewis et al. reviewed the experience at Mt. Sinai Medical Center in New York with two endoscopic techniques—push enteroscopy and small bowel enteroscopy—in 258 patients with obscure GI bleeding. Push enteroscopy uses a pediatric colonoscope that is passed orally and then pushed distally through the small intestine, facilitating intubation of the jejunum 60 cm distal to the ligament of Treitz. This technique established a diagnosis in 50% of patients examined. Small bowel enteroscopy, which uses a 120-degree, forward-viewing, 2,560-mm, balloon-tipped endoscope that is carried distally by peristalsis, permitted intubation of the terminal ileum in 77% of cases within 8 hours. Upper GI endoscopy, when performed to the ligament of Treitz, was diagnostic in eight of nine patients with duodenal malignancies reviewed by Ouriel and Adams in 2000.

Most retrospective studies report only moderate success in diagnosing small bowel neoplasms preoperatively, with large series reporting a correct preoperative diagnosis in only 50% of cases, the remainder diagnosed at laparotomy. Exploratory laparotomy remains the most sensitive diagnostic modality in evaluating a patient in whom small bowel neoplasm is suspected and should be considered in the diagnostic evaluation of a patient with occult GI bleeding, unexplained weight loss, or vague abdominal pain. Distally located small bowel adenocarcinoma at or near the ileum is diagnosed with laparotomy in 57% of patients, with UGI in 21% of patients, and CT scan in only 7% of patients. Because most tumors present as large, bulky lesions with lymph node metastasis, laparoscopy is potentially useful for establishing the diagnosis of malignancy when the workup is otherwise negative and for obtaining adequate tissue samples if a diagnosis of lymphoma is suspected. Early detection and treatment remain the most significant variables in improving outcome from small bowel malignancy, necessitating thoughtful and expedient diagnostic workup of patients presenting with vague abdominal symptoms.

Carcinoids

The diagnosis of carcinoid tumor is made using a combination of biochemical tests and imaging studies. Overall, approximately 50% of patients with carcinoids have elevated urinary levels of 5-HIAA, irrespective of whether they have symptoms of carcinoid syndrome. One study reported 100% specificity and 70% sensitivity of urinary 5-HIAA for the presence of carcinoid syndrome and 5-HIAA levels seem to correlate with tumor burden. Urinary 5-HIAA levels can be altered by medications and certain foods (e.g., bananas, walnuts, pineapples). When urinary 5-HIAA levels are nondiagnostic, a more extensive workup should be undertaken, consisting of measurement of urinary 5-hydroxytryptamine (5-HT, serotonin) and 5-hydroxytryptophan (5-HPT), plasma 5-HPT, platelet 5-HT, and serum levels of other secretory products such as chromogranin A, neuron-specific enolase (NSE), substance P, and neuropeptide K. In well-differentiated tumors, the sensitivity of serum chromogranin A is between 80% and 100% and also reflects tumor load. Chromogranin A can be used in the detection of functional and nonfunctional tumors. An overview of serotonin metabolism is shown in Figure 10.1.

Localization of the tumor may also help confirm the diagnosis. Bronchial carcinoids are best visualized with a chest radiograph or CT scan. Gastric, duodenal, colonic, and rectal carcinoids are usually seen on endoscopy and barium studies. Small intestine carcinoids are initially evaluated as described for other small bowel malignancies. Abdominal CT scan is useful for assessing involvement of the retroperitoneum and presence of liver metastasis. In addition, small bowel carcinoids have a spoke-wheel appearance on CT due to extensive mesenteric fibrosis, and 70% of cases demonstrate calcifications.

Nuclear medicine scans have also been used in localization. Scans using Indium 111 (^{111}In-penetreotide) or metaiodobenzylguanidine (MIBG) radiolabeled with iodine 131 (^{131}I) can identify primary or metastatic carcinoid tumors approximately 70% of the time, when MIBG is taken up by the tumor and stored in its neurosecretory granules. The combination of these two imaging modalities increases sensitivity to 95%. However, the sensitivity of detecting bone metastases is only 20% to 50%.

On occasion, a patient may benefit from angiography or selective venous sampling if other diagnostic maneuvers prove unsuccessful.

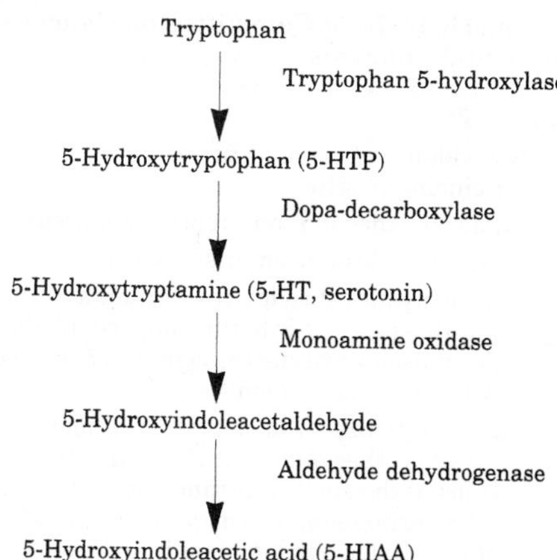

Figure 10.1. Biochemical steps in the production of 5-hydroxytryptamine (5-HT, serotonin) and 5-hydroxyindoleacetic acid (5-HIAA).

STAGING

The American Joint Committee on Cancer staging system for small bowel malignancies is shown in Table 10.4.

MALIGNANT NEOPLASMS

The distribution of small bowel malignancies (reported by Weiss and Yang in a 1987 review of nine population-based cancer registries participating in the National Cancer Institute's Surveillance, Epidemiology, and End Results Program) is shown in Table 10.5. Information on tumor biology, modes of lymphatic spread, and patterns of recurrence for small bowel malignancies is limited.

The most common histologic types of malignant tumors of the small intestine are adenocarcinoma (45.3%), carcinoid (29.3%), lymphoma (14.8%), and sarcoma (10.4%). Adenocarcinoma is the most common malignancy in the proximal small intestine, whereas carcinoid is the most common malignancy in the ileum. Sarcoma and lymphoma may develop throughout the small intestine but are more prevalent in the distal small bowel. Mutations of the Ki-*ras* gene are found in 14% to 53% of small intestine adenocarcinomas and are more prevalent in duodenal, rather than jejunal or ileal, adenocarcinomas. In contrast, mutations of the *APC* gene are uncommon in small bowel carcinomas, suggesting that these tumors arise through a different genetic pathway than colorectal carcinomas.

Adenocarcinoma

Pathology

Adenocarcinoma of the small intestine occurs most commonly in the duodenum, with 65% of these neoplasms clustered in the

Table 10.4. American Joint Committee on Cancer staging of small intestine malignancies

Primary tumor (T)

T0	No evidence of primary tumor
Tis	Carcinoma in situ
T1	Tumor invades lamina propria or submucosa
T2	Tumor invades muscularis propria
T3	Tumor invades through the muscularis propria into the subserosa or into the nonperitonealized perimuscular tissue (mesentery or retroperitoneum) with extension ≤2 cm
T4	Tumor perforates the visceral peritoneum or directly invades other organs or structures (includes other loops of the small intestine, mesentery, or retroperitoneum >2 cm, and abdominal wall by way of serosa; for duodenum only, invasion of the pancreas)

Regional lymph nodes (N)

N0	No regional lymph node metastasis
N1	Regional lymph node metastasis

Distant metastasis (M)

M0	No distant metastasis
M1	Distant metastasis

Staging

Stage 0	Tis	N0	M0
Stage I	T1-T2	N0	M0
Stage II	T3-T4	N0	M0
Stage III	Any T	N1	M0
Stage IV	Any T	Any N	M1

Adapted from Greene FL, Page DL, Fleming ID, et al., eds. *AJCC Manual for Staging of Cancer.* 6th ed. Philadelphia, Pa: Springer-Verlag, with permission.

Table 10.5. Distribution of primary malignant neoplasms in the small intestine by subsite of cancer and histologic type as percentages of total ($N = 1{,}413$)

Subsite Specified	Adenocarcinoma	Carcinoid	Lymphoma	Sarcoma
Duodenum	21.9	1.3	0.8	1.8
Jejunum	14.7	2.5	5.1	5.0
Ileum	8.7	25.5	8.9	3.6
Total	45.3	29.3	14.8	10.4

Adapted from NCI SEER Registries 1973–1982. In: Weiss NS, Yang C. Incidence of histologic types of cancer of the small intestine. *J Natl Cancer Inst* 1987;78:653, with permission.

periampullary region. These tumors infiltrate into the muscularis propria and may extend through the serosa and into adjacent tissues. Ulceration is common, causing occult GI bleeding and chronic anemia. Obstruction may develop from progressive growth of apple core lesions or large intraluminal polypoid masses. It can manifest as gastric outlet obstruction in cases of duodenal lesions or severe cramping pain in cases of more distally located lesions. Approximately 60% of tumors are well- or moderately differentiated tumors, and 37% are signet ring and poorly differentiated tumors.

Clinical Course

Adenocarcinoma of the small bowel follows a pattern of tumor progression similar to that of colon cancer, with similar survival rates when compared stage for stage. Seventy percent to 80% of small bowel lesions are resectable at the time of diagnosis, with a 5-year survival rate of 20% to 30% reported for patients undergoing resection. Approximately 35% of patients have metastasis to regional lymph nodes at the time of diagnosis, and an additional 20% have distant metastasis. Mural penetration, nodal involvement, distant metastasis, and perineural invasion correlate with a poor prognosis. Large tumor size and poor histologic grade were also associated with decreased survival in a study from the University of California, Los Angeles, but others have not found the same relationship.

Adenocarcinoma of the small bowel is known to be associated with Crohn disease, usually occurring in the distal ileum. Risk factors associated with development of a small bowel cancer in Crohn disease include duration of disease, male gender, associated fistulous disease, and the presence of surgically excluded bowel loops.

Treatment

Wide excision of the malignancy and surrounding zones of contiguous spread is performed to provide complete tumor clearance for lesions located in the jejunum and the ileum. A retrospective review of 217 patients diagnosed with small bowel adenocarcinoma treated at The University of Texas M. D. Anderson Cancer Center found that surgery was the primary definitive treatment modality in 67% of patients. Treatment strategies ranging from pancreaticoduodenectomy to local excision have been proposed for the management of duodenal adenocarcinoma. Pancreaticoduodenectomy has been touted as a superior operation for duodenal adenocarcinoma because of its more radical clearance of the tumor bed and regional lymph nodes. In fact, some authors, including Lai et al. in 1988, continue to recommend pancreaticoduodenectomy for all primary duodenal adenocarcinomas. However, segmental resection for adenocarcinoma of the duodenum satisfies the principles of en bloc resection, without the morbidity of a pancreaticoduodenectomy, and should be considered when technically feasible.

Unlike pancreatic cancer, which diffusely infiltrates into the surrounding soft tissues, adenocarcinoma of the duodenum extends into adjacent tissues as a more localized process. Therefore, tumor-free resection margins, critical to a curative extirpation, may be achieved without necessarily resecting a generous portion of the surrounding soft tissues and adjacent organs; however, the tumor-free status of resection margins must be confirmed on frozen-section evaluation of the resected specimen.

In a 1994 comparison of pancreaticoduodenectomy to segmental resection for management of duodenal adenocarcinoma at M. D. Anderson Cancer Center, Barnes et al. found no significant difference in survival rates, but did find a difference in 5-year local control rates—76% for pancreaticoduodenectomy and 49% for segmental resection. Several other reviews, including those of Lowell et al. in 1992, Joestling et al. in 1981, and van Ooijen and Kalsbeek in 1988, which compared survival following pancreaticoduodenectomy or segmental resection for lesions in the third and fourth portions of the duodenum, have demonstrated no significant difference in 5-year survival. In these studies, a more limited resection, with a lower rate of associated morbidity and mortality, provided a survival benefit equal to that of a more extensive resection.

At M. D. Anderson, a pancreaticoduodenectomy is performed for lesions involving the proximal duodenum to the right of the superior mesenteric artery (SMA). A segmental resection is performed for duodenal lesions to the left of the SMA. Local excision is considered for small lesions on the antimesenteric wall of the second portion of the duodenum. Two studies have found a higher rate of postoperative complications from pancreaticoduodenectomy in patients with periampullary malignancies than in those with pancreatic adenocarcinoma, although this did not result in a higher rate of perioperative mortality in either study. An increased pancreatic anastomotic leak rate was present in the group with duodenal carcinoma, presumably due to the fact that the pancreas in these patients would be normal with a soft texture, thereby increasing the technical difficulty of the pancreatic anastomosis.

Experimental Therapy

Electron-beam intraoperative radiation therapy and external-beam radiation therapy have been administered at M. D. Anderson in a limited number of cases of microscopic involvement of resection margins or unresectable disease. However, adenocarcinoma of the small intestine is generally considered to be radiation resistant. Chemotherapy, based on 5-fluorouracil (5-FU) and nitrosoureas, has been recommended in both the adjuvant setting and in cases of unresectable disease, yet most retrospective studies have failed to demonstrate a significant response to chemotherapy. Because most centers have only limited experience treating adenocarcinoma of the small intestine, the efficacy of chemotherapy needs further study, and patients should continue to be enrolled in prospective randomized clinical trials.

Carcinoid

Pathology

Carcinoids are known mainly for their ability to secrete serotonin and are the most common endocrine tumors of the GI system. They arise from enterochromaffin cells, which are located

Table 10.6. Biologically active substances that can be secreted by carcinoid tumors

Amines
5-HT
5-HIAA
5-HTP
Histamine
Dopamine
Tachykinins
Kallikrein
Substance P
Neuropeptide K
Others
Prostaglandins
Pancreatic polypeptide
Chromogranins
Neurotensin
hCGa
hCGb

5-HT, 5-hydroxytryptamine; 5-HIAA, 5-hydroxyindoleacetic acid; 5-HTP, 5-hydroxytryptophan; hCG, human chorionic gonadotropin.

predominantly in the GI tract and mainstem bronchi. In addition to serotonin, these tumors can secrete a number of biologically active substances (Table 10.6), including amines, tachykinins, peptides, and prostaglandins.

Carcinoid tumors occur most frequently in the appendix (40%), small intestine (27%), rectum (15%), and bronchus (11%). Small bowel carcinoids occur most commonly in the terminal 60 cm of the ileum as tan, yellow, or gray-brown intramural or submucosal nodules. The presence of multiple synchronous nodules in 30% of patients mandates careful inspection of the entire small intestine in these patients.

Clinical Course

Primary carcinoid tumors are indolent, slow-growing lesions that become symptomatic late in the course of the disease. Rarely ulcerative, these tumors infiltrate the muscularis propria and may extend through the serosa to involve the mesentery or retroperitoneum and to produce a characteristically intense desmoplastic reaction.

Metastatic disease, present in 90% of symptomatic patients, correlates not only with the depth of invasion, but also with the size of the primary lesion. For carcinoids less than 1 cm, the risk of metastasis is 2% for appendiceal, 15% to 18% for small bowel, and 20% for rectal primaries. If carcinoid tumors are greater than 2 cm, 33% of appendiceal, 86% to 95% of small bowel, and almost all rectal primaries have metastasized.

Distant sites of metastases include the liver and, to a lesser degree, the lungs and bone. There is no widely accepted histologic classification of carcinoids that accurately predicts metastatic behavior. Morphologic criteria such as mitotic activity, cytologic atypia, and tumor necrosis have been evaluated; however, these features can be affected by ischemia secondary to mesenteric sclerosis in GI carcinoids. An analysis of GI carcinoids by Moyana et al. in 2000 revealed that positive immunohistochemical staining for MIB-1 (a marker of proliferation) and p53 was associated with metastatic behavior. In addition, high levels of the nuclear antigen Ki-67 appears to correlate with decreased survival in patients with carcinoid tumors.

Treatment of Localized Disease

Surgical extirpation is the definitive treatment for localized primary carcinoid tumors. The extent of resection is determined by the size of the primary lesion and is based on the likelihood of mesenteric lymph node involvement. The incidence of metastasis depends on the location of the tumor, its depth of invasion, and its size.

Appendiceal carcinoids smaller than 1 cm rarely metastasize and are adequately treated by appendectomy alone unless the base of the appendix is involved, in which case a partial cecectomy may be necessary. Because the incidence of metastasis increases with primary tumor size, treatment of appendiceal carcinoids between 1 and 2 cm is more controversial. In general, most authors recommend appendectomy alone for lesions smaller than 1.5 cm and right hemicolectomy for lesions larger than 1.5 cm or for any lesion with invasion of the mesoappendix, blood vessels, or regional lymph nodes.

In contrast to appendiceal carcinoids, carcinoids of the small bowel are more likely to metastasize even when smaller than 1 cm. As a result, most surgeons recommend a wide en bloc resection that includes the adjacent mesentery and lymph nodes. Such a resection may be difficult at times; the small bowel mesentery is frequently fibrotic and foreshortened secondary to a desmoplastic reaction seen with these tumors. Although some surgeons advocate local excision for small midgut carcinoids, up to 70% of these tumors metastasize to the lymph nodes. Therefore, a wide resection may not only cure some of these patients, but should also provide better local disease control than local excision. Furthermore, a careful and thorough examination of the entire length of bowel is important because 20% to 40% of small bowel carcinoids are multicentric. Because of the slow-growing nature of these tumors, wide excision is advocated even when distant metastases are present. In addition, approximately 40% of patients with midgut carcinoids have a second GI malignancy. Therefore, the entire bowel and colon should be evaluated before any planned surgical intervention.

Rectal carcinoids less than 1 cm, which comprise two-thirds of all rectal carcinoids, are adequately treated by wide local excision alone. Tumors between 1 and 2 cm should be locally resected by a wide, local, full-thickness excision with abdominoperineal resection or low anterior resection recommended for tumors that invade the muscularis propria. The treatment of patients with rectal carcinoids greater than 2 cm remains controversial. Even though major oncologic operations were once recommended for rectal carcinoids greater than 2 cm, it is now appreciated that the risk of distant metastasis is so high that radical surgery should not be considered if the tumor can be removed by wide local excision. Every attempt should be made for sphincter preservation in patients with carcinoids of the rectum of greater than 2 cm because of the high likelihood of distant failure and the marginal benefit obtained from radical local therapy.

Long-term prognosis after surgical treatment of patients with GI carcinoids was evaluated in a study from the Mayo Clinic. With a median follow-up of 18 years, survival was significantly associated with embryologic origin of the tumor and patient age. Increased survival was found in those patients with midgut carcinoids, compared with those with foregut tumors, as well as in patients younger than 62 years. Overall survival rates at 5 and 10 years were 69% and 53%, respectively.

Treatment of Advanced Disease

The role of surgery for unresectable and metastatic disease is not clearly defined, but it appears that surgery may benefit some patients. When metastatic disease is present, it is necessary to establish whether the patient has symptoms of carcinoid syndrome and whether curative resection is possible. If the patient has no contraindications to surgery, then an attempt at complete extirpation should be made because it may lead to prolonged disease-free survival and symptomatic relief. Patients with metastatic carcinoid should all begin receiving octreotide therapy preoperatively to prevent a carcinoid crisis. Surgical resection of liver metastases has resulted in long-term relief of symptoms. Eighty-two percent of patients with midgut carcinoids metastatic to the liver who underwent resection demonstrated partial or complete relief of symptoms with a mean duration of 5.3 years. Patients in whom liver metastases from carcinoid tumor are suspected should undergo an abdominal CT scan. The study should be done before and after intravenous (IV) contrast material to better visualize carcinoid liver metastases, which are usually hypervascular and can be difficult to distinguish from normal liver after injection of IV contrast material.

Patients with mildly symptomatic carcinoid syndrome can be treated medically. Diarrhea can usually be controlled with loperamide, diphenoxylate, or the serotonin receptor antagonist cyproheptadine. Flushing can frequently be controlled with either adrenergic blocking agents (e.g., clonidine or phenoxybenzamine) or a combination of type 1 and 2 histamine receptor antagonists. Albuterol (a beta-adrenergic blocking agent) and aminophylline are effective in relieving bronchospasm and wheezing.

For patients whose symptoms cannot be controlled with these conservative measures or in whom a carcinoid crisis develops, the somatostatin analog octreotide has shown tremendous promise. A trial from the Mayo Clinic found that flushing and diarrhea could be controlled in the vast majority of patients with as little as 150 μg of octreotide administered subcutaneously three times per day. The duration of the responses was on the average more than 1 year. Interestingly, a number of studies have now shown that octreotide is also able to slow tumor growth significantly in more than 50% of patients and to cause tumor regression for variable periods in another 10% to 20% of individuals. Lanreotide, another long-acting somatostatin analog, is available in slow-release formulation. Treatment with lanreotide by injection every 10 to 14 days appears to be as effective as daily octreotide for malignant and nonmalignant endocrine disorders. Furthermore, treatment with a depot formulation of octreotide, 20 mg intramuscularly every 4 weeks, resulted in symptomatic relief and tumor regression in a patient with disseminated carcinoid who had progressed during treatment with lanreotide combined with interferon alfa.

Because such good results can be achieved with octreotide, interferon, or hepatic artery chemoembolization, surgical debulking procedures, which used to be recommended for patients with symptomatic carcinoid syndrome and liver metastasis, are rarely required. Patients with unresectable disease, if asymptomatic, should just be monitored. Local complications related to the tumor can be addressed if and when they develop. Our current indications for surgical intervention in unresectable and widely metastatic disease include complications of bulky carcinoid tumors such as obstruction and perforation. In addition, surgical debulking is considered for severe intractable symptoms unresponsive to medical treatment, if a dominant mass or liver metastasis can be identified. For patients who have undergone liver resection for metastatic carcinoid tumors, R2 (vs. R0) resection and pancreatic location of the carcinoid have been associated with poorer prognosis.

Despite the advanced stage of disease at presentation and the limited effectiveness of currently available therapies, the natural history of carcinoids affords affected patients a better prognosis than other malignancies of the small bowel. The 5-year survival rate for localized disease approaches 100% after complete resection. Resection of metastatic disease is associated with a 68% 5-year survival rate, whereas unresectable disease has a 38% 5-year survival rate.

Experimental Therapy

A number of chemotherapeutic agents have been studied in patients with carcinoid tumors. Results of chemotherapy trials with such agents as doxorubicin, dacarbazine, and streptozotocin, either alone or in combination, have been disappointing. Most chemotherapy trials show response rates of less than 30%, with responses lasting only a few months. The role of chemotherapy is still investigational, but for patients with advanced disease that cannot be controlled with standard measures, monitored clinical trials should be recommended.

One biological agent, interferon, in both alfa-2a and alfa-2b forms, has demonstrated promising results in diminishing urinary levels of 5-HIAA and symptoms of carcinoid syndrome. Most patients in various studies experienced either partial regression or stabilization of their disease for a prolonged period. Unfortunately, objective responses with reduction of tumor size occurred in only approximately 15% of patients.

In some centers, hepatic artery occlusion or embolization has been used with some success to diminish the size of liver metastases and decrease levels of biologically active mediators of carcinoid syndrome. However, duration of response is usually short, with median duration ranging from 7 months for hepatic artery occlusion alone to 20 months in a study using hepatic artery occlusion followed by systemic chemotherapy. Furthermore, side effects may be substantial. Liver embolization with Gelfoam performed in patients with neuroendocrine tumors resulted in serious complications in 10%, including renal failure, liver necrosis, and bowel ischemia. Another option for management of carcinoid hepatic metastases is radiofrequency ablation (RFA). In one small series, RFA was used as salvage therapy in patients with hepatic metastases who were not amenable to surgical resection and unresponsive to embolization. Although only three patients were treated, all three demonstrated decreases in both the size of the lesions and the severity of symptoms. Because RFA can be performed percutaneously or laparoscopically, this may be a useful treatment alternative for patients with disseminated carcinoid tumors.

Although external-beam radiation has not proven effective in treating carcinoid tumors, targeted radiation in the form of radioactive iodine coupled to either MIBG or octreotide is a therapeutic strategy that may hold some promise for the future.

Sarcoma

Pathology

Sarcomas of the small intestine are typically slow-growing lesions; they occur more frequently in the jejunum and ileum than in the duodenum. Sharing a similar growth pattern with other GI sarcomas, these malignancies invade adjacent tissues, with metastasis occurring predominantly via the hematogenous route to the liver, lungs, and bones. The most common clinical presentations are pain (65%), abdominal mass (50%), and bleeding. More than 75% of tumors exceed 5 cm in diameter at diagnosis, with extramural extension, rather than intramural or intraluminal extension, representing the typical growth pattern. For this reason, obstruction is rarely a manifestation of this disease process.

CT scan of these lesions typically demonstrates a heterogeneous mass with focal areas of necrosis where the tumor has outgrown its nutrient blood supply and formed localized abscesses.

Leiomyosarcoma and gastrointestinal stromal tumor (GIST) account for 75% of small intestine sarcomas; fibrosarcoma, liposarcoma, and angiosarcoma are seen less frequently. In summary, sarcoma represents only 10% of small bowel malignancies, yet the various subtypes encompass a broad range of biological behavior, the scope of which exceeds this review.

Treatment

Surgical resection is the primary treatment modality for sarcoma of the small bowel. Because sarcoma infrequently metastasizes to regional mesenteric lymph nodes, unlike adenocarcinoma and carcinoid, an extensive mesenteric lymphadenectomy is unnecessary and will not prolong survival. En bloc resection of the lesion with tumor-free margins is recommended for a potentially curative resection; however, at the time of diagnosis, 50% of lesions are unresectable and most exceed 5 cm in diameter. Local resection should be considered in the presence of widely metastatic disease for control of bleeding and relief of obstruction.

Experimental Therapy

Leiomyosarcomas of the small bowel are resistant to chemotherapy and radiation therapy. Combined chemotherapy and radiation therapy should be offered to patients with leiomyosarcomas only as part of an experimental protocol in an attempt to downstage the disease or possibly make an unresectable lesion resectable. Chemotherapy can be used in the treatment of recurrent or metastatic disease, but again, only as part of an experimental protocol. Currently at M. D. Anderson, chemoembolization with cisplatin is used in patients with metastatic disease to the liver. Sarcomas of other histologic subtypes, most importantly, the GISTs, are discussed in Chapter 5.

Lymphoma

Pathology

The distribution of lymphoma in the small intestine parallels the distribution of lymphoid follicles in the small intestine, with the lymphoid-rich ileum representing the most common location of small bowel lymphoma. Lymphoma arises from the lymphoid aggregates in the submucosa; infiltration of the mucosa can result in ulceration and bleeding. The tumor may also extend to the serosa and adjacent tissues, producing a large obstructing mass associated with cramping abdominal pain. Perforation occurs in as many as 25% of patients. Lymphoma may arise as a primary neoplasm or as a component of systemic disease with GI involvement. As with sarcoma, bulky disease is a characteristic of lymphoma, with approximately 70% of tumors larger than 5 cm in diameter.

Primary tumors are staged according to the Kiel classification (see Chapter 17) as low, intermediate, or high grade, with high-grade lesions being diagnosed most frequently. Prognostic factors include tumor grade, extent of tumor penetration, nodal involvement, peritoneal disease, and distant metastasis. The 5-year survival rate ranges from 20% to 33%.

Treatment

The initial treatment for primary lymphoma of the small bowel is chemotherapy. Unfortunately, chemotherapy is not always able to be administered due to intra-abdominal complications of the tumor, most notably obstruction and perforation. In addition, perforation of the bowel may result after initiating chemotherapy due to the inherent thin wall of the small intestine. In these clinical situations, extended surgical resection of the primary lesion may be a safer initial approach. Resection should extend to grossly normal bowel; there is no role for frozen-section evaluation of margins because potential microscopic disease will be adequately treated by adjuvant chemotherapy. Lymph node metastases are frequent; however, en bloc resection of the adjoining mesentery is only indicated if it is necessitated by the primary tumor mass for technical considerations. Otherwise, the tumor burden in the lymph nodes is better treated with adjuvant chemotherapy. The first-line chemotherapy regimen currently used at the M. D. Anderson Cancer Center is cyclophosphamide, doxorubicin, vincristine, and prednisone.

Experimental Therapy
Chemoradiation has been used at some institutions for nodal metastasis, positive resection margins, and unresectable disease. However, a survival benefit from such treatment regimens has not been demonstrated. The use of radiation therapy alone has been associated with significant tumor necrosis, bleeding, and bowel perforation, but may be considered in elderly patients unable to tolerate the toxicity of chemotherapy.

METASTATIC MALIGNANCIES

Pathology
Metastases are the most common form of malignancy in the small intestine and develop as a result of hematogenous or lymphatic spread from a primary tumor to the mucosa or submucosal lymphatics of the small intestine. The primary tumors that most commonly metastasize to the small bowel include ovarian, colon, lung, and melanoma. Metastatic melanoma is unique in that once localized in the small bowel, the metastatic focus may further disseminate to the small bowel mesentery and draining lymph nodes. In general, however, small bowel metastases remain localized to the bowel wall, and they may produce small bowel obstruction (frequently due to intussusception with melanoma metastases) or perforation.

Although the typical presentation of metastatic lesions is obstruction or perforation, the more common cause of obstruction and perforation in patients who have previously undergone resection of a GI primary tumor is related to the initial procedure—that is, either recurrence of the primary tumor or adhesions resulting from the initial exploration.

Segmental bowel resection is the primary treatment for small bowel metastases. Except for melanoma metastases, which may function as a source of further lymphatic dissemination, a regional lymphadenectomy is not performed for metastatic tumors of the small intestine.

Palliation

At the time of diagnosis, most small bowel malignancies are locally advanced, with significant bulky disease or metastases. When the advanced stage of disease precludes surgical resection, enteric bypass should be performed to prevent obstruction. In the event of bleeding from an unresectable small bowel malignancy, intra-arterial embolization of nutrient arteries may be considered, but the benefits must be weighed against the significant risks of this procedure. Our experience with this technique at M. D. Anderson Cancer Center has been discouraging because of the significant rate of bowel ischemia and perforation associated with embolization of the small bowel mesentery.

Chemotherapy or chemoradiation may offer effective control of locally advanced unresectable disease, particularly in the case of lymphoma, and should be considered as a palliative treatment option.

SURVEILLANCE

Routine follow-up for patients should include a complete history and physical examination, complete blood cell count, serum electrolyte determination, and liver function tests performed at regular intervals. A chest radiograph should be obtained every 6 months for the first 3 years after resection, followed by subsequent yearly examinations. Assessment of locoregional recurrence in patients who have undergone a right hemicolectomy for ileal malignancy or segmental resection for duodenal malignancy should include endoscopy at 6-month intervals. Assessment for recurrence at other sites may include CT scan, UGI/SBFT, angiography, or enteroscopy and must be directed by clinical suspicion based on patient history and physical and laboratory findings.

RECOMMENDED READING

Ajani JA, Carrasco H, Samaan NA, et al. Therapeutic options in patients with advanced islet cell and carcinoid tumors. *Reg Cancer Treat* 1990;3:235.

Arai M, Shimizu S, Imai Y, et al. Mutations of the Ki-*ras*, *p53* and *APC* genes in adenocarcinomas of the human small intestine. *Int J Cancer* 1997;70:390.

Ashley SW, Wells SA. Tumors of the small intestine. *Semin Oncol* 1988;15:116.

Barnes G, Romero L, Hess KR, et al. Primary adenocarcinoma of the duodenum: management and survival in 67 patients. *Ann Surg Oncol* 1994;1:73.

Bernstein D, Rogers A. Malignancy in Crohn's disease. *Am J Gastroenterol* 1996;91:3.

Bomanji J, Mather S, Moyes J, et al. A scintigraphic comparison of iodine-123 metaiodobenzylguanidine and iodine-labeled somatostatin analog (tyr-3-octreotide) in metastatic carcinoid tumors. *J Nucl Med* 1992;33:1121.

Carrasco CH, Charnsangavej C, Ajani J, et al. The carcinoid syndrome palliation by hepatic artery embolization. *AJR Am J Roentgenol* 1986;147:149.

Cattell RB, Braasch JW. A technique for the exposure of the third and fourth portions of the duodenum. *Surg Gynecol Obstet* 1960;11:379.

Cheek RC, Wilson H. Carcinoid tumors. *Curr Probl Surg* 1970;Nov:4.

Crist DW, Sitzman JV, Cameron JL. Improved hospital morbidity, mortality, and survival after the Whipple procedure. *Ann Surg* 1987;206:358.

Cubilla AL, Fortner J, Fitzgerald PJ. Lymph node involvement in carcinoma of the head of the pancreas area. *Cancer* 1978;41:880.

Dabaja BS, Suki D, Pro B, Bonnen M, Ajani J. Adenocarcinoma of the small bowel. *Cancer* 2004;101:518.

Dematteo RP, Lewis JJ, Leung D, et al. Two hundred gastrointestinal stromal tumors: recurrence patterns and prognostic factors for survival. *Ann Surg* 2000;231:51.

Donohue JH. Malignant tumors of the small bowel. *Surg Oncol* 1994;3:61.

Eriksson BK, Larsson EG, Skogseid BM, et al. Liver embolizations of patients with malignant neuroendocrine gastrointestinal tumors. *Cancer* 1998;81:2293.

Farouk M, Niotis M, Branum GD, et al. Indications for and the techniques of local resection of tumors of the papilla of Vater. *Arch Surg* 1991;126:650.

Feldman JM. Carcinoid tumors and syndrome. *Semin Oncol* 1987;14:237.

Godwin JD II. Carcinoid tumors: an analysis of 2837 cases. *Cancer* 1975;36:560.

Graadt van Roggen JF, van Velthuysen MLF, Hogendoorn PCW. The histopathological differential diagnosis of gastrointestinal stromal tumours. *J Clin Pathol* 2001;54:96.

Hanson MW, Feldman JE, Blinder RA, et al. Carcinoid tumors:

iodine-131 MIBG scintigraphy. *Radiology* 1989;172:699.

Joensuu H, Roberts PJ, Sarlomo-Rikala M, et al. Effect of the tyrosine kinase inhibitor STI571 in a patient with a metastatic gastrointestinal stromal tumor. *N Engl J Med* 2001;344:1052.

Joestling DR, Beart RW, van Heerden JA, et al. Improving survival in adenocarcinoma of the duodenum. *Am J Surg* 1981;141:228.

Johnson AM, Harman PK, Hanks JB. Primary small bowel malignancies. *Am Surg* 1985;51:31.

Kulke MH, Mayer RJ. Medical progress: carcinoid tumors. *N Engl J Med* 1999;340:858.

Kvols LK, Moertel CG, O'Connell MJ, et al. Treatment of the malignant carcinoid syndrome: evaluation of a long acting somatostatin analogue. *N Engl J Med* 1986;315:663.

Lai EC, Doty JE, Irving C, et al. Primary adenocarcinoma of the duodenum: analysis of survival. *World J Surg* 1988;12:695.

Lamberts SW, Bakker WH, Reubi JC, et al. Somatostatin-receptor imaging in the localization of endocrine tumors. *N Engl J Med* 1990;323:1246.

Lewis BS, Kornbluth A, Waye JD. Small bowel tumors: yield of enteroscopy. *Gut* 1991;32:763.

Lowell JA, Rossi RL, Munson L, et al. Primary adenocarcinoma of third and fourth portions of duodenum. *Arch Surg* 1992;127:557.

Maglinte DT, O'Connor K, Bessette J, et al. The role of the physician in the late diagnosis of primary malignant tumors of the small intestine. *J Gastroenterol* 1991;86:304.

Makridis C, Rastad J, Oberg K, et al. Progression of metastases and symptom improvement from laparotomy in midgut carcinoid tumors. *World J Surg* 1996;20: 900.

Martin RG. Malignant tumors of the small intestine. *Surg Clin North Am* 1986;66:779.

Moertel CG, Hanley JA. Combination chemotherapy trials in metastatic carcinoid tumor and the malignant carcinoid syndrome. *Cancer Clin Trials* 1979;2:327.

Moertel CG, Weiland LH, Nagorney DM, et al. Carcinoid tumor of the appendix: treatment and prognosis. *N Engl J Med* 1987;317:1699.

Motojima K, Tsukasa T, Kanematsu T, et al. Distinguishing pancreatic cancer from other periampullary carcinomas by analysis of mutations in the Kirsten-ras oncogene. *Ann Surg* 1991;214:657.

Moyana TN, Xiang J, Senthilselvan A, et al. The spectrum of neuroendocrine differentiation among gastrointestinal carcinoids. *Arch Pathol Lab Med* 2000;124:570.

Nave H, Mossinger E, Feist H, et al. Surgery as primary treatment in patients with liver metastases from carcinoid tumors: a retrospective, unicentric study over 13 years. *Surgery* 2001;129:170.

North JH, Pack MS. Malignant tumors of the small intestine: a review of 144 cases. *Am Surg* 2000;66:46.

O'Rourke MG, Lancashire RP, Vattoune JR. Lymphoma of the small intestine. *Aust N Z J Surg* 1986;56:351.

Oberg K. Carcinoid tumors: current concepts in diagnosis and treatment. *Oncologist* 1998;3: 339.

Oberg K, Eriksson B. The role of interferons in the management of carcinoid tumors. *Br J Haematol* 1991;79:74.

Ouriel K, Adams JT. Adenocarcinoma of the small intestine. *Am J Surg* 1984;147:66.

Patel SR, Benjamin RS. Management of peritoneal and hepatic metastases from gastrointestinal stromal tumors. *Surg Oncol* 2000;9:67.

Pidhorecky I, Cheney RT, Kraybill WG, et al. Gastrointestinal stromal tumors: current diagnosis, biologic behavior, and management. *Ann Surg Oncol* 2000;7:705.

Rothmund M, Kisker O. Surgical treatment of carcinoid tumors of the small bowel, appendix, colon and rectum. *Digestion* 1994;55(suppl 3):86.

Ryder NM, Ko CY, Hines OJ, et al. Primary duodenal adenocarcinoma. *Arch Surg* 2000;135:1070.

Sohn TA, Lillemoe KD, Cameron JL, et al. Adenocarcinoma of the duodenum: factors influencing long-term survival. *J Gastrointest Surg* 1998;2:79.

Stinner B, Kisker L, Zielke A, et al. Surgical management for carcinoid tumors of small bowel, appendix, colon and rectum. *World J Surg* 1996;20:183.

Strodel WE, Talpos G, Eckhauser F, et al. Surgical therapy for small bowel carcinoid tumors. *Arch Surg* 1983;118:391.

Talamini MA, Moesinger RC, Pitt HA, et al. Adenocarcinoma of the ampulla of Vater. A 28-year experience. *Ann Surg* 1997;225:590.

Thompson GB, van Heerden JA, Martin JK, Jr, et al. Carcinoid tumors of the gastrointestinal tract: presentation, management, and prognosis. *Surgery* 1985;98:1054.

Van Ooijen B, Kalsbeek HL. Carcinoma of the duodenum. *Surg Gynecol Obstet* 1988;166: 343.

Vinik AI, Thompson N, Eckhauser F, et al. Clinical features of carcinoid syndrome and the use of somatostatin analogue in its management. *Acta Oncol* 1989;28:389.

Wallace S, Ajani JA, Charnsangavej C, et al. Carcinoid tumors: imaging procedures and interventional radiology. *World J Surg* 1996;20:147.

Weiss NS, Yang C. Incidence of histologic types of cancer of the small intestine. *J Natl Cancer Inst* 1987;78:653.

Welch JP, Malt RA. Management of carcinoid tumors of the gastrointestinal tract. *Surg Gynecol Obstet* 1977;145:223.

Wessels FJ, Schell SR. Radiofrequency ablation treatment of refractory carcinoid hepatic metastases. *J Surg Res* 2001;95:8.

Willett CG, Warshaw AL, Connery K, et al. Patterns of failure after pancreaticoduodenectomy for ampullary carcinoma. *Surg Gynecol Obstet* 1993;176:33.

Yeo CJ, Cameron JL, Sohn TA, et al. Six hundred fifty consecutive pancreaticoduodenectomies in the 1990s: pathology, complications, and outcomes. *Ann Surg* 1997;226:248.

Younes N, Fulton N, Tanaka R, et al. The presence of K-12 *ras* mutations in duodenal adenocarcinomas and the absence of *ras* mutations in other small bowel adenocarcinomas and carcinoid tumors. *Cancer* 1997;79:1804.

Zuetenhorst JM, Taal BG. Metastatic carcinoid tumors: a clinical review. *Oncologist* 2005;10:123.

11

Cancer of the Colon, Rectum, and Anus

George J. Chang and Barry W. Feig

EPIDEMIOLOGY

Colorectal cancer is the fourth most common cancer and the second leading cause of cancer deaths. In 2005, there were an estimated 145,000 cases diagnosed in the United States, including 104,950 cases of colon cancer and 40,340 cases of rectal cancer. Colorectal cancer incidence rates have continued to decline since 1985, a decline partly believed to be due to improved screening and treatment of polyps before their progression to invasive cancers. However, colorectal cancer still accounts for 10% of cancer deaths. Estimates for the year 2005 show 54,290 deaths from colon and rectal cancer.

In the United States, the cumulative lifetime risk of developing colorectal cancer is about 6%. The mean age of onset is 65. The risk of colorectal cancer clearly increases with age. Except in the setting of hereditary forms of colorectal cancer, this disease rarely occurs before age 40. After age 50, there is a rapid increase in the rate of disease, and 90% of the cases occur in patients older than 50. These facts are responsible for the recommendations to begin screening at age 50.

When diagnosed, 39% of patients have localized disease, 38% have regional disease, 19% have distant metastasis, and 5% are unstaged. The survival rates for local, regional, and distant disease at 5 years are 90%, 66%, and 9.0%, respectively, and at 10 years are 85%, 58%, and 6.6%, respectively.

Approximately 75% of colorectal cancer cases are sporadic, with the remainder of cases occurring in patients who are at increased risk. The patients with increased risk include those with inflammatory bowel disease, familial adenomatous polyposis (FAP), and hereditary nonpolyposis colorectal cancer (HNPCC), as well as patients with a strong family history of colorectal cancer. Men are at slightly increased risk as the age-adjusted incidence is 58.5 per 100,000 in men and 44.2 per 100,000 in women.

RISK FACTORS

Diet

Many dietary factors have been studied regarding their effect on colorectal cancer. Consumption of red meat and animal fat, as well as the presence of high fecal levels of cholesterol, correlate with and may be causally related to an increased risk of colorectal carcinoma. Folate supplements have been shown to be protective against colorectal cancer. Calcium supplements have been shown to decrease the formation of new adenomas in patients with a history of adenomas. Vitamins with antioxidant properties including beta-carotene, vitamin C, and vitamin E have been studied, and at present there are no prospective data that demonstrate a protective effect from colorectal cancer with their use. Dietary fiber has also been studied and is epidemiologically associated with a decreased colorectal cancer risk; however, no prospective data support its use for protection from the development of colorectal cancer.

Medications

Several medications have demonstrated protective effects for colorectal cancer. Hormone replacement therapy has been shown to significantly decrease mortality from colorectal cancer in women. Aspirin and other nonsteroidal anti-inflammatory drugs have also demonstrated protective effects. Recent studies with sulindac and the selective cyclooxygenase-2 (COX-2) inhibitor celecoxib demonstrated the ability of these agents to cause regression of colon polyps in patients with FAP. However, the COX-2 inhibitors have been associated with an increased risk for cardiovascular complications; therefore, their role in chemoprevention remains unclear.

Polyps

Most colorectal cancers arise from polyps. Colorectal polyps are classified histologically as either neoplastic (adenomatous including serrated adenomatous) polyps (which may be benign or malignant) or nonneoplastic (including hyperplastic, mucosal, inflammatory, and hamartomatous) polyps. Adenomatous polyps are found in approximately 33% of the general population by age 50 and in approximately 50% of the general population by age 70. Most lesions are less than 1 cm in size, with 60% of people having a single adenoma and 40% having multiple lesions. Sixty percent of lesions will be located distal to the splenic flexure.

A genetic model for colon carcinogenesis has been developed from the genetic analysis of colorectal adenomas and carcinomas. This model demonstrates a sequence of genetic alterations responsible for the development of colorectal adenomas and their progression to invasive carcinoma. The National Polyp Study showed that colonoscopic removal of adenomatous polyps significantly reduced the risk of developing colorectal cancer.

Polyps coexist with colorectal cancer in 60% of patients and are associated with an increased incidence of synchronous and metachronous colonic neoplasms. Patients with a primary cancer and a solitary associated polyp have a lower incidence of synchronous and metachronous lesions when compared to patients with multiple polyps. The natural history of polyps supports an aggressive approach to their treatment: invasive cancer will develop in 24% of patients with untreated polyps at the site of that polyp within 20 years.

There are three histologic variants of adenomatous polyps. *Tubular adenomas* represent 75% to 87% of polyps and are found with equal frequency throughout all segments of the bowel. Less than 5% of tubular adenomas are malignant. *Tubulovillous adenomas* constitute 8% to 15% of polyps. They are also equally distributed throughout the bowel, and 20% to 25% are malignant. The remaining 5% to 10% of polyps are *villous adenomas,* which are most commonly found in the rectum; 35% to 40% of these polyps are malignant. Polyps may be pedunculated (usually tubular or tubulovillous) or sessile (usually tubulovillous or villous). Besides histologic characteristics, the size of a polyp and the degree of dysplasia has been associated with malignant potential. Malignancy was found in 1.3% of adenomas less than 1 cm, 9.5% between 1 and 2 cm, and 46% greater than 2 cm. Similarly, 5.7% of mild, 18% of moderate, and 34.5% of adenomatous polyps with severe dysplasia were found to have malignant cells on complete excision of the polyp. Therefore, although only 2% to 5% of adenomatous polyps harbor malignancy at the time of diagnosis, the histologic characteristics, size, and degree of dysplasia can help predict which polyps will be malignant.

The terms *carcinoma in situ*, *intramucosal carcinoma*, and *high-grade dysplasia* are used to describe severely dysplastic adenomas where the cancerous cells have not invaded through the muscularis mucosae and therefore have no risk of lymph node metastases. In an effort to avoid confusion, standardized use of the term *high-grade dysplasia* is advocated. Approximately 5% to 7% of adenomatous polyps contain high-grade dysplasia. If a polyp containing high-grade dysplasia is completely excised endoscopically, the patient should be considered cured.

Overall, 8.5% to 25% of polyps harboring invasive carcinoma will metastasize to regional lymph nodes. Unfavorable pathological features of malignant colorectal polyps increase the probability that regional lymph nodes will be involved with tumor and include (a) poor differentiation, (b) vascular and/or lymphatic invasion, (c) invasion below the submucosa, and (d) positive resection margin. Poorly differentiated lesions (grade 3) are associated with a higher incidence of lymphovascular involvement and recurrent disease when compared with well- and moderately differentiated lesions (grades 1 and 2, respectively). Approximately 4% to 8% of malignant polyps will be poorly differentiated. The presence of one or more of these adverse features should prompt evaluation for surgical resection. Depth of invasion is an important prognostic factor for mesenteric lymph node involvement with invasive cancer arising in a polyp. In 1985, Haggitt et al. classified the level of invasion from the head of the polyp to the submucosa of the underlying colonic wall (Table 11.1). In a multivariate analysis, only invasion into the submucosa of the underlying bowel wall (level 4) was a significant prognostic factor. This is in keeping with previous pathological studies that have shown that the lymphatic channels do not penetrate above the muscularis

Table 11.1. Haggitt's classification for colorectal carcinomas arising in adenomas

Classification	Depth of Invasion
0	Carcinoma confined to the mucosa
1	Head of polyp
2	Neck of polyp
3	Stalk of polyp
4	Submucosa of the underlying colonic wall

mucosa. Although these findings have been confirmed by other studies, there are frequently multiple adverse prognostic factors seen in patients with higher levels of invasion (i.e., levels 3 and 4), which makes it difficult to assign depth as the most important factor. A negative resection margin has consistently been shown to be associated with a decreased risk for adverse outcome (recurrence, residual carcinoma, lymph node metastases, decreased survival). Twenty-seven percent of patients with positive or indeterminate tumor margins will have adverse outcomes, compared with 18% with negative margins and poor prognostic features and 0.8% with negative margins and no other poor prognostic features. Therefore, a negative margin is only one component in risk factor assessment.

An additional classification system for malignant colorectal polyps has been popularized in Japan and may be applicable to malignant sessile polyps and was described by Kikuchi in 1995. It classifies invasive cancer as Sm1 (slight carcinoma invasion of the muscularis mucosa, 200–300 μm), Sm2 (intermediate invasion), or Sm3 (deep submucosal invasion extending to the inner surface of the muscularis propria). Sm1 depth of invasion is associated with a low risk for local recurrence or lymph node metastasis. Nascimbeni et al., have reported their series from the Mayo Clinic where Sm3 depth of invasion was associated with a 23% risk for lymph node metastasis.

Although clinical factors such as age, location, number of polyps, and gender are collectively known to be prognostic factors, only age of older than 60 years has been identified as an independent risk factor for invasion.

Treatment

When adenomatous polyps are found by sigmoidoscopy, we recommend complete colonoscopy with colonoscopic removal of the polyp and colonoscopic surveillance every 1 to 3 years until the examination result is normal. Colonoscopic polypectomy is a safe, effective treatment for nearly all pedunculated polyps. A biopsy is performed on those polyps not amenable to safe polypectomy; subsequently, surgical resection is recommended (usually for large sessile villous lesions). Fungation, ulceration, and distortion of the surrounding bowel wall indicate the presence of invasive cancer and are contraindications to polypectomy.

Colectomy is indicated for patients with residual carcinoma and for those at high risk for lymph node metastases despite complete endoscopic polypectomy. The high-risk pathological features previously described (margin <3 mm, poor differentiation, Haggitt level 4, and vascular or lymphatic invasion) and the resultant increased risk of lymph node metastasis should be weighed against the risk of surgical resection.

In a review of 17 studies to evaluate the frequency of lymph node metastases or residual carcinoma in low-risk patients with pedunculated polyps, only a 1% incidence was found. In sessile polyps with low-risk features, the incidence was increased to 4.1%. Because the incidence of nodal metastases is higher in sessile polyps with invasive cancer, those patients at low operative risk should be considered for resection even if no high-risk pathological features are observed. Stalk invasion in pedunculated polyps is not considered an adverse histologic feature, and treatment of polyps with stalk invasion is the same as that of polyps without stalk invasion (based on risk stratification). Polypoid cancers (almost all the polyp is invaded with carcinoma) are treated no differently from other malignant polypoid lesions. Large villous adenomas of the rectum may be amenable to transanal local excision. This provides a complete diagnostic evaluation for malignancy, and if excised with negative margins (with other favorable prognostic features), may be the only therapeutic procedure needed.

Hereditary Colorectal Cancer Syndromes

The majority of colorectal cancers are sporadic cancers that occur in patients without a significant family history of colorectal cancer. Approximately 5% to 10% of all colorectal cancers are associated with a familial colorectal rectal cancer syndrome, and an additional 15% to 20% are associated with a familial predisposition.

Familial adenomatous polyposis (FAP) is the best characterized of the syndromes; 1% to 2% of patients diagnosed with colon carcinoma will have FAP. Germ-line mutations in the adenomatous polyposis coli (APC) gene on chromosome 5q are characteristic of FAP. The majority of the mutations result in a truncated APC protein; however, some mutations do not and can only be identified with gene sequencing. The pattern of inheritance is autosomal dominant, with 90% penetrance. The incidence of new mutations in FAP patients is high; approximately 25% of all FAP cases are the result of a de novo germ-line mutation. In patients with FAP, thousands of polyps develop throughout the gastrointestinal (GI) tract but are most common in the colon. The median age of adenoma diagnosis is 15 years. Without prophylactic colectomy, colorectal cancer will develop in virtually all affected individuals by the end of the third decade of life. A milder phenotype known as *attenuated* FAP is associated with fewer polyps with the typical age of onset for colorectal cancer by the early fifties. Patients with FAP may also develop extracolonic manifestations including gastric polyps, duodenal adenomas and carcinomas, desmoid tumors, thyroid carcinoma, mandibular osteomas, congenital hypertrophy of the retinal pigmented epithelium, sebaceous and epidermoid cysts and fibromas (previously Gardner syndrome), or central nervous system tumors (Turcot syndrome). Commercial genetic testing can now identify the APC gene mutation by sequencing. Since the complete sequencing of the APC gene, studies have correlated the specific genetic mutations with the differing phenotypes of extraintestinal manifestations of FAP. Genetic testing and counseling should be offered to all patients in whom FAP is suspected. Surveillance for FAP should begin at the age of 10 to 12 with annual endoscopic evaluations. Once a mutation is identified within a family, unaffected individuals can be spared such an intensive surveillance regimen.

The primary treatment for FAP is prophylactic colectomy. Surgical options include abdominal colectomy with ileorectal anastomosis (IRA), restorative proctocolectomy with ileal-pouch anal anastomosis (IPAA), and less commonly proctocolectomy with end ileostomy. Patients who have polyp burdens within the rectum that cannot be endoscopically controlled should not undergo IRA.

It should be emphasized that after prophylactic colectomy or proctocolectomy, these patients must continue life-long surveillance because there remains a risk for cancer in the remaining rectum after IRA or at the anastomosis or within the ileal pouch itself after IPAA.

MYH (mutY homolog)-associated polyposis syndrome has recently been identified from subgroups of patients in FAP registries who have tested negative for APC gene mutations. The pattern or inheritance is autosomal recessive, and the phenotype demonstrates multiple colorectal polyps (>10) but typically fewer than in individuals with classic FAP. An age of onset of colorectal cancer in patients younger than 50 years has been reported in those with biallelic MYH mutations. Colorectal cancers in MYH polyposis syndrome are associated with G:C to T:A transversions resulting from defects in base excision repair. This colorectal cancer-associated polyposis syndrome continues to be defined.

Hereditary nonpolyposis colorectal cancer syndrome (HNPCC), also classically known as the Lynch I and II syndromes, is a nonpolyposis autosomal dominant disease that occurs five times more frequently than familial polyposis. HNPCC accounts for 5% to 7% of colon cancers. Isolated, early onset colorectal cancer occurs in the Lynch I syndrome. Colorectal cancer and tumors of the endometrium, ovary, stomach, small bowel, hepatobiliary tract, pancreas, ureter, and renal pelvis characterize the Lynch II syndrome. Penetrance is between 30% and 70%. There is an estimated 85% lifetime risk of colon cancer. Compared with patients with sporadic colon cancer, patients with HNPCC have cancers that are more right sided (60%–70% occur proximal to the splenic flexure), occur earlier (at about 45 years of age), have a lower stage, have better survival, and have an increased rate of metachronous and synchronous tumors (20%).

The genetic mutations causing HNPCC are in DNA mismatch repair (MMR) genes that prevent replication errors, and hence genetic instability. Five of the DNA MMR genes have been linked to HNPCC. These genes are hMSH2, hMLH1, hMSH6, hPMS1, and hPMS2. The first two genes account for the 50% and 39% of the cases of HNPCC, respectively. Mutations in tumor suppressor genes such as p53, DCC, and APC can be associated with HNPCC because replication errors are produced in these tumor suppressor genes. One of the main difficulties in the management of patients with HNPCC is the identification of those individuals who should be tested. A detailed family history should be obtained in all patients with colorectal cancer and may identify potentially affected individuals using Amsterdam criteria or Bethesda guidelines (Table 11.2). Although lacking in specificity, the use of these criteria and guidelines is associated with 60% to 94% sensitivity for identifying individuals with HNPCC. Furthermore, histopathological evaluation of the surgical specimen may reveal the presence of features associated with HNPCC, including a "Crohn's-like" inflammatory cell infiltrate and signet ring cells. At M. D. Anderson Cancer Center (MDACC), immunohistochemistry for mismatch repair gene protein expression is performed in the colorectal tumors of suspected individuals. If loss of one of the repair proteins is noted, genetic testing is performed.

Table 11.2. Amsterdam criteria and Bethesda guidelines

Amsterdam I	
At least three relatives must have histologically verified colorectal cancer	1. One must be a first-degree relative of the other two 2. At least two successive generations must be affected 3. At least one of the relatives must have received the diagnosis before age 50
Amsterdam II	
Similar to Amsterdam I, but may include any combination of cancers associated with HNPCC (e.g., colorectal, endometrial, gastric, ovarian, ureter or renal pelvis, brain, small bowel, hepatobiliary tract, sebaceous gland adenomas, keratoacanthomas)	
Bethesda guidelines	
1. Amsterdam criteria are met 2. Two colorectal or HNPCC-related cancers, including synchronous and metachronous presentation 3. Colorectal cancer and a first-degree relative with colorectal and/or an HNPCC-related cancer and/or a colonic adenoma; one of the cancers must be diagnosed before age 45 and the adenoma diagnosed before age 40 4. Colorectal or endometrial cancer diagnosed before age 45 5. Right-sided colorectal cancer with an undifferentiated pattern (solid/cribriform) on histopathology, diagnosed before age 45 6. Signet ring cell-type colorectal cancer diagnosed before age 45 (>50% signet ring cells) 7. Colorectal adenomas diagnosed before age 40	
Revised Bethesda guidelines	
1. Early onset colorectal cancer (before age 50) 2. Synchronous, metachronous, or other HNPCC-associated tumors, regardless of age 3. Colorectal cancer with high microsatellite instability diagnosed before age 60 4. Colorectal cancer diagnosed in one or more first-degree relatives with an HNPCC-related tumor, with one of the cancers being diagnosed before age 50 5. Colorectal cancer diagnosed in two or more first- or second-degree relatives with HNPCC-related tumors, regardless of age	

HNPCC, hereditary nonpolyposis colorectal cancer.

Other less common hereditary colorectal cancer syndromes may be associated with hamartomatous polyposis such as Peutz-Jeghers syndrome (PJS), juvenile polyposis syndrome (JPS), Cowden syndrome, and Bannayan-Ruvalcaba-Riley syndrome. Germ-line mutations in STK11 (LKB1) are associated with PJS, mutations in SMAD4 and BMPR1-A are associated with JPS, and PTEN mutations are associated with Cowden syndrome and Bannayan-Ruvalcaba-Riley syndrome. The hamartomatous polyposis syndromes are associated with a significantly increased risk for colorectal cancer and are present in <1% of colorectal cancer in North America.

People with a first-degree relative with colorectal cancer have a 1.8- to 8-fold higher risk of colorectal cancer than the general population. The risk is higher if more than one relative is affected, and higher if the cancer developed in the relative at a young age (<45). The role of inheritable genetic defects in predisposition to colorectal cancer in such patients is not well understood.

Inflammatory Bowel Disease

Chronic ulcerative colitis (CUC) carries a risk of colorectal carcinoma that is 30 times greater than that of the general population. The risk of cancer increases 0.5% to 1% per year after 10 years and is 18% to 35% at 30 years. The severity, extent, and duration of inflammation, as well as family history of colorectal cancer and history of primary sclerosing cholangitis, are risk factors for the development of cancer. In contrast to sporadic colorectal cancers, CUC-related cancers are more often multiple, broadly infiltrating, and poorly differentiated. It can be extremely difficult to identify small tumors in a CUC colon due to the chronic changes resulting from the inflammatory process. Therefore, random surveillance biopsies should be routinely performed in patients with CUC, and prophylactic colectomy or proctocolectomy should be recommended for high-grade dysplasia and considered for low-grade dysplasia. Crohn disease is also associated with an increased risk for colorectal cancer that is related to the duration and severity of disease. Its risk is similar to that with CUC. The risk associated with inflammatory bowel disease underscores the importance of surveillance in this patient population.

Previous Colon Carcinoma

A second primary colon carcinoma is three times more likely to develop in patients with a history of colon cancer than in the general population; metachronous lesions develop in 5% to 8% of these patients.

SCREENING

The value of routine screening of asymptomatic populations who lack high-risk factors for development of colorectal cancer has been established. Screening should be initiated at age 50. As many as 19% of the general population are at risk of developing adenomatous polyps, and 5% of sporadic polyps may progress to colorectal carcinoma. The goals of screening are detection of early cancers and prevention of cancer by finding and removing adenomas. Three randomized trials have shown that fecal occult blood screening followed by colonoscopy has been shown to detect cancers at an earlier stage. One of these trials, the Minnesota Colon Cancer Control Study, has demonstrated a significantly improved cancer-related survival, and a meta-analysis of the randomized trials indicates that Hemoccult testing is associated with a 19% reduction in the mortality rate from colorectal carcinoma. However, the sensitivity of fecal occult blood tests (FOBTs) has been reported to be 30% to 90%. Therefore, alternative methods have been investigated, including immunochemical FOBTs and fecal tests for DNA mutations. If FOBT is positive, total colonoscopy should be performed.

Four case-control studies have demonstrated that sigmoidoscopy is associated with a reduced mortality for colorectal cancer. The National Cancer Institute funded Prostate, Lung, Colorectal, and Ovarian screening trial and the UK FlexiScope Trial are being performed with an anticipated 250,000 subjects to evaluate screening flexible sigmoidoscopy, but outcomes data are not yet available. The utility of flexible sigmoidoscopy as a screening test for colorectal neoplasia is limited by the amount of colon visualized with a 70-cm sigmoidoscope. Therefore, flexible sigmoidoscopy should be used in conjunction with radiographic evaluation of the more proximal colon or annual fecal occult blood testing. As a screening test, flexible sigmoidoscopy, when normal, should be repeated every 5 years.

The value of colonoscopy in screening can be appreciated if one considers that approximately 40% of colon cancers arise proximal to the splenic flexure and that 75% of proximal colon cancers do not have an index lesion within reach of the flexible sigmoidoscope. All roads eventually lead to colonoscopy for diagnosis or therapy (as in the case of a lesion on barium enema). Most studies using screening colonoscopy in average-risk patients report an average of 30% of neoplastic lesions detected. Cost is an important issue, however, if colonoscopy is considered the ultimate screening tool. Currently, screening colonoscopy is cost-effective if a 10-year interval is used once the colon is cleared of polyps.

Double-contrast barium enema is used less frequently than colonoscopy for screening and can detect colorectal carcinoma and polyps greater than 1 cm with accuracy equal to that of colonoscopy. It has been used in patients who refuse or cannot have full colonoscopy to the cecum, as an adjunct to flexible sigmoidoscopy to evaluate the remainder of the colon, and for difficult-to-visualize turns in the colon. The difficulty with this method is that lesions detected by double-contrast barium enema require further evaluation, decreasing the cost-effectiveness of the method.

CT colonography (virtual colonoscopy) is an emerging technique for the diagnosis of colonic polyps in the screening population that uses three-dimensional reconstruction of the air distended colon. At the National Naval Medical Center, in 1,223 average-risk adults who subsequently underwent conventional (optical) colonoscopy, virtual colonoscopy was as good or better at detecting relevant lesions. However, it may be less accurate in surveillance populations, and subsequent multi-institutional studies have failed to confirm the excellent results from this series. The major limitations include uncertain accuracy, the need for full bowel preparation, and follow-up colonoscopy for tissue diagnosis of radiographic abnormalities. Because virtual colonoscopy is considerably time and labor intensive from the standpoint of the radiologist, active investigations into methods of automating the evaluation process are ongoing.

Carcinoembryonic antigen (CEA) is a glycoprotein found in the cell membranes of many tissues, including colorectal cancer. Some of the antigen enters the circulation and is detected by radioimmunoassay of serum; CEA is also detectable in various other body fluids, urine, and feces. Elevated serum CEA is not specifically associated with colorectal cancer; abnormally high levels are also found in sera of patients with malignancies of the pancreas, breast, ovary, prostate gland, head and neck, bladder, and kidney. CEA levels are high in approximately 30% to 80% of patients with cancer of the large intestine, but less than half of patients with localized disease are CEA positive. Therefore, CEA has no role in screening for primary lesions. False-positive results occur in benign disease (lung, liver, and bowel). The CEA level is also increased in smokers. Overall, 60% of tumors will be missed by CEA screening alone.

Screening Recommendations

Recently, the U.S. Multisociety Task Force on Colorectal cancer met to update the original 1997 consensus guidelines for colorectal cancer screening and surveillance and made recommendations regarding screening (Table 11.3).

PATHOLOGY

Histologically, more than 90% of colon cancers are adenocarcinomas. On gross appearance, there are four morphologic variants of adenocarcinoma. Ulcerative adenocarcinoma is the most common configuration seen and is most characteristic of tumors in the descending and sigmoid colon. Exophytic (also known as polypoid or fungating) tumors are most commonly found in the ascending colon, particularly in the cecum. These tumors tend to project into the bowel lumen, and patients often present with a right-sided abdominal mass and anemia. Annular (scirrhous) adenocarcinoma tends to grow circumferentially into the wall of the colon, resulting in the classic apple core lesion seen on barium enema radiologic study. Rarely, a submucosal infiltrative pattern can be observed that is similar to linitis plastica seen with gastric adenocarcinoma.

Other epithelial histologic variants of colon cancer that are occasionally seen include mucinous (colloid) carcinoma, signet-ring cell carcinoma, adenosquamous and squamous cell carcinoma (SCC), and undifferentiated carcinoma. Other rare tumors include carcinoids and leiomyosarcomas.

A commonly used grading system is based on the degree of formation of glandular structures, nuclear pleomorphism, and number of mitoses. Grade 1 tumors have the most developed glandular structures with the fewest mitoses, grade 3 is the least differentiated with a high incidence of mitoses, and grade 2 is intermediate between grades 1 and 3.

Table 11.3. Colorectal cancer screening recommendations

Risk Category	Screening Recommendations
Average risk, asymptomatic (age ≥50)	FOBT each year (full colonoscopy or DCBE/flex sig if +) Flex sig every 5 years (consider full colonoscopy if +) FOBT each year + flex sig every 5 years DCBE every 5 years Colonoscopy every 10 years
First-degree relative with CRC or adenomatous polyps at age ≥60 years, or two second-degree relatives affected with CRC	Same as for average risk but starting at age 40 years
Two or more first-degree relatives with CRC or single first-degree relative with CRC or adenomatous polyps diagnosed at age <60 years	Colonoscopy every 5 years beginning at age 40 or 10 years younger than the earliest diagnosis in the family
One second-degree or any third-degree relative with CRC	Same as for average risk
Gene carrier or at risk for FAP	Annual flexible sigmoidoscopy beginning at 10–12 years
Gene carrier or at risk for HNPCC	Colonoscopy every 1–2 years beginning at age 20–25 years or 10 years younger than the earliest case in the family

FOBT, fecal occult blood test; DCBE, double contrast barium enema; CRC, colorectal cancer; FAP, familial adenomatous polyposis; HNPCC, hereditary nonpolyposis colorectal cancer.

STAGING

The Dukes and TNM staging systems for colorectal carcinoma are presented in Tables 11.4 and 11.5. Although most clinicians are familiar with both staging systems, clinical trial and treatment planning should be based on the TNM staging system. The Dukes staging system is important for historical perspective.

CLINICAL PRESENTATION

Patients with colorectal cancer present with bleeding, anemia, abdominal pain, change in bowel habits, anorexia, weight loss, nausea, vomiting, fatigue, and anemia. Pelvic pain or tenesmus in rectal cancer may be associated with an advanced stage of disease indicating involvement of the pelvic floor muscles or nerves. Metastatic disease is suspected in patients with right upper quadrant pain, fevers and sweats, hepatomegaly, ascites, effusions,

Table 11.4. Modified Astler-Coller classification of the Dukes staging system for colorectal cancer

Stage	Description
A	Lesion not penetrating submucosa
B1	Lesion invades but not through the muscularis propria
B2	Lesion through intestinal wall, no adjacent organ involvement
B3	Lesion involves adjacent organs
C1	Lesion B1 invasion depth; regional lymph node metastasis
C2	Lesion B2 invasion depth; regional lymph node metastasis
C3	Lesion B3 invasion depth; regional lymph node metastasis
D	Distant metastatic disease

Table 11.5. TNM staging classification of colorectal cancer

Primary tumor (T)	
TX	Primary tumor cannot be assessed
T0	No evidence of primary tumor
Tis	Carcinoma in situ: intraepithelial or invasion of the lamina propria without invasion through the muscularis mucosae into the submucosa
T1	Tumor invades submucosa
T2	Tumor invades muscularis propria
T3	Tumor invades through the muscularis propria into the subserosa, or into nonperitonealized pericolic or perirectal tissues
T4	Tumor directly invades other organs or structures and/or perforates visceral peritoneum
Regional lymph nodes (N)	
NX	Regional lymph nodes cannot be assessed
N0	No regional lymph node metastasis
N1	Metastasis in one to three regional lymph nodes
N2	Metastasis in four or more regional lymph nodes
Distant metastases (M)	
MX	Distant metastasis cannot be assessed
M0	No distant metastasis
M1	Distant metastases present

and supraclavicular adenopathy. Central nervous system and bone metastases are seen in less than 10% of autopsy cases, and are very rare in the absence of advanced liver or lung disease. The incidence of complete obstruction in newly diagnosed colorectal cancer is 5% to 15%. In a large study from the United Kingdom, 49% of obstructions occurred at the splenic flexure, 23% occurred in the left colon, 23% occurred in the right colon, and 7% occurred in the rectum. Obstruction increases the risk of death from colorectal cancer 1.4-fold and is an independent co-variate in multivariate analyses. Perforation occurs in 6% to 8% of colorectal carcinoma cases. Perforation increases the risk of death from cancer 3.4-fold. Using TMN staging and Surveillance, Epidemiology, and End Results (SEER) Program data, 15% of patients present with stage I disease, 30% with stage II, 20% with stage III, and 25% with stage IV. The remainder have unknown staging.

DIAGNOSIS

Colon Cancer

Clinical evaluation of carcinoma of the colon should include colonoscopy and biopsy, air-contrast barium enema if the entire colon could not be visualized by colonoscopy, chest radiograph, complete blood cell count, CEA determination, urinalysis, and liver function tests (LFTs).

The use of computed tomography (CT) in the preoperative evaluation of patients with colon cancer is controversial. We evaluate the abdomen and pelvis with CT to detect involvement of contiguous organs, para-aortic lymph nodes, and the liver. Abnormal LFTs are present in only approximately 15% of patients with liver metastases and may be elevated without liver metastases in up to 40%; therefore, LFTs are not a useful screen for determining the need for obtaining a CT scan.

The preoperative CEA level can also reflect disease extent and prognosis: CEA levels surpassing 10 to 20 ng per mL are associated with increased chances of disease failure for both node-negative and node-positive patients. Fifteen to 20% of liver metastases will be nonpalpable at the time of surgery. However, up to 15% of lesions can be missed by combined preoperative and operative evaluation. Intraoperative ultrasonography has been shown to be the most accurate method of detecting liver metastasis. Approximately 20% of patients will have synchronous liver metastasis at the time of diagnosis; therefore, the preoperative identification of liver metastasis is necessary for the surgical planning of combined resections of the primary tumor and the liver metastasis or for the treatment of tumors involving contiguous organs. Magnetic resonance imaging (MRI) may be helpful in circumstances when intravenous contrast-enhanced CT scanning is contraindicated.

The role of routine preoperative urinary tract evaluation is controversial. Patients who are symptomatic or have large, bulky lesions should have a preoperative intravenous pyelogram, CT scan, or cystoscopy to evaluate the urinary tract.

Positron emission tomography (PET), and now PET-CT, has emerged as a potentially important imaging modality for colorectal cancer. The technique uses the glucose analog fluorodeoxyglucose, which accumulates in metabolically active tissues. The standardized uptake value can provide a semiquantitative determination to help discriminate benign from malignant disease. Although potentially useful in recurrent cancer, it has not been helpful in the primary evaluation of patients with colon cancer due to false positives and high costs.

Rectal Cancer

In addition to the history and physical examination, chest radiograph, complete blood cell count, and CEA, proctoscopic examination, endorectal ultrasound (ERUS), full colonoscopy, and CT scan of the abdomen and pelvis should be performed to accurately stage patients with rectal cancer. Symptomatic patients undergo evaluation of their urinary tract as described earlier for colon cancer.

Accurate preoperative staging tools are critical in rectal cancer because disease stage may influence treatment decisions such as transanal resection or preoperative multimodality therapy. ERUS is the most accurate tool in determining tumor (T) stage. Performed using rigid or flexible probes, the layers of the rectal wall can be identified with 67% to 93% accuracy. The ERUS characteristics of T1 and T3 tumors make them relatively easy to differentiate. However, the distinction between T2 and T3 tumors is more difficult, yet it is vital in determining treatment planning. ERUS is highly operator dependent, and it can be difficult to differentiate lymph nodes from blood vessels and other structures or peritumoral edema from tumor. Furthermore, ERUS is limited in its ability to evaluate tumors that are large or bulky, associated with large villous tumors, or have been treated with radiation therapy. As a result of these factors, overstaging occurs in approximately 20% of cases and understaging in approximately 10% to 20%. Stenotic lesions may make ERUS impossible secondary to the inability to pass the probe. ERUS evaluation of T stage is superior to that of CT scanning (52%–83% accuracy) and in recent reports compares to endorectal coil MRI (59%–95% accuracy). The relative accuracy of ERUS or MRI for rectal cancer staging is institution dependent, and ERUS is preferred at MDACC. CT and MRI can delineate the relationship of the tumor to surrounding viscera and pelvic structures. Neither CT nor MRI is more useful for the evaluation of locoregional disease after neoadjuvant chemoradiation treatment because radiation changes can be difficult to accurately differentiate from tumor.

Lymph node staging in rectal cancer has proven more difficult than primary tumor staging, with ERUS accuracies of 62% to 83%, CT accuracies of 35% to 73%, and MRI accuracies of 39% to 84% reported. Despite descriptions of methods to radiologically predict metastases in lymph nodes, only nodal enlargements can be detected with most current technologies. Fifty to 75% of positive lymph nodes in rectal cancer may be normal in size, thereby limiting accurate evaluation. Similarly, lymph nodes may be enlarged from inflammation, giving false-positive results. Combining size and ultrasonographic characteristics can increase accuracy. Lymph nodes that are greater than 3 mm and hypoechoic are more likely to contain metastatic deposits. In addition, it is possible to perform fine-needle aspiration of suspicious lymph nodes under ERUS guidance. ERUS is invaluable when evaluating patients for preoperative adjuvant therapy, but it cannot accurately assess response to preoperative adjuvant therapy due to the obliteration of tissue planes by edema and fibrosis.

Abdominopelvic CT scanning is important in assessing the presence of distant spread of disease and involvement of adjacent organs. In the management of rectal cancer, it is extremely important to accurately assess the local spread of disease, including the potential involvement of the levator muscles and other pelvic structures. Although ERUS is superior to CT in detecting depth of penetration, CT provides a better assessment of contiguous organ involvement. MRI is a useful adjunct in the evaluation of locally advanced rectal cancer by providing multiple views of the relationships of the tumor to adjacent pelvic structures.

The staging of recurrent rectal cancer is complicated by radiation and postoperative changes that are often difficult to distinguish from tumor. Due to the difficulty in distinguishing scar from tumor, the use of ERUS for postoperative surveillance is controversial and is not routinely performed. There is poor correlation of postradiation therapy ERUS in preoperative regimens to final pathological findings (postresection), indicating the limited value of ERUS in assessing tumor in an irradiated milieu. CT is useful to assess extent of disease and adjacent organ involvement if recurrent tumor is obvious. MRI may yield added information by providing sagittal images that give additional information on resectability. In cases where recurrence is unknown but suspected, CT is more useful if a baseline study is available for comparison. PET has recently been introduced with early reports of increased accuracy in distinguishing postoperative changes from recurrent tumor. In a selected series, it has been shown to be up to 95% sensitive, 98% specific, and 96% accurate in the detection of cancer recurrence. When used appropriately, it can help distinguish patients who would benefit from surgery for recurrent cancer from those who have unresectable disease, particularly when the other imaging modalities fail to localize the disease. However, further studies are required before this test can be recommended for use on a routine basis. Currently at MDACC, we obtain both a CT scan and an MRI of the pelvis in cases of isolated recurrent rectal carcinoma because we believe these studies are complementary in their provision of critical staging and resectability information.

MANAGEMENT OF COLON CANCER

The goal of primary surgical treatment of colon carcinoma is to eradicate disease in the colon, the draining nodal basins, and contiguous organs. Careful surgical planning is essential. The stage of disease, presence of synchronous colonic tumors, and the presence of underlying colorectal cancer syndromes are significant factors in determining the optimal surgical approach. The patient's general medical condition is also important because most perioperative deaths result from cardiovascular or pulmonary complications.

Anatomy

Thorough knowledge of the arterial, venous, and lymphatic anatomy of the colon and rectum is essential to appropriate surgical management (Fig. 11.1). The ascending and proximal transverse colons are embryologically derived from the midgut and receive their arterial blood supply from the superior mesenteric artery via the ileocolic, right, and middle colic arteries. The distal transverse, descending, and sigmoid colon are hindgut derivatives whose arterial blood supply arises from the inferior mesenteric artery (IMA) through the left colic and sigmoid arteries. The rectum, also a hindgut derivative, receives its blood supply to the upper third from the IMA via the superior hemorrhoidal artery. The middle and lower thirds of the rectum are supplied by the middle and inferior hemorrhoidal arteries, which are branches of the hypogastric artery. Collateral blood supply for the colon is provided through the marginal artery of Drummond. The venous drainage of the colon and rectum parallels the arterial supply, with the majority draining directly into the portal venous system. This provides a direct route for metastatic spread of tumor to the liver. The only minor anatomical variation in the venous drainage compared with the arterial supply is that the inferior mesenteric vein (IMV) joins the splenic vein before emptying into the portal system. The rectum has dual venous drainage; the upper rectum drains into the portal system, and the distal one-third of the rectum drains into the inferior vena cava via the middle and inferior hemorrhoidal veins, providing a direct route for hematogenous spread outside the abdomen.

The lymphatic drainage of the bowel is more complex than the vascular supply. Lymphatics begin in the bowel wall as a plexus beneath the lamina propria and drain into the submucosal and intramuscular lymphatics. The epicolic lymph nodes drain the subserosa and are located in the colon wall. This nodal group runs along the inner bowel margin between the intestinal wall and the arterial arcades. These nodes in turn drain into the paracolic nodes, which follow the routes of the marginal arteries. The epicolic and paracolic nodes represent the majority of the colonic lymph nodes and are the most likely sites of regional metastatic disease. The paracolic nodes drain into the intermediate nodes, which follow the main colic vessels. Finally, the intermediate nodes drain into the principal nodes, which begin at the origins of the superior and inferior mesenteric arteries and are contiguous with the para-aortic chain.

The route of lymphatic flow parallels the arterial and venous distribution of the colon. The right colon will drain to the superior mesenteric nodes through the intermediate nodes or to the portal system via the lymphatics of the superior mesenteric vein. The left colon's lymphatic drainage follows the marginal artery to the left colic intermediate nodes and finally to the inferior mesenteric nodes. The lymphatic drainage of the upper third of the rectum follows the IMV, whereas the lower two-thirds drain into the hypogastric nodes, which, in turn, drain into the para-aortic nodes. The lower third of the rectum can also drain along the pudendal vessels to the inguinal nodes.

Surgical Options

At resection, the primary tumor and its lymphatic, venous, and arterial supply are extirpated, as well as any contiguously involved organs. Our current use of intraoperative ultrasound is

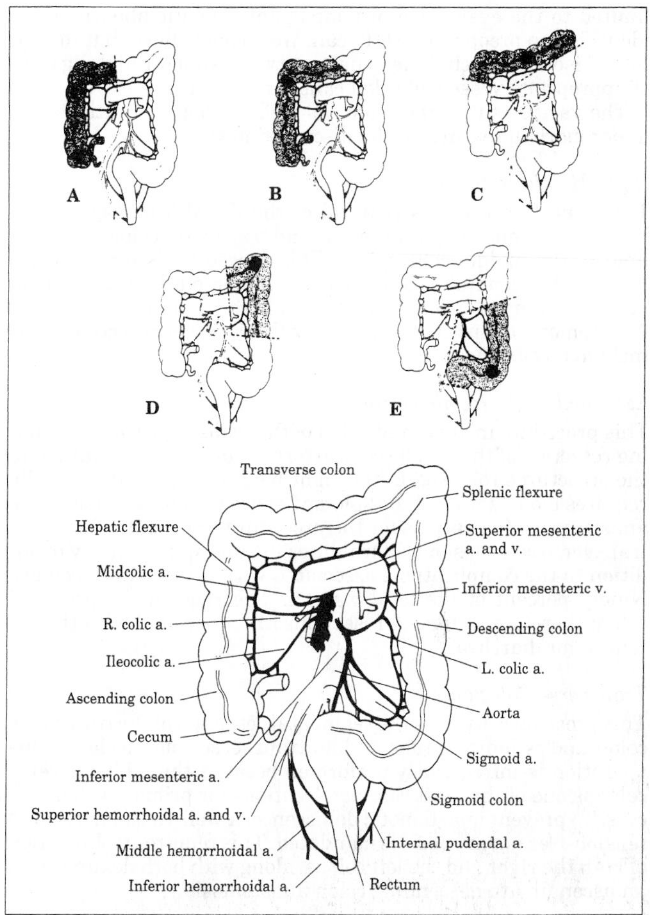

Figure 11.1. Anatomy of colonic blood supply along with a pictorial description of the various anatomical resections used for colon carcinoma. A: Right hemicolectomy. B: Extended right hemicolectomy. C: Transverse colectomy. D: Left hemicolectomy. E: Low anterior resection. (From Sugarbaker PH, MacDonald J, Gunderson L. Colorectal cancer. In: DeVita VT, Hellman S, Rosenberg SA, eds. *Cancer: Principles and Practice of Oncology.* 3rd ed. Philadelphia, Pa: Lippincott; 1984, with permission.)

limited to the evaluation of nonpalpable hepatic abnormalities identified on preoperative CT scan. We do not believe that the "no touch" isolation technique is necessary; we support high ligation of appropriate vessels in colon cancer resections.

The various surgical options, as well as their indications and major morbidities, are briefly discussed next.

Right Hemicolectomy

This operation involves removal of the distal 5 to 8 cm of the ileum, right colon, hepatic flexure, and transverse colon just proximal to the middle colic artery. This procedure is indicated for cecal and ascending colonic lesions. Major morbidities include ureteral injury, duodenal injury, and rarely bile acid deficiency. Anastomotic dehiscence is a risk with all bowel resections that include reconstruction.

Extended Right Hemicolectomy

This procedure includes resection of the transverse colon (including resection of the middle colic artery at its origin) in addition to the structures removed in the right hemicolectomy. It generally requires mobilization of the splenic flexure to allow a tension-free anastomosis. Indications for the procedure are hepatic flexure or transverse colon lesions. Morbidities include splenic injury in addition to the complications associated with right hemicolectomy. Ninety percent of the fecal water is absorbed in the proximal colon; therefore, extended resections are associated with the potential for diarrhea.

Transverse Colectomy

This procedure involves the segmental resection of the transverse colon and is indicated for middle transverse colon lesions. This operation is infrequently performed because the midtransverse colon is one of the least common locations for primary colon cancers. To prevent anastomotic dehiscence, a well-vascularized and tension-free anastomosis is mandated. This requires mobilization of both the right and the left colons, along with both flexures with an ascending-to-descending colon anastomosis.

Left Hemicolectomy

This resection involves the removal of the transverse colon distal to the right branch of the middle colic artery and the descending colon up to, but not including, the rectum and proximal ligation and division of the left colic vessels or IMA. This operation may be tailored to the location of the lesion. Indications for the procedure are left colon and splenic flexure lesions. Morbidities include splenic and ureteral injury.

Low Anterior Resection

When performed for lesions within the sigmoid colon or proximal rectum, this procedure includes removal of the sigmoid colon and the involved rectum, and ligation of superior rectal vessels at their origin. The splenic flexure is routinely mobilized and the reconstruction is performed using the descending colon. The use of the sigmoid colon is discouraged, especially for distal reconstruction as the thickened and hypertrophic muscle of the sigmoid is less compliant and well vascularized than the descending colon. To achieve a tension-free anastomosis, the IMA may need to be divided at its origin, along with the IMV at the inferior border of the pancreas. For lesions involving the rectum, the mesorectum should be divided at least 5 cm distal to the distal aspect of the tumor. Morbidities include anastomotic dehiscence, which is higher with more distal reconstruction and has been reported to be less than 10%, and bowel ischemia (secondary to inadequate flow through the marginal artery of Drummond). For routine low anterior resections for sigmoid or upper rectal lesions without radiation, a defunctioning ileostomy is not typically necessary.

Subtotal Colectomy

This resection involves the removal of the entire colon to the rectum with an ileorectal anastomosis. This procedure is indicated for multiple synchronous colonic tumors that are not confined to a single anatomical distribution, for selected patients with FAP with minimal rectal involvement, or for selected patients with HNPCC and colon cancer. Although an excellent quality of life can be achieved after ileorectostomy, frequent loose bowel movements are the norm. Patients should be counseled regarding a bowel regimen and perianal care. The risk for anastomotic leak after ileorectal anastomosis is approximately 5% or less.

The surgical treatment of the familial polyposis syndromes depends on the age of the patient and the polyp density in the rectum. Surgical options include proctocolectomy with Brooke ileostomy, total abdominal colectomy with IRA, or restorative proctocolectomy with IPAA. Proctocolectomy with continent ileostomy is rarely performed today. Total abdominal colectomy with ileorectal anastomosis has a low complication rate, provides good functional results, and is a viable option for patients with fewer than 20 adenomas in the rectum. These patients must be observed with 6-month proctoscopic examinations to remove polyps and detect signs of cancer. If rectal polyps become too numerous, completion proctectomy with Brooke ileostomy or IPAA, when technically possible, is warranted. The Cleveland Clinic Foundation recently evaluated their registry of patients with FAP who were treated with IRA or IPAA. Prior to the use of IPAA for patients with high rectal polyp burdens, the risk of cancer in the retained rectum was 12.9% at a median follow-up of 212 months. Because of the use of IPAA for patients with large rectal polyp burdens and the selected use of IRA for those with small rectal polyp burdens, no patient has developed rectal cancer in the remaining rectum at a median follow-up of 60 months. Restorative proctocolectomy with IPAA has the advantage of removing all or nearly all large intestine mucosa at risk for cancer, while preserving transanal defecation. Complication rates are low when this procedure is done in large centers. Morbidity from the procedure includes incontinence, multiple loose stools, impotence, retrograde ejaculation, dyspareunia, and pouchitis. Approximately 7% of patients have to be converted to a permanent ileostomy due to complications after the procedure.

Laparoscopic Resection for Colorectal Carcinoma

Recent studies have confirmed that laparoscopy for colorectal carcinoma resection is technically feasible and safe, yielding an equivalent number of resected lymph nodes and length of resected bowel when compared with open colectomy. Early concerns regarding port-site metastases have now been laid to rest. The first adequately powered randomized trial was conducted in Barcelona, Spain. This trial randomized 219 patients to laparoscopic versus open colectomy for cancer and demonstrated oncologic equivalency and a trend toward improved oncologic outcomes in a small subset of stage III patients.

The National Cancer Institute (NCI)-sponsored multicentered Clinical Outcomes of Surgical Therapy (COST) trial enrolled nearly 800 patients and validated the oncologic safety and efficacy of laparoscopy for colon cancer. Laparoscopic assisted colectomy for cancer was associated with equivalent recurrence-free and overall survival when compared with open surgery with no increase in wound recurrences. Patient related benefits included reduced length of hospital stay, decreased pain, faster resolution of ileus, improved cosmesis, and a small improvement in short-term quality of life.

The Medical Research Council-sponsored Conventional versus Laparoscopic-Assisted Surgery In patients with Colorectal Cancer (CLASICC) multicentered trial in the United Kingdom has finished accrual and has reported their short-term outcomes, which are oncologically equivalent for laparoscopic versus open colectomy for cancer. Similar patient-related benefits as in the COST trial were observed. The European Multicentered Colon Carcinoma Laparoscopic or Open Resection trial is still ongoing. An additional trial from Hong Kong demonstrated oncologic equivalency with laparoscopy for sigmoid and rectosigmoid tumors. The laparoscopic-assisted approach has consistently been associated with reductions in hospital stay, postoperative pain, and duration of postoperative ileus when compared with open surgery. However, the magnitude of these effects in randomized trials have been modest, approximately 20% to 35%, and remains the subject of further investigation. Unproven additional benefits of laparoscopy include potentially decreased morbidity, decreased convalescence, improved quality of life, and decreased costs.

With respect to clinical trials of laparoscopy for colorectal cancer, it should be noted that experienced surgeons who have demonstrated proficiency in laparoscopic colectomy for cancer obtained these results. Furthermore, although laparoscopic-assisted techniques have been validated for colon carcinoma, its use for rectal cancer has not yet been definitively established. Additional indications for laparoscopy include resection of polyps, creation of intestinal stomas, and diagnostic procedures.

The appeal of laparoscopic colon surgery is a simple one: minimally invasive techniques result in faster recovery and therefore may result in improved quality of life and lower health care costs when compared with open laparotomy. These benefits have been dramatically realized with surgery for other sites such as for benign gallbladder disease. When considering colectomy, reduction in postoperative pain and narcotic use, faster resolution of ileus, and shorter duration of hospitalization are unifying features of the laparoscopic approach. Added benefits may include the potential for improved short- and long-term complications and a reduction in costs. However, owing to the relatively increased complexity of laparoscopic colectomy and the ongoing evolution of the techniques, the magnitude of these benefits is still being determined.

Furthermore, the importance of these effects may in part depend on the underlying diagnosis. Most patients with colon cancer are candidates for laparoscopic-assisted techniques. Transverse colon tumors require extensive bilateral colonic mobilization and therefore are technically more difficult. Factors associated with an increased need for conversion include tumor-related factors such as proximal left-sided lesions and large bulky tumors, as well as patient obesity, adhesions, and the presence of an associated abscess that was not preoperatively identified. Cancers with perforation, obstruction, or invasion of the retroperitoneum or abdominal wall are not approached laparoscopically.

Obstructing Colorectal Cancers

Obstructing colorectal cancers are usually treated in two stages: resection and Hartmann's procedure, followed by colostomy takedown and anastomosis. An alternative is a one-stage procedure with either subtotal colectomy and primary anastomosis or a segmental resection and intraoperative colonic lavage for carefully selected patients. (Contraindications include multiple primary cancers, advanced peritonitis, hemodynamic instability, poor general health, steroid therapy, or immunosuppressed state.) In the SCOTIA prospective randomized trial using these two treatment modalities in 91 patients with malignant left-sided colonic obstruction, the morbidity and mortality rates were similar. Laser fulguration and endoscopic stenting of obstructive lesions can be used for palliation and to allow for bowel preparation and subsequent single-step resection. Obstructing right-sided cancers can be effectively treated with resection and anastomosis in one stage.

Survival

Nodal involvement is the primary determinant of 5-year survival. In node-negative disease, the 5-year survival rate is 90% for patients with T1 and T2 lesions and 80% for those with T3 lesions. For node-positive cancers, the 5-year survival ranges from 74% with N1 disease to 51% with N2 disease. These figures also vary depending on the number of lymph nodes evaluated in the surgical specimen, with improved survival associated with a higher number of lymph nodes evaluated. Other factors that are proven prognostic indicators include grade, bowel perforation, and obstruction. Patients who present with unresectable metastatic disease have historically had an 8% 5-year survival rate.

Adjuvant Therapy

Most patients with colon cancer present with disease that appears localized and can be completely resected with surgery. However, almost 33% of patients undergoing curative resection will relapse with recurrent disease secondary to unresected occult microscopic metastasis. Adjuvant therapy is administered to treat and hopefully eradicate this residual micrometastatic disease. Until recently, 5-fluorouracil (5-FU) was the only effective agent for colon carcinoma, with response rates of 15% to 30% in patients with advanced disease. In the past 5 years, several new agents have shown excellent activity in colorectal cancer, including irinotecan, oxaliplatin, and biological agents.

History

With the identification of the anticancer activity of 5-FU in patients with colorectal cancers, there have been numerous studies of 5-FU in combination therapies. Adjuvant trials using 5-FU and semustine (MeCCNU; Veterans Administration Surgical Oncology Group, VASOG no. 5) failed to demonstrate an overall survival benefit from adjuvant therapy with this combination. However, subset analysis of patients with one to four positive lymph nodes did reveal a significant improvement in 5-year survival in patients receiving surgery and 5-FU/semustine versus surgery alone (51%–31%, respectively). A second large trial was the National Surgical Adjuvant Breast and Bowel Project (NSABP) C-01 protocol, which compared surgery alone with surgery followed by MOF chemotherapy (MeCCNU, vincristine, and 5-FU). With more than 1,100 patients randomized, the study demonstrated an 8% improvement in 5-year survival in the adjuvant therapy arm. Although these initial results were positive, they were not sufficient to recommend adjuvant therapy for colorectal cancer. They did, however, stimulate further studies combining 5-FU with other agents.

5-Fluorouracil / Levamisole

The first major success of adjuvant therapy for colon cancer was demonstrated in trials of 5-FU in combination with levamisole, an antihelminthic agent with immunostimulatory properties. A pilot prospective randomized study comparing 5-FU/levamisole, levamisole, and surgery alone conducted by the North Central Cancer Treatment Group (NCCTG) demonstrated improved 5-year disease-free survival with levamisole and 5-FU/levamisole given for 1 year as compared with surgery alone. The improvement in the levamisole-only arm was less significant than that of the 5-FU/levamisole arm when examining overall 5-year survival. These results were confirmed by the National Cancer Institute Intergroup Trial (NCI-INT) protocol 035, a larger study comparing the same treatment arms. In this study, patients with stage III disease were shown to have a 41% reduction in the risk of recurrence when treated with 5-FU/levamisole. These patients also demonstrated a 33% improvement in overall 5-year survival. Interestingly, the levamisole-only arm failed to show any improvement in disease-free and overall 5-year survival rates compared with the surgery-only arm. In addition, the data suggested an improvement in disease-free and overall survival for patients with stage II colon carcinoma; however, statistical significance was not reached for this group of patients. Based on these results, the National Institutes of Health Consensus Conference in 1990 recommended that all patients with stage III colon carcinoma receive adjuvant chemotherapy with 5-FU and levamisole. Adjuvant chemotherapy for patients with stage II colon carcinoma remained of unproven benefit.

5-Fluorouracil / Leucovorin

The addition of leucovorin (LV) to 5-FU has been shown to increase antitumor activity in both in vitro and in vivo models. LV works by stabilizing the 5-FU thymidylate synthase complex, thus prolonging the inhibition of thymidylate synthase and increasing tumor cytotoxicity. In the United States, the two most commonly used regimens were the Mayo Clinic regimen of bolus 5-FU 425 mg/m^2/d and leucovorin 20 mg/m^2/d days 1 to 5 every 28 days and the Roswell Park regimen using bolus 5-FU 500 mg per m^2 and leucovorin 500 mg per m^2 weekly for 6 weeks every 8 weeks. These regimens showed efficacy in the metastatic cancer setting. These findings quickly led to study of this combination in the adjuvant setting. Initial efficacy of this combination was demonstrated in the NCI-INT protocol 089, which demonstrated a 30% improvement in 5-year survival when compared with surgery alone. An Italian study also demonstrated both improved disease-free and overall survival using the 5-FU/LV combination. More recent studies have compared 5-FU/LV to previously tested combinations. The NSABP C-03 trial compared 5-FU/LV to MOF chemotherapy (MOF was used in NSABP C-01). This study was reported early because 5-FU/LV was significantly superior to MOF in terms of overall survival, and it was much less toxic than MOF. NSABP C-04 compared 5-FU/LV with 5-FU/levamisole and 5-FU/LV/levamisole. Duration of therapy for this trial was 1 year. The results showed that the 5-FU/LV combination was superior to 5-FU/levamisole, with disease-free survival of 64% versus 60% and overall survival of 74% versus 69%, respectively ($p = 0.05$). The 5-FU/LV/levamisole combination did not improve outcome but had marked increased toxicity. Finally, NSABP C-05 compared 5-FU/LV with 5-FU/LV and interferon (IFN). No difference in disease-free and overall survival was demonstrated with the addition of IFN.

Oral Fluoropyrimidines

Two new oral agents, UFT and capecitabine, have been tested in large, well-designed trials. UFT, a combination of oral uracil and the 5-FU prodrug Tegafur, has been studied in the NSABP C-06 trial comparing 6 months of UFT with leucovorin to 5-FU and leucovorin using the Roswell Park regimen. No differences were seen in 5-year survival with these regimens.

Capecitabine is a drug with rapid GI absorption that undergoes a three-step enzymatic conversion to 5-FU in tumor tissue. When used in first-line treatment of metastatic colorectal cancer, it was associated with a better toxicity profile than 5-FU. The phase III "X-ACT" trial investigated the use of capecitabine in the adjuvant setting for resected stage III colon cancer and also noted an improved safety profile when compared with 5-FU and leucovorin using the Mayo Clinic regimen, with significantly less diarrhea, nausea/vomiting, stomatitis, and neutropenia. Capecitabine was associated with an increased risk for severe hand and foot syndrome.

Irinotecan

Irinotecan has shown significant activity in metastatic colorectal cancer and its use in the adjuvant setting has been studied by several trials. The most important are the Cancer and Leukemia Group B (CALGB) C89803 trial and European PETACC-3 trial. In the CALGB study, 1,260 patients with resected stage III colon cancer were randomized to Roswell Park regimen 5-FU and leucovorin with or without irinotecan (IFL). The IFL arm noted an increased 60-day mortality of 2.5% versus 0.8% in the control group, primarily due to gastrointestinal and thromboembolic toxicities. The PETACC-3 trial using two different schedules of 5-FU infusion alone or with irinotecan for 6 months in the adjuvant setting for stages II and III colon cancer has not yet reported its final data.

Oxaliplatin

Oxaliplatin, a new platinum derivative with activity against colorectal cancer, has shown impressive antitumor activity against advanced colorectal cancer. The Multicenter International Study of Oxaliplatin, 5-FU and leucovorin in the Adjuvant Treatment of Colon Cancer (MOSAIC) trial has recently published its results. This study enrolled 2,246 patients with completely resected stage II/III colorectal cancer to the infusional LV5-FU2 regimen or to FOLFOX-4, which is LV5-FU2 plus oxaliplatin (85 mg per m^2) given every 2 weeks for 12 cycles. The primary endpoint of 3-year disease-free survival was significantly better for the FOLFOX-4 arm (78.2% vs. 72.9%, $p = 0.002$). These results were more significant in stage III patients than in stage II patients. The NSABP C-07 trial is studying Roswell Park regimen bolus 5-FU and leucovorin with or without oxaliplatin.

Monoclonal Antibodies

One of the most important recent advances in the treatment of advanced colorectal cancer has been the availability of biological agents directed against tumor-specific targets. The epidermal growth factor receptor (EGFR)-mediated pathways are important for tumor proliferation and metastases. Monoclonal antibodies directed against EGFR include cetuximab, panitumomab, and others. Cetuximab is a chimeric antibody with activity against colorectal cancer that has been demonstrated by the European randomized phase II "BOND" trial, which randomized irinotecan failure patients to receive cetuximab and irinotecan or cetuximab monotherapy. The response rate was 10.8% with cetuximab alone and 22.9% with combination therapy. Currently, cetuximab is the only anti-EGFR antibody approved for use for colorectal cancer. Its role in the adjuvant setting has not yet been established.

The vascular endothelial growth factor (VEGF) family of glycoproteins is also important for tumor growth. Bevacizumab is a humanized monoclonal antibody that targets circulating VEGF. In previously untreated metastatic colorectal cancer, the addition of bevacizumab to IFL improved the response rate from 35% to 45% ($p = 0.0029$) and the overall survival from 15.6 to 20.3 months

(p = 0.00003). The ECOG 3200 trial compares FOLFOX with single-agent bevacizumab or FOLFOX and bevacizumab as second line for metastatic colorectal cancer. Addition of bevacizumab prolonged median survival from 10.7 months for FOLFOX to 12.5 months for the combination regimen. As with cetuximab, the role of bevacizumab in the adjuvant setting has not yet been established.

Duration of Therapy

Most of the adjuvant trials used 1 year of treatment for the adjuvant treatment arms. Optimal treatment duration was examined in two trials: the NCI-INT protocol 089 and an NCCTG trial. These studies examined 12- and 6-month treatment courses for 5-FU/LV and 5-FU/levamisole. Reduction of treatment from 12 to 6 months for 5-FU/levamisole resulted in an 8% increase in mortality. No increase in mortality was noted comparing 12- and 6-month treatment with 5-FU/LV. Overall, 6 months of 5-FU/LV was shown to be equivalent to 1 year of 5-FU/levamisole. For 5-FU/LV, maximal benefit of adjuvant therapy for the patient is achieved with 6 months of therapy. The method of administration has been under some debate. However, the bolus regimens have been associated with higher incidence of toxicity; therefore, the protracted regimens of intravenous 5-FU or the oral fluoropyrimidine, capecitabine, are currently favored.

Adjuvant Therapy for Stage II Disease

Although adjuvant therapy has been proven to benefit patients with stage III disease, the issue of benefit for patients with stage II disease remains controversial. Although many of the adjuvant trials included patients with stage II disease, subgroup analysis shows trends toward benefit without reaching statistical significance. This issue has been addressed in three meta-analyses from NSABP, NCCTG, and IMPACT (International Multi-center Pooled Analysis of Colon cancer Trials). All have suggested marginal improvements in disease-free and overall survival with 5-FU and leucovorin in stage II colon cancer patients. Adjuvant chemotherapy in stage II patients provides a relative improvement in overall 5-year survival that was comparable to that of stage III patients (approximately 30% relative improvement). However, the absolute improvement in overall survival is only 2% to 7%. Therefore, the routine use of adjuvant chemotherapy for stage II patients is still not common practice. Generally, patients with stage II disease are offered chemotherapy if adverse prognostic features such as lymphovascular invasion, T4 status, obstruction, or poor differentiation are present. The determination of molecular and genetic prognostic markers that will be useful in selecting those stage II patients who would benefit most from routine use of adjuvant therapy is an area of active investigation.

Treatment of Locally Advanced Colon Cancer

Colon cancers that are adherent to adjacent structures have a 36% to 53% chance of local failure after complete resection. Approximately 10% of carcinomas present in this fashion. Strategies designed to reduce local recurrence would benefit these patients.

Surgical Strategy

Resection of colorectal cancer that has invaded adjacent structures involves en bloc resection of all involved structures; failure to do so results in significantly increased local recurrence and decreased survival. Importantly, all adhesions between the carcinoma and adjacent structures should be assumed to be malignant and not taken down because 33% to 84% are malignant when examined histologically. The affected organ should have resection limited to the involved area with a rim of normal tissue. A patient who has a margin-negative multivisceral resection has the same survival as a patient with no adjacent organ involvement on a stage-matched basis.

Adjuvant Radiation Therapy

Retrospective series have shown subsets of patients who have benefited from postoperative radiation therapy with or without 5-FU–based chemotherapy. Unfortunately, there are no consistent criteria to use in assessing increased risk of local failure. The value of adjuvant radiation therapy after complete resection of high-risk colon cancer is currently being evaluated in a randomized prospective fashion (NCCTG 91-46-52). In this trial, patients with B3 or C3 (modified Astler-Coller) tumors are randomized to receive postoperative 5-FU/levamisole or 5-FU/levamisole and radiation therapy. Patients with subtotally resected cancers fare worse than those with positive microscopic disease, as one would expect. It has been found that radiation therapy is more effective in microscopic than in macroscopic disease, and that it is more effective when combined with 5-FU. In a recent retrospective Mayo Clinic study of 103 mostly stage B3 and C3 (modified Astler-Coller) patients, in which 49% had no residual disease, 17% had microscopic residual disease, and 34% had gross residual disease; the local failure rate was 10% for patients with no residual disease, 54% for those with microscopic residual disease, and 79% for those with gross residual disease. More recently, improved local control with adjuvant radiation has been demonstrated in a small set of patients with T4 cancers with perforation or fistula. If there is any question regarding the ability to achieve a margin-negative resection, surgical clips should be used to outline the area of the tumor bed. If the margin is positive on final pathological studies, radiation should be administered with concomitant 5-FU–based chemotherapy.

MANAGEMENT OF RECTAL CANCER

The primary principle in the management of localized rectal cancer is similar to that for colon cancer (i.e., complete oncologic resection). In line with this principle are the goals of cancer control (negative margin resection of tumor, and resection of all draining lymph nodes), restoration of intestinal continuity, and preservation of anorectal sphincter, sexual, and urinary function. Achieving these goals is made difficult due to the anatomical constraints of the bony pelvis. Local control is clearly related to the adequacy of the surgical procedure. Although local control is critical for increasing the chances of cure, many patient- and tumor-related factors are associated with overall outcome. Data suggest that there is a significant surgeon- and center-related variability in patient outcome after treatment for rectal cancer. The Stockholm Rectal Cancer Study Group found that "specialists" and centers with higher volumes of rectal cancer cases had lower local failure rates and increased survival rates. It is not unusual to see local recurrence rates ranging from 3.7% to 43% in various series for curative surgical resection, with or without adjuvant therapy. Obviously, other factors are involved, such as methods of adjuvant therapy, patient selection, and disease factors. These varying results have hindered an accurate assessment of the vital components of an adequate oncologic operation and prevented an accurate assessment of the value of adjuvant chemoradiation in rectal cancer. Consequently, there are some who believe that with an adequate oncologic procedure by an experienced surgeon, only large T3 and T4 (fixed) lesions need adjuvant chemoradiation treatment. Treating all other T3 patients and those with N1–N2 disease merely attempts to make up for "bad surgery." Others contend that the significant decrease in local recurrence and possibly some improvement in survival associated with adjuvant radiation or chemoradiation justify its application in all patients with tumors that are T3 or greater, or those with node-positive disease. Nevertheless, surgical technique is critical to the success of the treatment of rectal cancer.

When planning surgical treatment of a rectal cancer, the rectum can be generally divided into three regions: lower, middle, and upper thirds. The upper rectum is generally defined as extending 11 to 15 cm from the anal verge. The length of the rectum varies significantly, depending on the size of the individual, and therefore these distinctions should be individualized. Tumors of the proximal rectum, at the level of the sacral promontory, behave similarly to colonic cancers and are therefore generally considered to be "rectosigmoid" cancers. Tumors 6 to 10 cm from the anal verge are defined as middle rectal cancers, and tumors from 0 to 5 cm are defined as low rectal cancers. Note that low rectal cancers can be associated with the internal and external sphincters, anal canal, or levator muscles, or can be above the pelvic floor.

Surgical Aspects

In addition to understanding the anatomical site of the tumor, it is important to understand the principles influencing the extent of radical extirpative surgery, regardless of the type of resection planned.

Resection Margin

Optimal treatment of all malignancies requires an adequate margin of resection. Histologic examination of the bowel wall distal to the gross rectal tumor reveals that only 2.5% of patients will have submucosal spread of disease greater than 2.5 cm. However, the most important margin is the radial margin. For many, particularly distal, rectal cancers, this is the most difficult margin to achieve. In 1986 Quirke et al. were the first to characterize the critical importance of the negative radial margin in preventing rectal cancer recurrence. In their series, the rate of local recurrence was 86% in the setting of a positive radial resection margin.

At MDACC, we try to obtain a distal resection margin of at least 2 cm. Irrigation of the rectal stump has not shown to affect recurrence and is not mandatory.

Lymphadenectomy

An adequate lymphadenectomy should be performed for accurate staging and local control, and should include proximal vascular ligation at the origin of the superior rectal vessels from the IMA just distal to the origin of the left colic. Spread from the primary tumor occurs along the mesorectum and in a lateral and upward direction. Therefore, although a 2-cm bowel margin is considered adequate for rectal cancer, the mesorectal margin should be at least 5 cm distal to the inferior aspect of the tumor or to the end of the mesorectum at the pelvic floor. The technique of total mesorectal excision (TME) provides an adequate lymphadenectomy for rectal cancer. It involves sharp excision and extirpation of the mesorectum by dissecting outside the investing fascia of the mesorectum. TME optimizes the oncologic operation by not only removing draining lymph nodes, but also maximizing lateral resection margins around the tumor. Although no randomized prospective trial has compared TME with conventional mesorectal excision, some institutions have shown a significant decrease in the local recurrence rate compared with historical controls using conventional surgery (in the range of 6.3%–7.3%). The major morbidity associated with TME is an increased rate of anastomotic leak believed to be due to devascularization of the rectal stump. Leak rates of 11% to 16% have been reported for TME as compared with 8% for non-TME resections done by the same group of surgeons.

The TME dissection can be facilitated by ligation of the IMA (and IMV) at or near its origin ("high ligation"). This allows for maximal mobilization of the proximal bowel to facilitate a tension-free distal low pelvic or coloanal anastomosis. The data on whether high ligation results in a decreased local recurrence remain equivocal. It has been well documented that negative lateral (radial) margins are major determinants of local recurrence and survival, and may be more important than longitudinal resection margins. Lateral margin clearance can be maximized by sharp dissection between the fascia propria of the mesorectum and the endopelvic fascia. The bony pelvis, which inherently limits the maximal extent of lateral dissection, may serve as the best explanation of why distal rectal cancers have a higher local recurrence rate than their more proximal counterparts when comparing patients with tumors of similar stage. It is controversial whether the entire mesorectum must be excised for all rectal cancers or whether the mesorectum can be sharply divided at the distal resection margin. At MDACC, we perform a *tumor-specific* mesorectal excision. The mesorectum is transected 5 cm distal to the distal aspect of the tumor. This would include the entire mesorectum for the lower and lower-middle rectal cancers, while preserving a portion of the mesorectum for the upper and upper-middle rectal cancers. This *tumor-specific* mesorectal excision does not compromise an adequate oncologic operation and may decrease the risk for anastomotic dehiscence from devascularization of the rectum. No benefit in survival or local disease control has been attainable with the use of more extended lymphadenectomy (iliac/periaortic nodes, obturator), and the complication rates are higher with these more extensive surgical procedures.

Surgical Approaches to Rectal Cancer

Surgical approaches to the rectum include transabdominal procedures (abdominoperineal resection [APR], low anterior resection [LAR], coloanal anastomosis [CAA]), transanal approaches, and trans-sacral approaches (York-Mason, Kraske). These latter two approaches will be discussed in detail in the section on local treatment of rectal cancer. APR, an operation devised by Ernest Miles in the 1930s, was the only previous treatment for all rectal cancers. With the advent of better preoperative staging, neoadjuvant therapy, and improved surgical techniques and stapler technology, the use of APR has decreased significantly. APR is now reserved for patients with primary sphincter dysfunction and incontinence, patients with direct tumor invasion into the sphincter complex, and patients with large or poorly differentiated lesions in the lower third of the rectum that do not have adequate tumor clearance for sphincter preservation.

Sphincter Preservation Procedures

Besides local excision, sphincter preservation procedures include LAR and proctectomy/CAA either alone or combined with neoadjuvant radiation and chemoradiation. Another option includes the addition of a colonic reservoir for improved short-term function. These procedures can only be performed if the oncologic result is not compromised and the functional results are acceptable. It was demonstrated more than 20 years ago that there is no difference in local recurrence rate or survival in patients with midrectal cancers who undergo LAR rather than APR. The technical feasibility of LAR in this setting was increased with the advent of circular stapling devices and the knowledge that distal mucosal margins of resection of 2 cm were adequate. Survival was found to depend on the distance of the tumor from the anal verge, the presence of positive lymph nodes, and the lateral extent of dissection. An alternative to LAR is proctectomy with CAA. It is used in low rectal cancers, with the stapled or hand-sewn anastomosis just above or at the dentate line. Temporary fecal diversion is routinely performed. The use of proctectomy and CAA for low rectal cancers is usually in the context of preoperative radiation or chemoradiation. Using either LAR or proctectomy with CAA (and adjuvant therapy), local recurrence rates of 3% to 6.5% have been reported by MDACC and others. Functional results have been good, with 60% to 86% of patients attaining continence by 1 year, 10% to 15% requiring laxative use, and some with mild soiling at night. Preoperative chemoradiation does not seem to have a negative impact on these functional results. Obviously, the lower the anastomosis (i.e., coloanal), the greater the potential for bowel dysfunction. Many patient factors are related to the decision to avoid a colostomy; however, there have been no randomized comparative studies of quality of life after coloanal anastomosis versus APR.

Colonic J Pouch

Although continence can be maintained in patients with a CAA, there is a degree of incontinence in some patients, and others require antidiarrheal agents. This is partly due to lack of compliance in the neorectum. This led to the introduction of the colonic J pouch for low rectal cancers that showed better results in terms of stool frequency, urgency, nocturnal movements, and continence than straight coloanal anastomoses. These advantages are principally during the first 12 to 24 months after which time functional improvements after straight anastomosis improves. One potential problem, especially when the pouch is longer than 5 or 6 cm, is difficulty in pouch evacuation (approximately 20% of patients). As in anterior resection, the functional outcome of patients with CAA (with or without a J pouch) may take 1 to 3 years to stabilize and is related to the level of the anastomosis (lower anastomoses tend to have poorer function). Unfortunately, many patients with low rectal cancers do not have enough room within the pelvis to accommodate a colonic J pouch. An alternative approach is a transverse coloplasty pouch in which a longitudinal incision on the neorectum proximal to the anastomosis is closed in a transverse fashion. Some studies comparing colonic J pouch reconstruction to transverse coloplasty pouch have demonstrated both similar functional results but slightly increased complication rates following the transverse coloplasty; however, other studies have shown equivalent outcomes. Postoperative radiation therapy has not been shown to have a significant adverse effect on pouch function.

Proximal Diversion

Proximal diversion after sphincter preservation is indicated in the following circumstances: (a) anastomosis less than 5 cm above the anal verge, (b) patients who have received preoperative radiation therapy, (c) patients on corticosteroids, (d) when the integrity of the anastomosis is in question, and (e) any case of intraoperative hemodynamic instability.

Local Approaches to Rectal Cancer

Local treatment alone as definitive therapy of rectal cancer was first applied to patients with severe coexisting medical conditions unable to tolerate radical surgery. Currently, conservative, sphincter-saving local approaches are being more widely considered. Early studies of local excision demonstrate up to a 97% local control rate and 80% disease-free survival for properly selected individuals. Local treatment is best applied to rectal cancers within 10 cm of the anal verge, tumors less than 3 cm in diameter involving less than one-fourth of the circumference of the rectal wall, exophytic tumors, tumors staged less than T2 by EUS, highly mobile tumors, and tumors of low histologic grade. The decision to use local excision alone or to employ adjuvant therapy after local excision is based on the pathological characteristics of the primary cancer (with negative margins) and the potential micrometastases in draining lymph nodes. T1 lesions have positive lymph nodes in up to 18% of cases, whereas the rate for T2 and T3 lesions is up to 38% and 70%, respectively. T2 tumors treated with local resection alone can have local recurrence rates of 15% to 44%. T1 lesions with poor prognostic features and all T2 tumors should be resected with radical surgery; however, when local excision is performed, adjuvant chemoradiation and close surveillance should also be performed. Two phase II cooperative group studies evaluated local excision for T1 lesions and local excision with adjuvant chemoradiation using a 5-FU–based regimen for T2 lesions. The CALGB trial evaluated 177 patients with a median 48 months of follow-up. At a median follow-up of 48 months, 59 patients with T1 lesions and 51 patients with T2 lesions met eligibility criteria. Four of 59 patients with T1 lesions (2 local, 1 local and distant, 1 distant) and 10 of 51 patients with T2 lesions (5 local, 2 local and distant, 3 distant) had recurrences. Overall and disease-free survival rates were 85% and 78%, respectively, at 48 months. The RTOG protocol 89–02 used a similar strategy with a median follow-up of 6.1 years in 52 patients with T1/T2 rectal cancers and demonstrated a 4% local failure rate for T1 lesions and 16% local failure rate for T2 lesions. An additional 3 of 13 (23%) patients with T3 disease treated with local excision and chemoradiation were noted to have local failure. This data should be considered in the background of data from the University of Minnesota that revealed a recurrence rate of 18% and 37% in patients undergoing local excision alone for T1 and T2 tumors, respectively.

Local therapy of distal rectal cancers can be accomplished by transanal excision, posterior proctectomy, fulguration, or endocavitary irradiation.

Transanal excision is the most straightforward approach to removing distal rectal cancers. The deep plane of the dissection is the perirectal fat. Tumors should be excised with an adequate circumferential margin.

Posterior proctotomy (Kraske procedure) can be used for tumors in the middle and upper rectum and is more suitable for larger, low rectal lesions. In this procedure, a perineal incision is made just above the anus, the coccyx is removed, and the fascia is divided. The rectum can then be mobilized for a sleeve resection, or a proctotomy is performed for excision of the tumor. The disadvantages of this procedure are fistula formation and the potential to seed the posterior wound with malignant cells.

Fulguration uses either standard electrocautery or laser to ablate the tumor. *Endocavitary radiation* is a high-dose, low-voltage irradiation technique that applies contact radiation to a small rectal cancer through a special proctoscope. Fulguration and endocavitary radiation are used for palliation and do not have a role in treatments with curative intent.

Transanal endoscopic microsurgery (TEM) provides accessibility to tumors of the middle and upper rectum that would otherwise require a laparotomy or transsacral approach, with improved visibility and instrumentation. This approach can be used for selected lesions up to 15 cm from the anal verge. Caution must be taken with higher lesions because full-thickness excision can result in perforation into the abdomen that will result in leakage of gas into the abdominal cavity and loss of rectal insufflation, as well as potential for injury to intraperitoneal organs. The procedure is technically demanding and requires special equipment, which is expensive and therefore has limited its acceptance in the United States. This procedure is not recommended for tumors within 5 cm of the anal verge. These tumors are optimally treated with a standard transanal approach. Patient selection is important, and it is recommended that patients have preoperative EUS to select superficial lesions. Patients with deeper lesions and metastatic disease or comorbid conditions that would preclude laparotomy are also candidates. Although local procedures have become more commonly used, few randomized prospective trials have evaluated oncologic and functional outcomes compared with anterior resection or APR. In 1996, Winde et al. prospectively randomized 50 patients with T1 adenocarcinoma of the rectum to either anterior resection or TEM. Similar local recurrence and survival rates, as well as decreased morbidity rates for local excision, were found in the two study arms, confirming the advantages of local excision.

At MDACC, transanal excision is used for low rectal cancers, whereas a Kraske procedure is used for higher rectal lesions. Optimal local excision includes at least a 1-cm resection margin circumferentially, a full-thickness excision, and an excision that is not fragmented or piecemeal. An inadequate local excision mandates an alternate resection strategy, not merely the addition of adjuvant therapy. If preoperative T stage is increased after pathological evaluation following local excision, the appropriate standard resection is recommended. T1 tumors are treated with local therapy alone unless any of the following poor prognostic features are identified: tumor greater than 4 cm, poorly differentiated histologic type, lymphatic or vascular invasion, or clinical or radiologic evidence of enlarged lymph nodes. Those T1 tumors with poor prognostic features and tumors T2 and greater are treated with radical surgery. T2 and T3 lesions are treated with local excision alone only if the patient refuses standard resection. Adjuvant chemoradiation treatment followed by chemotherapy is strongly recommended postoperatively.

Treatment for Locally Advanced Rectal Cancer

Occasionally, patients will present with involvement of adjacent structures (bladder, vagina, ureters, seminal vesicles, sacrum). These patients benefit from multimodality therapy, including preoperative or postoperative chemoradiation treatment. Intraoperative radiation therapy (IORT) or brachytherapy has been shown to provide additional benefit. The goal of surgical therapy is resection of the primary tumor, with en bloc resection of adjacent involved structures to obtain negative margins. The confines of the pelvis and the proximity to nerves and blood vessels that cannot be resected decrease the resectability of rectal tumors compared with locally advanced colon cancer. Improved resectability and decreased locoregional recurrence have been demonstrated for locally advanced rectal cancers after preoperative chemoradiation treatment. As reported by Gunderson et al. from the Mayo Clinic, the addition of IORT to standard external-beam radiation therapy with 5-FU in patients with locally advanced rectal cancer has shown significantly improved local disease control and possibly some improvement in survival. Preoperative chemoradiation has also been shown to improve rates of sphincter preservation in patients who were initially believed to need APR for curative resection by as much as twofold when compared with postoperative chemoradiation regimens. The best chance of cure in patients with locally advanced disease appears to involve preoperative chemoradiation treatment, maximal surgical resection, and IORT in selected cases.

At MDACC preoperative chemoradiation is standard treatment for locally advanced rectal cancer. An evaluation of 40 patients (29 with locally advanced disease; 11 with recurrence) requiring pelvic exenteration for local disease control with negative margins demonstrated that chemoradiation may significantly improve survival and that chemoradiation response and S-phase fraction were important determinants of survival. Patients with low-risk factors had a 65% 5-year survival, whereas high-risk patients had only a 20% survival. Table 11.6 summarizes the treatment strategy for patients with rectal cancer at MDACC.

Survival after Surgical Therapy

Seventy-five percent to 90% of node-negative rectal cancers are cured by radical surgical resection. Five-year disease-free survival in stage III patients remains approximately 60% or less. Local failure still remains a significant problem, although its risk has decreased in the era of TME.

The survival rate after local therapy varies from 70% to 86%, with recurrence rates of 10% to 50%. The overall local recurrence rate is 30%, and increasing recurrence rates are seen with increasing stage of disease and decreasing distance from the anal verge. Many of these patients can be salvaged with radical surgery after a local recurrence; however, survival after salvage surgery may not be as good as after initial curative radical surgery. When considering local therapy for rectal cancer, patient selection is of paramount importance.

Complications of Surgical and Adjuvant Therapy for Rectal Cancer

Complications of surgical and adjuvant therapy for rectal cancer include all complications associated with major abdominal surgery (e.g., bleeding, infection, adjacent organ injury, ureteral injury, bowel obstruction), with the addition of some complications that are unique to pelvic surgery. Specifically, anastomotic leak occurs in 5% to 10% of cases overall, with increasing rates seen in lower anastomoses, those associated with immunocompromised states, and those associated with preoperative radiation therapy. A defunctioning stoma will decrease the consequences of such a leak and may decrease leak incidence. At MDACC, a defunctioning loop ileostomy is used in all anastomoses below the peritoneal reflection in patients who have received preoperative radiotherapy and in patients with CAA. Autonomic nerve preservation is always performed during pelvic dissections, unless tumor involvement necessitates the sacrifice of these structures. With careful dissection during TME, 75% to 85% of patients have a return to preoperative sexual and urinary function. Other complications include urinary dysfunction, stoma dysfunction, perineal wound complications, hemorrhage from presacral vessels,

Table 11.6. Recommended surgical treatment strategy for rectal cancer

Location	T Stage	N Stage	Resection	Mesorectal Excision to
Upper rectum	T1	N0	TEM or Kraske	—
	≥T2	N0	LAR	5 cm distal to tumor
	T1–T2	N1–N2	± CXRT followed by LAR	5 cm distal to tumor
	≥T3	N0–N2	± CXRT followed by LAR	5 cm distal to tumor
Middle rectum	T1	N0	TAE, Kraske	—
	T2	N0	LAR[a]	5 cm distal to resection margin or entire
	T1–T2	N1–N2	CXRT followed by LAR[a]	5 cm distal to resection margin or entire
	≥T3	N0–N2	CXRT followed by LAR[a]	5 cm distal to resection margin or entire
Low rectum	T1	N0	TAE	—
	T2	N0	Proctectomy/CAA,[b] (± J pouch), APR	Entire
	T1–T2	N1–N2	CXRT followed by proctectomy/CAA,[b] (± J pouch), APR	Entire
	≥T3	N0–N2	CXRT followed by proctectomy/CAA,[b] (± J pouch), APR	Entire

TEM, transanal endoscopic microsurgery; LAR, low anterior resection; CXRT, preoperative chemoradiation; TAE, transanal excision; CAA, coloanal anastomosis; APR, abdominoperineal resection.

[a]LAR distal bowel resection margin >2 cm.

[b]CAA with protective ileostomy.

and anastomotic stricture. The mortality rate from surgical resection varies from less than 2% to 6%.

The complications associated with chemoradiation treatment include radiation enteritis and dermatitis, autonomic neuropathy, hematologic toxicity, stomatitis (mostly with continuous 5-FU infusions), and venous access infections. The frequency and intensity of these complications depend on multiple factors, including radiation therapy total dosing, fractionation, field technique, and whether the radiation therapy is given preoperatively or postoperatively. There are no good predictors of which patients will have these complications and to what degree they will have them.

Adjuvant Therapy of Rectal Cancer

The two main components of adjuvant therapy for rectal cancer are radiation therapy to the pelvis and 5-FU–based chemotherapy. The goal of chemotherapy is to increase tumor radiation sensitivity and to decrease the chance of distant failure. The goal of radiation therapy is to increase local control, and in the preoperative setting, to increase margin-negative resection rates and sphincter preservation. It must be emphasized that successful multimodality treatment of rectal cancer requires close collaboration between radiation therapists, medical oncologists, and surgeons.

Postoperative Radiation

Three randomized trials have been performed comparing surgery alone with surgery plus postoperative radiation therapy for T3 or N1–N2 rectal cancer. The only trial to show a decrease in local recurrence rate was the NSABP R-01 trial. Local recurrence was decreased from 25% in the surgical arm to 16% in the postoperative radiation therapy arm ($p = 0.06$). Several nonrandomized trials have shown a decrease in local recurrence rates to the 6% to 8% level; the differences between these trials may reflect radiotherapy dosing and patient selection. These trials showed that postoperative radiation therapy could reduce local recurrence, but total radiation therapy dose and technique were important to achieve this effect. Despite the performance of several large prospective trials, survival, and extrapelvic recurrence rates have not been improved consistently by radiation doses of 45 to 50 Gy. This prompted the addition of chemotherapy to radiation therapy in the postoperative period. The subsequent NSABP R-02 study was developed to answer remaining questions about combined modality therapy and MOF chemotherapy versus 5-FU–based regimens. In the NASBP R-02 study, radiotherapy improved local control to 8% from 13% without radiotherapy ($p = 0.02$). However, as in previous studies, no differences were seen in disease-free or overall survival with addition of radiation to chemotherapy alone.

Postoperative Radiation Therapy and Chemotherapy

The addition of chemotherapy to radiation therapy has been used to enhance the radiation responsiveness of tumors and impact distant failure. Several studies have shown both improved local control and survival. The Gastrointestinal Tumor Study Group trial was an early trial that compared the following treatment arms: (a) surgery alone, (b) surgery followed by postoperative radiotherapy (40–48 Gy), (c) surgery followed by postoperative chemotherapy (bolus 5-FU and semustine), and (d) surgery followed by concurrent chemotherapy and radiotherapy. It demonstrated a decrease in pelvic failure for the group treated by surgery and postoperative chemoradiation therapy (11% vs. 24% for surgery alone). In addition, a statistically significant survival advantage was found at 7 years using the combination of resection, radiation, and chemotherapy. The NCCTG subsequently conducted a trial randomizing 204 patients to radiotherapy (45–50.4 Gy in 25–28 fractions) with or without concurrent chemotherapy (bolus 5-FU). There was a significant decrease in pelvic recurrence (14% vs. 25%) and a significant decrease in cancer-related deaths for the group treated by resection, radiation, and chemotherapy compared with the group treated with resection and radiation therapy.

The findings from these studies prompted the publication of a clinical advisory by the NCI Consensus Conference in 1990 recommending adjuvant treatment for patients with Dukes B2 and C rectal carcinoma (T3–T4, N0; T3–T4, N1–N3, now stage II–III) consisting of six cycles of fluorouracil-based chemotherapy and concurrent radiation therapy to the pelvis. This regimen has remained the standard by which all current adjuvant rectal cancer protocols are compared. In the United States, postoperative chemoradiation is by far the most common mode of delivering adjuvant therapy. This is usually given as a continuous infusion of 5-FU and approximately 50.4 Gy of irradiation delivered to the pelvis in 1.8 to 2.0 Gy fractions (6-week treatment). Although the trend in Europe has been treatment with radiation therapy and no chemotherapy, the addition of chemotherapy in the United States has been shown to decrease the rate of distant metastases, something not attainable with radiation therapy alone. In addition, there has consistently been a 10% to 15% survival advantage when radiotherapy with chemotherapy is compared to radiotherapy alone. The Intergroup 0114 trial was designed to study the effects of biochemical modulation of 5-FU during radiotherapy. It demonstrated no significant survival advantage to the addition of levamisole and/or leucovorin to adjuvant bolus 5-FU and pelvic radiation in the postoperative period. Protracted infusion 5-FU has been compared to bolus 5-FU by the NCCTG and has been demonstrated to result in improved disease-free and overall survival. This finding has been confirmed in subsequent studies.

Preoperative Radiation Therapy (± Chemotherapy)

Several advantages to the use of preoperative compared with postoperative radiation therapy have been identified:

1. A reduction in tumor size increases rates of sphincter preservation in those patients initially deemed to require an APR and improves overall resectability.
2. There is a decreased risk of local failure due to improved compliance with the chemoradiation regimen and improved tumor response in the preoperative setting.

3. There is a decreased risk of toxicity because the small bowel can more readily be excluded from the radiation field in a preoperative setting.
4. There is less bowel dysfunction because the colon used for reconstruction is not in the radiation field.
5. There is no delay of therapy as in some cases of postoperative therapy due to operative morbidity.

Until now, there have been several randomized trials evaluating the role of preoperative radiation therapy in resectable rectal cancer. Although most report significant decreases in local recurrence, only the 1997 Swedish Rectal Cancer Trial has shown a significant survival advantage for the total patient group. This trial gave short-course radiotherapy (25 Gy in five fractions, 1 week), followed by curative resection to the experimental group, and curative surgery alone to the control group. The local recurrence rate and 9-year disease-specific survival were 11% and 74%, respectively, versus 27% and 65% for the control group. One limitation of this study compared to more recent trials is the lack of surgical quality control, which is believed to be the reason for the high local recurrence rate in the control group. This was addressed in the Dutch Colorectal Cancer Group trial in which more than 1,800 patients with rectal cancer located within 15 cm from the anal verge were randomized to receive preoperative short-course radiotherapy followed by TME versus TME alone. The local recurrence rate in the surgery alone group was 8.2%. Preoperative radiotherapy improved this to 2.4%. However, there was no difference in overall survival. Also, subgroup analysis of data from this trial showed no significant benefit for irradiation of lesions located in the upper rectum greater than 10 cm from the anal verge ($p = 0.17$).

In the United States, preoperative radiation therapy trials have usually included chemotherapy in a more protracted course rather than using short-course radiotherapy alone. This practice has been based on data demonstrating the importance of the addition of chemotherapy to radiation in the adjuvant setting. Moreover, generally a 6-week interval is given after the completion of chemoradiation before surgery. Longer intervals after radiotherapy have been associated with improved pathological complete response rates. Two multicentered randomized trials have attempted to address the question of preoperative versus postoperative chemoradiation for rectal cancer, RTOG 94-01 and NSABP R-03. However, both have been closed due to a failure to accrue patients. The most definitive randomized data demonstrating the superiority of preoperative versus postoperative chemoradiation comes from the German Rectal Cancer Study Group. Four-hundred and twenty-one patients with tumors located within 16 cm from the anal verge were randomly assigned to preoperative long-course radiation (50.4 Gy in 28 fractions) with concurrent infusional 5-FU (1,000 mg/m^2/d) during weeks 1 and 5 followed by TME or to TME followed by postoperative radiation (45 Gy in 25 fractions) and concurrent infusional 5-FU. All patients in the preoperative group and those patients with stage II or greater disease in the postoperative group also received four cycles of bolus 5-FU in the adjuvant setting. Patients assigned to the preoperative arm had a lower 5-year cumulative risk of local failure (6% vs. 13%, $p = 0.006$), and decreased toxicity, both severe acute (27% vs. 40%, $p = 0.001$) and late (14% vs. 24%, $p = 0.01$). Moreover, improved sphincter preservation rates were noted in those patients who were initially deemed to require APR (39% vs. 19%, $p = 0.004$), preoperative versus postoperative, respectively. However, there was no difference in survival between the two arms.

The main disadvantage of the preoperative regimens is that approximately 20% of patients with rectal cancer will be preoperatively overstaged, and therefore may undergo potentially unnecessary radiation and chemotherapy. In the German study, 20% of the patients randomized to the postoperative arm were noted to actually have stage I disease once the specimen was available for evaluation. These patients do not need adjuvant therapy and would have been overtreated if they were treated preoperatively. Recently, a number of groups have demonstrated efficacy of the oral fluoropyrimidine, capecitabine, as the chemotherapeutic radiation sensitizer in neoadjuvant regimens. Capecitabine has the advantages of convenient oral administration and reduced toxicity when compared to intravenous 5-FU. The NSABP R-04 study hopes to address this issue in a multi-institutional trial.

Intraoperative Radiation Therapy

IORT is used for both recurrent and locally advanced rectal cancer. Its advantages include increased local control in high-risk cancers, accurate treatment of focal areas at risk, ability to adjust the depth of the radiation beam, and ability to shield sensitive structures. Even preoperative chemoradiation in high-risk tumors can result in high local recurrence rates. IORT allows treatment of areas with close or microscopically positive margins in this situation. At the Massachusetts General Hospital, IORT is used for focal areas of tumor adherence, close or positive margins, and areas of gross residual disease. IORT dosing depends on the clinical situation: 10 to 13 Gy is given for close margins (<5 mm), 15 Gy is given for microscopically positive margins, and 17 to 20 Gy is used for areas of gross residual disease. In a recent 2-year analysis of IORT in the RTOG study of locally advanced disease, the local control rate was 77%, with a 2-year survival of 88% and a complication rate of 16%. For facilities able to deliver this type of therapy, there is a clear advantage in local control in select patients with advanced and recurrent disease. An alternative approach is intraoperative brachytherapy. This allows radiation access in areas where the IORT beam cannot be focused due to anatomical constraints of the pelvis. At MDACC, intraoperative brachytherapy (10–20 Gy) is used selectively in patients with locally advanced or recurrent disease where there is a close or positive margin as demonstrated by frozen section.

M. D. Anderson Experience

Our preferred management of locally advanced rectal cancer (T3–T4, N0, or any T, N1–N2) includes preoperative radiation therapy with a protracted intravenous infusion of 5-FU or capecitabine.

We deliver 45 Gy of preoperative radiation therapy in 25 fractions with a boost to the tumor bed of 5.4 Gy in 3 fractions for a total of 50.4 Gy in 28 fractions. A continuous infusion of 5-FU at a dose of 300 mg/m^2/d or capecitabine 850 mg/m^2/d is given 5 days per week. Surgery is performed 6 to 8 weeks after completion of therapy. With this regimen, more than 60% of patients experience a T-stage decrease and 11% achieve a pathological complete response. In patients with T3 disease, 44% of patients with rectal cancers located within 3 cm of the anal verge are now able to undergo sphincter-preserving procedures, with a local control rate in excess of 90% and a 3-year survival rate of 88% in node-negative patients. In patients with fixed T3 and T4 tumors, the same regimen was used with the addition of an IORT boost for positive or close margins. The local control rate was 97% with an 82% 5-year survival.

Although some institutions will advocate TME alone for most rectal cancers, surgeons globally are now looking to identify those patients who will benefit most from adjuvant therapy and what therapy should be used (chemotherapy and radiation therapy dosing). Ongoing studies are investigating combinations of different agents and the timing of surgery following multimodal therapy in an effort to improve the pathological response rate. The role of local excision with multimodal therapy is still controversial, particularly in the era of newer biologically active chemotherapeutic agents. Some centers are exploring the use of IORT and brachytherapy as adjuncts to neoadjuvant chemoradiation treatments to increase the local disease control in select patients who are at high risk for local recurrence. Various molecular markers are being evaluated in fresh or archival specimens to aid in identifying patients who will benefit from treatment.

SURVEILLANCE

Patients with a history of colorectal carcinoma require close surveillance. The data to support this, however, are lacking. In a Danish prospective randomized study in 597 colorectal cancer patients, patients had either close follow-up (every 6 months for the first 3 years) or yearly for 3 years (including examination/stool heme test, colonoscopy, laboratory testing [except CEA], and chest radiograph). The frequency of recurrent cancer was the same in both groups, but it was diagnosed earlier in the close follow-up group. The close follow-up group had more resections for curative intent (local and distant), but cancer-specific survival differences have been more difficult to demonstrate. Multiple surveillance regimens have been advocated by several national societies. In general, close follow-up including CEA level determination during the first 2 years followed by less intensive follow-up during years 3 to 5 are advocated.

History and physical examination and laboratory tests including a CEA are performed at MDACC every 3 to 4 months for the first 2 years after surgery, every 6 months during years 3 through 5, and yearly thereafter. Colonoscopy should be performed after 1 year, and then at 3 years if normal. A baseline CT scan of the abdomen and pelvis is obtained preoperatively followed by annual intervals unless otherwise indicated by disease biology. A chest radiograph is obtained every 6 months for the first

2 years and yearly thereafter. It has traditionally been proposed that patients should be monitored closely for local recurrence during the first 2 years postoperatively (the time at which most local recurrences appear). Recent data show that the addition of adjuvant radiation therapy may extend this period of vulnerability such that 50% of local recurrences may occur more than 2 years from surgery. Finally, it should be noted that these are *general* guidelines that may need to be tailored to individual patients.

RECURRENT AND METASTATIC DISEASE

More than 50% of patients who undergo curative surgery for colorectal cancer have tumor recurrences. Of the patients who have recurrences, 85% do so during the first 2.5 years after surgery. The remaining 15% experience recurrence during the subsequent 2.5 years. Recurrence develops in less than 5% of patients who are disease-free at 5 years. The risk of recurrence is higher with stage II or III disease. Other recurrence risk modifiers include race, presentation, grade of tumor, aneuploidy, and adjacent organ invasion. Many molecular markers are currently being evaluated for their usefulness in predicting recurrence risk. Recurrences may be local, regional, or distant. Distant disease recurrence, the most common presentation, occurs either alone or concomitantly with locoregional recurrence. Local recurrence develops in 20% to 30% of patients who undergo initial curative resections for rectal cancer, and in 50% to 80% of these patients, the local recurrence is the only site of disease. For all recurrence sites, complete resection results in a 25% to 30% cure rate. Recurrence isolated to the anastomosis (intramural) is rare and can indicate inadequate surgical resection. Liver involvement occurs in approximately 50% of patients with colon cancer, whereas lung, bone, and brain involvement occurs in 10%, 5%, and less than 5%, respectively. Symptomatic recurrences present with a constellation of symptoms ranging from the vague and nonspecific to the clinically overt.

CEA is invaluable for postoperative monitoring. It is most useful in patients in whom levels are increased preoperatively and return to normal following surgery. Levels should be determined preoperatively, 6 weeks postoperatively, and then according to the schedule described in the surveillance section. The absolute level and rate of increase in CEA and the patient's clinical status are important in determining prognosis and treatment. Postoperative CEA levels that do not normalize within 4 to 6 weeks suggest incomplete resection or recurrent disease, although false-positive results do occur. CEA levels that normalize postoperatively and then start to increase are indicative of recurrence. This may represent occult or clinically obvious disease. A rapidly increasing CEA level suggests liver or lung involvement, whereas a slow, gradual rise is associated with locoregional disease. Despite the reliability of an increased CEA level in predicting tumor recurrence, 20% to 30% of patients with locoregionally recurrent tumors have a normal CEA level. Poorly differentiated tumors may not make CEA, which is one explanation for such false-negative results. In contrast, CEA is increased in 80% to 90% of patients with hepatic recurrences. A prospective randomized trial of the value of CEA in follow-up was undertaken in 311 patients and reported by McCall et al. The study followed asymptomatic patients with increased CEA levels until symptoms developed; then, a full workup was initiated. The purpose was to define the "natural history" of an elevated CEA. The sensitivity, specificity, and positive predictive values of an increased CEA level were 58%, 93%, and 79%, respectively. The median lead-time of the increased CEA to detection by other means was 6 months, a result found in other studies. Seven percent of patients who had an increased CEA failed to have identifiable recurrent disease on workup. Two meta-analyses have been performed pooling results from five randomized studies and found a survival advantage in patients allocated to intensive follow-up, including CEA. The German Colorectal Cancer Study Group evaluated follow-up CEA levels in 1,321 patients after curative resection. They determined that CEA monitoring was beneficial in 47% of patients with recurrence and 11% of patients overall; however, only 2.3% underwent a curative R0 resection of recurrent disease. A more recent analysis of data from a UK multicenter randomized prospective trial of protracted infusion 5-FU versus bolus 5-FU in the adjuvant setting demonstrated that both CT and CEA were valuable components for postoperative follow-up and resulted in improved survival.

In an effort to improve the detection of recurrences, *radiolabeled monoclonal antibodies* (mAb) directed against tumor-specific antigens and CEA have been used for imaging the extent and location of metastases with disappointing results. This modality is particularly useful in the evaluation of recurrent disease where postsurgical or postradiation changes are not easily differentiated from tumor on CT or MRI. One agent OncoScint CR/OV (Cytogen Corp., Princeton, NJ) is an indium-111–labeled mAb to B72.3 that targets the tumor-associated glycoprotein TAG-72, which is reactive with approximately 83% of colorectal tumors. A technetium labeled anti-CEA preparation is also available (CEA-Scan). These agents were found to be superior to CT in evaluating extrahepatic and pelvic disease, whereas CT was better for detecting metastatic disease to the liver. Most studies of labeled mAbs show a sensitivity range of 70% to 86%, with a higher specificity, and positive predictive values greater than 90%. These studies are most useful for the detection of recurrent disease in a patient with an increasing CEA level and negative radiographic workup, or to rule out metastatic disease in a patient with locoregional recurrence who may be suitable for surgical therapy (i.e., hepatic resection/cryotherapy, pelvic exenteration).

Recently, PET with 2-(^{18}F)fluorodeoxy-D-glucose (FDG) has been reported to have an 89% positive predictive value and 100% negative predictive value in patients who had a rising CEA and normal conventional radiography. FDG-PET imaging relies on the increased metabolic uptake of glucose (fluorine-labeled analog of 2-deoxyglucose or FDG) in tumors compared with normal tissues and may be able to distinguish postsurgical and postradiation changes from recurrent tumor. It has also been shown to be effective at identifying resectable recurrences in a prospective blinded study of second-look laparotomy.

Treatment of the asymptomatic patient with an increased CEA level can be challenging. An increased level should be confirmed by a repeat CEA determination. A thorough clinical investigation should include LFTs; CT scan of the chest, abdomen, pelvis, and brain (when indicated); and colonoscopy. At MDACC, we routinely monitor CEA values because of the potential to detect resectable metastases, especially within the liver, in a subgroup of patients who may benefit from early recurrence detection. PET scans are performed to evaluate patients with rising CEA values where conventional radiography is not able to identify the site of recurrence.

If the metastatic evaluation is negative in the face of an increased CEA level, a second-look laparotomy may be indicated. In older studies, approximately 60% to 90% of patients with asymptomatically increased CEA levels will have recurrent disease at laparotomy; 12% to 60% of these patients will have resectable disease at the time of laparotomy; and 30% to 40% will survive 5 years following resection of the recurrence. Early detection of asymptomatic disease results in a higher resectability rate than when resection is performed for symptomatic disease (60% vs. 27%). The liver is the most common site of recurrence, followed by adjacent organs, the anastomotic site, and the mesentery. Resectability rates correspond to the level of CEA elevation, with CEA levels less than 11 ng per mL being associated with higher resectability rates.

Treatment

The appropriate treatment of resectable recurrent disease depends on the location of disease. If two disease sites are detected that are completely resectable, the procedure is undertaken in select patients. Otherwise, individual treatment modalities are used as needed for palliation of pelvic symptoms. As in locally advanced disease, potentially resectable recurrent disease is treated in a multimodality fashion using preoperative chemotherapy (with our without radiation), surgery, IORT (if available), and brachytherapy. For recurrence involving the sacrum, en bloc sacral resection can sometimes result in 4-year survival rates of 30%. Contraindications to sacral resection include pelvic sidewall involvement, sciatic notch involvement, bilateral S2 involvement, encasement of iliac vessels, and extrapelvic disease. A review of pelvic recurrence at Memorial Sloan-Kettering Cancer Center revealed no predictors either in the initial tumor or in the recurrent tumor to indicate survival other than complete resection. Symptoms of recurrent disease could be adequately palliated with surgery. At MDACC, potentially resectable pelvic recurrences are treated with preoperative chemoradiation, followed by surgery and the use of IORT and brachytherapy as needed for close or positive margins. Using this approach in 43 patients, the overall resection rate was 77%, with an 88% margin-negative resection rate, a 64% local control rate, and a 58% 5-year survival rate. Although the usual surgical procedure for resectable recurrent rectal cancer is APR, select cases can be treated with sphincter preservation.

Median survival for metastatic colorectal cancer without systemic chemotherapy ranges from 6 to 9 months in early series.

The addition of 5-FU–based regimens improves survival to 10 to 12 months. The addition of irinotecan or oxaliplatin to 5-FU further improves survival to 14 to 17 months. As described previously, the addition of the monoclonal antibodies have improved median survival to greater than 20 months.

Liver

The liver is the most common site of visceral metastases, and it is the only site affected in up to 20% of patients. Recent data from MDACC demonstrates that surgical resection of hepatic metastases now offers the potential for 5-year survival up to 58%. Colorectal hepatic metastases are discussed in detail in Chapter 12.

Lung

Pulmonary metastases occur in 10% to 20% of patients with colorectal cancer. They are most commonly seen in the setting of a large hepatic tumor burden or extensive metastatic disease. Isolated pulmonary metastases occur most commonly with distal rectal lesions because the venous drainage of the distal rectum bypasses the portal system and allows metastasis to travel directly to the lungs.

The finding of a solitary lesion on a chest radiograph should prompt evaluation with thoracic CT scanning and, for a centrally located lesion, bronchoscopy with biopsy. Peripheral lesions may be amenable to CT-guided needle biopsy or video-assisted thoracoscopic surgery. Fifty percent of patients with solitary pulmonary nodules will have primary lung tumors rather than colorectal metastases.

Patients with locally controlled primary tumors, no evidence of metastases elsewhere, good pulmonary reserve, and good medical condition are candidates for resection. Patients with solitary metastases experience the best survival, but patients with as many as three lesions (unilateral or bilateral) can experience up to a 40% 5-year survival. The optimum surgical approach is a median sternotomy to allow for bilateral pulmonary exploration because contrast-enhanced CT scan has up to a 25% false-negative and false-positive rate for the detection of metastases. As in liver resection for metastatic disease, the optimum surgery involves the minimal procedure to obtain negative margins (i.e., wedge resection vs. pneumonectomy).

The overall 5-year survival rate following resection of pulmonary metastases ranges from 20% to 40%. In newer series involving only colorectal cancer metastases, the rate is closer to 40% to 43% 5-year survival. Age, gender, location of the primary disease, disease-free interval, or involvement of hilar or mediastinal lymph nodes does not seem to influence survival. The number of metastases in most series is inversely correlated with 5-year survival. Recurrence confined to the lung after resection is an indication by some for repeat resection.

Bone and Brain

Metastatic disease to the brain is uncommon and usually occurs after established lung involvement. Symptomatic solitary lesions can be treated by palliative craniotomy and resection. In a very small subpopulation of patients, cranial disease may be the only site of involvement, and excision in this setting may increase survival. Bone metastases are quite uncommon and are best managed with radiation therapy.

Ovary

Because 1% to 8% of women who undergo potentially curative resections subsequently develop ovarian metastases, prophylactic oophorectomy at the time of colectomy has been considered for female patients. However, prophylactic oophorectomy has not been shown to improve survival and therefore is not routinely performed. The preliminary results of a prospective randomized trial of 155 patients at the Mayo Clinic reported an initial trend toward improved survival with prophylactic oophorectomy; however, this difference did not persist at 5 years, and the trial results have not since been updated. When isolated metastatic disease to the one ovary is identified, a bilateral oophorectomy is performed because there is a high risk for bilateral involvement.

Pelvis

Local recurrence in the pelvis is a major problem after treatment for rectal cancer. Radical surgical procedures, including pelvic exenteration and sacrectomy, may benefit a select group of patients whose disease can be completely extirpated by these procedures. Preoperative chemoradiation, even in the setting of prior radiation, IORT, and brachytherapy, is useful in the setting of radical surgery for recurrent disease.

UNCOMMON COLORECTAL TUMORS

Lymphoma

Lymphoma is an uncommon tumor that occurs in 0.4% of patients with intestinal lymphoma presenting anywhere between the second and eighth decades. Almost all are non-Hodgkin lymphomas. Twenty-five percent of patients may present with fever, occult blood loss, anemia, a palpable mass, or an acute abdomen. The diagnosis is often made intraoperatively. A history of abdominal pain, fever, and weight loss in a patient who is younger than the expected age for a colorectal tumor should raise the suspicion of intestinal lymphoma.

Abdominal CT and endoscopy with biopsy are the most useful diagnostic tests because lesions are often missed on barium enema examination. A thickened bowel, adjacent organ extension, or nodal enlargement may be seen. If the lesion is intraluminal, endoscopic biopsy will facilitate the diagnosis. Most of these lesions are intermediate- to high-grade B-cell lymphomas. If a diagnosis is made preoperatively in an otherwise asymptomatic patient, bone marrow biopsy should be performed. A primary lesion is defined as a lesion with no associated organ or lymphatic involvement, negative chest CT, and a negative peripheral blood smear and bone marrow.

Surgery is performed in the clinical setting of obstruction, bleeding, perforation, or an uncertain diagnosis. In rare cases, surgery may be performed for complete resection of a primary lesion. A thorough exploration is performed, and all suspicious nodes or organs are biopsied to assess the stage of disease. The primary intestinal lesion should be resected with negative margins whenever possible. The bowel mesentery should be resected with the tumor so regional nodes can be assessed pathologically. Intestinal continuity should be restored whenever possible. If a large tumor is found to be unresectable and is not obstructing the bowel, a bypass can be performed. Surgical clips should be placed to facilitate identification of the tumor by the radiation oncologist.

Intestinal lymphoma requires a combined-modality approach using surgery and chemotherapy with or without radiation. For rectal lymphoma, complete resection is followed by radiation treatments to the pelvis. Chemoradiation is used if the resection was incomplete. The overall survival for stages I and II disease is approximately 80%. This decreases to 35% with advanced disease.

Gastrointestinal Stromal Tumors

Gastrointestinal stromal tumors (GISTs) account for most mesenchymal tumors arising in the wall of the colon or rectum. Primary colorectal GISTs are rare and comprise less than 1% of colonic tumors. GISTs have recently been characterized, but historically classified, as leiomyomas, leiomyosarcomas, neurofibromas, and schwannomas, and are further discussed in detail elsewhere in this text. In a review of 1,458 cases of malignant GISTs from 1992 to 2000 in the SEER database, 7% were located in the colon and 5% in the rectum. These tumors can present as small submucosal or as large intramural masses. Patients can present with pain, bleeding, obstruction, nausea, vomiting, anemia, tenesmus, or hematuria. Ulceration may be present in 30% to 50% of patients. A thorough clinical evaluation should be conducted to exclude metastatic disease. Excision with negative surgical margins is the treatment of choice. Colonic tumors are excised with adjacent mesentery. Wide nodal excision is not indicated in the absence of clinically evident disease. Small tumors of the rectum and anal canal can be removed transrectally or endoscopically. Criteria similar to GISTs elsewhere in the gastrointestinal tract are used for determining the need for adjuvant therapy with imatinib mesylate (STI-571, Gleevec), a monoclonal antibody to the tyrosine kinase receptor. Further details regarding GISTS are discussed in Chapter 5.

Carcinoid

Carcinoids are neuroendocrine tumors derived from Kulchitsky's cells, which are uncommonly found in the colon and rectum. Approximately 18% to 30% of intestinal carcinoids occur in the rectum or rectosigmoid, 4% to 15% occur in the colon, and 4% to 50% have been reported to occur in the appendix. They are usually discovered incidentally unless they are large. Size and depth of invasion are the best predictors of clinical behavior. Hindgut carcinoids almost never produce the carcinoid syndrome. Although large tumors may present with bleeding, obstruction, or constipation, tumors less than 2 cm are frequently asymptomatic. Diagnosis is made by endoscopic biopsy. In general, tumors less than 1 cm rarely metastasize, whereas those greater than 2 cm have increased metastatic potential; in the 1- to 2-cm range, 10% to 20% will metastasize. This makes treatment decisions for tumors in the 1- to 2-cm range problematic. Small lesions (<1 cm) are commonly well differentiated and can be adequately treated with endoscopic excision. Lesions less than 2 cm can be treated with full-thickness local excision. It is recommended that larger lesions, those that demonstrate invasion through the muscle wall, or inadequate resection margins be treated with standard resection techniques using either an anterior approach or APR. However, a recent retrospective review from this institution on 44 rectal carcinoids revealed that extensive surgery offered no survival advantage over local excision. At MDACC, we locally excise tumors less than 2 cm and resect those greater than 2 cm if sphincter preservation is possible. The experience with radiation therapy and chemotherapy in rectal carcinoids is currently inadequate to make recommendations regarding its use.

ANAL CANCER

Squamous Carcinoma of the Anus

Epidemiology and Etiology

Anal SCC is a relatively uncommon cancer with an annual incidence of approximately 9 per million in the United States and an estimated 3,400 new cases in 2000. However, this represents a near doubling in recent decades. Since the mid 1970s, the incidence has increased 96% in men and 39% in women. The incidence is of epidemic proportions in men who have sex with men (MSM), reaching 35/100,000, and among the HIV-positive population where the incidence is reported to be twice that of HIV-negative MSM (70/100,000). Other causes of immunocompromise such as transplantation or immunotherapy for autoimmune diseases are additional risk factors. Kidney transplant patients have at least a fourfold increased incidence of the disease. In the general population, elderly women and men in their sixties are at the highest risk for anal cancer, with women having the greater risk.

Population-based evidence has established that anal cancer is a sexually transmitted disease (STD) in much the same way that cervical cancer is an STD. Women with anal cancer are more likely to have had a history of genital warts or other STDs and men with anal cancer are more likely to have reported homosexual activity or to have a history of genital warts or gonorrhea. As with cervical cancer, anal cancer has been linked to human papillomavirus (HPV) infection. Studies have shown that 40% to 95% of anal cancers harbor HPV DNA, with the strongest association seen with nonkeratinizing squamous cell types originating from the squamous mucosa of the anal canal. This association has proven to be even stronger with advances in HPV detection techniques.

The national cancer registries in Denmark and Sweden identified 417 patients with anal cancer between 1991 and 1994 and compared them with 534 controls with rectal adenocarcinoma and 554 population controls. Using multivariate analysis adjusting for smoking and education, the lifetime number of sexual partners; history of anal intercourse; a history of anogenital warts, gonorrhea, or cervical neoplasia; testing for HIV; and a history of partners with STDs were all associated with a significantly increased risk for anal cancer in women. Risk factors for men included lifetime number of sexual partners, homosexuality, history of anal warts or syphilis, and being unmarried with or without a current sexual partner. The associations were similar when data from Denmark and Sweden were considered separately or together. When polymerase chain reaction for HPV DNA was performed on archived tissue specimens from these patients, 88% of patients overall were positive for HPV, and HPV-16 was identified in 83% of those with HPV. This compares to cervical cancer where HPV-16 is responsible for about 50% of cases, HPV 18, 31, and 45 is responsible for an additional 30% and additional HPV types account for the remaining 20% of cases. Analysis of the data from the SEER program revealed that the relative risks of anal cancer and vaginal cancer in women who had been diagnosed with invasive cervical cancer were 4.6 and 5.6, respectively. This increased risk for anal cancer in women with cervical dysplasia or cancer, and their sexual partners, is likely through autoinoculation by the virus that caused the cervical dysplasia.

Anal cancers can be located within the anal canal or in the perianal skin (anal margin). Anal canal cancers are three to four times more common in women than in men. Anal margin cancers (tumors of the hair-bearing perianal skin) are more common in males. There are significantly more cases of anal margin cancers in homosexual males.

Pathological Characteristics

More than 80% of malignant anal lesions are histologically SCCs. With the exception of melanoma, small cell carcinoma, and anal adenocarcinoma, all other histologic subtypes behave similarly and are treated according to their anatomical location. Basaloid carcinoma (basal cell carcinoma with a massive squamous component), mucoepidermoid carcinoma (originating in anal crypt glands), and cloacogenic carcinoma are all variants of squamous carcinoma. As with cervical cancer, SCC of the anus may be preceded by or coexist with premalignant dysplasia or anal intraepithelial neoplasia.

The prognosis of anal margin cancers is favorable. The rate of local recurrence is higher than the rate of distant metastases, which are rare. When they do occur, metastases are most commonly found in the superficial inguinal lymph nodes (approximately 15% of cases). It is unusual for anal margin cancers to metastasize to mesenteric or internal iliac nodes.

Anal canal cancers are associated with aggressive local growth and if untreated will extend to the rectal mucosa and submucosa, subcutaneous perianal tissue and perianal skin, ischiorectal fat, local skeletal muscle, perineum, genitalia, lower urinary system, and even the pelvic peritoneum and the broad ligament. Historically, mesenteric lymph node metastases have been detected in 30% to 50% of surgical specimens. More than 50% of patients will present with locally advanced disease. The most common sites of distant metastases are the liver, lung, and abdominal cavity. However, most cancer-related deaths are due to uncontrolled pelvic or perineal disease.

Diagnosis

The initial symptoms of anal cancer include bleeding, pain, and local fullness. These symptoms are similar to those caused by the common benign anal diseases, which accompany anal cancer in more than 50% of cases. A detailed history, including previous anal pathology and sexual habits, should precede a meticulous physical examination. Physical examination should attempt to identify the lesion, its size and anatomical boundaries, and any associated scarring or condylomata. It is also important to determine the resting and voluntary anal sphincter tone. Occasionally, an examination under general anesthesia may be necessary to complete the local evaluation. Pelvic and abdominal CT scans and a chest radiograph are important in assessing extent of local disease and distant spread. Proctosigmoidoscopy is essential to assess the proximal extent of disease and to obtain tissue for biopsy. Palpable inguinal lymph nodes should be evaluated by fine-needle aspiration.

Staging

The current American Joint Committee on Cancer (AJCC) staging system for anal margin and anal canal cancers is depicted in Tables 11.7 and 11.8.

Treatment

ANAL CANAL. Until the 1980s, APR with permanent colostomy was the recommended treatment for all SCCs of the anal canal. This treatment, however, was attended by low survival rates as a result of distant failure. Radiation therapy in the range of 50 to 60 Gy was also used as definitive treatment of these cancers, with recurrence and survival rates similar to those seen using APR. The pioneering chemoradiation protocol developed by Nigro et al. in 1983, which has since been confirmed and modified by others, has radically changed the approach to this disease. Currently, surgery is reserved for (a) T1 and small T2 lesions, which may be locally excised; (b) salvage treatment for patients with persistent disease (within 6 months of chemoradiation) or recurrent disease (after 6 months); (c) severely symptomatic patients (perineal sepsis, intractable urinary or fecal fistulae, intolerable incontinence); (d) inguinal lymph node dissection for persistent inguinal disease, recurrent inguinal disease (treated first with radiation therapy unless associated with local recurrence), or primary disease in the inguinal basin, where the disease is bulky or fungating; and (e) temporary fecal diversion in patients with nearly obstructing lesions.

Since the initial work of Nigro et al. in 1983, studies have been performed to dissect out the vital components and doses of the chemoradiation treatments to optimize treatment. There is evidence that (a) higher doses of radiation produce better local control rates using a constant mitomycin-C dose (Rich, 1997); (b) 5-FU and mitomycin-C with radiation therapy produces better local control rates than radiation therapy alone; (c) 5-FU, mitomycin-C with radiation therapy produces better local control rates than 5-FU with radiation therapy; and (d) cisplatin with 5-FU and radiation therapy produces local control and survival

Table 11.7. American Joint Committee on Cancer staging of anal canal cancer

Primary tumor (T)

TX	Primary tumor cannot be assessed
T0	No evidence of primary tumor
Tis	Carcinoma in situ
T1	Tumor $\leq$2 cm in greatest dimension
T2	Tumor >2 cm but not >5 cm in greatest dimension
T3	Tumor >5 cm in greatest dimension
T4	Tumor of any size invades adjacent organ(s)

Lymph nodes (N)

NX	Regional lymph nodes cannot be assessed
N0	No regional lymph node metastasis
N1	Metastasis in perirectal lymph node(s)
N2	Metastasis in unilateral internal iliac and/or inguinal lymph node(s)
	Metastasis in perirectal and inguinal lymph nodes and/or bilateral internal iliac and/or inguinal lymph nodes

Distant metastasis (M)

MX	Presence of distant metastasis cannot be assessed
M0	No distant metastasis
M1	Distant metastasis

Stage grouping

0	Tis	N0	M0
I	T1	N0	M0
II	T2	N0	M0
	T3	N0	M0
IIIA	T1	N1	M0
	T2	N1	M0
	T3	N1	M0
	T4	N0	M0
IIIB	T4	N1	M0
	Any T	N2	M0
	Any T	N3	M0
IV	Any T	Any N	M1

Table 11.8. AJCC staging of anal margin cancer

Primary tumor (T)			
TX	Primary tumor cannot be assessed		
T0	No evidence of primary tumor		
Tis	Carcinoma in situ		
T1	Tumor ≤2 cm in greatest dimension		
T2	Tumor >2 cm but not >5 cm in greatest dimension		
T3	Tumor >5 cm in greatest dimension		
T4	Tumor invades deep extradermal structures (i.e., cartilage, skeletal muscle, or bone)		
Lymph nodes (N)			
NX	Regional lymph nodes cannot be assessed		
N0	No regional lymph node metastasis		
N1	Regional lymph node metastasis		
Distant metastasis (M)			
MX	Presence of distant metastasis cannot be assessed		
M0	No distant metastasis		
M1	Distant metastasis		
Stage grouping			
0	Tis	N0	M0
I	T1	N0	M0
II	T2	N0	M0
	T3	N0	M0
III	T4	N0	M0
	Any T	N1	M0
IV	Any T	Any N	M1

rates similar to 5-FU, mitomycin-C, and radiation therapy, possibly with less toxicity.

The current regimen for primary treatment of SCC of the anal canal is chemoradiation therapy (Table 11.9). At MDACC, this has recently been changed from the 5-FU mitomycin-C–based chemoradiation therapy protocol to one that is 5-FU– and cisplatin-based, because of decreased toxicity, and similar response and survival data. Complete responses with this treatment can be expected in up to 90% of patients, with 5-year survival rates approaching 85%. Patients with advanced AIDS and anal cancer are poor candidates for high-dose radiation therapy and the use of mitomycin. Current research is being directed at different chemotherapy regimes with radiation for this group.

The presence of a persistent mass on examination 12 to 14 weeks after chemoradiation is an indication for biopsy because a persistent mass after therapy will demonstrate cancer on biopsy in 18% to 34% of cases. There are reports of positive biopsy specimen results 6 to 8 weeks after therapy (persistent disease), which will revert to negative biopsy results in patients

Table 11.9. Current and classic treatment protocols for anal canal cancer

Current	
	External-beam radiation therapy 5 d/wk for total dose of 45–55 Gy
	5-FU, 250 mg/m^2/day, M–F for the entire duration of radiation
	Cis-platin, 4 g/m^2/day, M–F for the entire duration of radiation
Classic	
Days 1–4	5-FU, 750–1,000 mg/m^2 over 24-h continuous IV infusion
Day 1	Mitomycin C, 10–15 mg/m^2, IV bolus
Days 1–35	Radiation therapy 5 d/wk for total dose of 45–55 Gy; boosts of up to 60 Gy may be given to the anus and/or inguinal basins
Days 29–32	5-FU, 750–1,000 mg/m^2 over 24-h continuous IV infusion

5-FU, 5-fluorouracil; IV, intravenous.

who have refused surgery. This implies that there may be a delayed radiation effect for up to several months after treatment. At MDACC, we do not routinely obtain a biopsy specimen of the treated tumor site unless obvious disease persistence exists; instead, we wait for clinical evidence of locally recurrent disease in follow-up visits.

Patients with local recurrence or persistent disease are salvaged with APR, with a resultant 50% 5-year survival. However, cisplatin-based chemotherapy with additional radiation therapy has been used successfully to salvage up to one-third of patients with locally recurrent disease and is currently under investigation.

ANAL MARGIN. SCC of the anal margin is defined currently by the AJCC as a lesion originating in an area between the anal margin and 5 cm in any direction onto the perianal skin and is classified with skin tumors. Note that the data supporting the treatment of these uncommon, heterogeneous lesions derive from small, single-institution, mostly retrospective studies. Moreover, many of these studies include lesions of the lower anal canal (dentate to anal verge) that were included previously in older definitions of the anal margin. The rationale for any modality of therapy derives from the proportional increase in chance of metastases with increasing tumor size; in tumors less than 2 cm, lymph node metastases are rarely found. For lesions between 2 and 5 cm, and those greater than 5 cm, the rates are 24% and 25% to 67%, respectively.

Small (<5 cm), superficial (T1–T2) anal margin cancers that do not invade the sphincter complex can be treated by a negative-margin wide local excision alone, with a 5-year survival rate greater than 80%. Wide local excision may include parts of the superficial internal and external anal sphincters without compromising anal continence.

Larger T2, T3 to T4, or T1 to T2, N-positive lesions are best treated with multimodality therapy, as in anal canal cancers, given the higher local recurrence rate. Prophylactic inguinal node radiation is given to patients with T3 to T4, N0 lesions, and higher doses of radiation are given to patients with positive inguinal nodes. Lymph node dissection is reserved for those patients with residual or recurrent disease. It is not known whether the treatment of inguinal disease translates into improved survival. Patients with T3 to T4 and poor sphincter function may require APR. For all patients, the 5-year disease-specific survival is 71% to 88%, and the local control rate after initial therapy is 70% to 100%.

Surveillance

Patients should be followed for detection of local and systemic failures and treatment complications. Local inspection, digital examination, anoscopy, and biopsy of any suspicious area are recommended every 3 months after chemoradiation treatment for 2 years, and twice a year thereafter. Early detection of local recurrence may enable less extensive salvage surgical procedures. Distant failures of epidermoid cancer are responsive to radiation therapy, and up to 30% of patients respond to second-line chemotherapy. Therefore, chest radiography, LFTs, and pelvic CT are recommended every 6 to 12 months for 2 to 3 years after initial therapy. Patients with anal margin cancers should have careful, close follow-up, given the indolent nature of these tumors and the benefits of further local therapy.

Anal Intraepithelial Neoplasia

Anal intraepithelial neoplasia (AIN) is a term used to describe squamous intraepithelial lesions (SILs) of the anus. This is an increasingly prevalent condition associated with HPV infection and condylomata that can occur both externally on the perianal skin and internally within the anal canal. Dysplasia in squamous intraepithelial lesions may be low-grade (LSIL) or high-grade (HSIL), an intermediate stage in the malignant transformation to SCC of the anus. Anal HSIL represents cytopathological and histopathological findings that have been referred to as AIN II/III, severe dysplasia, carcinoma in situ, or Bowen disease. The presence of HPV infection is the principal risk factor for anal neoplasia. Cofactors include anal-receptive intercourse and immunocompromise. Paralleling observations in the cervix (cervical cancer and cervical intraepithelial neoplasia), infection by oncogenic strains of HPV are causally related to the development of anal cancer and to the development of the precursor lesion, HSIL. Under the microscope, cervical SIL and anal SIL are virtually indistinguishable. The anatomical region at risk includes the anal transition zone and the distal rectum extending up to 8 cm proximal to the dentate line where immature squamous metaplastic cells are the most susceptible to oncogenic HPV, although the nonkeratinizing and keratinizing squamous epithelium of the surrounding tissues are also susceptible. There is also morphologic and histologic similarity between cervical and anal cancer.

The populations at greatest risk for AIN are the same as for anal cancer. Natural history studies have demonstrated that in HIV-negative MSM, the 4-year incidence of HSIL was 17%. It is higher in HIV-positive men, with receptive anal intercourse, the presence of condylomata, multiplicity of HPV serotype infections, injection drug abuse, cigarette smoking, depressed host immunity, and the presence of cervical, vulvar, or penile neoplasia.

Treatment

Patients with anal SIL often present with minor complaints related to anal condylomata, hemorrhoids, or pruritus ani. Physical exam may reveal anything from typical condylomatous lesions to normal-appearing anal and rectal mucosa. The perianal skin and the entire surgical anal canal, as defined by the AJCC and by the World Health Organization, extending through the length of the internal anal sphincter from the anal verge (2–4 cm in women, up to 6 cm in men), should be thoroughly examined.

Patients with low volume disease and no history of dysplasia may be treated with topical agents in the office, regardless of risk factors, with surveillance anal Pap smears. Patients with large volume disease are treated in the operating room with a combination of excisional biopsy or incisional biopsy and cautery destruction under monitored anesthetic care with a standard perianal block. Patients with a history of dysplasia, either from previous biopsy or Pap smear, may be "mapped" in the operating room with the operating microscope, acetic acid, and Lugol's solution or may be treated in the office if the lesions are readily visualized. HSIL demonstrates various characteristic vascular patterns allowing otherwise occult premalignant disease to be identified. The tissues may subsequently be painted selectively with Lugol's solution, but the Lugol's may obscure some of the acetic acid findings. The nonkeratinizing high-grade lesions of the anal canal do not readily take up Lugol's solution and stain either mahogany or yellow. HSIL may be destroyed with electrocautery by superficially "painting" the lesion and a small 2- to 10- mm rim of tissue trying to avoid injury that extends deep into the submucosa if a tissue diagnosis has been made. This strategy is safe and well tolerated, and has been shown to eradicate HSIL in HIV-negative patients. In HIV-positive patients, recurrence is high and treatment may need to be repeated; however, with close follow-up, transformation to invasive cancer can be prevented.

Bowen Disease

Bowen disease is an intraepithelial SCC (carcinoma in situ or intraepithelial high-grade dysplasia) that develops most commonly in middle-age women and is often discovered during histologic evaluation of an anal specimen obtained for an unrelated diagnosis. The lesion is raised, irregular, scaly, and plaquelike, with eczematoid features. Histologically, large atypical haloed cells (Bowenoid cells) are seen that stain PAS negative. Although it has previously been believed to have an association with other invasive carcinomas, the evidence for this is weak. The risk of progression to invasive cancer has been reported to be approximately

10%. Bowen disease has traditionally been treated with random biopsies and wide excision with flap reconstruction. However, even if normal tissue is sacrificed to obtain clear margins, the recurrence rate is 23%, and the patient may still be at risk for cancer development. This aggressive approach is associated with complications such as anal stenosis and fecal incontinence.

Bowen's disease is histologically and immunohistochemically indistinguishable from anal HSIL and has also been associated with HPV infection. There is increasing agreement that Bowen disease and anal HSIL should be treated in a similar fashion. Local recurrence may occur, but re-excision provides excellent local control. Other therapeutic modalities include topical 5-FU cream, topical imiquimod, photodynamic therapy, radiation therapy, laser therapy, and combinations of these. The reports are generally small series with limited follow-up, but there has been anecdotal success with each approach, and the options may be kept in mind for challenging cases.

Paget Disease

Paget disease is an intraepithelial adenocarcinoma that occurs mostly in elderly women. The lesion (a well-demarcated, eczematoid plaque) is usually characteristic; however, morphologic variations can occur, making the diagnosis difficult by inspection alone. The diagnosis is made histologically by the presence of large, vacuolated Paget cells, which stain periodic acid-Schiff (PAS) positive (from high mucin content). There is some evidence for the association of perianal Paget disease with other invasive carcinomas, but this relationship is not as strong as that seen with Paget disease of the breast. Invasion can develop in these lesions, and the prognosis is poor in those cases. Perianal Paget disease should be treated with wide local excision.

Anal Melanoma

Primary melanoma of the anus or rectum is a rare tumor, accounting for 0.4% to 1.6% of all melanomas and less than 1.0% of all anal canal tumors. The overall prognosis for patients with anorectal melanoma is very poor. Several reports in the literature have shown 5-year survival rates that are less than 25% and the median survival time is about 15 months. Mucosal melanoma is further discussed elsewhere in this text. This discussion focuses on anal melanoma.

Pathological Characteristics

The primary tumor may arise from the skin of the anal verge or the transitional epithelium of the anal canal. Inguinal nodal metastases are common at presentation. Prognosis is related to tumor thickness, as with cutaneous melanomas.

Diagnosis

Patients most commonly present with rectal bleeding. The incidental finding of a mass on digital examination may also lead to a workup that establishes the diagnosis. Melanoma may be an incidental pathological finding after hemorrhoidectomy. Physical examination should include evaluation of the rectal mass and palpation of the inguinal nodes. Radiographic staging should be performed as for melanomas elsewhere.

Treatment

Historically, APR has been the treatment of choice, but high failure rates have questioned the role for this radical approach. Wide local excision with at least 2 cm of normal surrounding tissue and sentinel lymph node biopsy of the inguinal lymph nodes is now performed whenever possible, reserving APR for large bulky tumors that cannot be locally excised. Therapeutic inguinal node dissection is indicated for nodal disease. Using this approach with hypofractionated adjuvant radiation therapy (30 Gy in five fractions) to the primary site and nodal beds, MDACC has reported a 5-year actuarial survival of 31%, local control rate of 74%, and a nodal control rate of 84% in 23 patients after a median follow-up of 32 months.

RECOMMENDED READING

A comparison of laparoscopically assisted and open colectomy for colon cancer. *N Engl J Med* 2004;350(20):2050–2059.

Abdalla EK, Vauthey JN, Ellis LM, et al. Recurrence and outcomes following hepatic resection, radiofrequency ablation, and combined resection/ablation for colorectal liver metastases. *Ann Surg* 2004;239(6):818–825, discussion 825–827.

Al-Tassan N, Chmiel NH, Maynard J, et al. Inherited variants of MYH associated with somatic G:C→T:A mutations in colorectal tumors. *Nat Genet* 2002;30(2):227–232.

Ballo MT, Gershenwald JE, Zagars GK, et al. Sphincter-sparing local excision and adjuvant radiation for anal-rectal melanoma. *J Clin Oncol* 2002;20(23):4555–4558.

Bedrosian I, Rodriguez-Bigas MA, Feig B, et al. Predicting the node-negative mesorectum after preoperative chemoradiation for locally advanced rectal carcinoma. *J Gastrointest Surg* 2004;8(1):56–62, discussion 62–63.

Bertagnolli M, Miedema B, Redston M, et al. Sentinel node staging of resectable colon cancer: results of a multicenter study. *Ann Surg* 2004;240(4):624–638, discussion 628–630.

Bonnen M, Crane C, Vauthey JN, et al. Long-term results using local excision after preoperative chemoradiation among selected T3 rectal cancer patients. *Int J Radiat Oncol Biol Phys* 2004;60(4):1098–1105.

Bowne WB, Lee B, Wong WD, et al. Operative salvage for locoregional recurrent colon cancer after curative resection: an analysis of 100 cases. *Dis Colon Rectum* 2005;48(5):897–909.

Burt RW. Colon cancer screening. *Gastroenterology* 2000;119(3):837–853.

Cawthorn SJ, Parums DV, Gibbs NM, et al. Extent of mesorectal spread and involvement of lateral resection margin as prognostic factors after surgery for rectal cancer. *Lancet* 1990;335(8697):1055–1059.

Chang GJ, Berry JM, Jay N, et al. Surgical treatment of high-grade anal squamous intraepithelial lesions: a prospective study. *Dis Colon Rectum* 2002;45(4):453–458.

Chau I, Allen MJ, Cunningham D, et al. The value of routine serum carcino-embryonic antigen measurement and computed tomography in the surveillance of patients after adjuvant chemotherapy for colorectal cancer. *J Clin Oncol* 2004;22(8):1420–1429.

Church J, Simmang C. Practice parameters for the treatment of patients with dominantly inherited colorectal cancer (familial adenomatous polyposis and hereditary nonpolyposis colorectal cancer). *Dis Colon*

Rectum 2003;46(8): 1001–1012.

Compton C, Fenoglio-Preiser CM, Pettigrew N, Fielding LP. American Joint Committee on Cancer Prognostic Factors Consensus Conference: Colorectal Working Group. *Cancer* 2000;88(7):1739–1757.

Cotton PB, Durkalski VL, Pineau BC, et al. Computed tomographic colonography (virtual colonoscopy): a multicenter comparison with standard colonoscopy for detection of colorectal neoplasia. *JAMA* 2004;291(14):1713–1719.

Crane CH, Skibber J. Preoperative chemoradiation for locally advanced rectal cancer: rationale, technique, and results of treatment. *Semin Surg Oncol* 2003;21(4):265–270.

Crane CH, Skibber JM, Birnbaum EH, et al. The addition of continuous infusion 5-FU to preoperative radiation therapy increases tumor response, leading to increased sphincter preservation in locally advanced rectal cancer. *Int J Radiat Oncol Biol Phys* 2003;57(1):84–89.

Crane CH, Skibber JM, Feig BW, et al. Response to preoperative chemoradiation increases the use of sphincter-preserving surgery in patients with locally advanced low rectal carcinoma. *Cancer* 2003;97(2):517–524.

de Gramont A, Figer A, Seymour M, et al. Leucovorin and fluorouracil with or without oxaliplatin as first-line treatment in advanced colorectal cancer. *J Clin Oncol* 2000;18(16):2938–2947.

Enker WE. Sphincter-preserving operations for rectal cancer. *Oncology (Huntingt)* 1996;10(11):1673–1684, 1689, discussion 1690–1692.

Farouk R, Nelson H, Gunderson LL. Aggressive multimodality treatment for locally advanced irresectable rectal cancer. *Br J Surg* 1997;84(6):741–749.

Fisher B, Wolmark N, Rockette H, et al. Postoperative adjuvant chemotherapy or radiation therapy for rectal cancer: results from NSABP protocol R-01. *J Natl Cancer Inst* 1988;80(1):21–29.

Frisch M, Glimelius B, van den Brule AJ, et al. Sexually transmitted infection as a cause of anal cancer. *N Engl J Med* 1997;337(19):1350–1358.

Garcia-Aguilar J, Mellgren A, Sirivongs P, et al. Local excision of rectal cancer without adjuvant therapy: a word of caution. *Ann Surg* 2000;231(3):345–351.

Gastrointestinal Tumor Study Group. Prolongation of the disease-free interval in surgically treated rectal carcinoma. *N Engl J Med* 1985;312(23):1465–1472.

Gerard A, Buyse M, Nordlinger B, et al. Preoperative radiotherapy as adjuvant treatment in rectal cancer. Final results of a randomized study of the European Organization for Research and Treatment of Cancer (EORTC). *Ann Surg* 1988;208(5):606–614.

Gill S, Sinicrope FA. Colorectal cancer prevention: is an ounce of prevention worth a pound of cure? *Semin Oncol* 2005;32(1): 24–34.

Guillem JG, Chessin DB, Cohen AM, et al. Long-term oncologic outcome following preoperative combined modality therapy and total mesorectal excision of locally advanced rectal cancer. *Ann Surg* 2005;241(5):829–836, discussion 836–838.

Gunderson LL, Nelson H, Martenson JA, et al. Locally advanced primary colorectal cancer: intraoperative electron and external beam irradiation ± 5-FU. *Int J Radiat Oncol Biol Phys* 1997;37(3):601–614.

Habr-Gama A, Perez RO, Nadalin W, et al. Operative versus nonoperative treatment for stage 0 distal rectal cancer following chemoradiation therapy: long-term results. *Ann Surg* 2004;240(4):711–717, discussion 717–718.

Haggitt RC, Glotzbach RE, Soffer EE, Wruble LD. Prognostic factors in colorectal carcinomas arising in adenomas: implications for lesions removed by endoscopic polypectomy. *Gastroenterology* 1985;89(2):328–336.

Hahnloser D, Haddock MG, Nelson H. Intraoperative radiotherapy in the multimodality approach to colorectal cancer. *Surg Oncol Clin N Am* 2003;12(4):993–1013, ix.

Harewood GC. Assessment of publication bias in the reporting of EUS performance in staging rectal cancer. *Am J Gastroenterol* 2005;100(4):808–816.

Havenga K, Enker WE. Autonomic nerve preserving total mesorectal excision. *Surg Clin North Am* 2002;82(5):1009–1018.

Heald RJ, Ryall RD. Recurrence and survival after total mesorectal excision for rectal cancer. *Lancet* 1986;1(8496):1479–1482.

Hida J, Yasutomi M, Maruyama T, et al. Lymph node metastases detected in the mesorectum distal to carcinoma of the rectum by the clearing method: justification of total mesorectal excision. *J Am Coll Surg* 1997;184(6):584–588.

Improved survival with preoperative radiotherapy in resectable rectal cancer. Swedish Rectal Cancer Trial. *N Engl J Med* 1997;336(14):980–987.

Jemal A, Murray T, Ward E, et al. Cancer statistics, 2005. *CA Cancer J Clin* 2005;55(1):10–30.

Jo WS, Chung DC. Genetics of hereditary colorectal cancer. *Semin Oncol* 2005;32(1):11–23.

Kikuchi R, Takano M, Takagi K, et al. Management of early invasive colorectal cancer. Risk of recurrence and clinical guidelines. *Dis Colon Rectum* 1995;38(12):1286–1295.

Korner H, Soreide K, Stokkeland PJ, Soreide JA. Systematic follow-up after curative surgery for colorectal cancer in Norway: a population-based audit of effectiveness, costs, and compliance. *J Gastrointest Surg* 2005;9(3):320–328.

Koura AN, Giacco GG, Curley SA, et al. Carcinoid tumors of the rectum: effect of size, histopathology, and surgical treatment on metastasis-free survival. *Cancer* 1997;79(7):1294–1298.

Lavery IC, Lopez-Kostner F, Pelley RJ, Fine RM. Treatment of colon and rectal cancer. *Surg Clin North Am* 2000;80(2):535–569, ix.

Le Voyer TE, Sigurdson ER, Hanlon AL, et al. Colon cancer survival is associated with increasing number of lymph nodes analyzed: a secondary survey of intergroup trial INT-0089. *J Clin Oncol* 2003;21(15):2912–2919.

Libutti SK, Alexander HR, Jr, Choyke P, et al. A prospective study of 2-[18F] fluoro-2-deoxy-D-glucose/positron emission tomography scan, 99mTc-labeled arcitumomab (CEA-scan), and blind second-look laparotomy for detecting colon cancer recurrence in patients with increasing carcinoembryonic antigen levels. *Ann Surg Oncol* 2001;8(10):779–786.

Lowy AM, Rich TA, Skibber JM, et al. Preoperative infusional chemoradiation, selective intraoperative radiation, and resection for locally advanced pelvic recurrence of colorectal adenocarcinoma. *Ann Surg* 1996;223(2):177–185.

Mamounas E, Wieand S, Wolmark N, et al. Comparative efficacy of adjuvant chemotherapy in patients with Dukes' B versus Dukes' C colon cancer: results from four National Surgical Adjuvant Breast and Bowel Project adjuvant studies (C-01, C-02, C-03, and C-04). *J Clin Oncol* 1999;17(5): 1349–1355.

Mendenhall WM, Zlotecki RA, Vauthey JN, Copeland EM III. Squamous cell carcinoma of the anal margin. *Oncology (Huntingt)* 1996;10(12):1843–1848, discussion 1848, 1853–1854.

Merg A, Lynch HT, Lynch JF, Howe JR. Hereditary colon cancer-part I. *Curr Probl Surg* 2005;42(4):195–256.

Merg A, Lynch HT, Lynch JF, Howe JR. Hereditary colorectal cancer-part II. *Curr Probl Surg* 2005;42(5):267–333.

Meterissian SH, Skibber JM, Giacco GG, et al. Pelvic exenteration for locally advanced rectal carcinoma: factors predicting improved survival. *Surgery* 1997;121(5):479–487.

Meyerhardt JA, Mayer RJ. Systemic therapy for colorectal cancer. *N Engl J Med* 2005;352(5): 476–487.

Meyerhardt JA, Tepper JE, Niedzwiecki D, et al. Impact of

hospital procedure volume on surgical operation and long-term outcomes in high-risk curatively resected rectal cancer: findings from the Intergroup 0114 Study. *J Clin Oncol* 2004;22(1):166–174.

Middleton PF, Sutherland LM, Maddern GJ. Transanal endoscopic microsurgery: a systematic review. *Dis Colon Rectum* 2005;48(2):270–284.

Moertel CG, Fleming TR, Macdonald JS, et al. Levamisole and fluorouracil for adjuvant therapy of resected colon carcinoma. *N Engl J Med* 1990;322(6):352–358.

Nascimbeni R, Burgart LJ, Nivatvongs S, Larson DR. Risk of lymph node metastasis in T1 carcinoma of the colon and rectum. *Dis Colon Rectum* 2002;45(2):200–206.

Nelson H, Petrelli N, Carlin A, et al. Guidelines 2000 for colon and rectal cancer surgery. *J Natl Cancer Inst* 2001;93(8):583–596.

Nigro ND, Seydel HG, Considine B, et al. Combined preoperative radiation and chemotherapy for squamous cell carcinoma of the anal canal. *Cancer* 1983;51(10):1826–1829.

NIH consensus conference. Adjuvant therapy for patients with colon and rectal cancer. *JAMA* 1990;264(11):1444–1450.

Nivatvongs S. Surgical management of malignant colorectal polyps. *Surg Clin North Am* 2002;82(5):959–966.

O'Connell MJ, Martenson JA, Wieand HS, et al. Improving adjuvant therapy for rectal cancer by combining protracted-infusion fluorouracil with radiation therapy after curative surgery. *N Engl J Med* 1994;331(8):502–507.

Papillon J. Intracavitary irradiation of early rectal cancer for cure. A series of 186 cases. 1975. *Dis Colon Rectum* 1994;37(1):88–94.

Pickhardt PJ, Choi JR, Hwang I, et al. Computed tomographic virtual colonoscopy to screen for colorectal neoplasia in asymptomatic adults. *N Engl J Med* 2003;349(23):2191–2200.

Pignone M, Rich M, Teutsch SM, et al. Screening for colorectal cancer in adults at average risk: a summary of the evidence for the U.S. Preventive Services Task Force. *Ann Intern Med* 2002;137(2):132–141.

Rabkin CS, Yellin F. Cancer incidence in a population with a high prevalence of infection with human immunodeficiency virus type 1. *J Natl Cancer Inst* 1994;86(22):1711–1716.

Rodriguez-Bigas MA, Boland CR, Hamilton SR, et al. A National Cancer Institute Workshop on Hereditary Nonpolyposis Colorectal Cancer Syndrome: meeting highlights and Bethesda guidelines. *J Natl Cancer Inst* 1997;89(23):1758–1762.

Rodriguez-Bigas MA, Stoler DL, Bertario L, et al. Colorectal cancer: how does it start? How does it metastasize? *Surg Oncol Clin N Am* 2000;9(4):643–652, discussion 653–654.

Rosen M, Chan L, Beart RW, Jr, et al. Follow-up of colorectal cancer: a meta-analysis. *Dis Colon Rectum* 1998;41(9):1116–1126.

Saltz LB, Cox JV, Blanke C, et al. Irinotecan plus fluorouracil and leucovorin for metastatic colorectal cancer. Irinotecan Study Group. *N Engl J Med* 2000;343(13):905–914.

Sanfilippo NJ, Crane CH, Skibber J, et al. T4 rectal cancer treated with preoperative chemoradiation to the posterior pelvis followed by multivisceral resection: patterns of failure and limitations of treatment. *Int J Radiat Oncol Biol Phys* 2001;51(1):176–183.

Sauer R, Becker H, Hohenberger W, et al. Preoperative versus postoperative chemoradiotherapy for rectal cancer. *N Engl J Med* 2004;351(17):1731–1740.

Schaffzin DM, Wong WD. Endorectal ultrasound in the preoperative evaluation of rectal cancer. *Clin Colorectal Cancer* 2004;4(2):124–132.

The SCOTIA Study Group. Single-stage treatment for malignant left-sided colonic obstruction: a prospective randomized clinical trial comparing subtotal colectomy with segmental resection following intraoperative irrigation. Subtotal colectomy versus on-table irrigation and anastomosis. *Br J Surg* 1995;82(12):1622–1627.

Scott N, Jackson P, al-Jaberi T, et al. Total mesorectal excision and local recurrence: a study of tumour spread in the mesorectum distal to rectal cancer. *Br J Surg* 1995;82(8):1031–1033.

Skibber J, Rodriguez-Bigas MA, Gordon PH. Surgical considerations in anal cancer. *Surg Oncol Clin N Am* 2004;13(2):321–338.

Steele GD, Jr, Herndon JE, Bleday R, et al. Sphincter-sparing treatment for distal rectal adenocarcinoma. *Ann Surg Oncol* 1999;6(5):433–441.

Tepper JE, O'Connell M, Niedzwiecki D, et al. Adjuvant therapy in rectal cancer: analysis of stage, sex, and local control–final report of intergroup 0114. *J Clin Oncol* 2002;20(7):1744–1750.

Umar A, Boland CR, Terdiman JP, et al. Revised Bethesda guidelines for hereditary nonpolyposis colorectal cancer (Lynch syndrome) and microsatellite instability. *J Natl Cancer Inst* 2004;96(4):261–268.

U.S. Preventative Task Force. Screening for colorectal cancer: recommendation and rationale. *Ann Internl Med* 2002;137(2): 129–31.

Vogelsang H, Haas S, Hierholzer C, et al. Factors influencing survival after resection of pulmonary metastases from colorectal cancer. *Br J Surg* 2004;91(8): 1066–1071.

Walsh JM, Terdiman JP. Colorectal cancer screening: clinical applications. *JAMA* 2003;289(10):1297–1302.

Walsh JM, Terdiman JP. Colorectal cancer screening: scientific review. *JAMA* 2003;289(10):1288–1296.

Wibe A, Eriksen MT, Syse A, et al. Effect of hospital caseload on long-term outcome after standardization of rectal cancer surgery at a national level. *Br J Surg* 2005;92(2):217–224.

Wilson SM, Beahrs OH. The curative treatment of carcinoma of the sigmoid, rectosigmoid, and rectum. *Ann Surg* 1976;183(5):556–565.

Winawer SJ, Zauber AG. Colonoscopic polypectomy and the incidence of colorectal cancer. *Gut* 2001;48(6):753–754.

Wolmark N, Rockette H, Fisher B, et al. The benefit of leucovorin-modulated fluorouracil as postoperative adjuvant therapy for primary colon cancer: results from National Surgical Adjuvant Breast and Bowel Project protocol C-03. *J Clin Oncol* 1993;11(10):1879–1887.

Young-Fadok TM, Wolff BG, Nivatvongs S, et al. Prophylactic oophorectomy in colorectal carcinoma: preliminary results of a randomized, prospective trial. *Dis Colon Rectum* 1998;41(3):277–283, discussion 283–285.

Zaheer S, Pemberton JH, Farouk R, et al. Surgical treatment of adenocarcinoma of the rectum. *Ann Surg* 1998;227(6):800–811.

12

Hepatobiliary Cancers

Eugene A. Choi, Steven E. Rodgers,
Syed A. Ahmad, and Eddie K. Abdalla

INTRODUCTION

The approach to patients with liver and biliary tumors is complex. Overall assessment of comorbidity and specific indications for hepatic surgery of the liver depend on both tumor factors and liver factors. Some tumors develop in otherwise normal underlying livers, while others arise in livers compromised by biliary obstruction or underlying liver disease, such as steatosis, fibrosis, or cirrhosis. The preoperative preparation, operative approach, surgical techniques, anticipated complications, and outcome relate to both the tumor and the liver factors. Careful attention to each of these issues is necessary to optimize outcome.

Advances in hepatobiliary surgery have come largely as a result of attention to these details, and data suggest the outcome can be improved by taking a multidisciplinary approach to the patient with liver or biliary cancers. In fact, both short- and long-term outcome are significantly better in "centers of excellence," where surgeons have specialized training and experience in hepatobiliary surgery and work as part of a specialized team of oncologists, radiologists, and gastroenterologists.

This chapter outlines treatment approaches to the major hepatobiliary cancers, addresses issues of anatomy, and describes preoperative preparation and the operative approach. For each disease type, the current literature is reviewed to provide an explanation of epidemiology, pathology, clinical presentation, diagnosis, staging, and issues regarding surgical therapy.

SURGICAL ANATOMY OF THE LIVER

Hepatic anatomy is highly variable. Ten separate types of hepatic arterial anatomy have been defined, and numerous portal and biliary segmental variations are important to the hepatic surgeon. A description of the major arterial variations is beyond the scope of this chapter, however an overview of hepatic anatomy, which is essential to the discussion of resection options for hepatic tumors is provided.

The portal and arterial vessels in the liver are the first level of complexity in the liver's anatomy. Based on portal segmentation, eight separate anatomical segments of the liver can be identified, and these are termed the Couinaud segments of the liver. This predominantly portal segmentation of the liver described by Couinaud in 1957 provides the surgeon with an anatomical approach to the liver, such that any of the eight segments can be resected while preserving the vascular inflow, venous outflow, and biliary drainage of the remaining segments.

The left and right livers are not symmetric. The right liver is typically two-thirds of the total liver volume, and the left liver is

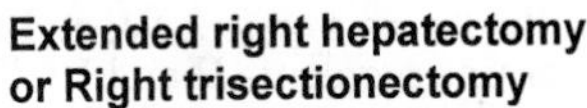

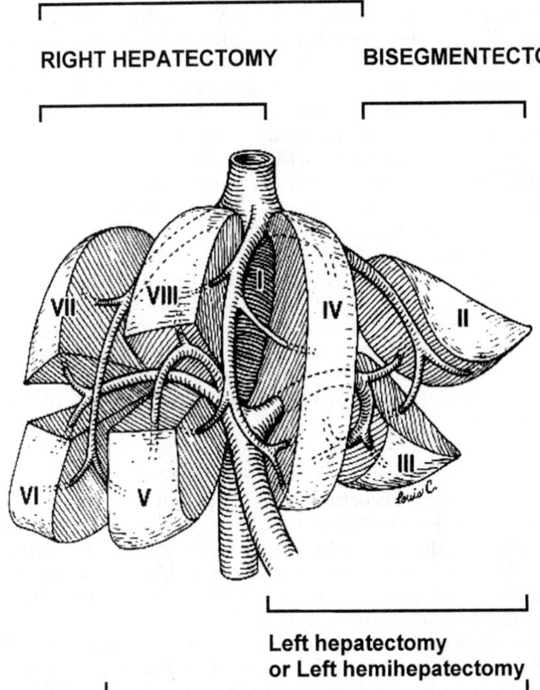

Figure 12.1. Segmental liver anatomy as originally described by Claude Couinaud, with the terminology that should be used to describe liver resection according to the Brisbane 2000 international consensus conference. (Adapted from Abdalla EK, Denys A, Chevalier P, Nemr RA, Vauthey JN. Total and segmental liver volume variations: implications for liver surgery. *Surgery* 2004;135:405, with permission.)

about one-third. The caudate or posterior liver, which is a single anatomical unit, represents about 1% the total liver volume (segment 1). The right liver can be divided into the right anterior and posterior sectors, and the left liver divided into the lateral and medial sectors. The left lateral liver is subdivided into segments II and III, and the medial left liver is also known as segment IV. The right anterior liver is subdivided into segment V inferiorly and segment VIII superiorly, and the right posterior liver is subdivided into segment VI inferiorly and segment VII superiorly (Fig. 12.1).

Three major hepatic veins are typically found: the right hepatic vein, which typically drains the right liver (segments V–VIII); the middle hepatic vein, which typically drains segment IV; and the left hepatic vein, which typically drains segments II and III. The left hepatic vein crosses the left lateral liver transversely, between segments II and III. The middle hepatic vein defines the main plane, or the division between the left and right livers, which is the plane on which right or left hepatectomy is undertaken. The caudate liver, because it arises embryologically as a separate anatomical unit from the remaining liver, has its own venous drainage, with short veins draining directly into the vena cava, and highly variable biliary and portal anatomy.

It is essential that the surgeon understand the many anatomical variations of the liver that can be identified on preoperative imaging and intraoperative ultrasound (US). Surgical techniques—including the Glissonian approach or dissection along the fibrous sheath that surrounds the portal triads—may enable the hepatic surgeon to identify important elements of the anatomy intrahepatically and thereby minimize the risk of injury to the remaining liver after resection of anatomical segments. Most liver surgeons consider intraoperative US essential for safe surgery because it permits real-time identification of the intrahepatic anatomy.

TERMINOLOGY FOR HEPATIC RESECTION

Terminology for hepatic resection has changed over time. Different definitions of the term "lobe" had been used in Europe and the United States, causing confusion. Accordingly, the Brisbane 2000 International Conference was held to establish a consensus on terminology used for liver resection. That revised terminology is used throughout this chapter (Fig. 12.1).

The terminology for hepatectomy is as follows: (a) resection of the right liver (or segments V–VIII) is termed a right hepatectomy or right hemihepatectomy; (b) resection of the left liver (or segments II–IV) is termed a left hepatectomy or left hemihepatectomy; (c) resection of the left lateral liver (or segments II and III) is termed a bisegmentectomy II + III or a left lateral sectionectomy; and (d) extended right hepatectomy, or right trisectionectomy, is the resection of segments IV to VIII, whereas extended left hepatectomy, or left trisectionectomy, is resection of segments II to V and VIII. Elimination of the term "lobe" has enabled much clearer communication among physicians worldwide when discussing and writing about hepatic resection.

PREDICTING LIVER REMNANT FUNCTION

Liver Volume Determination

Liver volume after major hepatic resection has been critically linked to liver function. Also, underlying liver disease will affect liver function so patients with normal underlying liver are treated differently than patients with diseased underlying liver. The realization that liver volume alone does not predict function leads to two additional conclusions: Large patients need large livers and small patients need small livers, and patients with diseased livers need to have a larger volume of liver preserved than patients with normal underlying livers. Careful analysis of outcome based on liver remnant volume stratified by underlying liver disease (or the absence of disease) has led to recommendations regarding the safe limits of resection. The liver remnant to be left after resection is termed the future liver remnant (FLR). For patients with normal underlying liver, complications, extended hospital stay, admission to the intensive care unit, and hepatic insufficiency are rare when the standardized FLR is >20% of the total liver volume (TLV) as compared to when it is ≤20%. For patients with marked underlying liver disease, a 40% liver remnant is necessary to avoid cholestasis, fluid retention, and liver failure. Patients with normal underlying liver and a small remnant have a greater complication rate but rarely die of those complications, whereas patients with cirrhosis and a small remnant are at risk for a cascade of complications that may culminate in liver failure and death.

When the liver remnant is normal or has only mild disease, the volume of liver remnant can be measured directly and accurately with three-dimensional computed tomography (CT) volumetry. However, CT volumetry is frequently not appropriate for determining the total functional liver volume when the goal is to use this volume to estimate the functionality of the FLR after resection. Inaccuracy may arise because the liver *to be resected* is often diseased, particularly in patients with cirrhosis or biliary obstruction; the total liver size can be large, normal, or small, or when multiple or large tumors occupy a large volume of the liver to be resected, subtracting tumor volumes from liver volume further decreases accuracy of CT volumetry. The calculated TLV, which has been derived from the close association between patient size and liver size (specifically the association between body surface area [BSA] and liver size), provides a standardizing estimate of the TLV. The following formula is used:

$$\text{TLV}(\text{cm}^3) = -794.41 + 1267.28 \times \text{BSA (square meters)}$$

Thus, the standardized FLR volume calculation uses the *measured* FLR volume from CT volumetry as the numerator and the *calculated* TLV as the denominator:

$$\text{Standardized FLR} = \text{measured FLR volume/TLV}$$

Calculating the standardized TLV corrects the actual liver volume to the individual patient's size and provides an individualized estimate of that patient's postresection liver function. This approach has been validated and used at The University of Texas M. D. Anderson Cancer Center, where it has enabled 127 consecutive extended hepatectomies with only a single mortality. Furthermore, use of this standardized approach to liver volume measurement enables the systematic use of preoperative liver preparation to increase the liver remnant volume prior to major resection when indicated based on the criteria described previously.

Several other tests have been used to evaluate liver function, including the urea-nitrogen synthesis rate, galactose elimination capacity, bromsulphalein and aminopyrine breath tests, and indocyanine green (ICG) clearance. ICG is a dye that is cleared from the circulation by the liver, and its clearance is an indicator of hepatocyte function. ICG clearance is the most studied test used to select cirrhotic patients for hepatic resection, although it is used mostly in Asia. Makuuchi et al. advocated selection of cirrhotic patients for *minor* resection based on the presence or absence of ascites, stratification according to the total serum bilirubin level and ICG 15 value (i.e., the percentage of dye clearance in 15 minutes). Patients with high bilirubin levels and low hepatic clearance of ICG are considered for limited resection or alternative locoregional ablative treatments. These studies are of limited value in selecting patients for major resection because they assess global hepatic function. Standardized FLR volume remains our sole approach at M. D. Anderson Cancer Center because it is a validated approach to assessment of liver remnant volume and guides treatment planning. The following section discusses strategies to increase the volume and function of an inadequate FLR prior to major hepatectomy.

Portal Vein Embolization

Portal vein embolization (PVE) is a preoperative procedure designed to increase the safety of major liver resections. The portal flow is diverted from the liver segments to be resected to the liver that will remain (the FLR) because this diversion of flow leads to increased size and better function of the FLR before resection. PVE was refined by Makuuchi after Kinoshita observed that embolization of the portal vein to prevent tumor extension led to hypertrophy of the contralateral liver. Since then, PVE techniques and indications have been standardized to increase the safety of major hepatectomy in patients with normal and diseased livers.

The indications for PVE are the same as those predicting postresection liver function as described in the previous section. In patients with normal underlying liver and a standardized FLR volume $\leq$20% of the TLV, PVE is indicated to increase the volume and function of the FLR. In patients with cirrhotic and fibrotic livers and a standardized FLR volume $\leq$40% of the TLV, PVE is also indicated. For patients who have undergone extensive chemotherapy, PVE should be considered when the standardized FLR is $\leq$30%.

Although several different approaches to embolization have been proposed, we at M. D. Anderson Cancer Center use the percutaneous ipsilateral approach to avoid puncturing or otherwise injuring the liver remnant. Then, using small particles followed by larger coils, the portal branches supplying the entire tumor-bearing liver, including segment IV (if this is to be resected), are occluded. This procedure diverts portal flow to the FLR. Studies have shown that hypertrophy-inducing factors are carried in the portal vein and not the hepatic artery, and so PVE leads to FLR hypertrophy. Hypertrophy occurs quite rapidly, and the normal liver can be reassessed by volumetry within 3 or 4 weeks. Surgery is undertaken when the target FLR volume is reached. In cirrhotics and diabetics, hypertrophy occurs more slowly; therefore, an interval of 5 or 6 weeks may be required to achieve the target volume. Numerous outcome studies have shown that this hypertrophy correlates with an improvement in hepatic function and reduces the risk of cholestasis, fluid retention, and ascites in patients with normal liver. It has also been shown to reduce the risk of these problems, as well as death due to hepatic failure, in cirrhotics.

Attention to the liver remnant, systemic volumetry for major resection, and systematic use of PVE based on carefully prescribed indications has enabled very safe extended hepatic resection in patients with normal liver function and major hepatectomy in patients with underlying liver disease.

PRIMARY HEPATOCELLULAR CARCINOMA

Epidemiology

Worldwide, hepatocellular carcinoma (HCC) is the fifth most common malignant neoplasm in men and the ninth most common in women, accounting for 500,000 to 1 million cancer cases annually. In the United States, HCC is comparatively rare, with an annual incidence of fewer than 5 cases per 100,000 persons, making it the 22nd most common type of cancer. However, the incidence of HCC in the United States is rising because of the increasing prevalence of hepatitis B (HBV) and hepatitis C (HCV) infection.

HCC occurs with greater frequency in regions of the world where viral hepatitis is endemic. There is, however, considerable variation in the prevalence of HCC, HBV, and HCV, depending on the patient's country of origin. It is estimated that one-fourth of patients with HCC in the United States have evidence of HCV infection, and HBV and HCV infections together account for no more than 40% of HCC cases. In contrast, in many Eastern countries where both HBV and HCV infections are endemic, the vast majority of HCC patients are seropositive for either HBV or HCV. Even within Eastern countries, however, there are geographic variations. For example, in contrast to Taiwan, China, and Korea, where HBV infection rates are high, HCV and HBV+HCV infections are predominant in Japan. Patients from the West (the United States and France) are more likely than patients from the East (Hong Kong and Japan) to have negative hepatitis serology.

Several other risk factors have been implicated in the development of HCC. Alcohol-related cirrhosis is the leading cause of HCC in the United States, Canada, and Western Europe. Chemicals such as nitrites, hydrocarbons, and polychlorinated biphenyls have also been associated with HCC. Dietary intake of aflatoxins is high in several countries with a high incidence of HCC. The common etiologic factor may be recurrent chronic hepatocellular injury and/or cirrhosis. HCC has also been reported in association with several metabolic disorders, such as hemochromatosis, Wilson disease, hereditary tyrosinemia, type I glycogen storage disease, familial polyposis coli, alpha-1 antitrypsin deficiency, and Budd-Chiari syndrome. HCC is more likely to develop in men than in women. In high-incidence areas, the male-to-female ratio is approximately 8:1, and in low-incidence areas, the ratio is 4:1. HCC develops early in life in the high-incidence areas, whereas it occurs predominantly in the elderly in low-incidence areas. More important than the patient's age is the chronicity of the infection or cirrhosis. Patients with HCV infections are often older and present with active chronic hepatitis and larger tumors.

Pathology

The histological variations of HCC are of little importance in determining treatment and prognosis, with two exceptions: fibrolamellar carcinoma is found in younger patients without cirrhosis and carries a better prognosis than standard HCC, and adenomatous hyperplasia is a premalignant lesion that can be cured by resection. HCC frequently spreads by local extension to the diaphragm and adjacent organs and into the portal and hepatic veins. Metastatic spread occurs most often to the lungs, bone, adrenal glands, and brain.

Clinical Presentation

Presentation depends on the stage of disease. In countries with systematic screening programs, HCC may be detected at an earlier stage. In the United States, where there is no systematic screening for HCC, patients usually present at a late stage, often with upper abdominal pain or discomfort, a palpable right upper quadrant mass, weight loss, ascites, or other sequelae of portal hypertension. Jaundice is relatively uncommon but ominous. The triad of abdominal pain, weight loss, and an abdominal mass is the most common clinical presentation in the United States. In fewer than 5% of cases, patients present with tumor rupture. In Eastern countries, including Taiwan, Hong Kong, Japan, and Korea, HCC is often diagnosed by surveillance abdominal US, helical CT scan, magnetic resonance imaging (MRI), or routine screening of blood for features such as elevated serum alpha-fetoprotein (AFP) before clinical symptoms are apparent. Numerous paraneoplastic complications have been described, including hypoglycemia, hypercalcemia, erythrocytosis, and hypertrophic pulmonary osteoarthropathy. Patients with HCV infection are more often screened and thus tend to present with signs and symptoms of cirrhosis and earlier-stage HCC tumors. Patients with HBV infection or no serological evidence of hepatitis infection tend to present with larger tumors and less cirrhosis.

Diagnosis

AFP is increased in 50% to 90% of all patients with HCC, with levels greater than 400 ng per mL usually found in those with large or rapidly growing tumors. Despite these general correlations, AFP is neither sensitive nor specific for HCC. A patient with a small HCC tumor may have minimal or no elevation of AFP. Moreover, transient increases in AFP may be seen with inflammatory hepatic disease or cirrhosis. Several studies have reported a correlation between AFP elevation, advanced tumor stage, and poor patient prognosis, or an association between highly elevated AFP and metastatic disease; AFP >200 ng per mL in association with characteristic imaging findings is nearly 100% sensitive for HCC.

Several imaging modalities can be used to diagnose HCC, including helical (CT) scanning, percutaneous US, and MRI. Both CT and MRI permit dynamic contrast-enhanced imaging. Each imaging modality has advantages and disadvantages. US is an inexpensive screening tool, but its sensitivity and specificity are low, with an overall false-negative rate of more than 50%.

At M. D. Anderson Cancer Center, helical thin-slice CT scanning is the preferred imaging technique. These CT scans have the advantage of speed when compared with MRI, and they effectively image the entire abdomen and the liver in four phases of contrast enhancement: precontrast, early vascular or arterial phases, a portal phase, and a delayed phase. HCCs, hepatic adenomas, and metastatic disease demonstrate arterial phase enhancement. Enhancement during the portal-dominant phase reveals hypovascular tumors, such as metastatic adenocarcinoma or cholangiocarcinoma (CCA). Multiphasic MRI is used selectively at our institution to provide additional information concerning the benign or malignant nature of a hepatic lesion or the anatomical relationship between a tumor and major vessels. MRI has an advantage over CT in that it does not require the use of contrast agents for detecting lesions, although HCC protocols typically use dynamic contrast enhancement. Many institutions prefer MRI to CT, but data that demonstrate superiority of one modality are lacking. In some regions, lipiodol, an oily derivative of the poppy seed, is combined with iodine contrast medium; the mixture is retained by the tumor and has been used with CT scanning to evaluate small HCCs.

More invasive imaging techniques are also used in the diagnosis of HCC, including CT with arterial portography (CTAP), CT hepatic arteriography (CTHA), and angiography. In CTAP, a contrast agent is injected into the superior mesenteric artery or the splenic artery prior to the scan. Delayed images are obtained when the contrast material has entered the portal venous system. Because it is not well perfused by the portal system, HCC appears as a low-density area against the surrounding liver parenchyma. Angiography of the hepatic artery is performed to further delineate aberrant blood supply to the liver or, more infrequently, prior to the placement of a hepatic artery infusion pump.

Diagnostic laparoscopy (DL), although invasive, may have a role in the workup for some patients with HCC. Patients most likely to benefit from DL are those with large or ruptured tumors, possible advanced cirrhosis, or indeterminate nodules in the FLR.

When the diagnosis of HCC is uncertain (e.g., when imaging findings are noncharacteristic and AFP is normal), the histologic diagnosis of HCC can be obtained by US-guided percutaneous needle biopsy or fine-needle aspiration (FNA) biopsy of the mass. Tumor seeding along the biopsy needle track rarely occurs when using modern techniques (<1% of cases). The risks of significant bleeding are low. The risks associated with major resection or transplantation for benign disease may be outweighed by the benefit of FNA biopsy in cases where the diagnosis is uncertain.

Staging

The current American Joint Committee on Cancer (AJCC) staging system for HCC is shown in Table 12.1. This system is unified with the Union Internationale Contre le Cancer (UICC) system and is derived from the analysis by Vauthey et al., of an international group of patients from the United States, France, and Japan who underwent complete resection of HCC. Tumor size per se has no effect on survival in patients who have solitary tumors without vascular invasion. The new system recognizes that the

Table 12.1. American Joint Commission on Cancer staging system for primary liver cancer

Primary tumor (T)			
TX	Primary cannot be assessed		
T0	No evidence of primary tumor		
T1	Solitary tumor without vascular invasion		
T2	Solitary tumor with vascular invasion or multiple tumors none more than 5 cm		
T3	Multiple tumors more than 5 cm or tumor involving a major branch of the portal or hepatic vein(s)		
T4	Tumor(s) with direct invasion of adjacent organs other than the gallbladder or with perforation of visceral peritoneum		
Regional lymph nodes (N)			
NX	Regional lymph nodes cannot be assessed		
N0	No regional lymph node metastasis		
N1	Regional lymph node metastasis		
Distant metastasis (M)			
MX	Distant metastasis cannot be assessed		
M0	No distant metastasis		
M1	Distant metastasis		
Stage groupings			
Stage I	T1	N0	M0
Stage II	T2	N0	M0
Stage IIIA	T3	N0	M0
Stage IIIB	T4	N0	M0
Stage IIIC	Any T	N1	M0
Stage IV	Any T	Any N	M1
Histological grade (G)			
GX	Grade cannot be assessed		
G1	Well differentiated		
G2	Moderately differentiated		
G3	Poorly differentiated		
G4	Undifferentiated		
Fibrosis score (F)			
F0	Fibrosis score 0–4 (no fibrosis to moderate fibrosis)		
F1	Fibrosis score 5–6 (severe fibrosis to cirrhosis)		

Adapted from Greene FL, Page DL, Fleming ID, Fritzag, Balch EM, Haller DG, Marrow M, editors. *AJCC Cancer Staging Manual*. 6th ed. New York, NY: Springer-Verlag; 2002, with permission.

prognosis for T1 tumors >10 cm in largest diameter is the same as that for smaller T1 tumors (T1 = any size, without vascular invasion). Tumors having evidence of microvascular invasion or multiple tumors less than 5 cm in diameter are designated as T2 disease. HCC with major vascular invasion or with multiple tumors, with at least one measuring 5 cm, are designated T3. Most important, the presence of severe fibrosis of the underlying liver has a negative impact on overall survival, regardless of the T classification. For stage I disease, the 5-year survival rate is 64% when there is no fibrosis (F0) and 49% when fibrosis is present (F1). For stage II disease, the 5-year survival rate is 46% for F0 disease and 30% for F1 disease. For stage IIIA disease, the 5-year survival rate is 17% for F0 disease and 9% for F1 disease. The AJCC staging manual recommends notation of fibrosis but has not yet formally incorporated the F classification into the staging system.

The majority of patients analyzed in the international study by Vauthey et al. had HCV-related HCC rather than HBV-related HCC; thus, Poon et al. undertook validation of the staging system with HBV-infected patients from Hong Kong. Despite the different clinicopathological features of patients with HCV and HBV, Poon et al. demonstrated that the new staging system provides reliable prognostic information for patients with hepatitis B, and showed that the new system is simpler to use than the previous AJCC staging system. Appropriate emphasis is placed on the most important prognostic features: vascular invasion within the tumor, and fibrosis of the nontumoral liver. Several other authors from Taiwan and Europe have independently validated the AJCC/UICC system, confirming its prognostic accuracy.

Patient Selection for Surgical Treatment

HCC typically occurs in the background of cirrhosis. Thus, after assessment of a patient's candidacy for surgery based on overall health and comorbidity, assessment of liver function is necessary.

The most widely used classification system for the assessment of liver function is the Child-Pugh (sometimes called the Child-Pugh-Turcotte) system. The parameters measured in this classification system are the total bilirubin and albumin levels, presence or absence of ascites, presence or absence of encephalopathy, and prothrombin time/international normalized ratio; together, these parameters give a rough estimate of the gross synthetic and detoxification capacity of the liver. Numerous studies have validated this system as an overall predictor of survival after surgery in cirrhotic patients (Table 12.2). Patients with Child-Pugh class A liver function generally tolerate hepatic resection. Patients with class B liver function may tolerate minor resection, but generally do not tolerate major resection. Patients with class C liver function are at significant risk from anesthesia and laparotomy.

Several other clinical staging systems have been developed to guide initial therapy for HCC. The Okuda staging system, developed in Japan, incorporates tumor size, ascites status, and albumin and bilirubin levels, accounting for both liver function and tumor extension. The Cancer of the Liver Italian Program

Table 12.2. Child-Pugh classification of hepatic functional reserve

Clinical or Laboratory Feature	1 Point	2 Points	3 Points
Encephalopathy (grade)	0 (absent)	1–2	3–4
Ascites	Absent	Slight	Poorly
Bilirubin (mg/dL)	<2.0	2.0–3.0	>3.0
Albumin (g/dL)	>3.5	2.8–3.5	<2.8
International normalized ratio	<1.7	1.7–2.2	>2.3

Each feature is assigned 1, 2, or 3 points.
Class A: 5–6 points; Class B: 7–9 points; Class C: 10–15 points.

(CLIP) group derived a system from a retrospective study of 435 patients diagnosed with HCC that incorporates the Child-Pugh score, data on tumor morphology and extension, presence or absence of portal vein thrombosis, and serum level of AFP. The Barcelona Clinic Liver Cancer (BCLC) system uses a clinical staging system based on tumor progression and liver function. The CLIP and Okuda systems may be useful to predict prognosis in patients who have advanced tumors and liver disease but are not useful for treatment selection. The BCLC system is highly criticized and has not been widely accepted because it allocates palliative treatment to patients who are candidates for curative resection. The BCLC system is generally considered to be more of a treatment algorithm than a staging system.

For anatomically resectable HCC without extrahepatic metastases, our approach to patient selection for major hepatectomy is first based on clinical parameters (performance status, Child-Pugh classification) and degree of portal hypertension. We require a platelet count ≥100,000 and exclude patients with gastric or esophageal varices. Next, systematic determination of the FLR volume, as described previously, is necessary. PVE is considered based on the previous criteria. We do not use ICG clearance or other tests of liver function in this assessment.

This approach enables resection in cirrhotics with low incidences of liver failure and death. In patients with normal livers, this approach enables extended hepatectomy with <1% mortality and very low morbidity. The systematic evaluation of patients using standardized volumetry is the key to low morbidity and mortality, despite extensive and aggressive hepatic surgery in our center.

Surgical Resection

The standard treatment for HCC is surgical resection or orthotopic liver transplantation (OLT). However, not all patients with HCC are candidates for surgical resection; of those presenting with HCC, only 10% and 30% will be eligible for surgery, and of those patients who undergo exploratory surgery, only 50% and

70% will have a resection with curative intent. Patients with cirrhosis may be candidates for limited surgical resection, OLT, or locoregional ablative treatment, depending on the severity of the cirrhosis.

The only absolute criterion that renders a tumor unresectable is the presence of extrahepatic disease (and even this exclusion has caveats in highly selected cases). Other relative contraindications to resection are evidence of severe hepatic dysfunction, an inadequate FLR, and tumor involvement of the portal vein or vena cava. Patients with normal liver parenchyma are usually eligible for extensive resection. Patients with compensated cirrhosis may be candidates for minor or major hepatectomy in selected cases.

Once the tumor has been determined to be resectable, the next decision is the extent of liver resection to be done. The extent of surgery will depend, in part, on the size of the mass, the number of nodules, the tumor's proximity to vascular structures, and as discussed previously, the severity of any underlying liver disease. Formerly, a 1-cm surgical margin was believed to be necessary to ensure long-term survival after resection. However, Poon et al. analyzed outcome based on resection margins in 288 patients who underwent hepatectomy for HCC and found that recurrence rates were similar between groups with narrow (<1 cm) and wide (≥1 cm) margins; only patients with histologically positive margins or satellites separate from the main tumor had relatively high recurrence rates. The authors noted that patients with margins positive for HCC had a higher incidence of intratumoral microvascular invasion than other patients. In addition, recurrences did not necessarily occur at the margin, but also sometimes appeared in the remaining liver, distant from the margin, reflecting tumor biology that was more likely to lead to a positive margin.

The operative approach to the patient with a potentially resectable HCC should begin with a thorough surgical exploration of the abdomen, searching for evidence of extrahepatic disease. In particular, care should be taken to evaluate the periportal lymph nodes in addition to the nodes in the hepatoduodenal ligament. The liver then should be completely mobilized to allow full examination of the organ. Intraoperative US should be used to define both the size of the tumor and its relationship to the major vascular and biliary structures. DL should be considered in patients with ruptured tumors, indeterminate nodules, or possible extrahepatic disease.

Anatomical resections are preferred over segmental resections, when feasible, based on the extent of underlying liver disease and because of the tendency of HCC to spread along portal tracts. In addition, portal-oriented resections have been shown to be associated with lower morbidity, mortality, and blood loss, as well as higher survival rates, than segmental resections. Regimbeau et al. demonstrated that the overall 5-year survival rate in patients who underwent anatomical resections (54%) exceeded that of those who had segmental resections (35%). Extended hepatectomy is generally not feasible in patients with cirrhosis, but major hepatectomy can be considered when PVE is used appropriately, as described previously, following systematic volumetry of the FLR.

A major pattern of recurrence after hepatic resection is intrahepatic failure with development of new disease. The concept of the field of cancerization—that is, the tendency of the remaining liver to generate new HCCs—partially explains the 30% to 70% recurrence rate after hepatic resection. Recurrence risk and survival vary, based on two dominant factors and several other minor factors. The most potent predictors of poor survival and high-risk recurrence of HCC are vascular invasion in the tumor and severe fibrosis in the underlying liver. Other correlates with poor outcome are absence of a tumor capsule and high-grade or poor tumor differentiation.

A recent study from our International Liver Tumor Study Group examined the risk factors for recurrence <1 year from resection. We identified tumor size greater than 5 cm, multiple tumors, and histology revealing more than five mitoses per ten high-power fields as being associated with risk of early death due to recurrence. We stress that these are not exclusion criteria—that is, the presence of multiple or large tumors that are resectable should not exclude patients from consideration for potentially curative resection. Rather, these factors help us move forward in identifying patients whose HCCs are likely to recur and who might benefit from adjuvant therapy, if that is developed for HCC.

Hepatitis serology has also been proposed as a factor related to the risk of HCC, but in another large study from our institution, we demonstrated that hepatitis serology, per se, is not a predictor of this outcome. Analysis of 446 patients in our international database who underwent complete resection for HCC demonstrated that patients with HBV infection or no infection tended to have larger tumors than patients with HCV or HBV+HCV infection. In addition, the serology-negative and HBV-infected patients had a higher incidence of vascular invasion; in contrast, they had lower incidence of severe, underlying liver fibrosis, which was predominant in the other two groups. However, the final analysis revealed that status of vascular invasion and fibrosis were equally predictive of poor outcome and that the other putative risk factors were not independent; that is, patients with HBV or no infection have larger tumors with vascular invasion but no fibrosis, whereas patients with HCV infection who are screened regularly tend to have smaller tumors and a lower incidence of vascular invasion but established cirrhosis.

Major vascular invasion, that is, invasion of a main portal trunk or hepatic vein, even extending to the vena cava, presents a difficult problem. Survival in patients with this feature has generally been poor; however, selected patients can derive a significant palliative benefit from hepatectomy with extraction of caval thrombi or hepatectomy in the presence of segmental portal vein thrombosis. Specific indications for such extensive surgery are beyond the scope of this chapter, but selected patients in this group can be treated with major hepatectomy, which can provide significantly better survival than other treatment options.

In the event of recurrence after resection, selected patients can be considered for repeat resection, depending on the pattern of recurrence. Both focal, intrahepatic, recurrent tumors and certain adrenal metastases can be resected. Solitary extrahepatic metastases at sites such as the lung, diaphragm, and abdominal wall can also be resected. In all these cases, median survival may be as high as 50 months, compared with survival on the order of 10 months for those treated without surgery.

Although some classification systems, such as the BCLC system, and some groups in the United States propose that patients with large tumors should not be considered for surgery, many authors recognize that tumor size alone does not predict biology. In fact, many studies have shown that patients with T1 tumors >10 cm in diameter have exactly the same survival pattern after resection as those with tumors <3 cm. We recently analyzed 300 patients undergoing resection for tumors >10 cm and found that, for the entire group, including some patients with vascular invasion, the 5-year survival was 27% and the 10-year survival was 18%. Perioperative mortality was 5%. There were long-term (≥10 years) survivors among patients who had more than one tumor in which the largest exceeded 10 cm in diameter. As would be expected, the best survival was achieved in patients who had tumors without vascular invasion and who did not have severe fibrosis. We also analyzed the utility of a clinical scoring system to select patients with large HCCs for resection, using AFP, tumor number, and presence or absence of major vascular invasion and fibrosis as the factors placed into the scoring system. Patients with no risk factors (high AFP, multiple tumors, major vascular invasion or fibrosis) had a 5-year survival rate of nearly 50%. Those with any risk factor had a 5-year survival rate in the 20% range, but even in the group of patients with three risk factors, there were 10-year survivors. AJCC T classification clearly stratifies survival; this has been validated in many studies, including that of Yamanaka et al., who found that resection of T1 tumors yielded a 5-year survival rate as high as 78%.

Orthotopic Liver Transplantation

Even in the case of margin-negative resection of HCC, recurrence remains a problem. Most published series report a median survival of 30 to 40 months with a 5-year survival rate of 30% to 40%, as well as a high incidence of recurrence, ranging from 30% to 70%. It has been suggested that the liver fibrosis and necrosis associated with chronic, active hepatitis caused by HBV and HCV provides a potential field for further HCC development (a field of cancerization); imaging studies of patients with chronic liver disease have led to the early detection of small HCCs (<5 cm). For these reasons, some have proposed that the only definitive treatment for HCC is orthotopic liver transplantation (OLT) to remove both the HCC tumors and the damaged liver parenchyma.

Once liver transplantation was established as a safe treatment for cirrhosis, it began to be considered as a treatment option for unresectable tumors of the liver, but early recurrence was the rule. The observation that the outcome following transplantation for liver failure in patients found *incidentally* to have small HCC suggested that better selection criteria might reinsert liver transplantation into the treatment strategy for HCC. These criteria were formalized after analysis of a study by Mazzaferro et al., who evaluated patients with cirrhosis and either a single tumor ≤5 cm or three tumors ≤3 cm in maximum diameter, who underwent liver transplantation. Survival at 5 years after transplantation exceeded 60%, with disease-free survival exceeding 50%. These criteria, based on the Milan Meeting, were then adopted as the criteria for appropriate selection of patients for OLT for HCC, although the study was small (48 patients) and no tumor had vascular invasion.

Interest exists in expanding these criteria so OLT can be considered in cases of larger and more numerous tumors, although biological selection criteria (e.g., tumor grade and AFP level) would be more attractive criteria for selection than the simple morphologic criteria of tumor size and number currently used. Furthermore, the effect of chronic immunosuppression on the course of recurrent cancer after transplantation is unclear.

Nonresectional Locoregional Therapies

For selected patients with HCC confined to the liver whose disease is not amenable to surgical resection or OLT, locoregional ablative therapies can be considered. Although these therapies may also be used in patients with resectable HCC, their efficacy has not been established as equivalent to resection. A discussion of ablation treatments follows.

The advantages of ablation techniques include destruction of tumors and preservation of a maximal volume of nontumorous liver, and the potential to combine ablation of small lesions with resection of larger lesions. The major disadvantages of any ablation technique are the limited ability to evaluate treatment margins and the need to obtain negative treatment margins in three dimensions. All ablation techniques have higher local recurrence rates than resection for virtually all tumors. Percutaneous ablation is particularly attractive for treatment of patients with severe underlying liver disease, for treatment of patients with a contraindication to laparotomy, or as a bridge to more definitive therapy, such as OLT.

Percutaneous Ethanol Injection

Percutaneous ethanol injection (PEI) is a treatment administered under US guidance through a fine (22-gauge) needle. Absolute ethanol (8–10 mL) induces cellular dehydration, necrosis, and vascular thrombosis, causing tumor cell death. Outpatient treatments are repeated once or twice a week, for up to 6 weeks. PEI is most effective for tumors <3 cm in diameter. Studies have demonstrated 100% necrosis in HCCs <2 cm in diameter. The treatment-related death rate has been reported to be 0.09% to 0.1% and the complication rate 1.7% to 3.2%. PEI is contraindicated in patients with gross ascites, coagulopathy, and obstructive jaundice, as well as in patients with large tumors, thrombosis in the main portal or hepatic vein, and extrahepatic metastasis. Complications that can occur with this method include minor adverse effects, such as pain and fever, as well as hemorrhage, liver abscess and failure, and cholangitis.

Several studies have documented post-PEI survival rates similar to those obtained with hepatic resection for extremely small tumors in well-selected patients, but HCC recurrence in the liver is frequent, with an incidence of 50% at 2 years; the majority of recurrences are new lesions in distant segments of the liver. Randomized trials suggest PEI is appropriate for tumors ≤2 cm in diameter because it has lower rates of morbidity but equivalent efficacy when compared with other ablation techniques, such as radiofrequency ablation (RFA).

Cryotherapy

Cryotherapy is no longer commonly used as an ablation technique. Serious complications that can occur with this method include intraoperative hemorrhage from the probe tract, bile duct fistula, freezing injury to adjacent structures, and renal failure related to myoglobinuria. For these reasons, cryotherapy has largely been supplanted by newer ablation techniques.

Radiofrequency Ablation

RFA uses heat to destroy tumors. Using US or CT guidance, a needle electrode with an uninsulated tip is inserted into the tumor. The electrode delivers a high-frequency alternating current, generating rapid vibration of ions, which leads to frictional heat and, ultimately, coagulative tissue necrosis. RFA can be performed percutaneously, laparoscopically, or through an open incision and is most effective in tumors <3 cm in diameter. Larger tumors generally require several insertions of the electrode.

RFA complications are rare but may include pneumothorax, pleural effusion, hemorrhage, subcapsular hematoma, hemobilia, biliary stricture, and liver abscess. The treatment-related death rate has been reported to be 0% to 1% and the complication rate 0% to 12%. Early tumor recurrence after RFA treatment is associated with large tumor size, poor histological differentiation, advanced stage of presentation, elevated serum AFP, and the presence of hepatitis. RFA may be more effective in patients with cirrhosis because the fibrotic liver permits a "baking effect" by confining the heat to the tumor. The safety and efficacy of RFA for HCC in cirrhotic patients were largely established at the M. D. Anderson Cancer Center.

Several studies have suggested that RFA may be effective for unresectable tumors. Two reports have directly compared percutaneous RFA and surgery for treatment of HCC. Despite having higher rates of local recurrence, patients treated with RFA had overall survival and recurrence-free survival rates similar to those of patients undergoing surgical resection. Hong et al. reported a series of 148 patients who presented with solitary small (<4 cm diameter) HCCs and either no evidence of cirrhosis or Child-Pugh class A hepatic function. The patients selected for RFA either refused surgery or were predicted to have insufficient postoperative hepatic reserve to justify the high operative risks, and were significantly older than those in the comparative resection group. The overall recurrence rates for RFA and surgery were 41.8% and 54.8%, respectively, but the rate of local recurrence (defined as occurring near the margin of the ablation) was higher in the RFA group (7.3%) than in the surgery group (0.0%). The rates of remote recurrence (defined as distant metastasis or intraheptic metastasis in the hepatic parenchyma, but somewhere other than the original tumor site) and of simultaneous local and remote recurrence were similar between the two treatment groups. The 1- and 3-year overall survival rates were 97.9% and 83.9%, respectively, in the surgery group and 100% and 72.7%, respectively, in the RFA group.

However, equivalence of RFA to surgery has not been consistently supported. Some studies have demonstrated that patients treated with surgical resection had significantly higher overall and disease-free survival rates. Furthermore, patients with significant underlying liver dysfunction had similar survival rates regardless of treatment, suggesting RFA may be a suitable alternative for patients with progressive hepatic dysfunction in livers already so impaired as to preclude safe surgical resection; nevertheless, surgical resection remains the gold standard for HCC. With the cooperation of two separate medical institutions, Vivarelli et al. reported 158 patients who underwent either RFA or surgical resection. The majority of patients in the surgery group had Child-Pugh class A liver function, whereas most patients treated with RFA had class B function. The RFA group did have a few patients with Child-Pugh A liver function with a single potentially resectable nodule. Furthermore, in both the RFA and surgery groups, a majority of patients had chronic hepatitis caused by HBV, HCV, or HCV+HBV infection. The overall and disease-free survival rates were significantly higher for patients treated with resection. One- and 3-year rates of overall survival were 78% and 33%, respectively, for surgical patients and were 60% and 20%, respectively, for RFA patients. Patients with Child-Pugh class A liver function and with solitary lesions, as well as lesions <3 cm in maximum diameter, had significantly higher rates of survival with surgery (overall 3-year survival = 79%) than with RFA (overall 3-year survival = 50%).

There is no consensus regarding the efficacy of RFA as a single therapy for HCC, but the ablative technique is generally accepted as the best treatment for small HCCs in the patient whose tumor cannot be resected safely or as a means of preventing tumor growth/spread prior to OLT. For patients who have a tumor recurrence after treatment and who are not candidates for resection, RFA is probably the best "salvage technique" and may enable long-term remission. Ablation techniques such as RFA clearly have an important role in the treatment of a subset of patients with HCC.

Chemotherapy

In general, systemic chemotherapy has little activity against HCC. Single-agent chemotherapy with 5-fluorouracil (5-FU), doxorubicin, cisplatin, vinblastine, etoposide, and mitoxantrone provides response rates of 15% to 20%, and the responses are usually short lasting. Combination chemotherapy does not seem to improve these results. The most active agent appears to be doxorubicin, with an overall response rate pooled from several trials of 19%.

Current treatment regimens for unresectable HCC combine conventional chemotherapy (specifically 5-FU) with immunomodulatory agents, such as alpha-interferon. Preclinical and clinical studies have demonstrated that the two drugs have synergistic activity against colorectal cancer. Despite its considerable toxic effects, including myelosuppression, the combination of doxorubicin, 5-FU, and alpha-interferon (PIAF) downstaged initially unresectable tumors to a size amenable for resection, and increased the overall median survival rate in an important study conducted in Hong Kong. The same investigators have reported sufficient tumor regression for subsequent resection, enabling long-term survival after PIAF.

Other therapies, including hormonally active (Tamoxifen), vitamin-based (retinoid), and molecular agents (angiogenesis inhibitors), are under investigation, but results so far are generally disappointing.

Transcatheter Arterial Embolization and Transarterial Chemoembolization

Transarterial chemoembolization (TACE) is a combination of intra-arterially infused chemotherapy and hepatic artery occlusion, whereas transcatheter arterial embolization (TAE) omits the chemotherapeutic agent. Chemotherapeutic agents may be either infused into the liver before embolization or impregnated in the gelatin sponges used for the embolization. Lipiodol also has been used in conjunction with TACE because this agent will remain selectively in HCCs for an extended period, allowing the delivery of locally concentrated therapy.

Two randomized control trials have shown that TACE provides a survival advantage for patients with unresectable HCC; thus, TACE is the standard of care for patients who are not candidates for resection, transplantation, or ablation. Furthermore, TACE can be used in combination with ablation or resection or as a bridge to transplantation.

Despite the favorable results of TACE therapy, this treatment modality has limitations. Morbidity rates have been reported to be as high as 23%, especially among patients with HCCs >10 cm in diameter. Moreover, postembolization syndrome, including fever, nausea, and pain, is common. Other side effects and complaints, such as fatal hepatic necrosis and liver failure, have rarely been reported. TACE is generally contraindicated in patients with ascites.

Lo et al. presented a randomized controlled trial of TACE and Lipiodol for unresectable HCC in patients with compensated liver failure and in patients with advanced disease (including segmental portal invasion). The chemotherapeutic agent was an emulsion of cisplatin in Lipiodol and gelatin-sponge particles, which was injected through the hepatic artery. The chemoembolization group (40 patients) received a median of 4.5 courses per patient and showed significant tumor response. For the chemoembolization group, the 1-, 2-, and 3-year survival rates were 57%, 31%, and 26%, respectively, while for the control group the rates were 32%, 11%, and 3%, respectively ($p = 0.005$).

Another investigator from the BCLC group performed a randomized trial comparing either TAE or TACE with symptomatic treatment in a much more selected group of patients, who had favorable characteristics compared with those studied by Lo et al. The 112 nonsurgical candidates with HCC and cirrhosis had Child-Pugh class A or B liver functional reserve. The TACE group received doxorubicin combined with Lipiodol and gelfoam. The trial was stopped when data review demonstrated that chemoembolization yielded survival rates significantly higher than those of conservative treatment. One- and 2-year survival rates were, respectively, 75% and 50% for the embolization group, 82% and 63% for the chemoembolization group, and 63% and 27% for the control group. Since publication of these trials, TACE has secured a role in the treatment of selected patients with HCC.

Radiation Therapy

External-beam radiation therapy has limited utility in the treatment of HCC. The dose that can be safely delivered to the liver is approximately 30 Gy; higher doses cause radiation hepatitis. Radiation therapy can, however, provide palliative, symptomatic relief among highly selected patients with HCC. Alternatively, locally concentrated doses of radiation can be delivered along with intra-arterially infused Lipiodol or antiferritin antibodies coupled to radioactive iodine. These therapies are considered investigational.

Multimodality Therapy

Combinations of surgical and nonsurgical therapies are the state-of-the-art for HCC. Some unresectable tumors can be rendered resectable by transarterial chemotherapy, portal vein embolization, or systemic chemotherapy. Various chemotherapeutic agents have been studied in the neoadjuvant setting, including doxorubicin, 5-FU, mitomycin C, and cisplatin. Furthermore, tumor recurrence may be prevented by the administration of adjuvant intra-arterial chemotherapy after surgical resection or PEI.

Strategies implementing TACE and PVE have allowed safe complete resection of HCCs in patients with marginal liver function. TACE inhibits tumor progression because HCCs derive the majority of their blood supply from the hepatic artery. Subsequent PVE induces hypertrophy of the contralateral liver without diverting blood through the tumor's arterial blood supply. This combined treatment modality may be particularly important for HCCs with vascular invasion of the portal or major hepatic vein.

METASTASES TO THE LIVER

Nearly all malignant tumors can metastasize to and proliferate in the liver. Most metastases originate from gastrointestinal primary tumors, and of these, most are from the colon and rectum. In general, 5-year survival is rare among patients who undergo resection for noncolorectal metastases to the liver. The exceptions are selected patients with, in particular, neuroendocrine tumors, Wilm's tumor, and to a lesser extent, renal cell carcinoma; 5-year survival rates of 40% to >70% have been reported after resection of their metastases. Hepatic resection may provide excellent palliation of the hormone syndrome in selected patients with hormone-secreting neuroendocrine tumors. Given that the vast majority of liver metastases that are considered for resection are from colorectal primary tumors, the remainder of this discussion is concerned with their management.

Epidemiology and Etiology

Colorectal cancer represents the third most common type of cancer for both men and women in the United States, with an estimated incidence of 150,000 cases per year. Approximately 85% of the patients will have malignancies that are amenable to surgical cure, but half of the resected cancers will recur within 5 years. Only 20% of these recurrences will be solely or predominantly in the liver, and fewer still will be amenable to surgical resection a second time. It has been estimated that 15,000 to 20,000 patients per year are potential candidates for resection of their liver metastases.

Clinical Presentation and Diagnosis

Symptoms or clinical signs suggesting metastatic disease in the liver usually are late occurrences. Consequently, findings such as ascites, jaundice, right upper quadrant pain, and increases in serum levels of factors associated with liver function are associated with a poor prognosis. In the vast majority of patients, metastases to the liver are found during routine postoperative carcinoembryonic antigen (CEA) screening or radiologic imaging after resection of a colorectal primary tumor. Patients with increasing CEA levels should undergo thorough diagnostic evaluation, including chest radiography and contrast-enhanced CT scan of the abdomen and pelvis. A slowly increasing CEA level usually indicates local or regional recurrence, whereas a rapidly increasing CEA level suggests hepatic metastases. Overall, 75% to 90% of patients with hepatic colorectal cancer metastases have an increased CEA level. In addition, colonoscopy should be performed to exclude a local recurrence or metachronous colon or rectal primary tumor as the source of the increasing CEA value.

Determining Resectability

Because indications for hepatic resection have been extended to include selected metastases from colorectal cancer, here, too, the FLR defines resectability. When all hepatic disease can be extirpated with a negative margin, leaving an adequate FLR (20% of the standardized TLV) with adequate vascular inflow, hepatic venous outflow, and biliary drainage, metastases from colorectal cancer should be deemed resectable. Specific recommendations with regard to response to chemotherapy are difficult to make, although patients with multiple metastases that continue growing during chemotherapy should probably be excluded from candidacy for hepatic resection; this same rule may not be applicable to patients with solitary lesions. Similarly, responsiveness to chemotherapy should not be a criterion for determining resectability. Clinical criteria such as CEA level, number of tumors, size of tumors, and location of the primary tumor, although prognostic, cannot be used to exclude patients from resection and a potential cure.

In cases of bilateral disease, multistage approaches to surgery should be considered. At the first stage, wedge or limited resection clears the planned FLR, preserving the major portion of the parenchyma in preparation for resection of the remaining liver. At the second stage, major hepatectomy or extended hepatectomy removes all remaining disease. Resection of dominant lesions and RFA of residual disease may be considered, but this approach yields poor survival compared with staged resection. Staged resection requires a certain level of excellence, an integrated multidisciplinary approach to disease management, and usually, interval PVE to increase the volume and function of the FLR after the first-stage resection. High tumor number, large tumor size, presence of limited extrahepatic disease, and extensive resection are no longer barriers to resection. Systemic chemotherapy can reduce the size and volume of tumors such that all tumor sites can be resected safely and provide long-term survival. Highly selected patients with extrahepatic disease—whether limited peritoneal carcinomatosis, minimal hilar lymphadenopathy, or metastatic disease to the lung—can undergo resection with acceptable survival.

Finally, the rule that a 1-cm margin is necessary to ensure long-term survival has been shattered. Analysis of nearly 500 patients in a multi-institutional database showed that the pattern and probability of disease recurrence and the rates of disease-free and overall survival were identical in patients with 1-mm and 1-cm resection margins. Thus, determining whether metastases from colorectal cancer are resectable requires a multidisciplinary approach and the participation of an experienced hepatic surgeon; otherwise, patients who have metastases that would otherwise be considered resectable will be relegated to noncurative therapy, such as systemic chemotherapy. A 1-cm margin remains the goal, but close margin-negative resection is also safe.

Evaluation of Operative Risk

Most patients with colorectal liver metastases (CRLM) have a normal underlying liver, although some will have injury due to prior therapy or more important patient factors (e.g., obesity and diabetes, which are associated with steatosis). Although some studies suggest that hepatic resection in patients with steatosis is associated with increased operative risk, blood loss, and complications, we have not found an increase in operative or postoperative complications related to chemotherapy. Most agree that mortality is equivalent to that for resection in patients without significant steatosis.

Patients who require extended hepatectomy should undergo systematic volumetry as described previously and if the FLR volume is <20% of the standardized TLV, they should undergo PVE of the entire tumor-bearing liver before resection. Some investigators have proposed that a larger remnant (e.g., 30% of the TLV) is necessary for patients who have received intensive chemotherapy; however, this group has not been studied systematically.

Particular to patients with metastases is the concern that tumor growth may be incited by the embolization. We have shown that complete embolization of the tumor-bearing liver is not associated with changes in tumor size that affect resectability; thus, we stress the importance of complete embolization of the liver to be resected and complete hepatic resection when this approach is used.

Other Methods of Preoperative Staging

High-quality imaging is critical to assessment of CRLM resectability. Although many modalities have been proposed, including MRI and positron emission tomography (PET) scanning, we use CT scanning almost exclusively at our institution; our published survival rates are equal to the best reported for resection of metastases from colorectal cancer, validating this approach. CT not only permits assessment of extrahepatic structures, but also accurately provides for liver volumetry, accurate localization of the tumors within the liver, and accurate lesion detection. Multiphase, thin-cut, spiral, hepatic CT is our modality of choice, and the information thus gained has been superior to that afforded by MRI and other approaches, resulting in our high rates of survival.

DL has a limited role in staging of CRLM; mainly because imaging is sensitive, full exploration by means of DL is often limited due to prior surgery, and additional findings at DL may *change* the operative approach, but typically do not lead to abandonment of resection.

Careful prelaparotomy staging must include colonoscopy to rule out local recurrence, plain radiography of the chest, and CT of the chest when indicated by the radiographic findings.

Although [^{18}F]fluoro-2-deoxy-D-glucose PET has been proposed by Fernandez et al. as necessary for staging, no study (including that by Fernandez et al., which did not use high-quality CT) has shown that PET improves outcome when high-quality cross-sectional imaging is used. However, false-negative PET is the rule after chemotherapy, limiting the utility of this technique alone. PET is likely to improve detection of extrahepatic disease, but has not yet become the standard of care.

Surgical Therapy

At exploratory laparotomy, a careful search for extrahepatic disease should be undertaken, and detection of enlarged portal and celiac lymph nodes may prompt biopsy when necessary. The colon should be examined for any local recurrence of the primary tumor. The liver is examined by visual inspection and palpation, and then by intraoperative US. US will help define the relationship of the tumor(s) to the portal veins, hepatic veins, and vena cava. In addition, it can identify small lesions that were not palpable or demonstrable on preoperative imaging studies. Suspicious areas can be sampled by FNA under US guidance. The type of resection to be performed will depend on what is needed to remove all disease and obtain microscopically disease-negative margins. Anatomical-oriented resection is favored over wedge resection because it is associated with less blood loss and lower likelihood of positive margins; this technique is often mandatory for patients with multiple lesions. However, it should be recognized that there is no oncologic indication for which anatomical resection is preferred to wedge resection, as long as the resection margin is negative for disease.

Survival After Resection of Colorectal Liver Metastases

Modern reports on series of patients undergoing hepatic resection for CRLM reveal that the new, gold standard 5-year survival rate is 53% to 58%. The 5-year survival rates have improved from earlier reported rates of 25% to 40%, despite the expansion of criteria, including resection of more and larger tumors and bilobar tumors, resection of synchronous CRLM, and resection with CRLM in the presence of limited extrahepatic disease. In select cases, it may be possible to resect synchronous liver metastases at the same time as the primary tumor. The complexity of the operation necessary to remove the primary tumor and the extent of hepatic resection that might be required for the primary tumor will affect decision making because the risk of adverse events from hepatic resection increases when the procedure is associated with extrahepatic surgery. Earlier studies demonstrated by univariate analysis that synchronous metastases were a predictor of poor prognosis. Solitary, small, peripherally located lesions in a healthy, hemodynamically stable patient can be excised adequately by nonanatomical resection or segmentectomy. Lesions that are larger or that will require a major hepatic resection are best approached during a second operation, after further evaluation and staging. A delay of weeks or months between surgeries has not been shown to negatively affect survival. At the time of the initial operation, a thorough exploration should be conducted to rule out the presence of extrahepatic metastases.

Prognostic Factors After Resection

Several modern studies have highlighted the improvement in survival over time with the use of improved operative techniques, anesthesia, patient selection, imaging, and probably chemotherapy. Figueras et al., who deemed all CRLMs resectable in patients who had an adequate FLR, regardless of tumor size or number, and who included patients with resectable extrahepatic disease, reported a 5-year survival rate of 53%. Choti et al. reported on a series of patients treated between 1984 and 1992 and compared the outcome with that of patients treated at the same institution between 1993 and 1999. They demonstrated a significant increase in the rate of 5-year overall survival, which was 31% in the early group and 58% in the later group, despite reductions in the hospitalization duration and the rate of perioperative blood transfusion and similar rates of morbidity and mortality. It is noteworthy that PET scanning was not routinely used in this study; <10% of the patients underwent PET scanning, although more patients received pre- or postoperative chemotherapy.

We subsequently published a report on the largest modern series of patients who underwent resection of CRLMs. Most patients required a major resection (64% underwent a hemihepatectomy or extended hepatectomy), and nearly one-fourth of the patients required a procedure in addition to the hepatic resection. Survival in our series was 58%, identical to that seen in the Choti et al. series. Fernandez et al. used PET rather than high-quality CT, and the outcome for the 100 patients in their series was similar, with survival of 58% at 5 years. Thus, despite an expansion in the indications for resection, clearly a new gold standard of 58% 5-year survival can be achieved because this rate has been validated in several series from different institutions around the world.

Despite the progressive improvement in survival after resection of CRLM, most patients (50%–70%) will have a tumor recurrence after hepatic resection. Several important studies have outlined the key prognostic factors.

The first is from Scheele et al., who analyzed 654 patients treated between 1960 and 1998. This is an important paper because none of the patients received chemotherapy. The 5-, 10-, and

20-year survival rates were 39%, 28%, and 24%, respectively. It is important to note that in this series, patients with only one tumor had the same survival rate as patients with three or more tumors despite the absence of chemotherapy. Scheele et al. emphasized the importance of margin-negative (R0) resection in this regard.

The second and most widely quoted study to outline prognostic factors is from Fong et al., who evaluated a series of 1,001 consecutive patients who underwent hepatic resection for metastatic colorectal cancer at the Memorial Sloan-Kettering Cancer Center. Seven independent factors were associated with poor outcome, including disease at the surgical margin, presence of extrahepatic disease, metastatic disease in the lymph nodes of the primary lesion, a short disease-free interval from resection of the primary tumor to detection of metastases, the number of hepatic tumors, hepatic tumor diameter >5 cm, and the elevation of the CEA level. These factors contribute to outcome in different degrees, and scoring of these factors is helpful in predicting prognosis after resection, but not in selecting patients for surgery.

A recent study from the M. D. Anderson Cancer Center clarified the importance of a margin-negative resection by examining the site of recurrence after resection for CRLM based on surgical margin status in a multi-institutional database. Patients with surgical margins positive for tumor cells had an overall recurrence rate of 52%, compared with 39% for patients with negative margins. Margin width (whether > or <1 cm) did not affect recurrence frequency, location, or overall survival. The overall recurrence rate for all 557 patients was 40%. The majority of patients who had recurrences developed them at an extrahepatic site (66%), whether alone (30%) or with simultaneous intrahepatic recurrence (36%). Only 3.8% of patients had a recurrence at the surgical margin. The recurrence rates were similar in patients with negative margins of 1 and 4 mm (39%), 5 and 9 mm (41%), and ≥1 cm (39%). This multi-institutional study confirmed the previously published 58% 5-year survival rate after resection of CRLM.

Pathobiological factors, such as proliferation-associated protein (Ki-67) and telomerase (hTERT), have been shown to be independent and more potent predictors of survival after resection than the previously mentioned clinical factors. Finally, the use of chemotherapy in conjunction with surgery, and the use of more effective chemotherapy, will undoubtedly alter the effects of clinical factors on outcome, as indicated by the steadily improving long-term survival rates that have been achieved despite the expanding indications for resection of CRLMs.

Ablative Therapy

RFA is used widely as a treatment for CRLM. Unfortunately, its use was widespread before true indications for ablation were defined. Initial, well-designed studies proved the safety, excellent side effects profile, and efficacy of RFA for CRLM. Initial studies from our institution and later from Europe and the Cleveland Clinic suggested a 78% 1-year survival rate could be attained by RFA, with 3-year survival at 46%. Unfortunately, >12% of patients had disease recurrence at 1 year. We were prompted to re-examine RFA as a treatment for CRLM and found that, although RFA provides a modest survival benefit over chemotherapy alone for CRLM at 4 years (22% vs. 7%), the outcome after RFA is vastly inferior to that after resection in terms of both overall and disease-free survival, whether single or multiple tumors are treated and regardless of tumor size. Furthermore, the overall recurrence rate after RFA (84%) in our study was much greater than that after resection (52%); intrahepatic-only recurrence was four times higher with RFA (44%) than with resection (11%), and the frequency of true local recurrences at the RFA site (9%) was 4.5 times that of margin recurrences after resection (2%). Although we ablated only unresectable tumors, these data strongly suggest RFA is inferior to resection as a treatment for CRLM.

Subsequent studies have supported our findings. In 2003, Livraghi et al. reported on percutaneous RFA of potentially resectable CRLMs. Despite the fact that the treatment was done at a center of excellence, and despite the investigators' experience with RFA, they reported a 40% treatment failure rate and a 70% recurrence rate in the 88 treated patients. This result can be contrasted with the 10% or less rate of recurrence in the case of positive-margin resection, and the 50% or less recurrence rate among patients who undergo hepatic resection with much more aggressive tumors, larger tumors, more lesions, and even patients with extrahepatic disease, suggesting that RFA is not equivalent to resection in patients with potentially resectable lesions.

The next important study compared RFA with resection in patients with solitary CRLMs, and was reported by Oshowo et al. in 2003. They, too, showed that RFA is inferior to resection as a treatment modality for the group of patients with probably the best prognosis—that is, those with solitary lesions. Although these investigators claimed that the RFA outcome was equivalent to that of resection, they reported only a 55% 3-year survival rate for patients with solitary metastases after resection (compared with 53% with RFA), which is inferior to the survival rate achieved by resection in virtually every other series, including our own (which yielded a 5-year survival rate >60%).

RFA may be used as an adjunct to resection, as proposed by Elias et al. and further analyzed by our group. Resection of dominant lesions may be supplemented with RFA of small, residual tumors in the FLR. Unfortunately, our series reveals that this approach is no more effective than RFA alone, and 5-year survival will be <20%. Furthermore, mortality rates are higher with this approach (2.3%) than with extended hepatectomy (0.8% in our series). Finally, several studies examining two-stage approaches to resection with PVE have demonstrated survival rates of 40% at 5 years, again proving the superiority of complete resection over ablation of CRLM.

Ablation may be used to treat disease that is unresectable because the patient is not a candidate for laparotomy (because of comorbidity) or because removal of the tumor-bearing liver with a negative margin would leave an insufficient FLR, particularly in patients with underlying liver disease. An alternative to RFA in some patients is staged hepatic resection and portal vein embolization. RFA may also have a role in treatment of the ill-placed recurrence after major hepatectomy when repeat resection is not safe.

The potential for ablation may be limited by a tumor's proximity to the confluence of the bile ducts because thermal injury to the bile ducts can lead to biloma and bile fistula; a 1-cm distance is required. Furthermore, the effect of thermal damage on the FLR can be more significant than that identified at the time of treatment; ablation at the time of resection must be performed with care.

RFA is safe. Curley et al. reported a treatment-related mortality rate of 0.5% and an early (<30 days) treatment-related complication rate of 7.1%. The late (>30 days) complication rate was 2.4%. The two most common early complications were symptomatic pleural effusion and perihepatic and RFA lesion abscesses. Late complications were bilomas in the RFA lesion or biliary fistulas. Open or laparoscopic RFA is contraindicated for lesions within 2 cm of the biliary confluence, in the presence of bilioenteric anastomosis, and near critical portal structures in the liver remnant after resection or at the time of combined resection and ablation. Close proximity to bowel or the diaphragm is a relative contraindication. Mullen et al. reported successful RFA using a transthoracic approach for a postresection recurrence adjacent to the diaphragm. Contraindications for percutaneous RFA include not only those for the open/laparoscopic approach, but also inability to adequately image or access the lesion percutaneously. Percutaneous RFA is associated with treatment failure and, consequently, a higher recurrence rate.

Thus, as for assessment of the resectability of CRLM, assessment for RFA of CRLM should be made jointly by a multidisciplinary team and a hepatic surgeon with considerable experience in this decision scenario.

Chemotherapy

Recent advances in chemotherapy for colorectal cancer have dramatically changed the outlook for patients with stage IV disease. The former standard was a combination of 5-FU and leucovorin (LV), which provided response rates from 12% to 40% and median survival of 10 to 17 months. Two new drugs that have shown promise are irinotecan (CPT-11) and oxaliplatin. Various combination therapies using these agents (5-FU or LV, with or without oxaliplatin, FOLFOX [5-FU, LV, folinic acid, and oxaliplatin], and FOLFIRI [5-FU, LV, folinic acid, and irinotecan]) have yielded overall response rates >50% and median survival times >20 months in the general population of patients with stage IV disease.

Of great interest is the potential for rendering unresectable tumors resectable with chemotherapy. Giacchetti et al., and subsequently Adam et al., showed that about 13% of patients who present with unresectable CRLM, with or without extrahepatic disease, can undergo resection after chemotherapy. Adam has shown a 33% rate of overall survival and a 22% rate of disease-free survival after resection in patients with previously unresectable disease treated using this approach. New biological agents that target angiogenesis have been approved for use and generally increase response rates from standard chemotherapy by about 10%.

It is hoped that these agents will be able to downstage disease and thereby permit resection in a greater proportion of patients who present with unresectable disease. Chemotherapy can be hepatotoxic; this problem is only now being recognized and studied in relation to subsequent resection and complications.

Regional Chemotherapy

Although patients with CRLM have systemic disease, the approximate 50% intrahepatic relapse rate led to investigation of liver-directed chemotherapy, alone or as an adjuvant to resection. Although 5-FU is the favored drug for use in systemic chemotherapy, its first-pass clearance by the liver is low. Consequently, the relative increase in hepatic exposure to the drug by hepatic arterial infusion (HAI) is estimated to be only five- to tenfold. A related pyrimidine antagonist, floxuridine (fluorodeoxyuridine [FUDR]), has a much higher extraction on the first pass through the liver. The estimated increase in the liver's exposure to this drug when delivered by HAI is 100- to 400-fold, making it ideal for this purpose.

The best reported response rates using HAI chemotherapy are 50% to 62% in studies that date from the late 1980s. Two recent European trials using 5-FU in patients with unresectable liver disease failed to demonstrate an improvement in survival and had a high complication rate. HAI therapy for unresectable disease has failed to keep pace with improving systemic chemotherapy including the emergence of new agents such as irinotecan and oxaliplatin that can yield high response rates (54%–56%) and median survival of 22 months with acceptable toxicity. The addition of biological agents (including bevacizumab and cetuximab) has increased response rates by 10% and increased median survival to 25 to 27 months. Use of the new chemotherapeutic and biological drugs has made it possible to downstage unresectable tumors to the point where surgical resection is possible. HAI therapy alone enables only 2% to 3% of patients with unresectable CRLM to downstage such that resection is possible; the rate is significantly lower than that obtained using systemic chemotherapy. Moreover, HAI chemotherapy makes the assessment of liver function and hepatectomy difficult, and may result in arterial thrombosis, an associated complication that can eliminate hepatectomy as a viable option or increase the probability of postresection liver failure. After HAI therapy, liver imaging underestimates the size and number of lesions, complicating further management. HAI chemotherapy can cause thrombosis of the hepatic artery and can make surgical resection of the liver more difficult technically. Other complications of the therapy include gastritis (25% of cases), ulcer (9%), diarrhea (5%), biliary sclerosis (11%), and death due to hepatic failure (2%–3%). At our institution, we have all but abandoned HAI therapy in any form for CRLM.

HAI chemotherapy has also been proposed as an adjuvant to liver resection, but prospective randomized studies of this approach showed no survival advantage. Furthermore, the treatment failed in the majority of patients, with extrahepatic disease as a component of recurrence. This locoregional strategy fails to address occult metastases, which are supplied by the portal vein, and distant extrahepatic disease, which occurs in the majority of patients with CRLM.

CANCER OF THE EXTRAHEPATIC BILE DUCT

Epidemiology and Etiology

Cancer of the extrahepatic bile duct (CCA) is extremely rare, comprising 2% of all cancers in the United States. In 2004, 3,000 new cases of CCA were diagnosed in the United States. In most reported series, males and females have nearly equal incidence (with the male:female incidence ratio at 1.2–1.5:1), and patients were ≥60 years old. The incidence of CCA is 1 case per 100,000 people in the United States, 5.5 cases to per 100,000 in Japan, and 7 cases per 100,000 in Israel. People of Asian descent are affected almost twice as often as whites and blacks, probably because of endemic chronic parasitic infestation.

The etiology of CCA is unknown. Several diseases are associated with an increased risk of such tumors—sclerosing cholangitis, ulcerative colitis, and choledochal cysts or Caroli disease (a congenital disease characterized by multiple intrahepatic biliary cysts). Exposure to Thorotrast and chronic typhoid carrier status has also been shown to increase risk. No strong evidence implicates gallstones or parasitic infection with *Ophisthorchis viverrini* or *Clonorchis sinensis* in CCA carcinogenesis, but there is an increased risk of CCA in patients who have parasitic infestation or hepatolithiasis. The common cancer-causing factor in these conditions is unclear, although chronic inflammation of the bile duct probably plays a role.

Pathological Characteristics

Adenocarcinoma is the most common histological type of biliary cancer; morphologically, CCA can be classified as papillary (<5% of cases), nodular (20%), or sclerosing (70%). Most papillary tumors are well differentiated and present with multiple lesions within the duct. Virtually all long-term survivors have papillary-type CCA. Conversely, most sclerosing-type CCAs are poorly differentiated, and this type is often associated with a poor prognosis. A tumor arising at the confluence of the right and left hepatic ducts is termed Klatskin's tumor, following the description of 13 such lesions by Klatskin in 1965.

CCAs are slow growing and most often spread by local intrabiliary ductal extension, peritoneal metastasis, or intrahepatic metastasis. Metastasis to regional lymph nodes occurs less frequently (30%–50% of cases), and perineural extension occurs as well. Distant metastases are present in approximately 25% to 30% of patients at the time of diagnosis, but hematogenous spread is rare. Lesions of the proximal and middle thirds of the extrahepatic bile duct can compress, constrict, or invade the underlying portal vein or hepatic artery. In addition, proximal tumors can invade the liver parenchyma. Hilar CCAs will involve the parenchyma of the caudate lobe in as many as 36% of patients; their appearance at this site usually occurs by means of biliary extension through the short caudate ducts that drain to the confluence, although they may emanate from a tumor located near the biliary confluence.

Intrahepatic Cholangiocarcinoma

Intrahepatic CCA is a different entity than hilar CCA, and forms of intrahepatic CCA can be grouped according to their growth patterns. These cancers can be mass-forming (MF), periductal-infiltrating (PI), or can grow within the duct lumens (intraductal growth). The MF type presents as a round mass within the liver parenchyma and can recur in the remnant liver after hepatic resection. The PI type of intrahepatic CCA grows longitudinally along the bile duct, often causing an obstruction or stricture. Several pathological findings are important in predicting the outcome of patients with CCA; poorer outcome is associated with tumor infiltration of the bile duct serosa, lymph node metastases, and vascular and perineural invasion. Intrahepatic CCAs have a higher propensity to metastasize to lymph nodes than hilar CCAs.

Clinical Presentation

The most common presenting symptoms in patients with hilar CCA are obstructive jaundice (which occurs in 90% of patients) and itching. Rarely, a very proximal tumor may block a segmental or lobar bile duct without causing jaundice. Other symptoms that may occur are weight loss (29% of cases), vague abdominal pain (20%), fatigue, and nausea. A patient may also present with cholangitis and sepsis resulting from bacterial contamination of the obstructed bile. In the case of middle or distal duct obstruction, a distended gallbladder may be palpable on abdominal exam; conversely hilar CCA is typically associated with a nondistended gallbladder. In addition to having elevated serum total bilirubin, patients with CCA will present with elevated alkaline phosphatase, gamma-glutamyltransferase, and possibly elevated tumor markers (carbohydrate antigen 19-9 [CA19-9] and CEA).

Diagnosis

The first radiologic test that should be performed when extrahepatic bile duct obstruction is suspected is US, which can provide information about the level and nature of an obstructing lesion. US can also give information regarding the morphology of the lesions, possible dilation of extrahepatic and intrahepatic bile ducts, portal vein and hepatic artery obstruction, and the presence of gallstones and gallbladder dilation.

Further imaging is necessary to delineate the cross-sectional and longitudinal (intrabiliary) extent of the tumor. Some centers use a combination of MRI and color or spectral Doppler US. At M. D. Anderson, multiphase helical thin-cut CT scanning is used in combination with prereferral endoscopic retrograde cholangiopancreatography (ERCP). Helical CT scanning has an overall accuracy of 76% to 100%, and MRI has an overall accuracy of 89% for staging CCA. We prefer CT because patients usually present to us after ERCP; also, the CT permits assessment of vascular encasement, cross-sectional assessment of tumor extent, and accurate delineation of the tumor's biliary extent in a single study.

CT is as sensitive as US in demonstrating biliary dilation, but in addition CT can give information about the local, regional, and distant extent of the disease. CT also gives information about the relationship between the tumor and surrounding structures (including the hepatic artery and portal vein and hepatic lobar atrophy), and may be used in the search for metastatic spread. If distant disease is demonstrated on CT, palliative percutaneous or endoscopic stent placement can be performed during cholangiography.

In the absence of distant disease, the actual location of the tumor and its proximal and distal extent must be defined before any intervention is planned. This information can be obtained using ERCP, magnetic resonance cholangiopancreatography (MRCP), or percutaneous transhepatic cholangiography (PTC). To evaluate lesions in the distal bile duct, ERCP is superior to the other techniques because it images both the bile and the pancreatic ducts. MRCP can also image the bile duct and provides information about surrounding vascular structures. MRCP usually has an advantage over ERCP because it is noninvasive. Both ERCP and MRCP overestimate the extent of bile duct involvement in about 40% of cases. Both imaging modalities may fail to define the extent of intrabiliary tumor proximally. If the point of obstruction is believed to be proximal to the perihilar region, PTC is the preferred method for defining the biliary tract. PTC also allows brush biopsies of the tumor, external drainage of obstructed biliary ducts, and palliative stent placement when indicated. The workup for a suspected CCA rarely requires visceral angiography or portography to assess vascular involvement because of the high quality of modern CT and MRI, with or without three-dimensional reconstruction.

Despite improved prelaparotomy imaging, 25% to 40% of patients are found to have unresectable disease at the time of surgery. DL is considered in most patients with large or extensive hilar tumors because of the frequency of metastases in the peritoneal cavity and because its use in selected cases results in fewer nontherapeutic laparotomies and shorter hospital stays.

For resectable CCA, obtaining tissue to confirm the diagnosis of bile duct cancer is not essential and may be difficult. In most instances, the decision to operate is based on the preoperative radiologic findings, not histologic confirmation. The sensitivity of brush biopsies is poor (well below 50%), although newer techniques such as fluorescence in situ hybridization assay and endoscopic US-guided FNA of the bile duct may improve diagnostic accuracy. Treatment is guided by anatomical findings (e.g., biliary obstruction, enhancing hilar mass, vascular encasement, liver atrophy).

Staging and Anatomical Classification

The current AJCC staging system for CCA is shown in Table 12.3. The anatomical classification of CCA is subdivided by the site of origin: intrahepatic (6%), distal extrahepatic (27%), or perihilar (67%). Extrahepatic CCA is typically classified according to the Bismuth-Corlette classification, which describes the common patterns of hilar CCA within the biliary tree, defines the surgical strategy, and provides the language used to describe such tumors (Fig. 12.2). Type I tumors obstruct the biliary confluence but do not touch the "roof" of the biliary confluence. Type II tumors are similar to type I tumors but *do* touch the roof. Type III lesions extend through the intrahepatic bile ducts to involve second-order

Table 12.3. American Joint Commission on Cancer staging system for cancer of the extrahepatic bile duct

Primary tumor (T)	
TX	Primary cannot be assessed
T0	No evidence of primary tumor
Tis	Carcinoma in situ
T1	Tumor confined to bile duct histologically
T2	Tumor invades beyond the wall of the bile duct
T3	Tumor invades the liver, gallbladder, pancreas, and/or unilateral branches of the portal vein (right or left) or hepatic artery (right or left)
T4	Tumor invades any of the following: main portal vein or its branches bilaterally, common hepatic artery, or other adjacent structures, such as the colon, stomach, duodenum, or abdominal wall
Regional lymph nodes (N)	
NX	Regional lymph nodes cannot be assessed
N0	No regional lymph node metastasis
N1	Regional lymph node metastasis
Distant metastasis (M)	
MX	Distant metastasis cannot be assessed
M0	No distant metastasis
M1	Distant metastasis

Stage groupings			
Stage 0	Tis	N0	M0
Stage IA	T1	N0	M0
Stage IB	T2	N0	M0
Stage IIA	T3	N0	M0
Stage IIB	T1–T3	N1	M0
Stage III	T4	Any N	M0
Stage IV	Any T	Any N	M1

Adapted from Greene FL, Page DL, Fleming ID, Fritzag, Balch EM, Haller DG, Marrow M, editors. *AJCC Cancer Staging Manual*. 6th ed. New York, NY: Springer-Verlag; 2002, with permission.

ducts to the right (type IIIa) or left (type IIIb) only, sparing contralateral ducts. Type IV tumors extend to second-order ducts on both the right and the left. Treatment is defined by location due to the fact that the liver drained by all involved ducts must be resected for cure.

RESECTABILITY CRITERIA

The definitive therapy for all extrahepatic bile duct carcinomas is complete resection. Overall resectability rates range from 10% to 85%, depending on whether distal cancers are present. Lesions of the lower third of the bile duct have the best rates of resectability

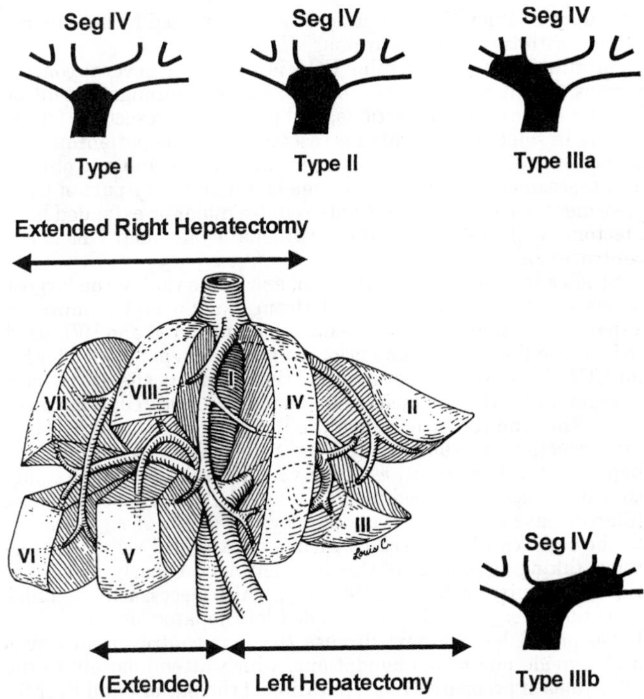

Figure 12.2. Classification of extrahepatic bile duct tumors according to the Bismuth-Corlette system, which describes the common patterns of hilar CCA within the biliary tree. The figure displays the surgical strategy for each tumor type and provides the language used to describe such tumors. Types I, II, and IIIa are treated by extended right hepatectomy, whereas type IIIb is treated by left or extended left hepatectomy.

by pancreaticoduodenectomy (considered in Chapter 13); middle-third obstructions of the bile duct are almost always due to gallbladder cancer, which is considered separately. Hilar CCAs and Klatskin's tumors are technically more challenging to resect, giving them the lowest rate of resectability among bile duct tumors. Standard criteria used to determine resectability relate to the biliary extent and vascular encasement by the tumor. Involvement of secondary bile ducts necessitates hepatic resection on the side involved. Vascular involvement of the portal vein or hepatic artery necessitates hepatic resection of the anatomical side involved as well. Thus, if secondary biliary extension and vascular encasement occur unilaterally, these tumors can be resected along with the hepatic resection. If secondary bile ducts are involved on one side and vascular encasement occurs on the opposite side, complete resection is not possible. Lymph node involvement outside the hepatic pedicle (N2) and distant metastases also preclude resection. Intrahepatic CCAs are treated by hepatic resection with tumor-free margins.

Surgical treatment of hilar CCA is subject to several controversies, which are described briefly: biliary drainage, extent of hepatic and caudate resections, and portal vein resection. Other factors in selecting patients for resection, such as patient performance status, are common between this disease and any others, and assessment of the FLR volume is a mandatory part of CCA treatment because most patients require major or extended hepatectomy with resection of the extrahepatic bile duct. This is not controversial.

Studies from our own institution, as well as that of the largest series of patients in the world (from Nagino and Nimura in Japan), show that FLR volume must be considered and PVE used to increase the FLR volume prior to extended hepatectomy for hilar CCA. Because the confluence of the bile ducts sits at the base of segment IV, this segment must usually be resected, regardless of whether the tumor is central, to the left, or to the right. Hepatic resection is usually to the right, to include extended right hepatectomy, because 97% of the variations in biliary anatomy that have been described include a long left hepatic duct. Thus, hilar disease extending even slightly to the left or significantly to the right can be cleared by means of extended right hepatectomy, taking advantage of this long left duct. Clearly, disease to the left requires a left hepatectomy, which necessarily includes resection of segment IV or extended left hepatectomy. Based on these principles, we next discuss the four controversial issues and provide our recommendations, which attend closely to the principles of preoperative preparation of the patient and liver for surgery.

Biliary Drainage

The need for preoperative biliary drainage has been debated at length in the literature, but most consider resolution of jaundice as a critical element in preparing the patient and liver for major hepatectomy. Prior studies evaluating stent placement and its associated morbidity and mortality, including six randomized studies (conducted during 1985–1994), reported only a single patient who subsequently underwent hepatectomy. Moreover, only one retrospective review demonstrated that stent placement was associated with an increase in infectious complications. At M. D. Anderson, routine placement of preoperative biliary drainage catheters is done for several reasons. The effect of hyperbilirubinemia is well known: It impairs liver regeneration and reduces resistance to systemic infection. Hepatic resection in a jaundiced patient is associated with increased rates of mortality (36% vs. 16% for those with bilirubin <2 mg per dL) and complications (50% vs. 15%). Cameron et al. advocated routine preoperative placement of biliary drainage catheters to facilitate identification and dissection of the bile duct during surgery and to aid the intraoperative placement of larger, softer Silastic transhepatic stents. In a Japanese series of 160 patients with hilar CCA, percutaneous intrahepatic biliary drainage was performed in 50 of the 52 patients who underwent combined liver and portal vein resection without complications. At the M. D. Anderson Cancer

Center, we universally drain the FLR, but drain the liver to be resected only if necessary to resolve jaundice, and do not leave transanastomotic biliary drains.

Extent of Hepatic Resection

In terms of outcome for surgical treatment of hilar CCA, patients in centers where major hepatic resection is performed (rather than duct excision) have the best prognosis. Resection of hilar CCA should be performed only when negative surgical margins (R0) can be achieved. The necessity of resecting the caudate lobe (segment I) en bloc with the bile duct is also a point of controversy. Pathological examination of resected specimens demonstrates direct invasion of tumor into the liver parenchyma or bile ducts of the caudate lobe in as many as 35% of patients. In addition, the caudate lobe is often the site of tumor recurrence following bile duct resection. Some surgeons believe the caudate lobe should be removed only if it has been invaded by the tumor, noting that survival data for those who had caudate resection are similar to data for those with similar CCA who did not undergo this procedure.

Jarnagin et al. reported a series of 80 patients who underwent resection for CCA; the operative mortality and 5-year survival rates were 10% and 27%, respectively. However, the 5-year survival after resection including hepatectomy (28% with caudate resection) was 37% vs. 0% after resection of the bile duct without hepatectomy. Ebata et al. later reported a series of 160 patients, all of whom underwent hepatic resection with caudate resection and reported a similar operative mortality (10%) and 5-year survival (37%), despite the need for portal resection in 52/160 patients. At our institution, we resect the liver including segment IV, the caudate process, and paracaval caudate lobe in all cases; Spiegel's lobe is resected when the dominant Spiegel's duct drains to the tumorous duct.

Lesions of the lower third of the bile duct do not require hepatic resection, but rather pancreaticoduodenectomy (Whipple procedure). The proximal bile duct should be resected to the point that the surgical margin is negative for tumor. Occasionally, this may require removal of most of the extrahepatic biliary tract with a high hepaticojejunostomy. The operative approach for pancreaticoduodenectomy at M. D. Anderson is outlined in Chapter 13.

Lesions of the middle third of the bile duct (termed type 0 tumors by Akeeb and Pitt) are exceedingly rare. Because of these tumors' proximity to the hepatic artery and the portal vein, these structures are typically invaded. When a type 0 tumor is deemed resectable, it is best treated by either hilar resection or pancreaticoduodenectomy. Clinically, most midduct obstructions are due to gallbladder cancer.

Limited regional lymphadenectomy is generally indicated for hilar CCAs during extrahepatic bile duct resection so staging and stratification for postoperative therapy and prognosis can be done.

Portal Vein Resection

There are two general approaches to portal vein (PV) invasion when considering resection of hilar CCA. Although some would consider portal invasion a contraindication to resection, long-term survival can be achieved by complete resection, even including PV resection (PVR).

Neuhaus et al. in Germany proposed a systematic approach to PVR, the "no touch technique." It involves PVR in all cases of hilar CCA. Analysis of these data reveals the tendency to perform portal vein resection and anastomosis. Although a better 5-year survival rate was attained with PV resection (65%) than without (0%), most patients with PVR underwent right-sided margin-negative resection (which, as described previously, enables a tumor-negative margin because of the long left duct). Furthermore, the operative mortality rate was 17%, perhaps unacceptably high. A second approach was proposed by Nimura et al. and updated by their group in a report from Ebata et al. This group recommended evaluating portal adherence to the region of the tumor at surgery. They validated their selective PVR approach (used in 52/160 patients) by demonstrating that 69% of those who underwent PVR had microscopic evidence of tumor invasion in the resected PV. Those in this series who did not undergo PVR had a better 5-year survival rate (37%) than those who did (10%), which reflects the different biologies in these cases and supports a selective approach.

At the M. D. Anderson Cancer Center, the surgical approach to proximal bile duct tumors depends on their location relative to the confluence of the right and left hepatic bile ducts and on their proximal extension. Lesions in this region are assessed according to the classification described by Bismuth and Corlette. Intrahepatic CCAs are managed with hepatic resection. Resectable lesions of the lower third of the bile duct are treated with a pancreaticoduodenectomy. Lesions of the middle third (type 0) are managed by pancreaticoduodenectomy or hepatectomy, depending on their location within the midduct. Type I, II, and IIIa CCAs are treated with an extended right hepatectomy, along with resection of the caudate process and paracaval caudate. The Speigel lobe is resected if the duct is involved. Type IIIb CCAs are treated with a left or extended left hepatectomy, along with resection of the entire caudate liver. The PV is resected and reconstructed when the vein is inseparable from the tumor and when resection of the vein will enable a margin-negative resection. Routine PVR is not performed at our institution.

Type IV lesions are generally not considered to be resectable. Several studies have reported OLT as a treatment option for CCA as a part of a multimodality protocol-based approach. The results have been consistently disappointing, with high tumor recurrence rates and low overall survival (5-year survival rate of 23%).

The sequence of open laparotomy for staging, intensive chemoradiation, and then OLT is being investigated primarily at the Mayo Clinic (Rochester, MN). The median follow-up after OLT was 42 months, and the 5-year actuarial survival rate was 87% in the highly selected patients treated using this investigational approach.

Despite aggressive surgical management, most patients with bile duct carcinoma will succumb to their tumors. Survival after resection of distal bile duct tumors has generally been better than that after resection of hilar CCAs. Reported 5-year survival rates range from 9% to 18% for proximal CCAs and 20% to 30% for distal lesions. Median survival is 18 to 30 months for patients without hilar involvement but only 12 to 24 months in patients with hilar involvement. Factors that are predictive of long-term survival after hepatic resection for CCA are T1 tumor stage, N0 lymph node stage, non–mass-forming histology, and R0 resection. Vascular invasion, N2 lymph node metastases, and lobar atrophy are associated with an adverse outcome. Lymph node metastases are found in 3% to 53% of patients; no data support extended lymphadenectomy.

The optimal palliation for patients with unresectable tumors is unclear. If the tumor has been deemed unresectable before exploration, the bile duct can be drained either percutaneously or endoscopically. The use of metallic in-dwelling stents, which are more durable than traditional stents, has made this option more appealing. If the tumor has been found to be unresectable at exploration, the duct can be intubated with either transhepatic Silastic stents or a T-tube after dilation of the lesion. Operative biliary bypass, with or without palliative tumor resection, is not generally recommended. Unresectable lesions at the bile duct confluence, especially Bismuth type III and IV lesions, can be particularly difficult to palliate and usually require percutaneous stenting, although the goal of tubefree palliation may be achieved by endoscopic or percutaneous methods.

Chemotherapy

No chemotherapeutic agents are clearly effective against CCA. Single-agent trials using 5-FU have demonstrated response rates less than 15%. Other agents, such as doxorubicin, mitomycin C, and cisplatin, used alone or in combination with 5-FU, have been no more successful. Newer agents, particularly gemcitabine and oxaliplatin, are showing some promise, particularly in combination. Toxicity remains a problem in patients with biliary obstruction and stents.

Radiation Therapy

Several studies have investigated the role of adjuvant radiation therapy after bile duct resection. Two separate studies from The Johns Hopkins University found no benefit from adjuvant radiation therapy. Kamada et al., however, showed radiation to be beneficial in patients with surgical margins histologically positive for disease. At M. D. Anderson, postoperative chemoradiation is given routinely to patients with resected bile duct cancers. If pathological analysis reveals positive margins or nodes, or peritoneal invasion, patients receive a continuous infusion of 5-FU concomitantly with 54 Gy of radiation to the tumor bed. Although patient numbers are small and follow-up duration is short, initial results suggest longer survival in treated patients than in untreated, historical controls. Radiation therapy has also been found to be effective in the palliation of unresectable bile duct cancers. Doses of 40 to 60 Gy have resulted in a median survival of 12 months, as well as reduced symptoms, probably because of improved stent patency. Palliative photodynamic bile duct therapy is also emerging.

GALLBLADDER CANCER

Epidemiology and Etiology

Although carcinoma of the gallbladder is rare, it was the most common malignant neoplasm among the estimated 6,950 cases of biliary tract cancer diagnosed in the United States in 2004 and is the sixth most common cancer of the gastrointestinal tract. The tumor has been reported in all age groups, but occurs most often in patients in their fifties and sixties. There is a striking difference in incidence of the tumor between the genders: females are affected three to four times as often as males. Examination of the Surveillance, Epidemiology, and End Results database reveals an incidence of 1.2 cases per 100,000 people per year in the United States.

The exact etiology of carcinoma of the gallbladder is not known; however, it has been associated with several conditions. Cholelithiasis is present in 75% and 92% of gallbladder carcinoma cases. Patients with larger stones (>3 cm in diameter) have a ten times greater risk of cancer than patients with small stones (<1 cm). In addition, gallbladder carcinoma can be found in 1% to 2% of all cholecystectomy specimens, a rate several times higher than that reported in autopsy studies. Chronic cholecystitis, including cases in which the gallbladder is calcified ("porcelain" gallbladder), is not associated with an increased risk of cancer, as was once believed. Towfigh et al. evaluated the pathology slides of 10,741 gallbladder specimens for evidence of calcification and gallbladder carcinoma. Among the specimens reviewed, none had gallbladder carcinoma.

The incidence of gallbladder cancer is higher in certain ethnic groups, such as Alaskan and American natives, mirroring the incidence of cholelithiasis. Other factors linked to gallbladder carcinoma include cholecystoenteric fistulas, anomalous pancreaticobiliary junction, exposure to chemical carcinogen exposure, inflammatory bowel disease, female gender, familial predisposition, chronic salmonella carrier status, and Mirizzi syndrome.

Pathological Characteristics

Adenocarcinoma of the gallbladder is a slow-growing tumor that arises from the fundus in 60% of cases. On gross examination, the gallbladder appears firm with thickened walls. The papillary adenocarcinoma subtype characteristically grows intraluminally and spreads intraductally. It is a less aggressive tumor that, consequently, carries a better prognosis when compared with other histological subtypes. Adenosquamous cancer is very rare and is treated like adenocarcinoma.

Gallbladder carcinoma spreads by metastasis to the lymph nodes and direct invasion of the adjacent liver. It can spread to the peritoneal cavity after bile spillage, and cells may be implanted in biopsy tracts or at laparoscopic port sites. Lymph node metastases are found in 56% of T2 gallbladder carcinomas and peritoneal disease has been found in 79% of patients with T4 gallbladder carcinoma. The cystic duct node, at the confluence of the cystic and hepatic ducts, is the usual initial site of regional lymphatic spread. Invasion of the liver, either by direct extension or via draining veins that empty into segments IV and V, is seen in >50% of patients. The most common site of distant extra-abdominal metastasis is the lung.

Clinical Presentation

In most series, abdominal pain is the most common presenting symptom. Nausea, vomiting, weight loss, and jaundice are other frequent symptoms. On physical examination, patients may have right upper quadrant pain with hepatomegaly or a palpable, distended gallbladder. Laboratory results are unremarkable unless the patient has developed obstructive jaundice. The tumor markers CEA and CA19-9 may be elevated in patients with gallbladder carcinoma but are neither sensitive nor specific for the disease.

Diagnosis

No laboratory or radiologic tests have shown consistent sensitivity in the diagnosis of gallbladder carcinoma. Furthermore, the paucity of clinical signs and symptoms makes preoperative diagnosis of this cancer difficult. The disease is usually diagnosed either incidentally after cholecystectomy or at an advanced stage, when presenting with a mass, jaundice, ascites, or peritoneal disease. A correct preoperative diagnosis of gallbladder carcinoma is made in fewer than 10% of cases in most series. In the Roswell Park experience, none of the 71 cases were diagnosed correctly preoperatively. The most common preoperative diagnoses are acute or chronic cholecystitis and malignancies of the bile duct or pancreas. Jaundice with a midleft bile duct stricture (type 0) is almost always related to gallbladder cancer.

In the case of gallbladder carcinoma, US may demonstrate an abnormally thickened gallbladder wall or the presence of a mass. Additional imaging by contrast-enhanced CT or MRI will help determine resectability and provide information about the local extent of disease, including portal vascular invasion, the presence of lymphadenopathy, and distant metastases.

Staging

Numerous staging systems have been described for gallbladder carcinoma. The original staging system, as described by Nevin, is based on the depth of invasion and the spread of tumor. The AJCC staging system for gallbladder carcinoma was revised recently (Table 12.4). The most significant change in the AJCC staging system is that there is no longer a distinction between T3 and T4 tumors based on the depth of liver invasion; instead, T3 tumors are defined as those that directly invade the liver and/or other adjacent organs and T4 tumors as those that invade the portal vein or hepatic artery.

Laparoscopy has a clear role in prelaparotomy staging of gallbladder carcinoma because DL complements high-quality imaging in detection of peritoneal disease, which is common with this cancer. Gallbladder carcinoma also spreads locally, metastasizing to the locoregional (N1) and distant parapancreatic/periaortic lymph nodes, often encasing the portal vein and hepatic artery precluding surgical resection. Two studies demonstrated that DL could prevent nontherapeutic laparotomy in 33% to 55% of

Table 12.4. American Joint Commission on Cancer staging system for gallbladder carcinoma

Primary tumor (T)	
TX	Primary cannot be assessed
T0	No evidence of primary tumor
Tis	Carcinoma in situ
T1	Tumor invades lamina propria or muscle layer
T1a	Tumor invades lamina propria
T1b	Tumor invades muscle layer
T2	Tumor invades perimuscular connective tissue; no extension beyond serosa or into liver
T3	Tumor perforates the serosa (visceral peritoneum) and/or directly invades the liver and/or one other adjacent organ or structure, such as the stomach, duodenum, colon or pancreas, omentum, or extrahepatic bile ducts
T4	Tumor invades main portal vein or hepatic artery or invades multiple extrahepatic organs or structures
Regional lymph nodes (N)	
NX	Regional lymph nodes cannot be assessed
N0	No regional lymph node metastasis
N1	Regional lymph node metastasis
Distant metastasis (M)	
MX	Distant metastasis cannot be assessed
M0	No distant metastasis
M1	Distant metastasis

Stage groupings

Stage 0	Tis	N0	M0
Stage IA	T1	N0	M0
Stage IB	T2	N0	M0
Stage IIA	T3	N0	M0
Stage IIB	T1–T3	N1	M0
Stage III	T4	Any N	M0
Stage IV	Any T	Any N	M1

Adapted from Greene FL, Page DL, Fleming ID, Fritzag, Balch EM, Haller DG, Marrow M, editors. *AJCC Cancer Staging Manual*. 6th ed. New York, NY: Springer-Verlag; 2002, with permission.

patients with metastatic disease. Laparoscopy was more accurate than CT in detecting peritoneal disease in patients with locally advanced tumors, suggesting that patients with T3 and T4 lesions may benefit from DL prior to surgery.

Surgical Therapy

Standard features that make a gallbladder tumor unresectable include (a) the presence of distant hematogenous or lymphatic metastases; (b) the presence of peritoneal implants; and (c) invasion of tumor into major vascular structures such as the celiac or superior mesenteric arteries, vena cava, or aorta. Gallbladder carcinoma in situ (Tis) and carcinoma limited to the mucosa (T1) can be treated adequately with a cholecystectomy alone, provided that the cystic duct margin is negative for disease. This approach can give 5-year survival rates as high as 100%. When carcinoma is suspected before surgery, open cholecystectomy with hepatoduodenal lymphadenectomy is advocated because the exact T classification cannot be determined at the time of surgery and because bile spillage is a significant risk factor for peritoneal or wound recurrence. Lymphadenectomy is performed primarily for staging purposes but may also improve local control of disease.

Surgical treatment for T2 tumors is somewhat controversial. Because the incidence of lymph node spread in the case of T2 tumors is 56%, optimal surgical treatment for these patients would consist of at least an extended cholecystectomy that includes resection of the gallbladder en bloc along with the portal lymph nodes. Addition of a wedge resection of the gallbladder bed (wedge resection of segments IVb and V) is controversial. Several recent studies evaluating extended resection for T2 tumors demonstrated significant improvements in 5-year survival rates (61%–100%) compared with simple cholecystectomy (19%–45%). Radical second operations for T2 tumors are also associated with improved 5-year survival rates (61%–75%). In contrast, other studies have reported similar survival rates after cholecystectomy when compared with more radical operations for T2 lesions. At the M. D. Anderson Cancer Center, we recommend extended cholecystectomy that includes a resection of the gallbladder en bloc along with the portal lymph nodes, and wedge or anatomical resection of the gallbladder bed (segments IVb and V) for T2 tumors.

Locally advanced tumors (T3 and T4) often present with lymph node metastases (75% of cases) and peritoneal metastases (79%) and are often associated with long-term (>5 year) survival rates in the range of 0% to 5%. However, recent studies have reported 5-year survival rates of 21% to 44% for series of patients with T3 and T4 tumors who underwent radical resection. The extent of hepatic resection is determined by the extent of tumor invasion into the gallbladder fossa and involvement of the right portal triad. To achieve a tumor-free margin, a right hepatectomy, extended right hepatectomy, or pancreaticoduodenectomy may be necessary. Pancreaticoduodenectomy has been proposed to optimize lymph node clearance, but it is generally not warranted unless the tumor extends into the head of the pancreas. Other studies have reported routine resection of the extrahepatic bile duct and pericholedochal and hilar lymph nodes, as well as en bloc resection of grossly involved adjacent structures to achieve R0 resections because there is a high incidence of occult, microscopic invasion of the hepatoduodenal ligament in cases of advanced gallbladder carcinoma. Tumors involving the hepatic artery or portal vein have been extirpated with en bloc vascular resection and subsequent reconstruction, but such an extensive procedure is not considered to be standard therapy because of the associated high morbidity and mortality rates. The most significant negative prognostic factor in gallbladder carcinoma is lymph node involvement, and vascular invasion has also been reported as indicative of poor prognosis. We recommend routine resection of the extrahepatic bile duct and portal lymph nodes.

Nonoperative Therapy

The use of single and multiple chemotherapeutic agents, either as primary or adjuvant therapy, has been disappointing. The response rate of locally advanced gallbladder cancer to 5-FU regimens is approximately 12%. 5-FU combined with doxorubicin has produced response rates of 30% to 40%. HAI chemotherapy produces response rates of 50% to 60% in patients with unresectable disease. These responses are short lived, however, and most patients die of progressive disease within 12 months; thus, HAI is not recommended.

Radiation therapy has shown some promise in the postoperative adjuvant setting, although most series have been small. Intraoperative radiation therapy has also been used with some success. External-beam radiation therapy at a dose of 45 Gy can reduce the tumor size in 20% to 70% of cases and relieves jaundice in up to 80% of patients. At M. D. Anderson, patients with gallbladder cancer are treated postoperatively with a combination of continuous-infusion chemotherapy and external-beam radiation therapy in an approach similar to that used in patients with CCA.

CONCLUSION

Many advances have been made in the surgical treatment of diseases of the liver. Advances in imaging, patient selection, and patient preparation for major hepatectomy have translated into longer and better survival of patients who undergo surgery. In particular, careful attention to volume measurement prior to major resection in patients with liver disease and extended resection in patients with normal liver, using such techniques as PVE, have enabled much lower morbidity and very low mortality for liver surgery. For HCC, the spectrum of treatments reflects the spectrum of the disease and/or underlying liver disease complex. Treatments range widely, including OLT, hepatic resection, tumor ablation, and transarterial embolization. For this disease, systemic therapy has a relatively small role in a highly selected group of patients.

For patients with CRLM, criteria for resection are expanding rapidly, to include larger, multiple, and bilateral tumors. Despite these expanded indications, survival is improving. Furthermore, rapidly evolving effective chemotherapy is expanding the population of patients eligible for definitive surgical treatment.

These benefits from adjuvant therapy have, unfortunately, not extended to patients with biliary tract cancer. Although a small group of patients with hilar CCA and gallbladder carcinoma benefit from major hepatic resection, most patients present with unresectable disease and limited treatment options, despite therapeutic advances in other areas.

In summary, the multidisciplinary approach to patients with liver tumors requires the involvement of specialists in hepatobiliary surgery; surgical, medical, and radiation oncology; gastroenterology; and radiology to enable optimal treatment today and advancement of treatment in the future.

RECOMMENDED READING

Abdalla EK, Barnett CC, Doherty D, Curley SA, Vauthey JN. Extended hepatectomy in patients with hepatobiliary malignancies with and without preoperative portal vein embolization. *Arch Surg* 2002;137(6):675–680.

Abdalla EK, Denys A, Chevalier P, Nemr RA, Vauthey JN. Total and segmental liver volume variations: implications for liver surgery. *Surgery* 2004;135(4):404–410.

Abdalla EK, Hicks ME, Vauthey JN. Portal vein embolization: rationale, technique and future prospects. *Br J Surg* 2001;88(2):165–175.

Abdalla EK, Vauthey JN. Focus on treatment of large hepatocellular carcinoma. *Ann Surg Oncol* 2004;11(12):1035–1036.

Abdalla EK, Vauthey JN, Couinaud C. The caudate lobe of the liver: implications of embryology and anatomy for surgery. *Surg Oncol Clin N Am* 2002;11(4):835–848.

Abdalla EK, Vauthey JN, Ellis LM, et al. Recurrence and outcomes following hepatic resection, radiofrequency ablation, and combined resection/ablation for colorectal liver metastases. *Ann Surg* 2004;239(6):818–825.

Ahmad SA, Bilimoria MM, Wang XM, et al. Hepatitis B or C virus serology as a prognostic factor in patients with hepatocellular carcinoma. *J Gastrointest Surg* 2001;5(5):468–476.

Bartlett DL, Fong Y, Fortner JG, Brennan MF, Blumgart LH. Long-term results after resection for gallbladder cancer. Implications for staging and management. *Ann Surg* 1996;224(5):639–646.

Belghiti J, Cortes A, Abdalla EK, et al. Resection prior to liver transplantation for hepatocellular carcinoma. *Ann Surg* 2003;238(6):885–892.

Bismuth H, Corlette MB. Intrahepatic cholangioenteric anastomosis in carcinoma of the hilus of the liver. *Surg Gynecol Obstet* 1975;140(2):170–178.

Bismuth H, Nakache R, Diamond T. Management strategies in resection for hilar cholangiocarcinoma. *Ann Surg* 1992;215(1):31–38.

Blumgart LH, Kelley CJ. Hepaticojejunostomy in benign and malignant high bile duct stricture: approaches to the left hepatic ducts. *Br J Surg* 1984;71(4):257–261.

Bruix J, Castells A, Bosch J, et al. Surgical resection of hepatocellular carcinoma in cirrhotic patients: prognostic value of preoperative portal pressure. *Gastroenterology* 1996;111(4):1018–1022.

Burke EC, Jarnagin WR, Hochwald SN, et al. Hilar cholangiocarcinoma: patterns of spread, the importance of hepatic resection for curative operation, and a presurgical clinical staging system. *Ann Surg* 1998;228(3):385–394.

Cady B, Stone MD, McDermott WV, Jr, et al. Technical and biological factors in disease-free survival after hepatic resection for colorectal cancer metastases. *Arch Surg* 1992;127(5):561–568.

Choti MA, Sitzmann JV, Tiburi MF, et al. Trends in long-term survival following liver resection for hepatic colorectal metastases.

Ann Surg 2002;235(6): 759–766.

Cillo U, Vitale A, Bassanello M, et al. Liver transplantation for the treatment of moderately or well-differentiated hepatocellular carcinoma. *Ann Surg* 2004;239(2):150–159.

Corvera CU, Weber SM, Jarnagin WR. Role of laparoscopy in the evaluation of biliary tract cancer. *Surg Oncol Clin N Am* 2002;11(4):877–891.

Curley SA, Izzo F, Delrio P, et al. Radiofrequency ablation of unresectable primary and metastatic hepatic malignancies: results in 123 patients. *Ann Surg* 1999;230(1):1–8.

Curley SA, Marra P, Beaty K, et al. Early and late complications after radiofrequency ablation of malignant liver tumors in 608 patients. *Ann Surg* 2004;239(4):450–458.

Ebata T, Nagino M, Kamiya J, et al. Hepatectomy with portal vein resection for hilar cholangiocarcinoma: audit of 52 consecutive cases. *Ann Surg* 2003;238(5):720–727.

Esnaola N, Vauthey JN, Lauwers G. Liver fibrosis increases the risk of intrahepatic recurrence after hepatectomy for hepatocellular carcinoma (*Br J Surg* 2002;89: 57–62). *Br J Surg* 2002;89(7): 939–940.

Farges O, Belghiti J, Kianmanesh R, et al. Portal vein embolization before right hepatectomy: prospective clinical trial. *Ann Surg* 2003;237(2):208–217.

Figueras J, Jaurrieta E, Valls C, et al. Resection or transplantation for hepatocellular carcinoma in cirrhotic patients: outcomes based on indicated treatment strategy. *J Am Coll Surg* 2000;190(5): 580–587.

Figueras J, Valls C, Rafecas A, et al. Resection rate and effect of postoperative chemotherapy on survival after surgery for colorectal liver metastases. *Br J Surg* 2001;88(7):980–985.

Fong Y, Fortner J, Sun RL, Brennan MF, Blumgart LH. Clinical score for predicting recurrence after hepatic resection for metastatic colorectal cancer: analysis of 1001 consecutive cases. *Ann Surg* 1999;230(3):309–318.

Gagner M, Rossi RL. Radical operations for carcinoma of the gallbladder: present status in North America. *World J Surg* 1991;15(3):344–347.

Grobmyer SR, Fong Y, D'Angelica M, et al. Diagnostic laparoscopy prior to planned hepatic resection for colorectal metastases. *Arch Surg* 2004;139(12):1326–1330.

Groupe d'Etude et de Traitement du Carcinome Hepatocellulaire. A comparison of lipiodol chemoembolization and conservative treatment for unresectable hepatocellular carcinoma. *N Engl J Med* 1995;332(19):1256–1261.

Hemming AW, Reed AI, Howard RJ, et al. Preoperative portal vein embolization for extended hepatectomy. *Ann Surg* 2003;237(5):686–691.

Imamura H, Seyama Y, Kokudo N, et al. Single and multiple resections of multiple hepatic metastases of colorectal origin. *Surgery* 2004;135(5):508–517.

Iwatsuki S, Starzl TE, Sheahan DG, et al. Hepatic resection versus transplantation for hepatocellular carcinoma. *Ann Surg* 1991;214(3):221–228.

Jarnagin WR, Bodniewicz J, Dougherty E, et al. A prospective analysis of staging laparoscopy in patients with primary and secondary hepatobiliary malignancies. *J Gastrointest Surg* 2000;4(1):34–43.

Jarnagin WR, Conlon K, Bodniewicz J, et al. A clinical scoring system predicts the yield of diagnostic laparoscopy in patients with potentially resectable hepatic colorectal metastases. *Cancer* 2001;91(6):1121–1128.

Jarnagin WR, Fong Y, Dematteo RP, et al. Staging, resectability, and outcome in 225 patients with hilar cholangiocarcinoma. *Ann Surg* 2001;234(4):507–517.

Kamada T, Saitou H, Takamura A, Nojima T, Okushiba SI. The role of radiotherapy in the management of extrahepatic bile duct cancer: an analysis of 145 consecutive patients treated with intraluminal and/or external beam radiotherapy. *Int J Radiat Oncol Biol Phys* 1996;34(4):767–774.

Kanematsu T, Matsumata T, Shirabe K, et al. A comparative study of hepatic resection and transcatheter arterial embolization for the treatment of primary hepatocellular carcinoma. *Cancer* 1993;71(7):2181–2186.

Kawai S, Okamura J, Ogawa M, et al. Prospective and randomized clinical trial for the treatment of hepatocellular carcinoma—a comparison of lipiodol-transcatheter arterial embolization with and without Adriamycin (first cooperative study). The Cooperative Study Group for Liver Cancer Treatment of Japan. *Cancer Chemother Pharmacol* 1992;31(suppl):S1–S6.

Kemeny N, Huang Y, Cohen AM, et al. Hepatic arterial infusion of chemotherapy after resection of hepatic metastases from colorectal cancer. *N Engl J Med* 1999; 341(27):2039–2048.

Klatskin G. Adenocarcinoma of the hepatic duct at its bifurcation within the porta hepatis. An unusual tumor with distinctive clinical and pathological features. *Am J Med* 1965;38:241–256.

Klempnauer J, Ridder GJ, von Wasielewski R, et al. Resectional surgery of hilar cholangiocarcinoma: a multivariate analysis of prognostic factors. *J Clin Oncol* 1997;15(3):947–954.

Lencioni R, Crocetti L, Cioni D, Della PC, Bartolozzi C. Percutaneous radiofrequency ablation of hepatic colorectal metastases: technique, indications, results, and new promises. *Invest Radiol* 2004;39(11):689–697.

Livraghi T, Bolondi L, Lazzaroni S, et al. Percutaneous ethanol injection in the treatment of hepatocellular carcinoma in cirrhosis. A study on 207 patients. *Cancer* 1992;69(4):925–929.

Livraghi T, Gazelle GS. Percutaneous radiofrequency ablation of liver metastases in potential candidates for resection—the "test-of-time" approach—reply. *Cancer* 2003;98(10):2304–2305.

Livraghi T, Solbiati L, Meloni F, et al. Percutaneous radiofrequency ablation of liver metastases in potential candidates for resection: the "test-of-time approach". *Cancer* 2003;97(12):3027–3035.

Llovet JM, Bruix J. Systematic review of randomized trials for unresectable hepatocellular carcinoma: chemoembolization improves survival. *Hepatology* 2003;37(2):429–442.

Llovet JM, Real MI, Montana X, et al. Arterial embolisation or chemoembolisation versus symptomatic treatment in patients with unresectable hepatocellular carcinoma: a randomised controlled trial. *Lancet* 2002;359(9319):1734–1739.

Llovet JM, Sala M, Castells L, et al. Randomized controlled trial of interferon treatment for advanced hepatocellular carcinoma. *Hepatology* 2000;31(1):54–58.

Lo CM, Ngan H, Tso WK, et al. Randomized controlled trial of transarterial lipiodol chemoembolization for unresectable hepatocellular carcinoma. *Hepatology* 2002;35(5):1164–1171.

Lorenz M, Muller HH, Schramm H, et al. Randomized trial of surgery versus surgery followed by adjuvant hepatic arterial infusion with 5-fluorouracil and folinic acid for liver metastases of colorectal cancer. German Cooperative on Liver Metastases (Arbeitsgruppe Lebermetastasen). *Ann Surg* 1998;228(6):756–762.

Madoff DC, Hicks ME, Abdalla EK, Morris JS, Vauthey JN. Portal vein embolization with polyvinyl alcohol particles and coils in preparation for major liver resection for hepatobiliary malignancy: safety and effectiveness—study in 26 patients. *Radiology* 2003;227(1):251–260.

Madoff DC, Hicks ME, Vauthey JN, et al. Transhepatic portal vein embolization: anatomy, indications, and technical considerations. *Radiographics* 2002;22(5):1063–1076.

Makuuchi M, Sano K. The surgical approach to HCC: our progress and results in Japan. *Liver*

Transpl 2004;10(2 suppl 1): S46–S52.

Mazzaferro V, Battiston C, Perrone S, et al. Radiofrequency ablation of small hepatocellular carcinoma in cirrhotic patients awaiting liver transplantation: a prospective study. *Ann Surg* 2004;240(5):900–909.

Mazzaferro V, Regalia E, Doci R, et al. Liver transplantation for the treatment of small hepatocellular carcinomas in patients with cirrhosis. *N Engl J Med* 1996;334(11):693–699.

McPherson GA, Benjamin IS, Hodgson HJ, et al. Pre-operative percutaneous transhepatic biliary drainage: the results of a controlled trial. *Br J Surg* 1984;71(5):371–375.

Meric F, Patt YZ, Curley SA, et al. Surgery after downstaging of unresectable hepatic tumors with intra-arterial chemotherapy. *Ann Surg Oncol* 2000;7(7):490–495.

Mullen JT, Walsh GL, Abdalla EK, et al. Transdiaphragmatic radiofrequency ablation of liver tumors. *J Am Coll Surg* 2004;199(5):826–829.

Nagino M, Kamiya J, Kanai M, et al. Right trisegment portal vein embolization for biliary tract carcinoma: technique and clinical utility. *Surgery* 2000;127(2):155–160.

Nagino M, Kamiya J, Uesaka K, et al. Complications of hepatectomy for hilar cholangiocarcinoma. *World J Surg* 2001;25(10):1277–1283.

Neuhaus P, Jonas S. Surgery for hilar cholangiocarcinoma—the German experience. *J Hepatobiliary Pancreat Surg* 2000;7(2):142–147.

Neuhaus P, Jonas S, Bechstein WO, et al. Extended resections for hilar cholangiocarcinoma. *Ann Surg* 1999;230(6):808–818.

Neuhaus P, Jonas S, Settmacher U, et al. Surgical management of proximal bile duct cancer: extended right lobe resection increases resectability and radicality. *Langenbecks Arch Surg* 2003;388(3):194–200.

Nevin JE, Moran TJ, Kay S, King R. Carcinoma of the gallbladder: staging, treatment, and prognosis. *Cancer* 1976;37(1):141–148.

Ng KK, Poon RT, Lo CM, et al. Impact of preoperative fine-needle aspiration cytologic examination on clinical outcome in patients with hepatocellular carcinoma in a tertiary referral center. *Arch Surg* 2004;139(2):193–200.

Oshowo A, Gillams A, Harrison E, Lees WR, Taylor I. Comparison of resection and radiofrequency ablation for treatment of solitary colorectal liver metastases. *Br J Surg* 2003;90(10):1240–1243.

Parikh AA, Gentner B, Wu TT, et al. Perioperative complications in patients undergoing major liver resection with or without neoadjuvant chemotherapy. *J Gastrointest Surg* 2003;7(8):1082–1088.

Pawlik TM, Esnaola NF, Vauthey JN. Surgical treatment of hepatocellular carcinoma: similar long-term results despite geographic variations. *Liver Transpl* 2004;10(2 suppl 1): S74–S80.

Pawlik TM, Poon RT, Abdalla EK, et al. Hepatectomy for hepatocellular carcinoma with major portal or hepatic vein invasion: results of a multicenter study. *Surgery* 2005;137(4): 403–410.

Pawlik TM, Poon RT, Abdalla EK, et al. Hepatitis serology predicts tumor and liver-disease characteristics but not prognosis after resection of hepatocellular carcinoma. *J Gastrointest Surg* 2004;8(7):794–804.

Pawlik TM, Scoggins CR, Zorzi D, et al. Effect of surgical margin status on survival and site of recurrence after hepatic resection for colorectal metastases. *Ann Surg* 2005;241(5):715–722, discussion.

Poon RT, Fan ST. Evaluation of the new AJCC/UICC staging system for hepatocellular carcinoma after hepatic resection in Chinese patients. *Surg Oncol Clin N Am* 2003;12(1):35–50, viii.

Poon RT, Fan ST. Hepatectomy for hepatocellular carcinoma: patient selection and postoperative outcome. *Liver Transpl* 2004; 10(2 suppl 1):S39–S45.

Poon RT, Fan ST, Lo CM, et al. Extended hepatic resection for hepatocellular carcinoma in patients with cirrhosis: is it justified? *Ann Surg* 2002;236(5):602–611.

Poon RT, Fan ST, Lo CM, et al. Improving survival results after resection of hepatocellular carcinoma: a prospective study of 377 patients over 10 years. *Ann Surg* 2001;234(1):63–70.

Poon RT, Fan ST, Lo CM, Liu CL, Wong J. Long-term survival and pattern of recurrence after resection of small hepatocellular carcinoma in patients with preserved liver function: implications for a strategy of salvage transplantation. *Ann Surg* 2002;235(3):373–382.

Poon RT, Fan ST, Ng IO, et al. Different risk factors and prognosis for early and late intrahepatic recurrence after resection of hepatocellular carcinoma. *Cancer* 2000;89(3):500–507.

Poon RT, Fan ST, Ng IO, Wong J. Significance of resection margin in hepatectomy for hepatocellular carcinoma: a critical reappraisal. *Ann Surg* 2000;231(4):544–551.

Poon RT, Fan ST, O'Suilleabhain CB, Wong J. Aggressive management of patients with extrahepatic and intrahepatic recurrences of hepatocellular carcinoma by combined resection and locoregional therapy. *J Am Coll Surg* 2002;195(3):311–318.

Poon RT, Fan ST, Tsang FH, Wong J. Locoregional therapies for hepatocellular carcinoma: a critical review from the surgeon's perspective. *Ann Surg* 2002;235(4):466–486.

Poon RT, Fan ST, Wong J. Selection criteria for hepatic resection in patients with large hepatocellular carcinoma larger than 10 cm in diameter. *J Am Coll Surg* 2002;194(5):592–602.

Poon RT, Ng IO, Fan ST, et al. Clinicopathologic features of long-term survivors and disease-free survivors after resection of hepatocellular carcinoma: a study of a prospective cohort. *J Clin Oncol* 2001;19(12):3037–3044.

Regimbeau JM, Abdalla EK, Vauthey JN, et al. Risk factors for early death due to recurrence after liver resection for hepatocellular carcinoma: results of a multicenter study. *J Surg Oncol* 2004;85(1):36–41.

Regimbeau JM, Kianmanesh R, Farges O, et al. Extent of liver resection influences the outcome in patients with cirrhosis and small hepatocellular carcinoma. *Surgery* 2002;131(3): 311–317.

Rosenberg PW, Friedman LS. Cirrhosis. In: Rakel R, Bope E, eds. *Conn's Current Therapy*. Philadelphia, Pa: WB Saunders; 1999:491.

Sala M, Varela M, Bruix J. Selection of candidates with HCC for transplantation in the MELD era. *Liver Transpl* 2004;10(10 suppl 2): S4–S9.

Saltz LB, Ahmad SA, Vauthey JN. Colorectal cancer: management of advanced disease. In: Kelsen DP, Daly JM, Kern SE, et al., eds. *Gastrointestinal Oncology: Principles and Practice*. Philadelphia, Pa: Lippincott Williams & Wilkins; 2002: 825–852.

Scaife CL, Curley SA, Izzo F, et al. Feasibility of adjuvant hepatic arterial infusion of chemotherapy after radiofrequency ablation with or without resection in patients with hepatic metastases from colorectal cancer. *Ann Surg Oncol* 2003;10(4):348–354.

Scheele J, Stang R, Altendorf-Hofmann A, Paul M. Resection of colorectal liver metastases. *World J Surg* 1995;19(1):59–71.

Shirabe K, Shimada M, Gion T, et al. Postoperative liver failure after major hepatic resection for hepatocellular carcinoma in the modern era with special reference to remnant liver volume. *J Am Coll Surg* 1999;188(3): 304–309.

Shirai Y, Yoshida K, Tsukada K, Muto T. Inapparent carcinoma of the gallbladder. An appraisal of a radical second operation after simple cholecystectomy. *Ann Surg* 1992;215(4):326–331.

Smith DL, Soria JC, Morat L, et al. Human telomerase reverse transcriptase (hTERT) and Ki-67 are better predictors of survival than established clinical indicators in patients undergoing curative hepatic resection for colorectal metastases. *Ann Surg Oncol* 2004;11(1):45–51.

Sugawara Y, Yamamoto J, Higashi H, et al. Preoperative portal embolization in patients with hepatocellular carcinoma. *World J Surg* 2002;26(1):105–110.

Townsend CM, Sabiston DC. *Sabiston Textbook of Surgery: The Biological Basis of Modern Surgical Practice*. 17th ed. Philadelphia, Pa: Elsevier; 2004.

Tuttle TM, Curley SA, Roh MS. Repeat hepatic resection as effective treatment of recurrent colorectal liver metastases. *Ann Surg Oncol* 1997;4(2):125–130.

Vauthey JN, Abdalla EK, Doherty DA, et al. Body surface area and body weight predict total liver volume in Western adults. *Liver Transpl* 2002;8(3):233–240.

Vauthey JN, Chaoui A, Do KA, et al. Standardized measurement of the future liver remnant prior to extended liver resection: methodology and clinical associations. *Surgery* 2000;127(5):512–519.

Vauthey JN, Lauwers GY, Esnaola NF, et al. Simplified staging for hepatocellular carcinoma. *J Clin Oncol* 2002;20(6):1527–1536.

Vauthey JN, Pawlik TM, Lauwers GY, et al. Critical evaluation of the different staging systems for hepatocellular carcinoma. *Br J Surg* 2004;91(8):1072.

Vauthey JN, Sobin LH. On the uniform use of the AJCC/UICC staging system for hepatocellular carcinoma. *Surgery* 2000;128(5):870.

Wayne JD, Lauwers GY, Ikai I, et al. Preoperative predictors of survival after resection of small hepatocellular carcinomas. *Ann Surg* 2002;235(5):722–730.

Yamamoto J, Sugihara K, Kosuge T, et al. Pathologic support for limited hepatectomy in the treatment of liver metastases from colorectal cancer. *Ann Surg* 1995;221(1):74–78.

Yamanaka N, Tanaka T, Tanaka W, et al. Correlation of hepatitis virus serologic status with clinicopathologic features in patients undergoing hepatectomy for hepatocellular carcinoma. *Cancer* 1997;79(8):1509–1515.

Yigitler C, Farges O, Kianmanesh R, et al. The small remnant liver after major liver resection: how common and how relevant? *Liver Transpl* 2003;9(9):S18–S25.

Yoo HY, Patt CH, Geschwind JF, Thuluvath PJ. The outcome of liver transplantation in patients with hepatocellular carcinoma in the United States between 1988 and 2001: 5-year survival has improved significantly with time. *J Clin Oncol* 2003;21(23):4329–4335.

Yoo HY, Thuluvath PJ. Outcome of liver transplantation in adult recipients: influence of neighborhood income, education, and insurance. *Liver Transpl* 2004;10(2):235–243.

13

Pancreatic Adenocarcinoma

Rosa F. Hwang, Ana M. Grau, Francis R. Spitz, Michael Bouvet, George M. Fuhrman, and David H. Berger

EPIDEMIOLOGY

Pancreatic cancer is the eighth most common malignancy and the fifth leading cause of adult cancer death in the United States. Only 1% to 4% of all patients diagnosed with pancreatic cancer can expect to survive for 5 years. In the year 2000, 28,300 new cases of adenocarcinoma of the pancreas were diagnosed in the United States, and 28,200 patients died of this aggressive malignancy. Thus, incidence rates are virtually identical to mortality rates. The incidence of pancreatic cancer in the United States steadily increased for several decades but has leveled off since the mid-1980s as a result of a steady decline in the rate for white men. In contrast, rates for white women, black men, and black women have not decreased and may have increased slightly, bringing the male-to-female ratio to 1.3:1.0. The risk of developing pancreatic cancer increases sharply after age 50, and most patients are between 65 and 80 years old at diagnosis.

The etiology of pancreatic adenocarcinoma is uncertain. Epidemiologic studies reported that cigarette smoking increases the risk of developing pancreatic cancer two- to threefold. The risk of pancreatic cancer increases as the amount and duration of smoking increase. The excess risk of developing pancreatic cancer persists for at least 10 years after smoking cessation. Coffee, alcohol, organic solvents, and petroleum products have been linked epidemiologically to pancreatic cancer. However, the data are conflicting, and none of these agents are conclusively causal. Diabetes mellitus has been implicated as both an early manifestation of pancreatic carcinoma and a predisposing factor. Recent studies have shown that pancreatic cancer occurs more frequently in patients with long-standing diabetes, which may increase the risk of pancreatic cancer by twofold. Reports have validated the epidemiologic association between chronic pancreatitis and pancreatic cancer, but the magnitude of the risk of pancreatic cancer attributable to pancreatitis remains controversial. All types of chronic pancreatitis are associated with an elevated risk of pancreatic cancer. Individuals with a history of idiopathic or alcoholic pancreatitis have a 15-fold increased risk. Tropical pancreatitis, which occurs in southern India and Africa and has no known etiology, is associated with a high risk of pancreatic cancer. Hereditary pancreatitis has been attributed to a germ-line defect on chromosome 7q35 that is inherited in an autosomal dominant pattern with 80% penetrance. These patients develop chronic pancreatitis at a young age and have a lifetime risk of pancreatic cancer of approximately 30% to 40%. Approximately 5% to 10% of pancreatic cancer cases have been associated with a familial predisposition.

Table 13.1. Presenting signs and symptoms of patients with carcinoma of the head of the pancreas

Sign or Symptom	Percentage of Patients
Weight loss	90
Pain	75
Malnutrition	75
Jaundice	70
Anorexia	60
Pruritus	40
Courvoisier's sign	33
Diabetes mellitus	15
Ascites	5
Gastric outlet obstruction	5

The most common inherited gene that has been linked to pancreatic cancer is the BRCA2 tumor suppressor gene, which has also been implicated in familial breast cancer. Germ-line BRCA2 mutations may be found in about 12% to 20% of patients with hereditary pancreatic adenocarcinoma. It is likely that risk factors such as familial predisposition and smoking may interact to result in early onset of pancreatic cancer.

CLINICAL PRESENTATION

The presenting signs and symptoms of patients with pancreatic cancer are shown in Table 13.1. The most common presenting symptoms are weight loss, pain, and jaundice. Pain is initially of low intensity, is visceral in origin, and is poorly localized to the upper abdomen. This pain may mimic peptic ulcer disease. Severe pain localized to the lower thoracic or upper lumbar area is more characteristic of advanced disease due to invasion of the celiac and superior mesenteric plexus.

Anorexia and weight loss are common in pancreatic cancer patients. Weight loss results from malabsorption and decreased caloric intake. The sudden onset of diabetes mellitus in nonobese adults older than 40 years warrants evaluation for pancreatic cancer.

Painless jaundice as the sole presenting symptom is more frequently seen with ampullary or distal bile duct tumors, but can be present with adenocarcinoma of the head or uncinate process of the pancreas. Small tumors of the pancreatic head may obstruct the intrapancreatic portion of the bile duct and cause the patient to seek medical attention when the tumor is still localized and potentially resectable. In the absence of extrahepatic biliary obstruction, few patients present with potentially resectable disease. Courvoisier's sign, a palpable gallbladder at presentation, is seen in less than one-third of patients.

NATURAL HISTORY

Pancreatic cancer spreads early to regional lymph nodes, and microscopic involvement of the liver is frequently present at diagnosis. Patients who undergo surgical resection for localized adenocarcinoma of the pancreatic head have a median survival of 13 to 20 months. Survival and local control are improved with either preoperative or postoperative chemoradiation. With improved locoregional control, the liver has become the most frequent site of recurrence for these patients. Patients with locally advanced disease and patients with metastatic disease have median survivals of 6 to 10 and 3 to 6 months, respectively. Therefore, improvements in systemic or regional therapy directed to the liver and the development of screening strategies for earlier diagnosis will be necessary to change the natural history of this disease.

PREOPERATIVE EVALUATION

Radiologic Studies

An algorithm for the current diagnostic and therapeutic management of pancreatic adenocarcinoma at the M. D. Anderson Cancer Center is presented in Figure 13.1. When pancreatic cancer is suspected, radiologic confirmation should be attempted. Several large reviews of pancreatic cancer noted delays of more than 2 months from the onset of symptoms to diagnosis in most patients.

Multidetector thin-section computed tomography (CT) scanning using a pancreas-specific protocol is the test of choice to evaluate the extent of disease and to assess tumor resectability. Using this technology, high-resolution images can be displayed to provide detailed information regarding the primary tumor, locoregional extension, lymph node involvement, and vascular invasion. In addition, these images can be converted into three-dimensional reconstructions. Local tumor resectability is most accurately assessed before surgery. Laparotomy should be therapeutic, not diagnostic. At M. D. Anderson, we use objective and reproducible radiologic criteria to operate only on patients with potentially resectable disease. Resectability is defined as the absence of extrapancreatic disease; the absence of direct tumor extension to the superior mesenteric artery (SMA) and celiac axis, as defined by the presence of a fat plane between the low-density tumor and these arterial structures; and a patent superior mesenteric-portal vein confluence. The accuracy of this form of radiographic staging is supported by previous work at M. D. Anderson and validated by a high resectability rate (94 of 118, 80%) and low rate of microscopic retroperitoneal margin positivity (17%). The accuracy of CT in predicting unresectability and the inaccuracy of intraoperative assessment of resectability are both well established. Furthermore, high-resolution pancreas protocol CT scans are usually able to demonstrate aberrant arterial anatomy prior to surgical exploration. The use of standardized, objective radiologic criteria for preoperative tumor staging allows physicians to develop detailed treatment plans for their patients, avoid unnecessary laparotomy in patients with locally advanced or metastatic disease, and improve rates of resectability at laparotomy. Therefore, we recommend a system for clinical (radiologic) staging as illustrated in Table 13.2.

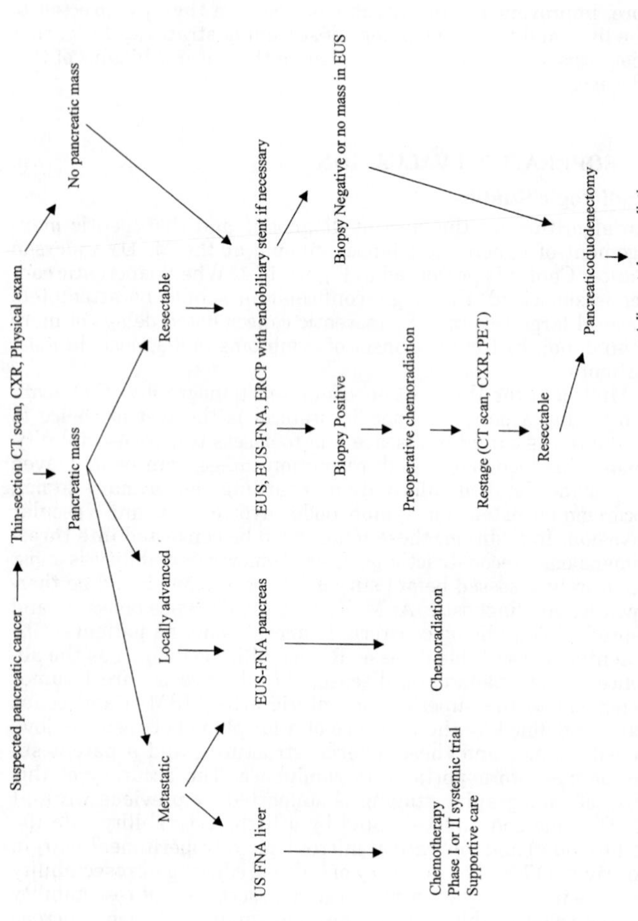
Suspected pancreatic cancer
Thin-section CT scan, CXR, Physical exam
No pancreatic mass
Pancreatic mass
Resectable
Locally advanced
Metastatic
EUS, EUS-FNA, ERCP with endobiliary stent if necessary
EUS-FNA pancreas
US FNA liver
Biopsy Negative or no mass in EUS
Biopsy Positive
Preoperative chemoradiation
Chemoradiation
Chemotherapy
Phase I or II systemic trial
Supportive care
Restage (CT scan, CXR, PET)
Resectable
Pancreaticoduodenectomy
Adjuvant chemoradiation

Table 13.2. Clinical/radiologic staging of pancreatic cancer

Stage	Clinical/Radiologic Criteria
I	Resectable (T1–T3, NX, M0) No encasement of the celiac axis or SMA Patent SMPV confluence No extrapancreatic disease
II	Locally advanced (T4, NX–1, M0) Arterial encasement (celiac axis or SMA) or venous occlusion (SMV or portal vein) No extrapancreatic disease
III	Metastatic (T1–T4, NX–1, M1) (liver, peritoneum, lungs)

SMA, superior mesenteric artery; SMPV, superior mesenteric-portal vein; SMV, superior mesenteric vein.

Other imaging modalities such as positron emission tomography (PET) using 18F-fluorodexoglucose (FDG) and magnetic resonance imaging (MRI) are used less frequently for the management of pancreatic cancer. FDG PET takes advantage of the increased glucose utilization of malignant cells to detect carcinomas; however, inflammatory conditions such as pancreatitis also accumulate FDG and can result in false-positive PET images. Moreover, elevated serum glucose can lower the sensitivity of FDG PET due to competitive inhibition and decreased FDG uptake in tumors. In several studies, the sensitivity of FDG PET in hyperglycemic patients was lower than in euglycemic patients, and it has been suggested that the standardized uptake value be adjusted to account for serum glucose level for more accurate interpretation of FDG PET images. MRI with intravenous gadolinium is useful for patients with a contraindication to CT contrast agents, and three-dimensional images can be constructed for noninvasive imaging of the biliary tree (magnetic resonance cholangiopancreatography).

American Joint Committee on Cancer Staging System

The current American Joint Committee on Cancer (AJCC) staging system for pancreatic cancer is listed in Table 13.3. In the sixth edition of the *AJCC Staging Manual*, there are two main changes from the previous edition. The T classification is modified to distinguish between potentially resectable (T3) and locally advanced (T4) primary pancreatic tumors. In addition, the grouping of the stages is changed such that stage III characterizes unresectable, locally advanced pancreatic cancer, while stage IV is reserved for patients with metastatic disease. The AJCC staging

Figure 13.1. Algorithm for the management of pancreatic carcinoma. CT, computed tomography; CXR, chest x-ray; US, ultrasound; FNA, fine-needle aspiration; EUS, endoscopic ultrasound; EUS-FNA, endoscopic ultrasound with fine-needle aspiration; ERCP, endoscopic retrograde cholangiopancreatography; PET, positron emission tomography.

Table 13.3. American Joint Committee on Cancer staging of pancreatic cancer

Primary tumor (T)

Tis	Carcinoma in situ
T1	Tumor limited to the pancreas ≤2 cm in greatest dimension
T2	Tumor limited to the pancreas >2 cm in greatest dimension
T3	Tumor extends beyond the pancreas but without involvement of the celiac axis or the superior mesenteric artery
T4	Tumor involves the celiac axis or the superior mesenteric artery (unresectable primary tumor)

Regional lymph nodes (N)

N0	No regional lymph node metastasis
N1	Regional lymph node metastasis

Distant metastasis

M0	No distant metastasis
M1	Distant metastasis

Stage grouping

Stage IA	T1	N0	M0
Stage IB	T2	N0	M0
Stage IIA	T3	N0	M0
Stage IIB	T1–T3	N1	M0
Stage III	T4	Any N	M0
Stage IV	Any T	Any N	M1

system provides only one system for both clinical (radiographic) and pathological staging. Pathological staging can be applied only to patients who undergo pancreatectomy; in all other patients, only clinical staging, based on radiographic examinations, can be performed. Without surgery, the histologic status of the regional lymph nodes cannot be determined. Optimal assessment of a pancreaticoduodenectomy specimen should include histologic evaluation of at least ten regional lymph nodes, which include peripancreatic nodes along the hepatic artery, celiac axis, and splenic and pyloric regions. In addition, treatment and prognosis are based on whether the tumor is potentially resectable, locally advanced, or metastatic, definitions that may not directly correlate with TNM status.

Endoscopy

Endoscopic ultrasound with fine-needle aspiration biopsy (EUS-FNA) has emerged as a helpful diagnostic tool that has proven to be safe and accurate. Pretreatment confirmation of malignancy is mandatory in patients with locally advanced or metastatic disease prior to chemotherapy or external-beam radiation therapy (EBRT) and before initiation of neoadjuvant therapy in patients with resectable pancreatic cancer. In our experience, EUS-FNA has a specificity and positive predictive value of 100%, while sensitivity and negative predictive values are 90% and 38%, respectively. In addition to patients with large tumors, EUS-FNA is successful in most patients with small, resectable tumors, allowing for the delivery of protocol-based neoadjuvant therapy. Negative results with EUS-FNA should not be interpreted as definitive proof that a malignancy does not exist.

Although pretreatment pancreatic fine-needle aspiration (FNA) biopsy is frequently performed, physicians should be cautioned about the use of intraoperative pancreatic biopsy. In patients with resectable disease, there is no indication for routine intraoperative pancreatic biopsy and the use of preoperative EUS-FNA should be limited to those patients receiving preoperative chemoradiation for whom cytologic confirmation of malignancy is needed. Unlike FNA, surgical manipulation and intraoperative large-needle biopsy during surgery increases the risk of peritoneal dissemination of tumor cells. Having undergone a previous laparotomy with tumor biopsy prior to definitive pancreaticoduodenectomy is the only factor associated with an increased risk of locoregional tumor recurrence. Furthermore, intraoperative pancreatic biopsy has been associated with significant complications, such as pancreatitis, pancreatic fistula, and hemorrhage.

Endoscopic retrograde cholangiopancreatography (ERCP) is used to differentiate choledocholithiasis and chronic pancreatitis from malignant obstruction of the distal common bile duct when CT does not see a mass. To prevent cholangitis in patients who undergo diagnostic ERCP because of extrahepatic biliary obstruction, endoscopic stents are routinely placed. Endoscopic stents are also placed in patients with elevated bilirubin levels who are enrolled in preoperative chemoradiation protocols. At our institution, expandable metallic stents have demonstrated a superior patency rate with fewer episodes of cholangitis and no difference in intra- or postoperative complications compared with plastic biliary stents.

Laparoscopy

Laparoscopy has been advocated for the identification of potential extrapancreatic disease in patients with radiologic evidence of localized disease. Recent investigations suggest that extrapancreatic disease not visible by CT is uncommon, being found in only 4% to 15% of patients with pancreatic tumors considered resectable following high-quality CT. Laparoscopy before laparotomy (during a single anesthesia induction) is a reasonable approach in patients with biopsy-proven or suspected potentially resectable pancreatic cancer in whom a decision has been made to proceed with pancreaticoduodenectomy. However, data are not available to support the cost effectiveness of routinely using laparoscopy as a staging procedure under a separate anesthesia induction prior to treatment planning.

Tumor Markers

Currently, the gold standard serologic marker for pancreatic cancer is CA19-9. Originally described as a marker for colon cancer, the CA19-9 antigen is a sialylated lacto-N-fucopentaose II related to the Lewis^a blood group antigen. The sensitivity and specificity of CA19-9 in the diagnosis of pancreatic cancer has been reported to be as high as 90% and 98%, respectively. A significant limitation of the use of CA19-9 as a marker for pancreatic cancer is its elevation in the setting of benign, as well as malignant, biliary obstruction. Biliary decompression usually results in a decrease in CA19-9 levels corresponding to a fall in serum bilirubin. To improve the usefulness of CA19-9 for the jaundiced patient, some investigators have proposed using an "adjusted CA19-9" by dividing the serum CA19-9 by the total bilirubin when the bilirubin is greater than 2.0 mg per dL. The utility of CA19-9 is also limited in the 5% to 15% of the population that is Lewis^{ab} negative who lack the enzyme specified by the *Le* gene involved in the synthesis of CA19-9. In these individuals, CA19-9 will be falsely low even with an extensive pancreatic tumor burden.

CA19-9 is commonly used not only to diagnose pancreatic cancer, but it may also help identify patients with resectable tumors. Virtually all patients with a CA19-9 greater than 200 U per mL will have a pancreatic malignancy, and when CA19-9 is greater than 300 U per mL, resection is rarely possible. Serum CA19-9 is an independent predictor of recurrence and survival after resection and has recently been shown to correlate with response to therapy.

PATHOLOGY

Approximately 90% of pancreatic exocrine tumors arise from the pancreatic ductules, and 80% of these tumors are adenocarcinomas. Pancreatic adenocarcinomas arise in the head of the gland in 60% to 70% of cases. The rest of the tumors are located in the body or tail, or diffusely throughout the pancreas.

In gross histologic examination, pancreatic adenocarcinoma is firm and white with poorly defined margins. An associated surrounding area of pancreatitis is often present and can make pathological diagnosis difficult. An intense desmoplastic reaction is identifiable on both gross and microscopic examination. Histologic identification of mucin production is helpful in diagnosing an adenocarcinoma. Perineural invasion can be identified in most specimens. The degree of differentiation reported on microscopic examination is based on the degree of formation of tubular glandular structures.

SURGICAL TREATMENT

Surgical resection of carcinoma of the pancreatic head remains the only potentially curative treatment modality. Five surgical techniques are used to resect pancreatic cancer: (a) the standard pancreaticoduodenectomy, modified from Whipple's initial description in 1935; (b) pylorus-preserving pancreaticoduodenectomy; (c) total pancreatectomy; (d) regional pancreatectomy; and (e) the M. D. Anderson extended resection. Thorough abdominal exploration should precede resection. There is no role for resection of adenocarcinoma in the presence of metastatic disease. Exploration should include intraoperative inspection and palpation of the liver, peritoneal surfaces, para-aortic lymphatics, and root of the mesentery to define the tumor's extent.

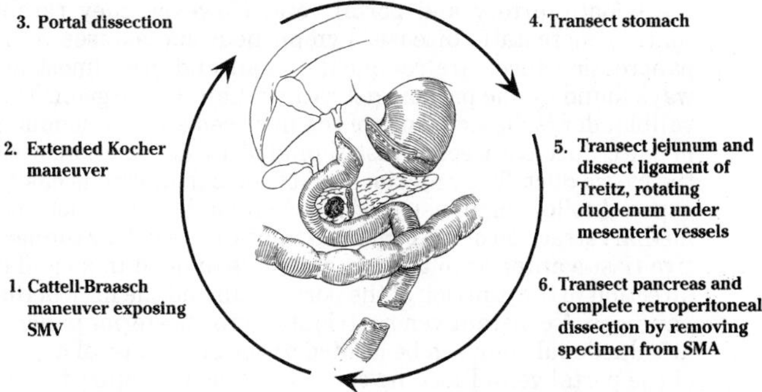

Figure 13.2. Six surgical steps of pancreaticoduodenectomy (clockwise resection). SMV, superior mesenteric vein; SMA, superior mesenteric artery. (From Tyler DS, Evans DB. Reoperative pancreaticoduodenectomy. *Ann Surg* 1994;219:214, reprinted with permission.)

The surgical resection is divided into the following six clearly defined steps (Fig. 13.2):

1. A Cattell-Braasch maneuver is performed by mobilizing the right colon and incising the visceral peritoneum to the ligament of Treitz. When complete, this maneuver allows cephalad retraction of the right colon and small bowel, exposing the third and fourth portions of the duodenum. Mobilization of the retroperitoneal attachments of the mesentery is of particular importance in patients who require venous resection and reconstruction. The omental bursa is entered by taking the greater omentum from the transverse colon. The middle colic vein is identified, ligated, and divided before its junction with the SMV. Routine division of the middle colic vein allows greater exposure of the infrapancreatic SMV and prevents iatrogenic traction injury during dissection of the middle colic vein-SMV junction.
2. The Kocher maneuver is begun at the junction of the ureter and right gonadal vein. The right gonadal vein is ligated and divided, and all fibrofatty and lymphatic tissue overlying the medial aspect of the right kidney and inferior vena cava is removed with the tumor specimen. The gonadal vein is again ligated at its entrance into the inferior vena cava. The Kocher maneuver is continued to the left lateral edge of the aorta, with careful identification of the left renal vein.
3. The portal dissection is initiated, exposing the common hepatic artery proximal and distal to the gastroduodenal artery. The gastroduodenal artery is then ligated and divided. Two large lymph nodes are commonly encountered during portal dissection: one along the inferior border of the common hepatic artery, and one behind the portal vein seen after transection of the common bile duct. Removal of these lymph nodes (en bloc with the specimen) is necessary to mobilize

the hepatic artery and portal vein. However, they rarely contain metastatic disease. Lymph node metastases from pancreatic cancer are commonly small and are almost always found by the pathologist rather than the surgeon. The gallbladder is dissected out of the liver bed and the common hepatic duct transected just cephalad to its junction with the cystic duct. The anterior wall of the portal vein is easily exposed following division of the common hepatic duct and medial retraction of the common hepatic artery. This connective tissue anterior to the portal vein is divided in a caudal direction to the junction of the portal vein and the neck of the pancreas. A constant venous tributary, the posterior pancreatic duodenal vein, can be located at the supralateral aspect of the portal vein. Bleeding caused by traction injury to this venous tributary may be difficult to control at the time of the operation. The portal dissection is made more difficult in the presence of anomalous hepatic artery circulation. Rarely, the hepatic artery (distal to the origin of the gastroduodenal artery) courses posterior to the portal vein. More commonly, an accessory or replaced right hepatic artery arises from the proximal SMA and lies posterior and lateral to the portal vein. The common hepatic artery may arise from the SMA (type IX hepatic arterial anatomy). Fatal hepatic necrosis can result if this is unrecognized and the vessel is sacrificed. Identification of aberrant arterial anatomy is generally not difficult, except in reoperative portal dissections.

4. The stomach is transected at the level of the third or fourth transverse vein on the lesser curvature and at the confluence of the gastroepiploic veins on the greater curvature. The omentum is divided at the level of the greater curvature transection.
5. The jejunum is transected approximately 10 cm distal to the ligament of Treitz, and its mesentery is sequentially ligated and divided. The duodenal mesentery is similarly divided to the level of the aorta; the duodenum and jejunum are then reflected beneath the mesenteric vessels.
6. After traction sutures are placed on the superior and inferior borders of the pancreas, the pancreas is transected using electrocautery at the level of the portal vein. If there is evidence of tumor adherence to the portal vein or SMV, the pancreas can be divided at a more distal location in preparation for segmental venous resection. The specimen is separated from the SMV by ligating and dividing the small venous tributaries to the uncinate process and the pancreatic head. Complete removal of the uncinate process combined with medial retraction of the superior mesenteric-portal vein confluence facilitates exposure of the SMA, which is then dissected to its origin at the aorta. Total exposure of the SMA avoids iatrogenic injury and ensures direct ligation of the inferior pancreaticoduodenal artery. Reconstruction proceeds in the counterclockwise direction, and again in a stepwise and orderly fashion (Fig. 13.3).
7. The pancreatic remnant is mobilized from the retroperitoneum and splenic vein for a distance of 2 to 3 cm. Failure to adequately mobilize the pancreatic remnant results

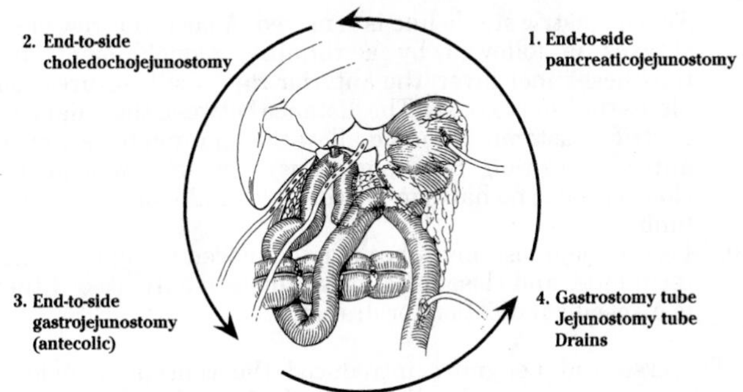

Figure 13.3. Four surgical steps of counterclockwise reconstruction following standard pancreaticoduodenectomy. (From Tyler DS, Evans DB. Reoperative pancreaticoduodenectomy. *Ann Surg* 1994;219:214, reprinted with permission.)

in poor suture placement at the pancreaticojejunal anastomosis. The transected jejunum is brought through a small incision in the transverse mesocolon to the right or left of the middle colic vessels. A two-layer, end-to-side, duct-to-mucosa pancreaticojejunostomy is performed over a small Silastic stent. Following completion of the posterior row of 3-0 seromuscular sutures, a small, full-thickness opening in the bowel is made. The anastomosis between the pancreatic duct and small bowel mucosa is completed with 4-0 or 5-0 monofilament sutures. Each stitch incorporates a generous bite of pancreatic duct and a full-thickness bite of jejunum. The posterior knots are tied on the inside, and the lateral and anterior knots are tied on the outside. Prior to the anterior sutures being tied, the stent is placed across the anastomosis so it extends into the pancreatic duct and into the small bowel for a distance of approximately 2 to 3 cm. The anastomosis is completed with a placement of an anterior row of 3-0 seromuscular sutures. When the pancreatic duct is not dilated and/or the pancreatic substance is soft (not fibrotic), a two-layer anastomosis that invaginates the cut end of the pancreas into the jejunum is recommended. The outer posterior row of 3-0 sutures is placed as outlined earlier. The bowel is then opened to a length equivalent to the transverse diameter of the pancreatic remnant. Using a running, double-armed, 4-0 nonabsorbable monofilament suture, the pancreatic remnant is sewn to the jejunum. The anastomosis is completed with placement of an anterior row of 3-0 seromuscular sutures.

8. A single-layer biliary anastomosis is performed using interrupted, 4-0 absorbable monofilament sutures. It is important to align the jejunum with the bile duct to avoid tension on the pancreatic and biliary anastomosis. A stent is rarely used in the construction of the hepaticojejunostomy.
9. An anticolic, end-to-side gastrojejunostomy is constructed in two layers. Starting from the greater curvature, 6 to

8 cm of gastric staple line is removed. A posterior row of silk sutures is followed by a running, monofilament, full-thickness inner layer; the anterior row of silk sutures completes the anastomosis. The distance between the biliary and gastric anastomosis should allow the jejunum to assume its anticolic position (for the gastrojejunostomy) without tension. There is no harm in making a long (25–35 cm) afferent limb.

10. Feeding jejunostomy tubes may be placed using the Witzel technique, and closed suction drains are only used if there is a specific indication for drainage.

Traverso and Longmire introduced the concept of pylorus-preserving pancreaticoduodenectomy in 1978, in an attempt to eliminate the postgastrectomy syndromes seen after antrectomy. This operation technically differs from a standard Whipple procedure only in the preservation of the blood supply to the proximal duodenum. This can be accomplished by carefully preserving the right gastroepiploic arcade after ligation of the right gastroepiploic artery and vein close to their origin. The right gastric artery can be spared in some cases to provide additional blood supply to the duodenum. The most significant morbidity of pylorus preservation is transient gastric stasis. Operative time and blood loss are slightly reduced compared with those of classic pancreaticoduodenectomy. Pylorus preservation should not be performed in patients with bulky tumors or tumors involving the first and second portion of the duodenum.

Some authors have advocated routine total pancreatectomy as definitive therapy for adenocarcinoma of the head of the pancreas. They cite the possible multicentric nature of pancreatic cancer and the avoidance of a pancreatic anastomosis as justification for this approach. However, the incidence of pathological documentation of multicentricity of pancreatic adenocarcinoma is less than 10% and does not justify the additional operative morbidity and lifelong insulin dependence that results from total pancreatectomy. The significant operative morbidity and mortality from pancreaticoduodenectomy is historically attributed to pancreaticojejunal anastomotic leak. However, anastomotic complications are rare at institutions experienced with this operation. Also, more effective management of pancreatic anastomotic leakage with hyperalimentation, percutaneous drainage, and somatostatin analog has reduced the magnitude of this problem. Total pancreatectomy is only indicated if there is tumor at the pancreatic margin on serial frozen sections or if the pancreas is not suitable for an anastomosis.

Regional pancreatectomy includes extensive retroperitoneal and hepatoduodenal lymph node dissection and sleeve resection of the SMV-portal venous confluence. Superior mesenteric and hepatic arterial resections have also been included by proponents of this more radical approach. The potential oncologic advantages of regional pancreatectomy are offset by its increased morbidity and mortality.

Venous resection should be considered when the lesion has been deemed resectable, the pancreatic neck is divided, and, while dissecting the uncinate process from the SMV, the tumor is found to be adherent to the posterior-lateral portion of the vein. Vein resection is preferable to shaving the tumor from the portal-superior mesenteric venous confluence. In addition, venous resection for any tumor involving the SMV-portal venous confluence should be performed as long as the vein has been demonstrated to be patent by preoperative CT. An interposition internal jugular vein graft is our preferred method of reconstruction. Unlike other recent reports, data from our institution suggest that resection of the SMV at pancreaticoduodenectomy can be performed safely, is not associated with retroperitoneal margin positivity (when high-quality preoperative imaging is performed), and does not negatively influence patient survival. In a review of 141 patients at our institution who underwent pancreaticoduodenectomy with major vascular resection, a R0 resection was possible in 78%. Vascular resection was considered only when there was isolated tumor involvement of the SMV or portal vein without extension to the celiac axis or SMA. The median survival of 110 patients with pancreatic adenocarcinoma who underwent vascular resection was 23 months.

Intraoperative decision making in the surgical treatment of pancreatic cancer can challenge the most experienced surgeon. The morbidity and mortality associated with pancreaticoduodenectomy are greater than those seen with many other procedures and should be performed only by experienced surgeons. This conclusion was supported by Lieberman et al. in 1995, who reported the experience with pancreaticoduodenectomy in New York State from 1984 to 1991. More than 75% of patients who underwent pancreaticoduodenectomy had their operations performed at hospitals that reported less than seven of these operations per year. For patients who received their surgical care at those hospitals, mean perioperative hospital stay was more than 1 month, and the risk-adjusted perioperative mortality was 12% to 19%. Patients and their families must be informed preoperatively of the required complex postoperative care and potential complications of pancreaticoduodenectomy. This is most critical when there is no preoperative histologic confirmation of the diagnosis. Neoplasms of the pancreatic head can obstruct the pancreatic duct, resulting in pancreatitis, which makes definitive histologic diagnosis difficult. An intraoperative transduodenal biopsy specimen that reveals inflammation does not exclude the possibility of malignancy. Because of this, many experienced pancreatic surgeons do not routinely perform intraoperative biopsies if malignancy is suspected. In our institution, we do not routinely perform intraoperative biopsies in patients with radiographic (CT or ERCP) studies consistent with malignancy. Occasionally, a surgeon suspects that a malignancy exists but cannot establish radiologic or histologic confirmation. Every large series of pancreatic resections includes a few patients resected for benign disease. The potential morbidity of an unnecessary pancreatic resection is preferred to leaving a potentially curable lesion in situ. Repeated biopsies to obtain histologic confirmation of malignancy are inadvisable because of the risk of pancreatic fistula, pancreatitis, and hemorrhage. Patients should be aware of the potential need to perform a resection without histologic confirmation of malignancy.

RESULTS OF SURGERY

Aggressive surgical resection of pancreatic head tumors has come under intense scrutiny, although, presently, pancreaticoduodenectomy remains the only procedure capable of curing adenocarcinoma of the pancreatic head. Postoperative morbidity rates that were greater than 50% in the late 1960s are now less than 25% in the most recently reported series. Postoperative mortality rates have also decreased, from a high of more than 20% to as low as 3% in the most recent reviews.

The presence of fever after postoperative day 3 or 4 should prompt careful evaluation. Potential sources of fever include those common to all abdominal surgeries and intra-abdominal abscess as a result of pancreaticojejunostomy leak. Gastric and biliary anastomoses rarely leak. The study of choice is CT scan of the abdomen, with CT-guided drainage of any localized fluid collection. Pancreaticojejunostomy anastomotic leaks generally close when adequately drained. The use of octreotide in this setting should be individualized. Postoperative gastrointestinal or drain tract bleeding should prompt immediate angiography to evaluate for arterial-enteric fistula. The most common cause is pancreaticojejunostomy leak followed by a herald bleed due to rupture of the ligated gastroduodenal artery stump. This is a rare complication and should be managed by embolization at the time of diagnostic angiography.

Despite the improvement in morbidity and mortality, there has been little change in long-term patient survival. The 5-year survival rate following curative pancreaticoduodenectomy for carcinoma of the pancreatic head remains less than 25%, with a median survival of 20 to 25 months.

Body and tail tumors are often considered to have a poorer prognosis than lesions of the pancreatic head because the former frequently go undetected until they are locally advanced or metastatic. At our institution, these lesions account for only 2% of the pancreatectomies performed. However, a Mayo Clinic report suggested that the few patients with body or tail lesions amenable to resection for cure have long-term survival rates similar to those patients who have undergone complete resection of the more common carcinoma of the pancreatic head.

ADJUVANT THERAPY

Because the 5-year survival rate of patients with resected pancreatic cancer is poor, it is imperative to examine the potential benefit of adjuvant therapy for this disease. Autopsy series have indicated that 85% of patients will experience recurrences in the field of resection. Furthermore, approximately 70% of patients will develop metastasis to the liver. Therefore, adjuvant therapy must address the possibilities of distant disease (chemotherapy) and locoregional recurrence (radiation therapy). The initial studies examining adjuvant therapy of pancreatic cancer were based on results from studies on patients with advanced disease.

Most widely used chemotherapeutic agents have limited activity against pancreatic cancer. 5-Fluorouracil (5-FU) is the only active agent, and its effect is marginal. Most studies report an overall response rate of 15% to 28% in patients with advanced disease. Studies of 5-FU have also demonstrated the ability of this agent to act as a radiation sensitizer. Gemcitabine, a deoxycytidine analog capable of inhibiting DNA replication and repair, has demonstrated activity against pancreatic cancer. In a randomized trial of patients with advanced disease, patients treated with gemcitabine experienced a modest but statistically significant improved response rate and median survival and an improved quality of life compared with patients treated with 5-FU.

Combined 5-FU and radiation therapy have been reported to significantly increase survival in patients with locally advanced disease. In a study by the Gastrointestinal Tumor Study Group (GITSG), patients with unresectable pancreatic cancer were randomized to receive high-dose postoperative radiation therapy (60 Gy) alone, high-dose postoperative radiation therapy (60 Gy) plus concomitant 5-FU, or standard-dose postoperative radiation therapy (40 Gy) and 5-FU. Patients receiving 5-FU and radiation therapy experienced a significant survival advantage compared with patients who received radiation therapy alone. The higher dose of radiation therapy did not confer an additional survival advantage.

The combination of postoperative EBRT and concomitant 5-FU as adjuvant therapy after resection was also investigated by the GITSG. Patients were randomized to receive surgery alone or surgery followed by radiation therapy (40 Gy delivered in two 20-Gy courses) and 5-FU (500 mg per m^2 by intravenous bolus delivered daily for the initial 3 days of each radiation therapy course and then weekly for 2 years). Median survival was 20 months in the group that received adjuvant therapy; this was significantly longer than the 11-month median survival seen in patients treated with surgery alone.

Unlike surgery for adenocarcinoma of the esophagus, stomach, or colorectum, pancreaticoduodenectomy requires complete reconstruction of the upper gastrointestinal tract, including reanastomosis of the pancreas, bile duct, and stomach. The magnitude of the operation and its associated morbidity may result in a lengthy recovery, preventing the timely delivery of postoperative therapy. In most large series, approximately 25% of patients who undergo pancreaticoduodenectomy do not receive postoperative chemoradiation because of prolonged recovery.

The risk of delaying adjuvant therapy, combined with small preliminary experiences of successful pancreatic resection following EBRT, prompted many institutions to initiate studies of chemoradiation before pancreaticoduodenectomy for patients with potentially resectable or locally advanced adenocarcinoma of the pancreas. The preoperative use of chemoradiation is supported by the following considerations:

1. Radiation therapy is more effective on well-oxygenated tumors that have not been devascularized by surgery.
2. Peritoneal spread of tumor cells as a result of surgery may be prevented by preoperative chemoradiation.
3. The high frequency of positive-margin resections recently reported supports the concern that the retroperitoneal margin of excision, even when negative, may be only a few

millimeters. Surgery alone may therefore be inadequate for local tumor control.

4. Patients with disseminated disease evident on restaging studies after chemoradiation will not be subjected to laparotomy and therefore will be spared the associated morbidity and risk of treatment-related mortality. Repeat staging CT after chemoradiation reveals liver metastases in approximately 25% of patients. It is probable that the liver metastases were already present subclinically at diagnosis, and if these patients had undergone pancreaticoduodenectomy, then they would have had a major surgical procedure only to have liver metastases found soon after surgery.
5. Because radiation therapy and chemotherapy are given first, long postoperative recovery will have no effect on the delivery of all components of the multimodality treatment, a frequent problem in postoperative adjuvant therapy studies.

The standard-fractionation preoperative chemoradiation regimen at M. D. Anderson was delivered over 5.5 weeks to a total dose of 50.4 Gy (1.8 Gy per fraction) concurrently with continuous-infusion 5-FU at a dosage of 300 mg/m^2/day, 5 days per week, through a central venous catheter. To avoid the gastrointestinal toxicity seen with this standard 5.5-week program, a rapid-fractionation program of chemoradiation was designed. Rapid-fractionation chemoradiation is delivered over 2 weeks to a total dose of 30 Gy (3 Gy per fraction) for 5 days per week. 5-FU is given concurrently by continuous infusion at a dosage of 300 mg/m^2/day, 5 days per week. This program is based on the principle that the total radiation dose required to obtain a given biological effect decreases as the dose per fraction increases. Restaging with chest radiography and abdominal CT is performed 4 weeks after chemoradiation. Patients with localized disease on restaging undergo pancreaticoduodenectomy with electron-beam intraoperative radiation therapy (EB-IORT). In our recently published series, patients with radiographically resectable localized adenocarcinoma of the pancreatic head were entered onto this preoperative protocol. Thirty-five patients received this treatment, 27 had surgery, and 20 (74%) underwent successful pancreaticoduodenectomy. Local tumor control and patient survival were equal to the results reported with standard-fractionation (5.5-week) chemoradiation: Locoregional recurrence developed in only 2 (10%) of the 20 patients who underwent resection, and the median survival time for all 20 patients was 25 months. This protocol had minimal toxicity, maximized the proportion of patients who received all components of therapy, was significantly shorter than standard therapy, and avoided pancreaticoduodenectomy on patients with metastatic disease on restaging.

The role of preoperative rapid-fractionation EBRT and concomitant gemcitabine for patients with resectable adenocarcinoma of the pancreatic head is currently being evaluated. A dose of 400 mg per m^2 of gemcitabine is administered weekly for 7 weeks. A total radiation dose of 30 Gy in 10 fractions over 2 weeks (Monday to Friday) is given beginning 4 days after the first dose of gemcitabine. Pancreaticoduodenectomy is performed 4 weeks after completion of therapy if restaging CT demonstrates

Table 13.4. Recent chemoradiation therapy studies of patients with resectable pancreatic cancer

Author (year)	No. of Patients	EBRT (Gy)	Chemotherapy	Median Survival (mo)
Postoperative				
Kalser (1985)	21	40	5-FU	20
Surgery alone	22	—	—	11
GITSG (1987)	30	40	5-FU	18
Yeo (1997)	120	40–57.6	5-FU	19.5
Surgery alone	53	—	—	13.5
Klinkenbijl (1999)	60	40	5-FU	17.1
Surgery alone	54	—	—	12.6
Preoperative				
Breslin (2000)	132	30–50.4	5-FU, paclitaxel or gemcitabine	21

EBRT, external beam radiation therapy; 5-FU, 5-fluorouracil; GITSG, Gastrointestinal Tumor Study Group.

resectable disease. So far, 69 patients have been entered in this study, and 65 have completed preoperative therapy. Fifty patients have had surgery, and 42 had resection. No treatment-related mortality has been observed. Table 13.4 summarizes the most recent published reports of adjuvant and neoadjuvant therapy for pancreatic cancer.

One potential barrier to neoadjuvant therapy for pancreatic cancer is the need for stent placement for biliary decompression. At the M. D. Anderson Cancer Center, the rates of biliary stent-related complications and mortality were evaluated in 300 patients undergoing preoperative chemoradiation therapy, 207 of whom received stents. On multivariate analysis, stent placement was associated only with an increased rate of wound infection after pancreaticoduodenectomy. Stents did not result in prohibitive morbidity during preoperative chemoradiation therapy.

Investigators from our institution studied a regimen of preoperative EBRT (50.4 Gy in 28 fractions or 30 Gy in 10 fractions) and concomitant protracted-infusion 5-FU (300 mg/m^2/day), followed by pancreaticoduodenectomy and EB-IORT (10–20 Gy) to the resection bed. EB-IORT was delivered with minimal morbidity after preoperative chemoradiation and pancreaticoduodenectomy. The median survival duration in our most recent report was 25 months. Disease recurred in 70% of the patients at a median follow-up of 37 months; 86% of the recurrences were distant, and only 14% were locoregional. The results of these studies indicated that EB-IORT can be safely combined with pancreaticoduodenectomy and current chemoradiation regimens. Although EB-IORT appears to improve local control, marked improvements in survival have not been demonstrated. At present, the use of EB-IORT should be limited to investigational protocols. EB-IORT for locally advanced unresectable tumors has been reported to reduce symptoms from advanced disease and to prolong survival. A National Cancer Institute controlled prospective trial of adjuvant radiation therapy for pancreatic cancer examined the benefit of EB-IORT (20 Gy) in addition to EBRT (50 Gy) after resection. Although EB-IORT did not have an impact on overall survival in this small study, patients who received EB-IORT experienced prolonged disease-free survival and improved local control.

SURVEILLANCE

Patients should be seen at 3 to 4 months after potentially curative resection of pancreatic adenocarcinoma or earlier if symptoms develop. Follow-up visits should include a thorough history, chest radiograph, and abdominal CT.

There have been numerous attempts to identify a tumor marker for pancreatic cancer. The most frequently measured antigens are carcinoembryonic antigen, CA19-9, and pancreatic-oncofetal antigen. Some encouraging results have been reported with use of CA19-9 to predict recurrence following resection of pancreatic adenocarcinoma.

Postoperatively, all patients receive some form of enteral nutritional supplementation via a jejunostomy tube for at least 6 weeks. Nutritional status, including serum albumin level, dietary history, and general body habitus, should be carefully assessed at each clinic visit. Patients must also be evaluated for signs of malabsorption resulting from pancreatic enzyme insufficiency. This is readily treatable with pancreatic enzyme replacement.

PALLIATION

Patients with unresectable or recurrent pancreatic cancer frequently require palliative treatment for biliary obstruction, gastric outlet obstruction, and pain. Historically, palliation for these patients was undertaken at laparotomy after a tumor was deemed unresectable. Operative biliary bypass, gastric bypass, and splanchnicectomy are effective methods of palliation. However, with current improved diagnostic techniques, unresectability should be determined before laparotomy. Biliary diversion can then be achieved either endoscopically or percutaneously. Gastric outlet obstruction occurs in only 10% to 15% of patients and is often a preterminal event, and so does not mandate surgical correction. CT-guided alcohol splanchnicectomy is an effective option for the palliation of pain in the occasional patient unresponsive to narcotics. Therefore, the surgeon can avoid laparotomy in most patients who have a limited life expectancy.

BILIARY OBSTRUCTION

Jaundice is a common presenting symptom in patients who have carcinoma of the head of the pancreas. Prolonged biliary obstruction leads to coagulopathy, hepatic dysfunction, malabsorption, and altered bile salt metabolism. Patients often complain of severe, disabling pruritus. Relief of biliary obstruction significantly palliates these problems and improves overall patient well-being. It is helpful to group patients with pancreatic cancer into four separate categories when considering operative versus nonoperative biliary decompression:

1. Patients in poor health who would not tolerate laparotomy and are clearly best served by nonoperative palliative measures
2. Patients with concomitant gastric outlet obstruction who require laparotomy for palliation of that symptom and for whom the benefit of avoiding the complications of a stent or transhepatic drain warrants the limited additional morbidity of a surgical biliary bypass
3. Patients undergoing operation for resection but who are found to have unsuspected unresectable disease; these patients are also best served by an operative biliary bypass
4. Patients who have unresectable pancreatic cancer on diagnostic evaluation and are an acceptable medical risk for laparotomy; these patients are candidates for operative or nonoperative management, depending on the judgment of the surgeon and the expertise of the available endoscopist or invasive radiologist (At M. D. Anderson, these patients are treated successfully with nonoperative palliative measures.)

Surgical biliary diversion can be accomplished by either choledochoenteric or cholecystenteric bypass. Constructing a Roux limb requires an additional anastomosis and longer operative time than making a simple loop of small bowel for biliary bypass. Roux reconstruction is necessary when an unresectable tumor prevents a loop from reaching the right upper quadrant without tension. Most authorities advocate either loop choledochojejunostomy or cholecystojejunostomy for surgical palliation of malignant biliary obstruction. Cholecystojejunostomy has the advantage of being simple to perform; however, there is the possibility of recurrent biliary obstruction after this procedure. The advantage of choledochojejunostomy is that it provides a more proximal biliary anastomosis and therefore obstruction by progressive extension of the tumor is less likely. The high operative mortality and short median survival associated with each procedure are due to the aggressive nature of the malignancy rather than to the technique used. The choice of surgical option ultimately depends on local tumor considerations and the surgeon's experience.

Nonoperative palliative biliary decompression can be accomplished endoscopically or percutaneously. Experienced endoscopists report a success rate of greater than 90%. In randomized studies comparing endoscopic biliary decompression with conventional surgical bypass, the procedures have resulted in identical survival times and relief of jaundice. Total hospital stay is also similar for the two procedures because of the need for occasional readmissions to change stents after endoscopic decompression. Percutaneous transhepatic biliary drainage has provided successful palliation in 80% to 90% of patients. External catheters are being replaced by newer indwelling endoprostheses, which are associated with a lower rate of infectious complications. Although endoscopic biliary decompression is the preferred method of nonoperative palliation, the choice of technique depends on the expertise available.

We use a selective approach to biliary decompression. Outpatient endoscopic stenting is performed in all patients who are not candidates for pancreaticoduodenectomy. In patients with a life expectancy of 3 to 5 months (i.e., those with poor performance status or liver or peritoneal metastases), an 11.5F polyethylene stent is placed. In patients with a life expectancy of 6 to 12 months (i.e., those with locally advanced, nonmetastatic disease), a self-expanding metal stent is preferred. However, patients in whom early stent occlusion or migration develops or who by clinical criteria appear to do poorly with endoscopic biliary decompression are quickly referred for operative biliary bypass. A multidisciplinary approach to these patients is critical—the medical oncologist, gastroenterologist, and surgeon must communicate and avoid overly dogmatic approaches to palliative care.

GASTRIC OUTLET OBSTRUCTION

Patients with pancreatic cancer rarely present with duodenal obstruction. Furthermore, less than 15% of patients will require operative correction of gastric outlet obstruction before death. Clearly, patients with unresectable disease and gastric outlet obstruction require a gastrojejunostomy for palliation. There is controversy about whether all patients undergoing palliative laparotomy should undergo prophylactic gastroenterostomy. Complications resulting from the longer surgery and the additional anastomosis are minimal. However, the incidence of subsequent duodenal obstruction in asymptomatic patients who undergo only biliary bypass is low. In addition, gastric outlet obstruction often occurs shortly before death and does not require treatment. In general, we do not perform prophylactic surgery in patients with pancreatic cancer.

If a patient is found to have unresectable disease during surgery for planned pancreaticoduodenectomy, gastrojejunostomy is considered when clinical symptoms or anatomical findings suggest impending obstruction. However, in patients with locally advanced or limited metastatic disease with good performance status, prospective randomized data would support the creation of a gastrojejunostomy.

NONINVASIVE PANCREATIC LESIONS

Several types of noninvasive lesions of the pancreas have been characterized that can be precursors to invasive adenocarcinoma of the pancreas. These lesions include pancreatic intraepithelial neoplasia (PanINs), intraductal papillary mucinous neoplasms (IPMNs), and mucinous cystic neoplasms. Only recently have these lesions been clearly defined by an internationally accepted set of diagnostic criteria. A more thorough understanding of the molecular nature of these lesions may provide a means of early diagnosis and more effective treatment.

Pancreatic Intraepithelial Neoplasia

PanINs are characterized as microscopic pancreatic duct lesions without invasion through the basement membrane. The grade of PanIN lesions ranges from 1 through 3, based on factors such as the presence of a papillary component, nuclear abnormality, presence of mitoses, and necrosis. The PanIN-1 lesions are often incidental findings and can be identified in 40% of individuals without pancreatic carcinoma. However, PanIN-3 lesions are found in 30% to 50% of individuals with invasive pancreatic ductal adenocarcinoma, suggesting that high-grade PanIN lesions are precursors of invasive carcinoma. A series of molecular aberrations have been identified with PanIN lesions to form a model for the development and progression of pancreatic cancer.

Intraductal Papillary Mucinous Neoplasm

IPMNs are intraductal neoplasms arising in the main pancreatic duct, pancreatic side branches, or both, with cystic formation and variable degrees of mucin secretion. The current World Health Organization grading system classifies IPMNs as adenomas, borderline tumors, or intraductal papillary mucinous carcinoma based on the degree of dysplasia, nuclear abnormality, and other pathological features. Although IPMNs and PanINs share many pathological characteristics, most IPMNs are clinically detectable, whereas PanINs are often incidental findings detected microscopically. IPMN lesions are usually greater than 1 cm in diameter and can be typically identified radiographically by pancreatic ductal dilatation. Furthermore, IPMNs often produce large amounts of mucin that can be visualized endoscopically. IPMNs, particularly those arising from the main pancreatic duct, can be associated with invasive carcinoma. When IPMN is associated with an invasive carcinoma, the prognosis is significantly worse than IPMN with invasive carcinoma.

Cystic Neoplasms

Cystic neoplasms of the pancreas account for approximately 1% of all pancreatic cancers and 10% of all pancreatic cystic lesions. These tumors are typically large, are located in the distal pancreas, and affect women three times more frequently than men. The diagnosis of a cystic neoplasm or IPMN must be considered in patients with radiographic evidence of a pancreatic cyst and no prior symptoms or history of pancreatitis. Mucinous cystic neoplasms should be distinguished from IPMNs by the presence of ovarian-type stroma and the absence of ductal involvement.

Cystic neoplasms with a cuboidal epithelial lining (serous cystadenoma) have no malignant potential. When a columnar epithelial lining is present in the cyst wall, the lesion is frankly malignant (mucinous cystadenocarcinoma) or premalignant (mucinous cystic neoplasm).

It is often impossible to distinguish malignant from benign cystic neoplasms preoperatively or intraoperatively because the epithelial lining is often incomplete. Therefore, all cystic neoplasms should be resected for potential cure. Patients with malignant cystic neoplasms who undergo complete resection have a 40% to 60% 5-year survival rate. Table 13.5 offers clinical and laboratory tools to help differentiate inflammatory pseudocysts from neoplastic cystic lesions of the pancreas.

Table 13.5. Differentiation of inflammatory pseudocysts from cystic neoplasms of the pancreas

Patient History, CT and FNA Findings	Mucinous Neoplasm (Adenoma or Carcinoma)	Serous Cystadenoma	Inflammatory Pseudocyst
History of pancreatitis, alcohol abuse, complicated biliary disease	No	No	Yes
CT	Small number ($\leq$6) of large cysts (>2 cm)	Many small cysts	No loculations
Cyst fluid analysis/cytology	Positive for mucin; malignant (if carcinoma)	No mucin; positive for glycogen	Negative
Cyst fluid CEA (ng/mL)	Usually >500; highly variable	<5	>50% elevated, but usually <400
Cyst fluid amylase (U/mL)	50% >2,000; variable	<5,000	>5,000

CT, computed tomography; FNA, fine-needle aspiration; CEA, carcinoembryonic antigen.

RECOMMENDED READING

Bold RJ, Charnsangavej C, Cleary KR, et al. Major vascular resection as part of pancreaticoduodenectomy for cancer: radiologic, intraoperative, and pathologic analysis. *J Gastrointestinal Surg* 1999;3(3):233.

Breslin TM, Hess KR, Harbison DB, et al. Neoadjuvant chemoradiotherapy for adenocarcinoma of the pancreas: treatment variables and survival duration. *Ann Surg Oncol* 2000;8(2):123.

Burris HA, Moore MJ, Andersen J, et al. Improvements in survival and clinical benefit with gemcitabine as first-line therapy for patients with advanced pancreas cancer: a randomized trial. *J Clin Oncol* 1997;15(6):2403.

Crist DW, Sitzman JV, Cameron JL. Improved hospital morbidity, mortality, and survival after the Whipple procedure. *Ann Surg* 1987;206:358.

Dalton RR, Sarr MG, van Heerden JA. Carcinoma of the body and tail of the pancreas: is curative resection justified? *Surgery* 1992;111:489.

Evans DB, Abbruzzese JL, Cleary KR, et al. Rapid-fractionation preoperative chemoradiation for malignant periampullary neoplasms. *J R Coll Surg Edinb* 1995;40:319.

Evans DB, Abbruzzese JL, Willet CG. Cancer of the pancreas. In: DeVita VT, Jr, Hellman S, Rosenberg SA, eds. *Cancer: Principles and Practice of Oncology*. 6th ed. Philadelphia, Pa: Lippincott; 2000.

Foo ML, Gunderson LL, Nagorney DM, et al. Patterns of failure in grossly resected pancreatic ductal adenocarcinoma treated with adjuvant irradiation +5 fluorouracil. *Int J Radiat Oncol Biol Phys* 1993;26:483.

Fortner JG. Regional pancreatectomy for cancer of the pancreas, ampulla, and other related sites. *Ann Surg* 1984;199:418.

Fuhrman GM, Charnsangavej C, Abbruzzese JL, et al. Thin-section contrast-enhanced computed tomography accurately predicts the resectability of malignant pancreatic neoplasms. *Am J Surg* 1994;167:104.

Fuhrman GM, Leach SD, Staley CA, et al. Rationale for en bloc vein resection in the treatment of pancreatic adenocarcinoma adherent to the superior mesenteric-portal venous confluence. *Ann Surg* 1996;223:154.

Gastrointestinal Tumor Study Group (GITSG). Further evidence of effective adjuvant combined radiation and chemotherapy following curative resection of pancreatic cancer. *Cancer* 1987;59:2006.

Geer RJ, Brennan MF. Prognostic indicators for survival after resection of pancreatic adenocarcinoma. *Am J Surg* 1993;165:68.

Hruban RH, Adsay NV, Albores-Saavedra J, et al. Pancreatic intraepithelial neoplasia (PanIN): a new nomenclature and classification system for pancreatic duct lesions. *Am J Surg Pathol* 2001;25:579.

Hruban RH, Takaori K, Klimstra DS, et al. An illustrated consensus on the classification of pancreatic intraepithelial neoplasia and intraductal papillary mucinous neoplasms. *Am J Surg Pathol* 2004;28(8):977.

Itani KM, Coleman RE, Akwari OE, et al. Pylorus-preserving pancreaticoduodenectomy: a clinical and physiologic appraisal. *Ann Surg* 1986;204:655.

Kwon RS, Brugge WR. New advances in pancreatic imaging. *Curr Opin Gastroenterol* 2005;21(5):561.

Leach SD, Rose JA, Lowy AM, et al. Significance of peritoneal cytology in patients with potentially resectable adenocarcinoma of the pancreatic head. *Surgery* 1995;118:472.

Lieberman MD, Kilburn H, Lindsey M, et al. Relation of perioperative deaths to hospital volume among patients undergoing pancreatic resection for malignancy. *Ann Surg* 1995;222:638.

Longnecker DS, Adler G, Hruban RH, et al. Intraductal papillary-mucinous neoplasms of the pancreas. In: Hamilton SR, Aaltonen LA, eds. *WHO Classification of Tumors of the Digestive System*. Lyon France: IARC Press; 2000:237.

Moertel CG, Frytak S, Hahn RG, et al. Therapy of locally unresectable pancreatic carcinoma: a randomized comparison of high dose (6000 rads) radiation alone, moderate dose radiation and 5-fluorouracil. *Cancer* 1981;48:1705.

Montgomery RC, Hoffman JP, Riley LB, et al. Prediction of recurrence and survival by post-resection CA19-9 values in patients with adenocarcinoma of the pancreas. *Ann Surg Oncol* 1997;4:551.

Pisters PWT, Abbruzzese JL, Janjan NA, et al. Rapid-fractionation preoperative chemoradiation, pancreaticoduodenectomy, and intraoperative radiation therapy for resectable pancreatic adenocarcinoma. *J Clin Oncol* 1998;16:3843.

Pisters PWT, Hudec WA, Lee JE, et al. Preoperative chemoradiation for patients with pancreatic cancer: toxicity of endobiliary stents. *J Clin Oncol* 2000;18:860.

Rumstadt B, Schwab M, Schuster K, et al. The role of laparoscopy in the preoperative staging of pancreatic carcinoma. *J Gastrointestinal Surg* 1997;1(3):245.

Safi F, Schlosser W, Faldenreck S, et al. Prognostic values of CA19-9 serum course in pancreatic cancer. *Hepatogastroenterology* 1998;45:253.

Shepherd HA, Royle G, Ross APR. Endoscopic biliary endoprosthesis in the palliation of malignant obstruction of the distal common bile duct: a randomized trial. *Br J Surg* 1988;75:1166.

Sindelar WF, Kinsella TJ. Randomized trial of intraoperative radiotherapy in resected carcinoma of the pancreas. *Radiat Oncol Biol Physiol* 1986;12:148.

Spitz FR, Abbruzzese JL, Lee JE, et al. Preoperative and postoperative chemoradiation strategies in patients treated with pancreaticoduodenectomy for adenocarcinoma of the pancreas. *J Clin Oncol* 1997;15:928.

Tseng JF, Raut CP, Lee JE, et al. Pancreaticoduodenectomy with vascular resection: margin status and survival duration. *J Gastrointest Surg* 2004;8(8):935.

Warshaw AL, Compton CC, Lewandrowski K, et al. Cystic tumors of the pancreas. *Ann Surg* 1990;212:432.

Wasan SM, Ross WA, Staerkel GA, et al. Use of expandable metallic biliary stents in resectable pancreatic cancer. *Am J Gastroenterol* 2005;100:2056.

Yeo CJ, Abrams RA, Grochow LB, et al. Pancreaticoduodenectomy for pancreatic adenocarcinoma: postoperative adjuvant chemoradiation improves survival. A prospective, single-institution experience. *Ann Surg* 1997;225(3):621.

Yeo CJ, Cameron JL, Lillemoe KD, et al. Pancreaticoduodenectomy for cancer of the head of the pancreas: 201 patients. *Ann Surg* 1995;221:721.

Pancreatic Endocrine Tumors and Multiple Endocrine Neoplasia

Jeffrey T. Lenert, Richard J. Bold, Jeffrey J. Sussman, and Douglas S. Tyler

PANCREATIC ENDOCRINE TUMORS

Pancreatic endocrine tumors are relatively rare, with approximately five clinically recognized cases occurring per one million people annually. However, some series of carefully performed, unselected autopsies have demonstrated an incidence as high as 0.5% to 1.5%. Many of these tumors are functional and patients present with symptoms attributable to excess hormone production and secretion. The tumors tend to arise in the islet cells of the pancreas but can also be located in the small bowel, especially the duodenum, and in other intraabdominal sites. Although the islet cells have long been thought to be of neural crest origin because of metabolic characteristics shared with other cells of neuroectodermal origin, specifically the amine precursor uptake and decarboxylation (APUD) cells, more recent studies suggest they may be of endodermal origin (e.g., pancreatic ductal epithelium).

Islet cell tumors are usually divided into functioning and nonfunctioning tumors. More than 75% of the islet cell tumors diagnosed clinically are functioning and frequently produce, and often secrete, more than one hormone. The tumors are categorized by the major hormone producing the clinical syndrome. The hormones may include gastrin, insulin, glucagon, somatostatin, neurotensin, pancreatic polypeptide (PP), vasoactive intestinal polypeptide (VIP), growth hormone-releasing factor (GRF), and adrenocorticotropic hormone (ACTH). The tumors are considered entopic, or orthoendocrine, if they produce hormones or peptides usually found within the pancreas (e.g., insulinomas, glucagonomas, somatostatinomas, and PPomas) or ectopic (paraendocrine) if the hormones or peptides are not native to the normal pancreas (e.g., gastrinomas, VIPomas, GRFomas, neurotensinomas, and ACTHoma). An overview of the characteristics of pancreatic endocrine tumors is shown in Table 14.1.

The diagnosis of pancreatic endocrine tumors is usually made by the recognition of the clinical syndrome caused by excess hormone secretion. The specific hormone excess also allows assessment of a patient's response to therapy and provides a mechanism for observing the long-term status of the disease. However, PPomas and nonfunctioning islet cell tumors do not secrete clinically apparent hormones and hence are diagnosed as a result of mass-effect symptoms or as an incidental finding on computed tomography (CT) scans of the abdomen for unrelated reasons. Unlike in patients with functioning neuroendocrine tumors, response to treatment and long-term follow-up of patients with

Table 14.1. Characteristics of pancreatic endocrine neoplasms

Tumor Name	Hormone Secreted	Pancreatic Cell Type	Clinical Syndrome	Malignant (%)	Association with MEN 1 (
Gastrinoma	Gastrin	D or D variant	Peptic ulcers, diarrhea, GERD	60–90	25–30
Insulinoma	Insulin	β	Hypoglycemia, neurologic symptoms, adrenergic excess symptoms	5–15	10
VIPoma	Vasoactive intestinal peptide	H	Watery diarrhea, achlorhydria, hypokalemia	60–80	Rare
Glucagonoma	Glucagon	α_2	Hyperglycemia dermatitis (necrolytic migratory erythema), cachexia, thrombophlebitis	60–70	Rare
Ppoma	Pancreatic polypeptide	PP	None	>60	Occasional
Somatostatinoma	Somatostatin	δ or α	Hyperglycemia Steatorrhea Gallstones	90	Never
GRFoma	Growth hormone-releasing factor		—	—	—
ACTHoma	Adrenocorticotropic hormone		—	—	—
PTHrp-oma	Parathyroid hormone-related protein		—	—	—
Nonfunctioning	None		None	>60	Frequent

GERD, gastroesophageal reflux disease; MEN 1, multiple endocrine neoplasia type 1.

Table 14.2. Anatomic distribution of pancreatic endocrine tumors within the pancreas (head, body, and tail) as well as the extrapancreatic tissue, including the duodenum

Tumor	Head (%)	Body (%)	Tail (%)	Extrapancreatic/ Duodenal (%)
Gastrinoma	30	12	14	44[a]
Insulinoma	25	41	33	1
Glucagonoma	23	37	40	0
PP-secreting tumor	52	14	14	20
Somatostatinoma	62	4	12	22

Adapted from Howard TJ, Stabile BE, Zinner MJ, et al. Anatomic distribution of pancreatic endocrine tumors. *Am J Surg* 1990;159:258.
[a]More recent series show that two-thirds are extrapancreatic.

nonfunctioning tumors is not aided by measurement of hormones specific to the tumor in question; however, more general tumor markers can be used. Functioning and nonfunctioning pancreatic neuroendocrine tumors secrete several tumor markers, including chromogranins, PP, and subunits of human chorionic gonadotropin. Chromogranin A (CgA) in particular may be a useful marker to supplement specific markers in functioning tumors and may be useful by itself or with other general markers when tumors are nonfunctioning. Histologic diagnosis of the islet cell tumor can be obtained with CT-guided fine-needle aspiration, although this is often not required, given the syndrome of pancreatic hormonal excess and a localizing study. (See Table 14.2 for the distribution of these tumors within the pancreas.)

In general, pancreatic endocrine tumors are more indolent than ductal adenocarcinoma and carry a better prognosis; even patients with hepatic metastasis may have a mean survival time of 5 years.

Gastrinoma: Zollinger-Ellison Syndrome

In 1955, Zollinger and Ellison described a syndrome characterized by the triad of severe, atypical peptic ulceration; gastric hypersecretion and hyperacidity; and a non-insulin–producing islet cell tumor of the pancreas. They theorized that a humoral factor arising from the tumor was responsible for the syndrome. Several years later, the hormone gastrin was discovered and found to be the underlying cause of the peptic hyperacidity, and the term Zollinger-Ellison syndrome (ZES) was applied to the clinical complex.

Epidemiology

At least 0.1% of patients with duodenal ulcer disease and approximately 2% of patients with recurrent ulcers after appropriate medical therapy are found to have a gastrinoma, making it the most common functioning malignant pancreatic endocrine tumor. Approximately 75% of gastrinomas occur sporadically; the remaining 25% are associated with the multiple endocrine neoplasia type 1 syndrome (MEN 1). The mean age at onset of symptoms is 50 years, and approximately 60% of those diagnosed with ZES are men. Gastrinomas that occur as part of MEN 1 are more often benign, multicentric, and extrapancreatic and occur at an earlier age than sporadic gastrinomas. In more than half of the patients with MEN 1 syndrome, the pancreatic tumors are gastrinomas.

Clinical Presentation

High levels of gastrin stimulate the parietal cells within the stomach to secrete excess acid in an unregulated state. This leads to severe ulcer diathesis and injury to the small bowel mucosa well past the ligament of Treitz, resulting in varying degrees of malabsorption. Profuse watery diarrhea occurs in up to 50% of patients because of the combination of acid hypersecretion and small bowel mucosal injury. In addition to secreting gastrin, the majority of gastrinomas secrete at least one other peptide hormone, such as insulin, PP, glucagon, or even ACTH.

The clinical manifestations of gastrinomas are almost invariably due to hypergastrinemia. Ninety percent of patients have endoscopically documented ulcerations of the upper gastrointestinal (GI) tract. Most of these ulcers are accompanied by abdominal pain, which is the most frequent single symptom. Bleeding occurs in 30% to 50% of patients and perforation in 5% to 10%. Secretory diarrhea is the only clinical manifestation of the syndrome in 20% of patients, although diarrhea and pain in combination is more frequent than either symptom alone. Symptoms of gastroesophageal reflux disease are also being recognized more often in association with ZES. The syndrome is often initially misdiagnosed due to the frequency of typical peptic ulcer disease (PUD) and a broad differential diagnosis. The mean duration of symptoms before diagnosis is often several years. Clinical situations in which ZES should be suspected and the differential diagnoses are listed in Tables 14.3 and 14.4.

Table 14.3. Clinical situations warranting further evaluation for gastrinoma

Recurrent peptic ulcers after appropriate medical or surgical therapy
Failure of peptic ulcer to heal on appropriate medical therapy, including treatment for *H. pylori* if present
Multiple UGI ulcers or ulcers in atypical locations
Family history of PUD
Peptic ulcer or GERD with diarrhea
Persistent diarrhea without clear etiology
Peptic ulcer in the absence of *H. pylori*
Personal or family history of MEN 1 tumors or endocrinopathies
Prominent gastric rugae with PUD
PUD resulting in complication (bleeding, perforation, obstruction)

GERD, gastroesophageal reflux disease; MEN 1, multiple endocrine neoplasia type 1; PUD, peptic ulcer disease; UGI, upper gastrointestinal.

Table 14.4. Differential diagnosis of hypergastrinemia and gastric hypersecretion

H. pylori infection
Gastric outlet obstruction
Antral G-cell hyperfunction/hyperplasia
Chronic renal failure
Retained gastric antrum syndrome
Short bowel syndrome
Zollinger-Ellison syndrome

Adapted from Jensen RT. Zollinger-Ellison syndrome. In: Doherty GM, Skögseid B, eds. *Surgical endocrinology.* Philadelphia: Lippincott Williams & Wilkins, 2001.

Biochemical Diagnosis

The diagnosis of gastrinoma requires confirmation with laboratory studies. A fasting serum gastrin measurement should be the first test obtained and is increased in greater than 90% of patients with gastrinoma (normal is 100–200 pg/mL). A level greater than 1,000 pg/mL is usually diagnostic of a gastrinoma and is seen in approximately 30% of patients. Most patients with gastrinomas have more moderate elevation of fasting gastrin levels (in the 200–1,000 pg/mL range). In addition to hypergastrinemia, gastric acid hypersecretion is required for the diagnosis of gastrinoma because hypergastrinemia is a normal physiologic response to achlorhydria or hypochlorhydria. Documentation of a gastric pH less than 2.5 rules out this physiologic response as the cause of hypergastrinemia. One third of patients with gastrinoma will have serum gastrin levels greater than 1,000 pg/mL and a gastric pH less than 2.5, which confirms the diagnosis. In the remaining two thirds, measurement of gastric acid output is required. Typically, patients with gastrinomas have a basal acid output of more than 15 mEq/hour or greater than 5 mEq/hour if they have had a previous ulcer operation aimed at reducing gastric acid secretion. A basal acid output/maximal acid output ratio greater than 0.6 also helps support the diagnosis of gastrinoma.

Provocative testing using the secretin stimulation test helps confirm the diagnosis in patients with more moderate hypergastrinemia (200–1,000 pg/mL) and gastric acid hypersecretion. After an overnight fast, the patient is given 2 units of secretin per kilogram of body weight intravenously. Serum gastrin levels are measured at 15 and 2 minutes before secretin injection and 0, 2, 5, 10, and 20 minutes following injection. A paradoxical increase in the serum concentration of gastrin by more than 200 pg/mL over baseline levels is diagnostic of gastrinoma. Patients with either antral G-cell hyperplasia or hypertrophy do not respond to secretin injection, although they do have postprandial gastrin elevation.

Tumor Localization

Tumor localization has become increasingly important in recent years with the demonstration that resection of gastrinomas is associated with an excellent prognosis and is frequently curative. Historically, numerous tests have been used to localize gastrinomas preoperatively, often without a well-designed strategy. This approach has used any, and frequently many, of the following modalities: CT scans, magnetic resonance imaging (MRI), transabdominal ultrasound, selective visceral angiography, selective venous sampling of portal venous tributaries, intraarterial secretin with hepatic venous sampling for gastrin, and conventional upper endoscopy. Two newer diagnostic methods—somatostatin receptor scintigraphy (SRS) and endoscopic ultrasonography (EUS)—are now complementing, and often replacing, the more traditional localization techniques. SRS, which takes advantage of the presence of high-affinity somatostatin receptors on the majority of pancreatic endocrine tumors, has been shown to have a sensitivity and specificity as high as 90% and 80%, respectively, equal to or greater than those for all other conventional localizing techniques combined (CT, MRI, US, angiography). The one relative weakness of SRS is in detecting small duodenal gastrinomas: it has been reported to miss up to one third of such lesions ultimately identified surgically. Because more than half of all lesions in recent surgical series have been duodenal gastrinomas, EUS has shown promise in complementing the information gained by SRS. Endoscopic ultrasound can localize up to half of duodenal lesions as well as most pancreatic gastrinomas. The combination of SRS and EUS should allow preoperative localization of most extrahepatic gastrinomas. When both of these studies are negative, an intraarterial secretin injection with hepatic venous sampling for gastrin is recommended by some because of its high sensitivity (approximately 89%) and ability to detect lesions independent of size, a drawback with SRS and EUS. CT and MRI can be used to address specific questions, if necessary (e.g., extent of liver metastases).

The introduction of SRS and EUS has clearly improved preoperative localization; still, up to one third of patients at experienced institutions will undergo exploration when preoperative imaging is negative. Although somewhat controversial, surgical exploration is warranted in patients with sporadic gastrinoma without diffuse liver metastases, even without successful preoperative localization. This scenario underscores the need for a careful operative strategy to ensure identification of the lesions to be resected.

Because most gastrinomas are found in the gastrinoma triangle (an anatomic area bounded by the junction of the body and neck of the pancreas medially, the junction of the second and third portion of the duodenum inferiorly, and the junction of the cystic duct and common bile duct superiorly), the operative focus is on this region. However, one must remember that primary gastrinomas can be found in numerous sites, including the lymph nodes, stomach, jejunum, mesentery, liver, ovary, and kidney. The combined use of an extensive Kocher maneuver for bimanual palpation of the pancreatic head and intraoperative ultrasonography detects virtually all intrapancreatic lesions. Detection of duodenal lesions requires more effort. Intraoperative endoscopy with duodenal transillumination will increase the duodenal gastrinoma detection rate above that of palpation and intraoperative ultrasound, but the key—some would advocate mandatory—maneuver is duodenotomy with careful palpation of the duodenal wall. The use of these intraoperative techniques has resulted in the ability to identify nearly all gastrinomas (including fairly small tumors, <5 mm) and essentially eliminated the nonproductive laparotomy. A final intraoperative technique using the gamma probe and radiolabeled octreotide to detect microscopic and otherwise undetected abdominal neuroendocrine tumors is currently being evaluated.

Treatment

Once the diagnosis of gastrinoma is suspected, the first step is to control the gastric acid hypersecretion and its end-organ effects. After initiation of appropriate medical therapy, definitive diagnosis and evaluation may proceed. Total gastrectomy warrants only a historical note and is rarely indicated because effective medical treatment is now readily available. Historically, total gastrectomy served as the only modality to eliminate the potentially lethal sequelae of gastric hypersecretion. H_2-blockers initially control acid secretion in most patients with gastrinomas, but over time most of these individuals require increasing dosages. In addition, up to 65% of patients, depending on the series, will fail to respond to this form of medical therapy. On the other hand, omeprazole, a gastric proton pump inhibitor, is associated with a considerably lower failure rate (0%–7.5%) and a more convenient dosing schedule. Omeprazole, or one of the newer proton pump inhibitors (e.g., lansoprazole, pantoprazole), is currently the drug of first choice. Long-term use may lead to drug-induced achlorhydria or hypochlorhydria with resultant vitamin B12 deficiency. Similarly, the question of increased incidence of gastric carcinoids—particularly in patients with MEN 1—has yet to be resolved satisfactorily. The somatostatin analogue, octreotide acetate, or the longer-acting lantreotide, may also be useful for symptomatic relief by decreasing the release of gastrin and other peptide hormones from gastrinomas and directly inhibiting gastric parietal cells.

In a patient with a sporadic gastrinoma, surgical exploration with attempted curative resection should follow localization studies regardless of whether the tumor is identified preoperatively. Because as many as 10% to 40% of tumors may not be localized before surgery, a standardized approach to exploration should be undertaken. The exploration should be done through a bilateral subcostal incision and the abdomen completely explored for evidence of metastasis, especially the regional lymph nodes and the liver, because up to 50% of gastrinomas are malignant with demonstrable disease at exploration. A complete mobilization of the pancreas is essential to allow inspection and palpation of the gland. Any suspicious lymph node or mass should be evaluated by frozen-section examination, as it is unclear whether surgical resection in the presence of metastasis prolongs survival or alleviates medical management of gastric hypersecretion. Some groups do recommend aggressive debulking of all tumor deposits if they are unresectable because survival may be improved and medical management of the acid disease may be better controlled. Intraoperative ultrasound may help identify intrapancreatic lesions, while intraoperative endoscopy with transillumination of the duodenal wall may help to identify duodenal gastrinomas. If no tumor is identified, a longitudinal duodenotomy should be made in the second portion of the duodenum. Careful bimanual examination of the bowel wall, along with its eversion, helps identify duodenal gastrinomas, which are frequently located submucosally with decreasing frequency from the proximal to the distal duodenum. When the tumor is small (<2 cm), duodenal gastrinomas can be resected with a small margin of normal tissue, whereas pancreatic gastrinomas should be enucleated, if possible, particularly in the head of the pancreas. Larger tumors often require pancreatic resection, either distal pancreatectomy or pancreaticoduodenectomy, particularly with tumors that are clearly invasive or abut critical ductal or vascular structures.

Despite extensive preoperative localizing studies and careful surgical exploration, the tumor of some patients cannot be identified even at laparotomy. "Blind" pancreatic head resection is controversial, especially given the dichotomous nature of gastrinoma whereby 75% of tumors pursue a fairly nonaggressive course. Patients with ZES in whom no tumor is found have an excellent prognosis, with 5- and 10-year survival rates of more than 94% and 87%, respectively. If gastric hypersecretion remains problematic despite maximal medical management, consideration may be given to performing a highly selective vagotomy. Total gastrectomy should be considered in patients who have had previous life-threatening complications from their ulcer disease despite appropriate medical management.

Medical management of ZES in patients with MEN 1 can be more difficult because of decreased sensitivity to antisecretory drugs, especially H_2-blockers. Parathyroidectomy and control of hypercalcemia can increase the potency of both proton pump inhibitors and H_2-blockers. The role of surgery in patients with ZES and MEN 1 is controversial. Resection of gastrinomas in patients with MEN 1 rarely results in normal serum gastrin levels, suggesting that the probability of curing these patients with surgery is extremely low. However, patients with MEN 1 tend to experience the less aggressive disease process and have a considerably long survival time even without complete surgical resection. As a result, many authorities have recommended that patients with MEN 1 and gastrinomas do not undergo exploration. Other groups think that resection of localized, larger (>2.5–3 cm) tumors may help reduce the risk of distant metastatic disease and presumably alter the natural history of the disease; therefore, they recommend that patients with MEN 1 undergo exploration. More extensive resections are generally discouraged because of the more favorable natural history, in addition to the problematic presence of multiple, synchronous, nonfunctioning pancreatic endocrine tumors, the prognostic effect of which is unclear.

Metastatic Disease

Now that medical treatment of gastric acid hypersecretion in ZES is so effective, patients rarely die from complications related to PUD. As a result, they live longer, only to die from metastatic disease. Given the propensity of malignant gastrinomas to metastasize to the liver, it is not surprising that patients ultimately die of liver failure. When feasible (approximately 15% of the time), cytoreductive hepatic resection can play a significant role in palliation of metastatic gastrinoma, often improving symptoms and extending life expectancy. When debulking procedures are not practical, nonsurgical therapy is often targeted directly at the liver in the form of peripheral hepatic artery embolization or chemoembolization and, in very selected cases, hepatic transplantation. Hepatic artery embolization with or without chemotherapeutic or radiotherapeutic agents takes advantage of the hypervascular morphology of pancreatic endocrine tumors derived preferentially from the hepatic artery. The nature of systemic therapy is to treat the entire body at risk for metastases and any currently manifest lesions. Systemic strategies include traditional chemotherapy, interferon-alpha, and somatostatin analogues used with and without radioisotopes (e.g., ^{90}yttrium). The larger series of gastrinoma patients report a 50% to 90% incidence of metastatic disease. Chemotherapy rarely results in cure, although some regimens have reasonable rates of response. The most promising regimen appears to be a combination of streptozocin and 5-fluorouracil, with or without doxorubicin; this combination gives response rates of 50% to 70%. Importantly, although many gastrinomas may not decrease demonstrably in volume, patients may have a symptomatically significant biochemical response. The somatostatin analogues appear effective in controlling symptoms of gastrinomas but show a disappointing objective tumor response rate of 10% to 20%. Interferon-alpha has also been studied alone and in combination with chemotherapy and somatostatin therapy. It also may result in biochemical response, with fewer patients realizing a reduction in tumor volume. Generally, traditional chemotherapy is considered first-line nonsurgical therapy.

When to initiate therapy for metastatic disease remains a controversial topic. Metastatic gastrinoma appears to follow at least three distinct clinical courses. In patients with rapidly progressing symptomatic disease, there would be little disagreement regarding the need to initiate potentially toxic therapy. However, in patients with slowly progressing, or even stable disease with easily controlled symptoms, the decision becomes less clear. Ultimately, the decision must be individualized to maximize the quality of the patient's remaining life.

Insulinoma

Epidemiology

In most series, insulinomas are the most common islet cell tumors of the pancreas, with a reported incidence estimated between less than one and four cases per 1 million people per year. These tumors occur slightly more often in women than in men. The average patient age at presentation is between 40 and 50 years. These tumors are almost always benign and overwhelmingly small (<2 cm), solitary lesions within the pancreas unless associated with MEN 1, when they tend to occur in a multicentric fashion.

Table 14.5. Symptoms associated with an insulinoma and their respective frequency

Symptoms	Frequency (%)
Neuroglycopenic symptoms	
Visual disturbances	59
Confusion	51
Altered consciousness	38
Weakness	32
Seizures	23
Symptoms related to hypoglycemic catecholamine release	
Sweating	43
Tremulousness	23
Tachycardia	23

Clinical Presentation

The original diagnostic criteria for an insulinoma are known as Whipple's triad and were proposed by Whipple, who initially described the syndrome. This triad consists of symptoms of hypoglycemia at fasting, documentation of blood glucose levels less than 50 mg/dL, and relief of symptoms following administration of glucose. However, Whipple's triad has proven not to be very specific, underscoring the importance of clinical suspicion and careful, systematic evaluation. The clinical symptoms of insulinomas are due to the hypoglycemia induced by excess insulin secretion and are commonly characterized as either neuroglycopenic or autonomic adrenergic. No truly hypoglycemic disorder presents with exclusively excess adrenergic symptoms. Many patients learn to recognize their specific symptom onset and thus avoid them by frequent meals or snacks. This is reflected in the often long duration of symptoms before diagnosis, frequently measured in months if not years. A list of the common symptoms and their frequency is shown in Table 14.5. Hunger, nausea, weight gain, and vomiting are also reported occasionally.

Biochemical Diagnosis

The measurement of normal serum glucose concentration documented during characteristic symptoms eliminates the diagnosis of insulinoma. The most reliable method of diagnosing an insulinoma is the provocative 72-hour supervised fast. Blood glucose and insulin levels are measured every 4 to 6 hours during the fast until serum glucose levels decrease below 60 mg/dL, at which time the frequency is increased to every 1 to 2 hours. Eighty percent of patients with insulinoma become symptomatic within 24 hours of starting the fast, and almost all are symptomatic if the fast is continued for 72 hours. The presence of hypoglycemia with concurrent elevation of serum insulin concentrations higher than 6 μU/mL (lack of appropriate suppression) and an insulin to glucose ratio of more than 0.3 confirm the diagnosis. One large series found, however, that 19% of patients with excised insulinomas had insulin to glucose ratios less than 0.3, pointing out the potential diagnostic weakness of the ratio. Measurement of the beta cell products C-peptide and proinsulin is important because both are usually increased in patients with insulinoma. In fact, the half-life of C-peptide is roughly twice that of insulin; therefore measurable C-peptide in a hypoglycemic patient is indicative of an endogenous insulin source. Patients who surreptitiously administer insulin to themselves usually have low levels of C-peptide and proinsulin, because commercial insulin does not contain the insulin precursor or its cleavage fragments. Patients taking oral hypoglycemic agents have normal or elevated levels of C-peptide and proinsulin, so differentiation from an insulinoma is made by measurement of plasma levels of sulfonylureas. Occasionally, ancillary tests such as the C-peptide suppression test and the tolbutamide test may provide evidence to support the diagnosis of insulinoma in equivocal cases.

Tumor Localization

Most insulinomas are small (<2 cm in diameter), and only approximately 10% of insulinomas are multicentric. There are no histologic criteria of malignancy for insulinomas; therefore, the diagnosis of a malignant tumor is based on the demonstration of metastatic disease, which is noted in 10% of cases. As with gastrinomas, all of the different modalities noted have also been used in an attempt to preoperatively localize insulinomas. Historical experience has demonstrated that, as with gastrinomas, no single technique is consistently reliable in localizing insulinomas short of exploration. Dynamic CT scanning is often the first localizing study performed, because it can detect approximately two thirds of the primary tumors and most metastatic lesions. When no tumor is seen with the CT scan, visceral angiography with digital subtraction techniques is successful in visualizing lesions approximately 60% to 90% of the time, although over the past decade the sensitivity of this study has fallen considerably in several reports. Selective portal venous sampling is reserved mainly for patients whose tumors cannot be visualized with CT or angiography. Portal venous sampling is able to define the general area of the tumor in 90% of patients overall and in approximately 75% of patients in whom other localizing tests are negative. The perfect study does not exist and thus the decision of which technique(s) will be used should revolve around institutional expertise and expected yield, the risk to the patient, and the cost of the total evaluation relative to its expected yield. In some experienced hands, preoperative localization is limited to transabdominal ultrasound.

Newer modalities are encouraging but continue to undergo definitive evaluation. Endoscopic ultrasound has shown promise, as it has with intrapancreatic gastrinomas, although its success becomes more limited when evaluating more distal pancreatic lesions. Lesions in the head of the pancreas can be visualized up to 95% of the time, while those in the body and tail were visualized in 78% and 60%, respectively, in one series. Unfortunately, insulinomas often (30%–90% of cases) do not possess appropriate somatostatin receptors, limiting the benefit of SRS in insulinomas as compared with other pancreatic endocrine tumors.

Regardless of preoperative imaging, intraoperative ultrasound has been uniformly helpful in locating lesions not identified before exploration or by manual palpation alone and for ruling out or identifying multiple tumors.

Treatment

At exploration, reddish-purple or white tumors may be visible on the surface of the gland; however, the pancreas must be completely mobilized as described previously for intrapancreatic gastrinomas. Small insulinomas located away from the main pancreatic duct can be enucleated. Small lesions in proximity to the main pancreatic duct can also be enucleated, and such a procedure is aided by intraoperative ultrasound guidance to avoid injury to the duct. Distal pancreatectomy is recommended for small lesions near the pancreatic duct to minimize the risk of a pancreatic fistula. Large lesions in the head of the pancreas may require pancreaticoduodenectomy, whereas those in the body and tail can be treated with a distal pancreatectomy. Resection is also preferred when signs of malignancy are present (e.g., hard tumors, puckering of adjacent tissue, infiltration, or tumors causing distal ductal obstruction). Intraoperative ultrasound can help identify tumors that could not be localized preoperatively using standard imaging techniques. Insulinomas are identified approximately 95% of the time at initial exploration. As with gastrinomas, blind resection of the pancreas is not recommended when no tumor is identified. Given the fairly uniform distribution of insulinomas throughout the pancreas, the logic behind "blind" resection is unclear, although there are those that would consider a "regionalizing" transhepatic portal venous sampling study adequate localization, particularly after an initial failed exploration and inadequate control of symptoms by appropriate medical therapy. If no tumor is identified at exploration, then pancreatic biopsy to rule out beta cell hyperplasia and adult nesidioblastosis is advisable. Beta cell hyperplasia or adult nesidioblastosis can generally be successfully treated by subtotal pancreatectomy.

Metastatic Disease

Patients with successful resection of insulinomas can expect an otherwise normal life expectancy. However, in those patients whose tumors are not found at exploration, are unsuitable for operative exploration, or have metastatic disease, symptoms can often be managed pharmacologically with diazoxide, verapamil, phenytoin, propranolol, or octreotide. Nonetheless, patients with metastatic disease should be considered for resection of the primary tumor and accessible metastatic lesions. Median disease-free survival is approximately 5 years in patients with malignant insulinoma who undergo curative resection. Approximately 65% of patients with malignant tumors will have recurrences at a mean of about 2.8 years. Although the chances for cure after resection are low in patients with malignant insulinoma, 10-year survival rates are 29%. Tumor debulking may improve control of hypoglycemic symptoms, but is recommended only if greater than 90% of disease can be resected.

Palliation can be achieved with medical therapy as well as surgery. Diazoxide can control the endocrine symptoms of insulinomas in 50% to 70% of patients by inhibiting the release of insulin from islet cells directly and by enhancing glycogenolysis indirectly. Octreotide controls symptoms in 40% to 60% of patients; however, its effect may be unpredictable in individual patients with tumors having atypical beta granules or none at all. Of the chemotherapeutic agents used for patients with metastatic disease, streptozocin, 5-fluorouracil, and doxorubicin have shown the best response rates.

Vasoactive Intestinal Polypeptidoma

Epidemiology

Although not a normal product of pancreatic islet cells, VIP can be secreted by islet cell tumors. The syndrome of excessive VIP secretion is associated with watery diarrhea, hypokalemia, and either hypochlorhydria or achlorhydria. First described in association with islet cell tumors in 1958, the syndrome has many names, including Verner-Morrison syndrome, pancreatic cholera, and WDHA (watery diarrhea, hypokalemia, and achlorhydria). Subsequently, it has been realized that 80% to 90% of so-called VIPomas are located in the pancreas, most often the body and tail (75%). Extrapancreatic tumors are often located in the chest and retroperitoneum (lung, esophagus, adrenal medulla [as ganglioblastomas, neuroblastomas, and ganglioneuromas], and along the autonomic nervous system). Ten percent of cases are due to islet cell hyperplasia. To date, approximately 200 well-documented cases of VIPoma have been described, and in most cases the tumor is malignant. An interesting bimodal distribution is noted, with younger patients (<10 years old) having less aggressive and extrapancreatic tumors.

Clinical Presentation / Tumor Localization

Patients usually present with excessive secretory diarrhea, often greater than 3 L/day that is aggravated by oral food intake and persists despite fasting. The patients become hypokalemic secondary to fecal potassium loss and acidotic from loss of fecal bicarbonate. The presence of a VIPoma is confirmed by demonstrating an increased fasting serum VIP level (>200 pg/mL) in the setting of secretory diarrhea with the presence of a mass. There are no provocative or inhibitory confirmatory studies. Pancreatic VIPomas are usually solitary, are greater than 3 cm in diameter, and most often are located in the tail of the pancreas. Diarrhea is such a nonspecific symptom that the evaluation should focus on eliminating more common causes (i.e., infectious, inflammatory, mechanical, even gastrinoma) before proceeding to serum VIP levels or localization studies. Typically, preoperative localization is easily achieved by abdominal and chest CT scans or by SRS. Mesenteric arteriography and hepatic portal venous sampling (HPVS) may be useful if the tumor location is still in question.

Treatment

Surgical excision remains the only effective method of cure. Preoperative preparation should include adequate rehydration and correction of electrolyte imbalances. The first-line therapy for control of the diarrhea is the use of long-acting somatostatin analogues. However, administration of steroids, nonsteroidal antiinflammatory drugs, or phenothiazines may also be helpful. At exploration, most tumors are located in the distal pancreas and are amenable to a complete resection by a distal pancreatectomy. A careful evaluation of both adrenal glands is mandatory if no tumor is found in the pancreas. Approximately 50% of the time, metastatic disease is found outside the pancreas at exploration. If curative resection is not possible, surgical debulking is often indicated to help palliate symptoms.

Long-term survival is relatively poor at approximately 15%. Streptozocin and interferon are currently the most active chemotherapeutic agents for advanced disease, and these are generally believed to be more effective against VIPomas than against other pancreatic endocrine tumors. Octreotide and other somatostatin analogues are useful for symptomatic relief from diarrhea in patients with metastatic disease and have been shown by some investigators to have some effect on tumor growth.

Glucagonoma

Glucagonomas arise from the A cells in the pancreatic islets of Langerhans. The syndrome caused by this tumor is due to excess secretion of glucagon. In contrast to other pancreatic endocrine tumors, glucagonomas are frequently fairly large at diagnosis (>5 cm) and are rarely found outside the pancreas. Approximately 70% of these tumors are malignant.

Clinical Presentation/Diagnosis

The most common and usually initial symptom in patients with glucagonoma is mild glucose intolerance (occurring in >90% of patients) that rarely requires insulin administration. The most striking and characteristic feature is a severe dermatitis called necrolytic migratory erythema, seen in approximately 70% of patients. The skin rash is most often located on the lower abdomen, perineum, perioral area, or feet. Other symptoms include a catabolic state, hypoaminoacidemia, stomatitis, anemia (normochromic/normocytic), weight loss, glossitis, depression, and venous thrombosis.

The diagnosis is confirmed by documenting the presence of an increased fasting serum glucagon level; levels greater than 1,000 pg/mL (normal, 0–150 pg/mL) are virtually diagnostic. Other conditions may cause hyperglucagonemia (e.g., hepatic insufficiency, severe stress, bacteremia, and starvation), but serum glucagon levels rarely exceed 500 pg/mL. In addition, the diagnosis can be confirmed by the characteristic findings on biopsy of the skin rash.

Tumor Localization

CT scanning is the first localization study. Most tumors are large at the time of diagnosis, ranging from 5 to 10 cm, and occur most often in the body and tail of the pancreas. As with the other pancreatic endocrine tumors, SRS localizes glucagonomas very reliably. Given the large size of these lesions, additional localization studies are rarely needed, although angiography and portal venous sampling may be required for glucagonomas that are difficult to identify.

Treatment

Surgical exploration should be undertaken in any patient whose tumor is thought to be resectable. Preoperative preparation of patients to reverse catabolism should include the use of somatostatin analogues and replenishment of amino acids—helping to ameliorate the catabolic state and often leading to resolution of the associated dermatitis. Sixty-eight percent of patients will have metastatic disease diagnosed by preoperative studies or at the time of exploration. Patients who are symptomatic due to metastatic disease frequently benefit from surgical resection. Patients with widely metastatic disease in whom surgical debulking is impossible can often benefit from medical therapy. Octreotide has been successful in controlling the diabetes and dermatitis in 60% to 90% of patients. Dacarbazine and streptozocin have been successfully used to treat some unresectable or recurrent glucagonomas. Although glucagonomas are rarely cured, long-term survival of up to 50% at 5 years is reported due to the frequent resectability and slow-growing nature of the lesions.

Somatostatinoma

Somatostatinomas arise from the D cells of the islets of Langerhans and are among the rarest endocrine neoplasms, with an estimated yearly incidence of one in 40 million. Generally mild hyperglycemia, cholelithiasis, steatorrhea, and diarrhea mark the somatostatinoma syndrome associated with these tumors. This "classic" syndrome is seen in patients with pancreatic tumors, while it is typically absent in those with duodenal somatostatinomas. Although duodenal tumors are not often associated with the classic somatostatinoma syndrome, they have been noted retrospectively to be often associated with neurofibromatosis. This has resulted in the proposal of a new MEN syndrome and should cause the clinician to be aware of the possibility of concurrent pheochromocytoma.

Early detection is difficult because symptoms are frequently mild and nonspecific. Diagnosis is often serendipitous during cholecystectomy, exploratory laparotomy, or radiologic or endoscopic evaluation of nonspecific abdominal symptoms. Confirmation of diagnostic suspicion can be achieved by demonstration of serum somatostatin levels 50-fold higher than normal. Provocative testing is not routinely available, although tolbutamide has been reported to cause an increase in serum levels in patients with somatostatinomas and not in controls. Most of these lesions are large and solitary and located in the head of the pancreas, and they are easily localized by CT scan or ultrasound (duodenal lesions are usually smaller but can be confirmed by esophagogastroduodenoscopy or radiography). Up to 90% of the lesions are malignant, and metastatic disease is found in most cases. In the absence of distant metastatic disease, resection is the treatment of choice; debulking, when possible, can offer symptomatic relief. Patients undergoing surgery for attempted resection should also have a cholecystectomy performed because of the high incidence of cholelithiasis. Medical therapy has proven disappointing, with 13% 5-year survival and only 48% 1-year survival reported.

Miscellaneous Functioning Tumors

Many islet cell tumors previously thought to be nonfunctioning have been found to secrete PP. Because this substance can now be measured, these tumors are referred to as *PPomas*. (Interestingly, 28%–70% of all functioning pancreatic endocrine tumors also secrete PP, the most likely being VIPomas and least likely insulinomas.) When an increased level of PP (>300 pmol/L) is detected in conjunction with a pancreatic mass, the diagnosis of PPoma is made by excluding the possibility of other functioning islet cell tumors. The excess secretion of PP is not associated with any clearly defined clinical syndrome; thus these tumors are usually large at diagnosis, presenting with symptoms related to local growth. Nonspecific symptoms such as diarrhea and weight loss may be present, however, possibly due to the inhibitory nature of PP on pancreatic secretion and gallbladder contraction. Surgical excision is the treatment of choice for resectable tumors, which can usually be easily localized by CT scan. PPomas are usually located in the head of the pancreas and are almost always malignant, though often slow-growing. Sixty percent are metastatic at the time of diagnosis. As with other pancreatic endocrine tumors, streptozocin is the chemotherapy of choice; however, because of the absence of hormonally related symptoms, no specific role for somatostatin analogues has been identified. The 5-year overall survival rate is 44%.

Growth hormone–releasing factor (GRF) is another hormone that has recently been identified as a tumor product. Referred to as GRFomas, tumors that secrete GRF are located in the pancreas 30% of the time, the lung 55% of the time, and the intestine 15% of the time. Approximately 30% of these lesions are malignant. Patients usually present with acromegaly, but these tumors also may secrete other products. In addition to GRFomas, 40% of patients have ZES, and 40% have Cushing's syndrome. Although octreotide can significantly suppress the levels of circulating growth hormone in this syndrome, surgical excision, if possible, is the treatment of choice.

Other uncommon islet cell tumors include those that secrete neurotensin, ACTH, or a parathyroid hormone–like peptide.

Carcinoid

The classic carcinoid tumor of the pancreas is extremely rare, although anecdotal cases have been reported. Pancreatic carcinoids are grouped with foregut carcinoids, and patients with these tumors may have normal serum levels of serotonin (may be increased or tumor stain for 5-hydroxytryptamine) but commonly have elevated urinary levels of 5-hydroxyindolacetic acid. Furthermore, the typical carcinoid syndrome is more common than in other foregut carcinoids. Pancreatic carcinoids generally are larger than midgut, hindgut, or other foregut carcinoids and therefore patients often present with mass-effect symptoms such as epigastric pain, weight loss, or jaundice from common bile duct compression. Localization has traditionally been by CT scan because most of these tumors are several centimeters in diameter at the time of diagnosis, although octreotide scanning has shown promise as a method to diagnose the disease and follow these patients after resection. Generally, carcinoid tumors grow slowly and invade adjacent organs late in the course of the disease, making resection possible in most patients. Unfortunately, at least 70% of patients have distant metastases at the time of diagnosis, minimizing the likelihood of long-term survival. However, in the absence of distant metastases, complete resection of the primary tumor offers an excellent possibility of long-term survival.

Nonfunctioning Tumors

Recent series report that 35% to 50% of pancreatic islet tumors are nonfunctioning, that is, they do not secrete detectable levels of functional hormones. Instead of a well-defined clinical syndrome, the presentation of these tumors is similar to that of pancreatic ductal adenocarcinoma. Since many nonfunctioning pancreatic tumors stain for one or many known hormones or precursor hormones, several hypotheses have been proposed to account for the lack of manifest symptoms. First, the hormones secreted in excess may not produce signs or symptoms. Second, a clinically active hormone may be secreted in clinically irrelevant amounts. Finally, the secreted hormone product may actually be either a precursor hormone or one that has yet to be identified. Common symptoms include abdominal pain, weight loss, and jaundice. Most of these tumors are found in the head of the pancreas, and most are malignant.

Diagnosis can be made by CT-guided fine-needle aspiration as well as by the characteristic hypervascular appearance on arteriography. However, conventional CT scans may have features characteristic of pancreatic islet cell tumors in contrast to adenocarcinoma of the pancreas. These features include a high degree of enhancement, cystic degeneration, and calcification. Additionally, endocrine tumors are less likely to encase vascular structures or obstruct the pancreatic duct. Following localization studies, operative exploration for attempted curative resection is often indicated.

The prognosis for patients with nonfunctioning islet cell tumors is significantly better than that for patients with pancreatic ductal adenocarcinoma, with the overall median survival rate in the former group reported at over 3 years. In patients with localized and completely resected disease, however, median overall survival is as long as 7 years. Even when localized disease is unresectable, the prognosis can remain fairly good, with a median survival of over 5 years. Chemotherapy with streptozocin and 5-fluorouracil has shown some favorable results and should be considered early in the course of the disease because median survival for unresectable metastatic disease is less than 2 years.

MULTIPLE ENDOCRINE NEOPLASIA

There are currently three well-defined MEN syndromes (MEN 1, MEN 2A, and MEN 2B), characterized by a familial predisposition to the development of tumors (often multiple) in various endocrine glands. Recognition of the individual components of

Table 14.6. Features of multiple endocrine neoplasia syndromes and the associated tumors (approximate incidence of tumor with each syndrome)

	MEN 1	MEN 2A	MEN 2B
Acronym	Werner's syndrome	Sipple's syndrome	None
Genetic mutation	Chromosome 11q13	RET proto-oncogene chromosome 10q11.2	RET proto-oncogene chromosome 10q11.2
Tumors	Parathyroid (90%)	MTC (100%)	MTC (100%)
	Pancreas (80%)	Pheo (20%–50%)	Pheo (20%–50%)
	Pituitary adenoma (55%)	Parathyroid (20%–35%)	Neuromas (~100%)
	Adrenal adenomas (30%)	Cutaneous lichen amyloidosis	Skeletal deformities
	Thyroid nodules (10%)	Hirschprung's disease	Megacolon
		Enlarged peripheral nerves	

MEN, multiple endocrine neoplasia; MTC, medullary thyroid carcinoma; Pheo, pheochromocytoma.

each syndrome may be synchronous but more often is over a long period of follow-up. Typically, not all of the clinical manifestations of the "classic" syndromes are expressed. A descriptive overview of the three syndromes is given in Table 14.6. Recently, specific genetic mutations have been identified as the likely causal event resulting in the clinical phenotypes associated with the development of the MEN syndromes.

MEN 1 was mapped by linkage analysis to the long arm of chromosome 11 (11q13). In 1997, positional cloning identified the specific gene. The MEN 1 gene encodes a 610-amino acid protein designated *menin*. Menin is principally a nuclear protein known to repress JUN-D–mediated RNA transcription, supporting the hypothesis that MEN 1 is caused by a tumor-suppressor gene.

Conversely, the gene responsible for MEN 2 is a proto-oncogene. It is located on chromosome sub-band 10q11.2 and is known as the RET proto-oncogene. This gene encodes the protein RET (rearranged during transfection), which is a receptor tyrosine kinase.

MEN 1

MEN 1, also known as Wermer's syndrome, has historically been characterized by the development of multigland parathyroid hyperplasia, pancreatic islet cell tumors, and pituitary tumors.

Patients with MEN 1 also have a high incidence of foregut carcinoid tumors, adrenocortical tumors, and thyroid adenomas and carcinomas. In addition to endocrine gland abnormalities, patients with MEN 1 often have subtle skin lesions, including lipomas, facial angiofibromas, and skin collagenomas. MEN 1 is found in approximately one of every 30,000 in the general population. Various combinations of tumors develop, with 94% penetrance by age 50 years. The inheritance pattern is autosomal dominant, although the mechanism of tumorigenesis at the cellular level is recessive. A particular individual inherits a germline mutation to one allele at 11q13 (most often encoding truncated, inactive protein); a subsequent somatic mutation to the other allele at the MEN 1 locus results in loss of heterozygosity and eventual phenotypic expression. The clinical manifestations vary and are generally apparent by the third or fourth decade, although with careful screening most known carriers show evidence of tumorigenesis by their mid-twenties.

Hyperparathyroidism

Hyperparathyroidism is the most common endocrine abnormality seen in MEN 1 and is usually the first to develop (in 60%–90% of affected patients). Almost all hyperparathyroidism develops secondary to asymmetric, four-gland hyperplasia. The clinical presentation is similar to that seen in sporadic hyperparathyroidism, with most patients being asymptomatic. Measurement of serum calcium, phosphate, and intact-PTH levels leads to the diagnosis. Increased serum calcium in the face of inappropriately elevated intact-PTH and an elevated 24-hour urinary calcium collection confirm the diagnosis of hyperparathyroidism. As with sporadic hyperparathyroidism, treatment is surgical excision. Pre-excision imaging is of little value prior to initial exploration because of the multi-gland nature of the pathophysiology of MEN 1. In recurrent or persistent hyperparathyroidism, however, noninvasive imaging and often invasive modalities (e.g., angiography and venous sampling) may aid in guiding successful re-exploration. The frequency of synchronous thyroid neoplasms (15%) dictates that a careful evaluation of the thyroid gland be part of any neck exploration in patients with MEN 1.

There continues to be controversy over the appropriate surgical procedure for hyperparathyroidism in the setting of MEN 1. Many surgeons perform a three-and-one-half gland parathyroidectomy, while others advocate total parathyroidectomy with autotransplantation. There is considerable overlap in the reported incidence of recurrent or persistent hyperparathyroidism, as well as permanent hypoparathyroidism with either technique. Theoretically, total parathyroidectomy minimizes the likelihood of recurrent or persistent disease, although adding to the potential risk of permanent hypoparathyroidism. Our preferred technique is to perform a four-gland excision with autotransplantation of pieces of the least hyperplastic gland into the brachioradialis muscle of the non-dominant forearm. Graft-dependent hyperparathyroidism may develop in up to 50% of patients and can be effectively managed by removing several pieces of parathyroid tissue from the forearm under local anesthesia, precluding the need for neck re-exploration and its attendant increased risk of recurrent nerve paresis/paralysis and permanent hypoparathyroidism. Either procedure should include cervical thymectomy because MEN 1 is associated with an increased incidence of supranumery parathyroid glands, which are often located within the thymus, in up to 20% of patients. In general, hyperparathyroidism associated with MEN 2A is much easier to control and is associated with a less frequent recurrence rate after surgery than is MEN 1. Hyperparathyroidism should be addressed before therapy for pancreatic islet cell tumors because control of calcium-dependent hormone release from these tumors may be improved.

Pancreatic Tumors

The second most common neoplasms associated with MEN 1 are the pancreatic islet cell tumors, which occur in approximately 60% of patients with MEN 1. The clinical syndrome associated with these tumors results from the specific hormone secreted by each. The most common islet cell tumors are gastrinomas, followed by insulinomas. Rarely, glucagonomas, VIPomas, and somatostatinomas are found. MEN 1–associated pancreatic endocrine tumors are multifocal and may be located outside the pancreas, as is typical with gastrinomas. It is important to recognize that any particular radiographically demonstrable pancreatic mass may not be specifically responsible for a clinically apparent syndrome. However, the risk of malignancy remains even, and often especially, for clinically silent pancreatic masses. Details of the treatment of these tumors have been discussed previously. One must keep in mind that although biochemical cure is often not a realistic goal, prevention of the lethal consequences of malignant transformation and metastatic disease may be possible by aggressive surgical intervention.

Thompson et al. (1988) have advocated a strategy with this in mind, including the following: distal pancreatectomy at the level of the superior mesenteric vein, regardless of tumor location in the pancreas or duodenum; duodenotomy even without palpable duodenal lesions when faced with elevated serum gastrin and a positive secretin-stimulation test; peripancreatic lymph node dissection for duodenal or pancreatic neuroendocrine masses greater than 3 cm; and enucleation of pancreatic head or uncinate process tumors identified by palpation or intraoperative ultrasound. This aggressive approach remains controversial.

Pituitary Neoplasms

Pituitary neoplasms occur in 30% to 50% of patients with MEN 1; benign prolactin-producing adenomas are most common. Symptoms may be related directly to tumor mass effect (i.e., headache, diplopia, and hypopituitism) or be related to specific hormone overproduction. Excess prolactin causes galactorrhea and amenorrhea in women and impotence in men. Tumors may also produce growth hormone (30%) or ACTH (>10%), leading to acromegaly or Cushing's disease, respectively. Bromocriptine, a dopamine agonist, can be used to treat prolactinomas medically. Transsphenoidal hypophysectomy is reserved for patients who do not respond to bromocriptine and who have nonprolactin-secreting tumors. All patients with MEN 1 should be observed periodically with measurement of serum prolactin and growth hormone levels.

MEN 2

MEN 2 consists of three subtypes, each inherited in an autosomal dominant pattern with 100% penetrance but variable expression; all are marked by the presence of medullary thyroid carcinoma (MTC). MEN 2A and MEN 2B are defined by the presence of MTC and pheochromocytoma. Additionally, in MEN 2A (90% of all cases MEN 2), hyperparathyroidism often develops secondary to four-gland hyperplasia. Patients with MEN 2B (5% of cases of MEN 2) almost invariably have characteristic facies and marfanoid habitus. MEN 2B is also marked by the presence of multiple neuromas on the lips, tongue, and oral mucosa. In addition, patients with MEN 2B have a high incidence of skeletal abnormalities as well as diffuse ganglioneuromatosis of the GI tract, which can lead to a number of GI motility problems, most frequently involving the colon. Megacolon, associated with severe constipation, is the most common GI manifestation. Familial MTC is believed to be the most indolent of the three subtypes and is characterized by the absence of consistent phenotypic manifestations in addition to MTC.

Medullary Thyroid Carcinoma

MTC comprises approximately 5% to 10% of all thyroid malignancies. The vast majority—approximately 80%—of these tumors occur sporadically; the remaining 20% are familial. MTC can occur in the familial setting without any other associated syndromes. Some features of sporadic and familial MTC are shown in Table 14.7. In the setting of MEN 2, MTC is usually the first endocrine abnormality to occur. MTC arises from the parafollicular or C cells of the thyroid gland and as a result can secrete not only calcitonin but also a variety of other hormonally active substances, such as serotonin, ACTH, prostaglandins, melanin, and carcinoembryonic antigen.

CLINICAL PRESENTATION. MTC is often detected by genetic or biochemical screening when it is clinically occult. Most index cases, or patients who are not identified by screening, present with a palpable neck mass. Approximately 30% of the patients with MTC present with watery diarrhea, usually secondary to the stimulatory effect of high plasma calcitonin levels on intestinal fluid and electrolyte secretion. Symptoms such as hoarseness, dysphagia, and respiratory difficulty may be related to locally advanced disease. Presenting symptoms may also be secondary to

Table 14.7. Comparison of features of sporadic versus familial medullary thyroid carcinoma

Feature	Sporadic	Familial
Proportion of cases	80%	20%
Age at onset	40–60 yr	10–30 yr
Location	Unilateral	Bilateral

metastatic disease, which is most commonly seen in the lungs, liver, and bones.

DIAGNOSIS. Historically, demonstrating elevated calcitonin levels using provocative testing in at-risk individuals has made the diagnosis of MTC. This strategy required multiple tests over many years to establish a diagnosis of MTC, and thus MEN 2. Because of the autosomal-dominant pattern of inheritance, 50% of at-risk patients using this strategy would undergo considerable inconvenience, be subjected to undue anxiety, and be exposed to some degree of risk from provocative testing. The application of genetic screening for the RET proto-oncogene has allowed earlier and more reliable diagnosis of MEN 2 while obviating long-term biochemical screening in those patients lacking the RET gene. Thus, early screening for the RET gene is the preferred method of diagnosis in at-risk patients. The appropriate timing of screening is still a topic of debate, but it is generally accepted that children of patients with MEN 2B should be screened in infancy. Metastatic MTC has been reported in infants less than 1 year old and warrants early and aggressive treatment. Affected children of patients with MEN 2A may have a more indolent disease course, but childhood MTC can develop and should be screened for by age 5 to 6 years.

Otherwise, when patients present with a palpable mass, fine-needle aspiration biopsy should be performed. Histologically, MTC frequently shows sheets of uniformly round or polygonal cells separated by fibrovascular stroma. Immunohistochemical staining for calcitonin in the tumor cells is the most reliable way to confirm the diagnosis. Laboratory measurements for serum calcitonin are also important as a baseline measurement and are usually markedly increased. Patients with clinically occult tumors, however, may have normal or minimally elevated serum calcitonin levels.

Provocative tests still can be useful for follow-up of patients previously treated for MTC. Generally, patients with MTC will have a demonstrable increase in serum calcitonin level; however, up to 30% of patients may have normal levels. By using pentagastrin (with or without calcium infusion) as a calcitonin secretagogue, the diagnosis of recurrence can be made.

TREATMENT. Once the diagnosis of MTC is made, the presence of pheochromocytoma should be excluded before definitive surgical treatment or intervention. Similarly, hyperparathyroidism should be diagnosed, if present, before surgery. If a pheochromocytoma is found, it should be treated first (see Chapter 15). If hyperparathyroidism is diagnosed, it can be treated at the time of neck exploration for the MTC. Important points to keep in mind with regard to treatment of MTC are its aggressive nature relative to well-differentiated thyroid cancer, its inability to concentrate radioactive iodine, the ineffectiveness of radiation and chemotherapy, its frequent multicentricity, and the high probability of nodal metastases.

With the above points in mind, the appropriate treatment for MTC is total thyroidectomy and central neck dissection (levels VI and VII). In patients with MEN 2 syndromes, MTC is frequently multicentric and bilateral and metastasizes early to the cervical lymph nodes. The central neck dissection, which removes the lymphatic tissue between the jugular veins laterally, the hyoid bone superiorly, and the innominate vessels inferiorly, helps eradicate microscopic metastatic disease. Some authors argue that in patients with palpable primary tumors, the high frequency of microscopic disease in the lymph nodes bilaterally warrants bilateral functional neck dissections in addition to central nodal dissection. Intraoperative nodal evaluation is believed to be an inadequate predictor of nodal involvement. Others contend that only patients with palpable lymphadenopathy should undergo a concomitant functional neck dissection on the side of the enlarged pathologic nodes.

Intraoperative management of the parathyroid glands is an important consideration during operation for MTC and is controversial as well. Some surgeons are content to identify the glands and leave them in situ, while others advocate four-gland resection with autotransplantation into the non-dominant forearm (MEN 2A [possibility or presence of hyperparathyroidism]) or the sternocleidomastoid muscle (MEN 2B and sporadic MTC).

Patients can be followed postoperatively with provocative testing to identify residual or recurrent MTC. Overall, the prognosis of MTC is good, with 10-year survival rates of 60% to 80% reported for patients with MEN 2A. Patients with MEN 2B usually present with more advanced disease (i.e., extrathyroidal extension or macroscopic nodal metastasis), and long-term survival is less common. In general, the course of the MTC determines the prognosis for patients with MEN 2. The average life expectancy for this group of patients is more than 50 years.

Metastatic Disease

Controversy exists over the appropriate treatment of patients with stimulated elevations of plasma calcitonin levels in the postoperative period. Such a finding implies the presence of residual disease in the neck or mediastinum or undetected metastatic disease. Some clinicians prefer to simply follow these patients with observation because of the relatively slow rate of progression of MTC, while the chances for cure with repeat neck exploration are low and the risks of exploration are increased. Others recommend a repeat neck exploration after selective catheterization of the neck veins and determination of stimulated plasma calcitonin levels. In experienced hands, and with careful patient selection to exclude the presence of distant metastases (often including laparoscopic liver evaluation), a 30% to 40% normalization of plasma calcitonin levels by provocative testing can be achieved after repeat exploration. Radiation therapy may be useful when surgical options are exhausted for residual or recurrent disease in the neck, but such treatment is generally ineffective. Likewise, chemotherapy is generally ineffective in treating metastatic disease; however, doxorubicin, alone or in combination, may result in a partial response. Because of the indolent nature of the tumor, many physicians do not treat metastatic disease aggressively.

Pheochromocytoma

Usually, pheochromocytoma associated with MEN 2 appears between the ages of 10 and 30 years and is diagnosed concurrently with, or shortly after, MTC. The pheochromocytomas associated with MEN 2 are usually bilateral (60%–80% of the time), limited to the adrenal medulla, and almost always benign. The adrenal gland appears to become hyperplastic before the pheochromocytoma develops. Further discussion of pheochromocytoma can be found in the chapter on adrenal tumors (Chapter 15).

The workup and management of pheochromocytoma are discussed in more detail in Chapter 15. MEN 2 is typically diagnosed by catecholamine screening (urinary epinephrine, norepinephrine, and total metanephrines) before the onset of characteristic symptoms. A cross-sectional imaging study (CT or MRI) that demonstrates a unilateral adrenal mass or bilateral adrenal masses is generally adequate for preoperative localization in most cases. When cross-sectional imaging or catecholamine screening is equivocal ^{131}I metaiodobenzylguanidine (MIBG) scanning and additional localizing studies can help confirm the diagnosis. MIBG scintigraphy is also useful to further eliminate the possibility of bilateral pheochromocytomas.

Because many years (10 or more) can separate the appearance of pheochromocytomas in the opposite adrenal gland in patients with MEN 2, if a subsequent tumor develops at all, some controversy exists about the optimal surgical procedure for patients who are initially found to have a unilateral pheochromocytoma. Although some surgeons recommend bilateral adrenalectomy in patients with MEN 2 because bilateral tumors will develop in up to 80% of these patients, a more conservative approach is followed by most to avoid as long as possible the need for lifetime glucocorticoid and mineralocorticoid replacement. This approach involves unilateral adrenalectomy and examination of the contralateral adrenal gland at the time of exploration. If no abnormality is found, the unaffected adrenal gland is left intact and the patient is observed closely for evidence of a contralateral tumor, which develops in approximately 50% of patients after 10 years of follow-up. In the event of bilateral pheochromocytoma, cortical-sparing adrenalectomy has been demonstrated to be an effective alternative to bilateral adrenalectomy, avoiding chronic steroid replacement and the risk of Addisonian crisis. Long-term follow-up is indicated in all patients with MEN syndromes for the recurrence of any endocrine lesion.

Although laparoscopic adrenalectomy has become increasingly popular for benign adrenal lesions, the role of laparoscopy in the surgical treatment of pheochromocytoma has yet to be fully defined. Several groups have demonstrated the safety of laparoscopic adrenalectomy, although patients with pheochromocytoma may experience significant hypertensive crises during laparoscopy, even in the face of adequate preoperative medical treatment. This issue is further discussed in the chapter on adrenal tumors (Chapter 15).

Hyperparathyroidism

Hyperparathyroidism is the third and most variable component of the MEN 2A syndrome. Most often, patients are asymptomatic and the diagnosis is made on routine follow-up laboratory tests. Occasionally, patients present with kidney stones. In patients with MEN 2, a workup for hyperparathyroidism should be undertaken before neck exploration for MTC. In the vast majority of cases, the hyperparathyroidism is secondary to hyperplasia or multiple gland disease. As previously discussed, many surgeons prefer total parathyroidectomy with autotransplantation at the time of thyroidectomy whether or not concurrent hyperparathyroidism exists. However, surgeons who prefer a selective approach may choose not to perform a parathyroidectomy if, at the time of exploration, the calcium levels are normal and the parathyroid glands appear normal. If the calcium and serum PTH levels are elevated, or if the glands appear grossly abnormal or are hyperplastic on biopsy, a total parathyroidectomy should be performed.

Approximately one-half of the most normal-appearing parathyroid gland should be transplanted into the forearm. If normal parathyroid tissue becomes devascularized during total thyroidectomy for MTC in a patient with MEN 2, parathyroid autotransplantation should also be performed. Patients with MEN 2A should have the autotransplant performed into the brachioradialis muscle of the forearm, because the gland could become hyperplastic in the future and this placement facilitates later removal. In patients with MEN 2B, because hyperparathyroidism rarely develops, the devascularized parathyroid glands can be transplanted into the sternocleidomastoid muscle in the neck.

RECOMMENDED READING

Pancreatic Endocrine Tumors

Adams S, Baum RP, Hertel A, et al. Intraoperative gamma probe detection of neuroendocrine tumors. *J Nucl Med* 1998;39:1155.

Alexander HR, Fraker DL, Norton JA, et al. Prospective study of somatostatin receptor scintigraphy and its effect on operative outcome in patients with Zollinger-Ellison syndrome. *Ann Surg* 1998;228:228.

Arnold R, Simon B, Wied M. Treatment of neuroendocrine GEP tumours with somatostatin analogues. *Digestion* 2000;62(suppl 1):84.

Bieligk S, Jaffe BM. Islet cell tumors of the pancreas. *Surg Clin North Am* 1995;75:1025.

Delcore R, Friesen SR, Gastrointestinal neuroendocrine tumors. *J Am Coll Surg* 1994;178:187.

Doherty GM, Doppman JL, Shawker TH, et al. Results of a prospective strategy to diagnose, localize, and resect insulinomas. *Surgery* 1991;110:989.

Doherty GM, Skögseid B (eds). *Surgical oncology,* Philadelphia: Lippincott Williams & Wilkins, 2001.

Eriksson B, Oberg K, Stridsberg M. Tumor markers in neuroendocrine tumors. *Digestion* 2000;62 (suppl 1):33.

Eriksson BK, Larsson EG, Skogseid BM, et al. Liver embolizations of patients with malignant neuroendocrine gastrointestinal tumors. *Cancer* 1998;83:2293.

Evans DB, Skibber JM, Lee JF, et al. Nonfunctioning islet cell carcinoma of the pancreas. *Surgery* 1993;114:1175.

Fraker DL, Alexander HR. The surgical approach to endocrine tumors of the pancreas. *Semin Gastrointest Dis* 1995;6:102.

Gibril F, Doppman JL, Jensen RT. Recent advances in the treatment of metastatic pancreatic endocrine tumors. *Semin Gastrointest Dis* 1995;6:114.

Gibril F, Reynolds JC, Doppman JL, et al. Somatostatin receptor scintigraphy: its sensitivity compared with that of other imaging methods in detecting primary and metastatic gastrinomas. *Ann Intern Med* 1996;125:26.

Gower WR, Fabri PJ. Endocrine neoplasms (non-gastrin) of the pancreas. *Semin Surg Oncol* 1990;6:98.

Grant CS. Surgical aspects of hyperinsulinemic hypoglycemia. *Endocrinol Metab Clin North Am* 1999;28:533.

Harmon JW, Norton JA, Collen MJ. Removal of gastrinomas for the control of Zollinger-Ellison syndrome. *Ann Surg* 1984;200:396.

Heitz PU, Kasper M, Polak JM, et al. Pancreatic endocrine tumors: immunocytochemical analysis of 125 tumors. *Hum Pathol* 1982;13:263.

Howard TJ, Stabile BE, Zinner MJ, et al. Anatomic distribution of pancreatic endocrine tumors. *Am J Surg* 1990;159:258.

Jensen RT. Zollinger-Ellison syndrome. In: Doherty GM, Skögseid B, eds. *Surgical oncology.* Philadelphia: Lippincott Williams & Wilkins, 2001.

Krejs GJ. Gastrointestinal endocrine tumors. *Scand J Gastroenterol* 1996;220(suppl):121.

Lam KY, Lo CY. Pancreatic endocrine tumour: a 22-year clinico-pathological experience with morphological, immunohistochemical observation and a review of the literature. *Eur J Surg Oncol* 1997;23:36.

Lee JE, Evans DB. Advances in the diagnosis and treatment of gastrointestinal neuroendocrine tumors. *Cancer Treat Res* 1997;90:227.

Legaspi A, Brennan MF. Management of islet cell carcinoma. *Surgery* 1988;104:1018.

Le Treut YP, Delpero JR, Dousset B, et al. Results of liver transplantation in the treatment of metastatic neuroendocrine tumors: a 31 case French multicentric report. *Ann Surg* 1997;225:355.

Mao C, El Attar A, Domenico D, et al. Carcinoid tumors of the pancreas: status report based on two cases and review of the world's literature. *Int J Pancreatol* 1998;23:153.

Maton PN. The use of long-acting somatostatin analogue, octreotide acetate, in patients with islet cell tumors. *Gastroenterol Clin North Am* 1989;18:897.

Maurer CA, Baer HU, Dyong TH, et al. Carcinoid of the pancreas: clinical characteristics and morphologic features. *Eur J Cancer* 1996;32A:1109.

Meko JB, Norton JA. Endocrine tumors of the pancreas. *Curr Opin Gen Surg* 1994;2:186–194.

Nguyen HN, Backes B, Lammert F, et al. Long-term survival after diagnosis of hepatic metastatic VIPoma: report of two cases with disparate courses and review of therapeutic options. *Dig Dis Sci* 1999;44:1148.

Norton JA. Intraoperative methods to stage and localize pancreatic and duodenal tumors. *Ann Oncol* 1999;110(suppl 4):182.

Norton JA. Neuroendocrine tumors of the pancreas and duodenum. *Curr Probl Surg* 1994;31:77.

Norton JA, Doppman JL, Collen MJ, et al. Prospective study of gastrinoma localization and resection in patients with Zollinger-Ellison syndrome. *Ann Surg* 1986;204:468.

Norton JA, Doppman JL, Jensen RT. Curative resection in Zollinger-Ellison syndrome: results of a 10 year prospective study. *Ann Surg* 1992;215:8.

Norton JA, Fraker DL, Alexander HR, et al. Surgery to cure the Zollinger-Ellison syndrome. *N Engl J Med* 1999;341:635.

Oberg K. Neuroendocrine gastrointestinal tumors. *Ann Oncol* 1996;7:453.

Orbuch M, Doppman JL, Jensen RT. Localization of pancreatic endocrine tumors. *Semin Gastrointest Dis* 1995;6:90.

Pasieka JL, McLeod MK, Thompson NW, et al. Surgical approach to insulinomas: assessing the need for preoperative localization. *Arch Surg* 1992;127:442.

Perry RR, Vinik AI. Diagnosis and management of functioning islet cell tumors. *J Clin Endocrinol Metab* 1995;80:2273.

Phan GQ, Yeo CJ, Hruban RH, et al. Surgical experience with pancreatic and peripancreatic neuroendocrine tumors: review of 125 patients. *J Gastrointest Surg* 1998;2:473.

Proye C, Malvaux P, Pattou F, et al. Non-invasive imaging of insulinomas and gastrinomas with endoscopic ultrasonography and somatostatin receptor scintigraphy. *Surgery* 1998;124:1134.

Ricke J, Klose K-J. Imaging procedures in neuroendocrine tumors. *Digestion* 2000;62 (suppl 1):39.

Service FJ. Hypoglycemic disorders. *N Engl J Med* 1995;332:1144.

Sloan DA, Schwartz RW, Kenady DE. Surgical therapy for endocrine tumors of abdominal origin. *Curr Opin Oncol* 1993;5:100.

Tanaka S, Yamasaki S, Matsushita H, et al. Duodenal somatostatinoma: a case report and review of 31 cases with special reference to the relationship between tumor size and metastasis. *Pathol Int* 2000;50:146.

Termanini B, Gibril F, Reynolds JC, et al. Value of somatostatin receptor scintigraphy: a prospective study in gastrinoma of its effect on clinical management. *Gastroenterology* 1997;112:335.

Thompson GB, van Heerden JA, Grant CS, et al. Islet cell carcinomas of the pancreas: a twenty-year experience. *Surgery* 1988;104:1011.

Veenhof CHN. Pancreatic endocrine tumors, immunotherapy and gene therapy: chemotherapy and interferon therapy of endocrine tumors. *Ann Oncol* 1999;10(suppl.4):S185.

Venkatesh S, Ordonez NG, Ajani J, et al. Islet cell carcinoma of the pancreas. *Cancer* 1990;65:354.

Weber HC, Venzon DJ, Lin J-T, et al. Determinants of metastatic rate and survival in patients with Zollinger-Ellison syndrome: a prospective long-term study. *Gastroenterology* 1995;108:1637.

Wymenga ANM, Eriksson B, Salmela PI, et al. Efficacy and safety of prolonged-release Lantreotide in patients with gastrointestinal neuroendocrine tumors and hormone-related symptoms. *J Clin Oncol* 1999;17:1111.

Yu F, Venzon DJ, Serrano J, et al. Prospective study of the clinical course, prognostic factors, causes of death, and survival in patients with long-standing Zollinger-Ellison syndrome. *J Clin Oncol* 1999;17:615.

Zollinger RM, Ellison EC, O'Dorisio T, et al. Thirty years' experience with gastrinoma. *World J Surg* 1984;8:427.

Multiple Endocrine Neoplasia

Cance WG, Wells SA. Multiple endocrine neoplasia type IIa. *Curr Probl Surg* 1985;22:1.

Carlson KM, Dou S, Chi D, et al. Single missense mutation in the tyrosine kinase catalytic domain of the RET protooncogene is associated with multiple endocrine neoplasia type 2B. *Proc Natl Acad Sci USA* 1994;91:1579.

Chandrasekharappa SC, Guru SC, Manickam P, et al. Positional cloning of the gene for multiple endocrine neoplasia-type 1. *Science* 1997;276:404.

Clark OH. What's new in endocrine surgery. *J Am Coll Surg* 1997;184: 126.

Eng C. RET proto-oncogene in the development of human cancer. *J Clin Oncol* 1999;17:380.

Gagner M, Breton G, Pharand D, et al. Is laparoscopic adrenalectomy indicated for pheochromocytomas? *Surgery* 1996;120:1076.

Herfarth KK, Bartsch D, Doherty GM, et al. Surgical management of hyperparathyroidism in patients with multiple endocrine neoplasia type 2A. *Surgery* 1996;120:966.

Howe JR, Norton JA, Wells SA. Prevalence of pheochromocytoma and hyperparathyroidism in multiple endocrine neoplasia type 2A: results of long-term follow-up. *Surgery* 1993;114:1070.

Jensen RT. Management of the Zollinger-Ellison syndrome in patients with multiple endocrine neoplasia type 1. *J Intern Med* 1998;243:477.

Lairmore TC, Ball DW, Baylin SB, et al. Management of pheochromocytomas in patients with multiple endocrine neoplasia type 2 syndromes. *Ann Surg* 1993;217:595.

Lee JE, Curley SA, Gagel RF, et al. Cortical-sparing adrenalectomy for patients with bilateral

pheochromocytoma. *Surgery* 1996;120:1064.
Marx SJ, Agarwal SK, Heppner C, et al. The gene for multiple endocrine neoplasia type 1: recent findings. *Bone* 1999;25:119.
Moley JF, Debenedetti MK, Dilley WG, et al. Surgical management of patients with persistent or recurrent medullary thyroid cancer. *J Intern Med* 1998;243:521.
Moley JF, Debenedetti MK. Patterns of nodal metastases in palpable medullary thyroid carcinoma. *Ann Surg* 1999;229:880.
NIH Conference. Multiple endocrine neoplasia type 1: clinical and genetic topics. *Ann Intern Med* 1998;129:484.
Pipeleers-Mirichal M, Somers G, Willems G, et al. Gastrinomas in the duodenums of patients with multiple endocrine neoplasia type I and the Zollinger-Ellison syndrome. *N Engl J Med* 1990;322:723.
O'Riordain DS, O'Brien T, Crotty TB, et al. Multiple endocrine neoplasia type 2B: more than an endocrine disorder. *Surgery* 1995;118:936.
Thompson JC, Lewis BG, Wiener I, et al. The role of surgery in Zollinger-Ellison syndrome. *Ann Surg* 1983;197:594.
Thompson NW. Current concepts in the surgical management of multiple endocrine neoplasia type 1 pancreatic-duodenal disease. Results in the treatment of 40 patients with Zollinger-Ellison syndrome, hypoglycemia or both. *J Intern Med* 1998;243:495.
Wolfe MM, Jensen RT. Zollinger-Ellison syndrome: current concepts in the diagnosis and management. *N Engl J Med* 1987;317:1200.

15

Adrenal Tumors

Ricardo J. Gonzalez and Jeffrey E. Lee

The diagnosis and treatment of adrenal tumors have undergone a significant transformation with advances in diagnostic imaging and minimally invasive approaches to surgical resection. However, treatment of the patient with an adrenal mass still requires a thorough understanding of adrenal endocrine physiology and sound clinical judgment. Appropriate biochemical evaluation and radiographic assessment of an identified adrenal mass are crucial before surgical intervention. Common nonfunctional adrenal adenomas or "incidentalomas" must be differentiated from functioning adrenal tumors (cortisol-producing adenomas, aldosteronomas, and pheochromocytomas), the occasional metastasis to the adrenal gland, and the rare adrenocortical carcinoma.

ALDOSTERONOMA

Primary hyperaldosteronism (Conn syndrome) is a clinical syndrome that results from hypersecretion of aldosterone. This condition is caused by bilateral adrenal hyperplasia in approximately 40% of cases and by an adrenal adenoma in approximately 60% of cases. Other rare causes of primary aldosteronism include glucocorticoid-suppressible hyperaldosteronism, adrenocortical carcinoma, and aldosterone-secreting ovarian tumors. Primary hyperaldosteronism is responsible for approximately 0.5% to 2.0% of all cases of hypertension and represents 5% to 10% of surgically correctable cases of hypertension.

Clinical Manifestations

The main difficulty in diagnosing primary hyperaldosteronism is that the symptoms are usually mild and nonspecific. The most common symptoms are headache, fatigue, polydipsia, polyuria, and nocturia. Hypertension is almost always present but is frequently mild, with diastolic blood pressures less than 120 mm Hg in more than 70% of cases.

Diagnosis

Initial laboratory findings that support a diagnosis of primary hyperaldosteronism include hypertension and spontaneous hypokalemia. Before further biochemical testing, diuretics should be discontinued for at least 2 to 4 weeks. A plasma aldosterone/plasma renin ratio greater than 30 (ng/dL:ng/mL/h), along with a plasma aldosterone level greater than 20 ng per dL, is sensitive and specific in the screening and diagnosis of primary hyperaldosteronism. The plasma renin level is typically very low in patients with primary hyperaldosteronism, and a plasma aldosterone–plasma renin activity ratio of greater than 30 (ng/dL:ng/mL/h), along with a plasma aldosterone concentration less than 20 ng per dL, have been shown to be very sensitive and specific for the diagnosis of primary hyperaldosteronism.

Confirmation of hyperaldosteronism can be obtained using the saline suppression test or the 3-day sodium loading test. In the saline suppression test, 2 L of normal saline is infused intravenously over 4 hours and plasma aldosterone is measured. Confirmation of hyperaldosteronism is obtained when the plasma aldosterone level is greater than 10 ng per dL. In the 3-day sodium loading test (100 mmol NaCl per day), a 24-hour urine collection is obtained on the third day of the test to measure aldosterone, sodium, and potassium, and serum is obtained to measure sodium and potassium. Confirmation of hyperaldosteronism is obtained when the urinary aldosterone is greater than 14 μg per 24 hours. In the latter test, it is important to demonstrate adequate salt loading; therefore, urinary sodium should be greater than 200 mEq per 24 hours.

Once the diagnosis of hyperaldosteronism is established, it is critical to differentiate unilateral adrenal adenoma (60% of cases) from bilateral hyperplasia of the zona glomerulosa (idiopathic hyperaldosteronism; 40% of cases). In patients with an aldosterone-producing adenoma, unilateral adrenalectomy corrects the hypokalemia and decreases the blood pressure in 70% of surgically treated patients. However, surgery is of little value in patients with idiopathic hyperaldosteronism. Patients with a unilateral adenoma usually have more severe hypertension, higher plasma aldosterone levels, and therefore more profound hypokalemia; however, these findings cannot accurately differentiate patients with unilateral adenoma from those with idiopathic hyperaldosteronism. Computed tomography (CT) and magnetic resonance imaging (MRI) can help confirm the presence of a unilateral adrenal nodule, while iodocholesterol (NP-59) imaging and selective venous sampling for aldosterone determinations can localize the hyperfunctioning adrenal tissue to the right or left side. The high frequency of nonfunctioning adenomas in the normal population (2%–8%) means that the finding of a small adrenal mass on CT or MRI is not necessarily diagnostic of a unilateral aldosterone-producing adenoma. Because selective venous sampling is invasive and cannulation of the right adrenal vein is often difficult and occasionally results in adrenal vein thrombosis with adrenal infarction, we now often combine adrenal imaging (CT or MRI) with iodocholesterol imaging to confirm the presence of a unilateral functioning adrenal mass. Our current approach to the evaluation of patients suspected of having primary hyperaldosteronism is shown in Figure 15.1.

Treatment

The treatment of primary hyperaldosteronism depends on the cause. Bilateral adrenal hyperplasia is best managed medically using the aldosterone antagonist spironolactone. Most patients can achieve adequate control of their blood pressure with this medication alone or in conjunction with other antihypertensives. When an aldosterone-producing adenoma is diagnosed, the appropriate therapy remains surgical resection. Preoperatively, patients should be placed on spironolactone and given potassium supplementation to help normalize fluid and electrolyte balance over a 3- to 4-week period.

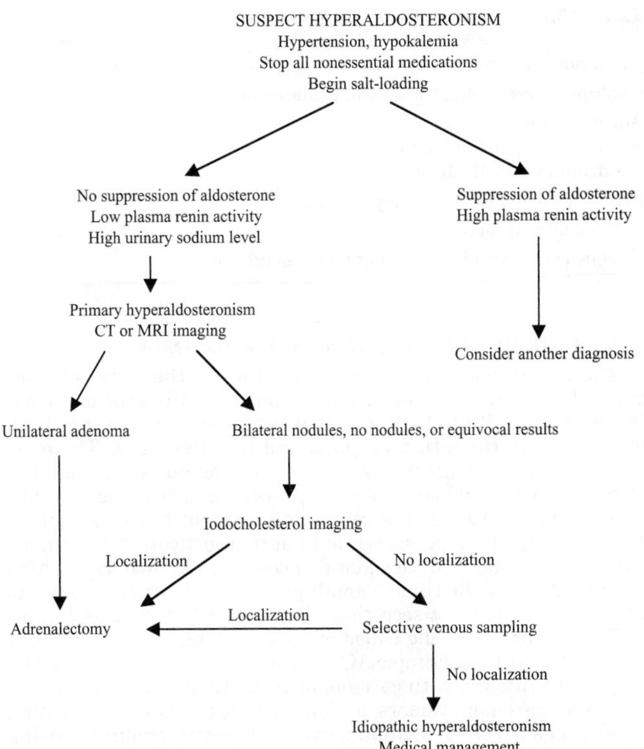

Figure 15.1. Algorithm for the evaluation of the patient with suspected primary hyperaldosteronism. CT, computed tomography; MRI, magnetic resonance imaging.

Although surgical resection can be performed either through an open or a laparoscopic approach because nearly all patients with aldosteronomas have relatively small tumors, they are usually excellent candidates for a laparoscopic approach, and laparoscopic adrenalectomy has become the standard surgical approach for patients with aldosterone-producing adenomas due to its lower morbidity, fewer postoperative complications, and equal results in cure rates compared with open adrenalectomy. As noted previously, the early results from surgical resection of an aldosterone-producing adenoma are good, and the long-term cure rate is approximately 70%. Nearly all patients will have resolution of hypokalemia with adrenalectomy, while 30% will require continued management with antihypertensive medications.

Approximately 2% or less of adrenocortical carcinomas cause isolated hyperaldosteronism. In the very rare situation of a patient presenting with hyperaldosteronism and a large adrenal mass, an open anterior approach should be taken to facilitate complete resection.

Table 15.1. Causes of Cushing syndrome

Exogenous steroids
Cushing disease (due to pituitary adenoma)
Adrenal tumors
Adrenal cortical adenoma
Adrenal cortical carcinoma
Primary adrenal cortical hyperplasia
Ectopic adrenocorticotropin syndrome
Ectopic corticotropin-releasing factor syndrome

CORTISOL-PRODUCING ADRENAL ADENOMA

Cushing syndrome is the term used to refer to the state of hypercortisolism that can result from a number of different pathological processes (Table 15.1). Cortisol regulation involves feedback loops through the pituitary gland and hypothalamus. The most common cause of Cushing syndrome is exogenous steroid administration. After exclusion of patients taking exogenous steroids, approximately 70% of the remaining cases of hypercortisolism are secondary to hypersecretion of adrenocorticotropic hormone (ACTH) from the pituitary gland, a condition known as Cushing disease. Most of the time, a small pituitary adenoma is found to be the cause. Ectopic secretion of ACTH, referred to as ectopic ACTH syndrome, is the cause of approximately 15% of cases of Cushing syndrome. Ectopic ACTH syndrome is usually caused by malignant tumors, with carcinoma of the lung, carcinoma of the pancreas, carcinoid tumors, and malignant thymoma accounting for 80% of such cases. Ectopic secretion of corticotropin-releasing factor is exceedingly rare but has been reported in a few cases.

Hypersecretion of cortisol from the adrenal glands accounts for approximately 10% to 20% of cases of Cushing syndrome. The underlying cause is an adrenal adenoma 50% to 60% of the time and an adrenocortical carcinoma 20% to 25% of the time. Bilateral adrenal hyperplasia accounts for the remaining 20% to 30% of cases.

Clinical Manifestations

Weight gain is the most common feature of hypercortisolism and occurs predominantly in the truncal area. Centripetal obesity combined with muscle wasting in the extremities, fat deposition in the head and neck region ("moon facies"), and dorsal kyphosis ("buffalo hump") gives the patient a characteristic habitus. Abdominal striae, hypertension, and hyperglycemia are three other common findings.

Diagnosis

The evaluation for Cushing syndrome should be aimed at establishing the diagnosis first and then determining the etiology. To establish the diagnosis, a state of hypercortisolism must be documented. The adult adrenal glands secrete on average 10 to 30 mg of cortisol each day. The secretion follows a diurnal variation–cortisol levels tend to be high early in the morning and low in the evening. The most sensitive initial screening test for hypercortisolism in patients with an adrenal mass is an overnight 1-mg dexamethasone suppression test. Documentation of lack of cortisol suppression following 1 mg of dexamethasone should be followed by measurement of 24-hour urinary free cortisol; the normal level is generally below 80 μg per day. In addition, to determine the etiology of an elevated cortisol level, plasma ACTH levels must be checked. ACTH secretion also follows a diurnal variation, preceding that of cortisol by 1 to 2 hours. Suppressed levels of ACTH are seen in patients with adrenal adenomas, adrenocortical carcinomas, or autonomously functioning adrenal hyperplasia. In such cases, autonomous secretion of cortisol by the pathological process within the adrenal gland inhibits pituitary ACTH release. Patients with Cushing disease (i.e., a pituitary adenoma secreting ACTH) usually have plasma ACTH levels that are elevated or within the upper limits of normal. When there is an ectopic source of ACTH secretion, for example, a metastatic tumor process, the plasma ACTH level is usually markedly increased.

The most sensitive method for detecting hypercortisolism is the overnight low-dose dexamethasone suppression test. One milligram of dexamethasone is taken orally at 11:00 p.m.; normal individuals have a cortisol level less than 5 mg per dL at 8:00 a.m. the following morning. Failure to suppress the 8:00 a.m. cortisol level to less than 5 mg per dL is consistent with hypercortisolism; however, although this test has a false-negative rate of only 3%, the false-positive rate is 30%. Therefore, although a normal overnight dexamethasone suppression test excludes clinically significant hypercortisolism, an abnormal test result requires further investigation. Twenty-four-hour urine collection for urinary free (unmetabolized) cortisol is somewhat less sensitive than overnight dexamethasone suppression but more specific. Salivary cortisol can also be used as a screening test for the presence of hypercortisolism.

To confirm the presence of Cushing syndrome following abnormal screening test results, low-dose and high-dose dexamethasone suppression tests can be performed. However, these tests are usually unnecessary in patients with a unilateral adrenal mass with hypercortisolism identified by the overnight 1-mg dexamethasone suppression test and confirmed by 24-hour urine collection. Likewise, although the metyrapone test is occasionally used to differentiate between the various etiologies of Cushing syndrome, this test is rarely helpful in patients with hypercortisolism and an adrenal mass.

All patients with an incidentally identified adrenal mass should undergo an evaluation to exclude Cushing syndrome. Initial screening involves the 1-mg overnight dexamethasone suppression test. Patients with suppressed cortisol levels do not have Cushing syndrome and do not require further evaluation for this condition. Patients without suppressed cortisol levels should undergo a 24-hour urine collection for measurement of free cortisol level. In selected cases of patients with hypercortisolism and equivocal abdominal cross-sectional imaging studies, imaging of the adrenal glands with radiolabeled iodocholesterol can help distinguish primary adrenal hyperplasia (which should demonstrate bilateral uptake) from a cortisol-secreting adenoma (which suppresses the contralateral gland and thus limits uptake to only the side containing the adenoma).

Treatment

The appropriate management of Cushing syndrome depends on the underlying etiology. Patients with Cushing disease should undergo transsphenoidal hypophysectomy of the pituitary adenoma when it is believed to be resectable. Bilateral adrenalectomy is rarely indicated for patients with Cushing syndrome and should be reserved for those patients who fail to respond to standard management, including medical therapy and transsphenoidal hypophysectomy, and who experience end organ injury from the consequences of overt hypercortisolism. If bilateral adrenalectomy is performed, patients require not only perioperative steroid coverage (Tables 15.2 and 15.3), but also lifelong replacement of both glucocorticoids and mineralocorticoids. Patients with autonomously functioning bilateral adrenal hyperplasia usually require bilateral adrenalectomy. Patients with ectopic ACTH syndrome should have the underlying malignant condition identified and treated. Bilateral adrenalectomy in this setting should be reserved for the small group of patients whose primary tumor is unresectable and whose symptoms of cortisol excess cannot be controlled medically. Bilateral adrenalectomy can be performed laparoscopically, via a posterior approach, or via laparotomy; our current preferred approach to the majority of these patients is via a posterior approach.

Patients with a cortisol-producing neoplasm of the adrenal gland, whether adenoma or carcinoma, should undergo resection of the involved side. Although almost all adenomas can be resected, adrenocortical carcinomas that secrete cortisol are resectable in only 25% to 35% of patients. Chemotherapy has been disappointing in patients with unresectable or metastatic adrenocortical carcinoma. Symptoms related to hypercortisolism in

Table 15.2. Recommendations for perioperative glucocorticoid coverage

Surgical Stress	Examples	Hydrocortisone Equivalent (mg)	Duration (d)
Minor	Inguinal herniorrhaphy	25	1
Moderate	Open cholecystectomy Lower-extremity revascularization Segmental colon resection Total joint replacement Abdominal hysterectomy	50–75	1–2
Major	Pancreaticoduodenectomy Esophagogastrectomy Total proctocolectomy Cardiac surgery with cardiopulmonary bypass	100–150	2–3

Table 15.3. Comparison of steroid preparations

Steroid	Half-life (h)	Glucocorticoid Activity (Relative to Cortisol)	Mineralocorticoid Activity (Relative to Cortisol)
Cortisol	8–12	1	1
Cortisone	8–12	0.8	0.8
Prednisone	12–36	4	0.25
Prednisolone	12–36	4	0.25
Methylprednisolone	12–36	5	0
Triamcinolone	12–36	5	0
Betamethasone	36–72	25	0
Dexamethasone	36–72	30–40	0

patients with metastatic or unresectable functioning tumors can sometimes be minimized with various agents, including mitotane, aminoglutethimide, metyrapone, or ketoconazole.

PHEOCHROMOCYTOMA

Pheochromocytomas represent a potentially curable form of endocrine hypertension that, if undetected, places patients at high risk for morbidity and mortality, particularly during surgery and pregnancy. In large series of hypertensive patients, less than 0.1% of patients are found to have pheochromocytomas. These neuroectodermal tumors arise from the chromaffin cells of the adrenal medulla. Approximately 10% of pheochromocytomas are bilateral, with some patients presenting with multiple tumors. Ten percent of pheochromocytomas can be found in extra-adrenal sites, where they are more appropriately called paragangliomas because of their close association with ganglia of the sympathetic nervous system. The most common extra-adrenal sites include the organ of Zuckerkandl (located between the inferior mesenteric artery and the aortic bifurcation), the urinary bladder, the thorax, and the renal hilum.

Histologic evidence of malignancy in pheochromocytomas can be demonstrated approximately 10% of the time; malignancy is more commonly seen with extra-adrenal lesions than with those arising in the adrenal glands. Documenting malignancy can be difficult because invasion of adjacent organs or metastatic disease must be present. Furthermore, both benign and malignant lesions may show tumor penetration of the gland's capsule, invasion of veins draining the gland, cellular pleomorphism, mitoses, and atypical nuclei.

Familial pheochromocytomas have been estimated to account for approximately 10% of cases; however, recent data suggest that up to 25% of unselected cases of apparently sporadic pheochromocytomas are in fact hereditary. Hereditary pheochromocytomas are almost always benign. The familial syndromes associated with pheochromocytomas include multiple endocrine neoplasia

(MEN) types IIA and IIB, in which bilateral tumors are common, as well as the neuroectodermal dysplasias consisting of neurofibromatosis, tuberous sclerosis, Sturge-Weber syndrome, and von Hippel-Lindau disease. The risk for inherited pheochromocytomas is very low in neurofibromatosis type 1 ($<1\%$) and MEN 1 syndrome ($<1\%$). Pheochromocytoma can also occur in hereditary paraganglioma syndrome (mutations in *SDHD, SDHB,* and *SDHC* genes). Hereditary paraganglioma syndrome predisposes to both extra-adrenal and adrenal paragangliomas. Patients with familial pheochromocytoma syndromes require follow-up and periodic screening for pheochromocytoma, especially before any planned surgical procedure.

Clinical Manifestations

The clinical manifestations of pheochromocytoma can be varied and at times quite dramatic. Hypertension, sustained or paroxysmal, is the most common clinical presentation. Paroxysmal elevations in blood pressure can vary markedly in frequency and duration, and can be initiated by various events, including heavy physical exertion and eating foods high in tyramine (e.g., chocolate, cheese, red wine). Other common symptoms include excessive sweating, palpitations, tremulousness, anxiety, and chest pain. More than half of patients with pheochromocytomas have impaired glucose tolerance, and may have symptoms of diabetes mellitus, including polydipsia or polyuria. These signs and symptoms are secondary to the excess catecholamine secretion by the tumors, and resolve with tumor resection. Patients with functioning tumors are rarely asymptomatic; an exception is patients with hereditary pheochromocytomas. Nonfunctioning pheochromocytomas are rare; extra-adrenal paragangliomas, however, may be nonfunctioning.

Diagnosis

The diagnosis of pheochromocytoma is made by documenting the excess secretion of catecholamines. Plasma free metanephrine determination is a very sensitive screen for the presence of catecholamine elevation and is more convenient than timed urine collection. Twenty-four-hour urine collection for free catecholamine levels (dopamine, epinephrine, and norepinephrine) and their metabolites (normetanephrine, metanephrine, vanillylmandelic acid) should be used to confirm suspected catecholamine elevation identified by plasma screen. Increased levels of catecholamines or their metabolites are seen in more than 90% of patients with pheochromocytoma. The adrenal glands and the organ of Zuckerkandl produce the enzyme phenylethanolamine-*N*-methyl-transferase, which converts norepinephrine to epinephrine. Pheochromocytomas that arise elsewhere do not contain this enzyme and thus do not produce much, if any, epinephrine. As a result, extra-adrenal pheochromocytomas secrete predominantly dopamine and norepinephrine.

Once the diagnosis of pheochromocytoma is made, localization studies can be carried out. A review of preoperative imaging in a large series of histologically confirmed pheochromocytomas found that MRI was the most sensitive modality (98%), followed by CT scans (89%) and ^{131}I-metaiodobenzylguanidine (MIBG) scanning

(81%). Our experience indicates that high-quality spiral CT scans can depict up to 95% of adrenal masses larger than 6 to 8 mm and is usually the initial imaging study. MRI may be useful in selected cases because the T2-weighted images can identify chromaffin tissue; the T2-weighted adrenal mass-to-liver ratio of pheochromocytomas or paragangliomas is usually more than three. This ratio is higher than that of adrenal cortical adenomas, adrenal cortical carcinomas, or metastases to the adrenal gland. Thus, the MRI may provide potentially useful functional or biochemical information. MIBG imaging is another procedure that is helpful in localizing extra-adrenal, metastatic, or bilateral pheochromocytomas. This radiolabeled amine is selectively picked up by chromaffin tissue and can identify the majority of pheochromocytomas, regardless of their location. Therefore, MIBG scanning is useful in patients with biochemical evidence of pheochromocytoma whose tumors cannot be localized by CT or MRI and in the follow-up evaluation of patients with suspected or documented recurrent or metastatic disease. Using these techniques, it is rare to have a patient whose pheochromocytoma cannot be localized preoperatively.

Treatment

After diagnosis and localization of the pheochromocytoma, careful preoperative preparation is required to prevent a cardiovascular crisis during surgery caused by excess catecholamine secretion. The main focus of the preoperative preparation is adequate alpha-adrenergic blockade and complete restoration of fluid and electrolyte balance. Phenoxybenzamine is the alpha-adrenergic blocking agent of choice and is usually begun at a dose of 10 mg twice a day. The dosage is gradually increased over a 1- to 3-week period until adequate blockade is reached. The total dosage used should not exceed 1 mg per kg per day. Beta blockade following alpha blockade may help prevent tachycardia and other arrhythmias. Beta blockade should not be instituted unless alpha blockade has been established; otherwise, the beta-blocker will inhibit epinephrine-induced vasodilation, leading to more significant hypertension and left heart strain. In addition to requiring pharmacologic preparation, patients with pheochromocytoma require correction of fluid volume depletion and any concurrent electrolyte imbalances.

The perioperative management of patients with pheochromocytoma can be difficult. Rarely is alpha-adrenergic blockade complete. The anesthesiologist should be prepared to treat a hypertensive crisis with sodium nitroprusside, and tachyarrhythmias with either a beta-blocker or antiarrhythmics. If preoperative imaging suggests a modestly sized, benign-appearing unilateral pheochromocytoma with a radiographically normal contralateral gland, we currently prefer a unilateral laparoscopic approach. A laparoscopic approach is also appropriate for patients with MEN II or von Hippel-Lindau disease with a small, unilateral pheochromocytoma; for patients with MEN II or von Hippel-Lindau disease with bilateral disease, a bilateral laparoscopic approach may also be appropriate. Cortical-sparing adrenalectomy, either open or laparoscopic, has been performed successfully in patients with MEN II or von Hippel-Lindau disease with bilateral pheochromocytomas, avoiding chronic steroid hormone replacement and the risk of Addisonian crisis in most patients. Whatever the operative approach, the surgeon should manipulate the tumor as little as possible, and ligate the tumor's venous outflow via the adrenal vein as early in the procedure as possible.

Postoperatively, patients should be monitored carefully for 24 hours so they can be observed for arrhythmias, as well as hypotension secondary to compensatory vasodilation. Occasionally, hypertension remains a problem postoperatively, especially in those patients who had sustained hypertension preoperatively. Following surgical treatment for pheochromocytoma, all patients should undergo yearly evaluation to include plasma free metanephrine level or timed urine collection for catecholamine determination to exclude recurrence.

The most common sites of metastases from malignant pheochromocytoma are bone, liver, and lungs, and less commonly, regional lymph nodes. Patients with known or suspected malignant pheochromocytoma should be staged with standard imaging studies and MIBG scanning. Therapy should be individualized based on extent of disease. Palliative therapy may include treatment with alpha-methyltyrosine, as well as α- and β-blockade. Resection of malignant pheochromocytoma, including resection of metastases, may be considered in good risk individuals if the metastases are limited in extent. The most commonly used chemotherapy regimens for pheochromocytoma are high-dose streptozocin and a combination of cyclophosphamide, vincristine, and dacarbazine. The overall response rates with these regimens are approximately 50%. Radiation therapy has been effective only for bony metastases. There has been some interest in treating metastatic lesions with therapeutic doses of ^{131}I-MIBG. Unfortunately, a high percentage of metastatic pheochromocytomas do not take up ^{131}I-MIBG; therefore, the response rate, as manifested by a reduction in urinary catecholamines, is only approximately 50%. Objective responses as determined by imaging studies are seen even less frequently. The 5-year survival rate for patients with malignant pheochromocytoma is approximately 43%, as compared with a 97% 5-year survival rate for benign lesions.

ADRENAL CORTICAL CARCINOMA

Adrenal cortical carcinoma is a rare malignancy, with approximately 150 to 200 new cases reported each year in the United States. There is a bimodal age distribution, with incidence peaking in young children and then again between 40 and 50 years of age.

Clinical Manifestations

Patients with adrenal cortical carcinoma usually present with vague abdominal symptoms secondary to an enlarging retroperitoneal mass or with clinical manifestations of overproduction of one or more adrenal cortical hormones. Most of these tumors are functional as measured by biochemical parameters. Fifty percent secrete cortisol, producing Cushing syndrome. The workup and treatment of patients with Cushing syndrome are described in that section in this chapter. Another 10% to 20% of adrenocortical carcinomas produce androgens, estrogens, or aldosterone, which can cause virilization in females, feminization in males, or hypertension, respectively.

Diagnosis

The preoperative evaluation of these patients involves biochemical screening for cortisol overproduction; the results of this screening serve to guide perioperative replacement therapy. Screening to exclude pheochromocytoma should also be performed. Standard preoperative staging in patients with suspected adrenal cancer includes high-resolution abdominal CT or MRI. MRI may be especially helpful in delineating tumor extension into the inferior vena cava. Chest radiography is helpful in ruling out pulmonary metastasis. The various staging systems for adrenocortical carcinomas are shown in Table 15.4.

Treatment

Complete surgical resection is currently the only potentially curative therapy for localized adrenal cortical cancer. Approximately 50% of the tumors are localized to the adrenal gland at the time of initial presentation. We recommend an open transabdominal approach to facilitate maximal exposure for complete resection, minimize the risk of tumor spillage, and allow for vascular control of the inferior vena cava, aorta, and renal vessels when necessary. Radical en bloc resection that includes adjacent organs, if necessary, provides the only chance for long-term survival. Patients who undergo a complete resection of their tumor have a 5-year survival rate of approximately 40% and a median survival of 43 months; those who undergo incomplete resection have median survival duration of less than 12 months. Therefore, the strongest predictor of outcome in this disease is the ability to perform a complete resection. Laparoscopic resection of adrenal cortical carcinoma, although technically potentially feasible in the rare patient with a small, localized adrenal cortical carcinoma, has been associated with a very high rate of tumor recurrence and peritoneal carcinomatosis, presumably due to tumor fracture and peritoneal contamination. For this reason, we continue to prefer open adrenalectomy for patients with known or suspected adrenal cortical carcinoma, including adrenal incidentaloma (see Adrenal Incidentaloma section in this chapter).

Common sites of metastasis of adrenal cortical carcinoma include lungs, lymph nodes, liver, peritoneum, and bone. Complete resection of recurrent disease, including pulmonary metastases, is associated with prolonged survival in some patients and can help control symptoms related to excess hormone production. After a potentially curative resection, patients whose tumors were hormonally active should be monitored with interval urinary steroid measurement and abdominal and chest imaging studies. Adjuvant therapy for adrenocortical carcinoma (mitotane) has had minimal impact, if any, on disease progression.

Radiation therapy can provide palliation for bony metastases. No chemotherapeutic agent or combination of agents has been shown to be consistently effective against unresectable or metastatic adrenal cortical cancer. Mitotane has been one of the most commonly used systemic agents because of its ability to

Table 15.4. Staging systems for adrenal cortical carcinoma

Stage	MacFarlane (1958)	Sullivan et al. (1978)	Icard et al. (1992)	Lee et al. (1995)
I	T1 (≤5 cm), N0, M0	T1 (≤5 cm), N0, M0	T1 (≤5 cm), N0, M0	T1 (≤5 cm), N0, M0
II	T2 (>5 cm), N0, M0	T2 (>5 cm), N0, M0	T2 (>5 cm), N0, M0	T2 (>5 cm), N0, M0
III	T3 (local invasion without involvement of adjacent organs) or mobile positive lymph nodes, M0	T3 (local invasion), N0, M0 or T1–T2, N1 (positive lymph nodes), M0	T3 (local invasion) and/or N1 (positive regional lymph nodes), M0	T3/T4 (local invasion as demonstrated by histologic evidence of adjacent organ invasion, direct tumor extension to IVC, and/or tumor thrombus within IVC or renal vein) and/or N1 (positive regional lymph nodes), M0
IV	T4 (invasion of adjacent organs) or fixed positive lymph nodes or M1 (distant metastasis)	T4 (local invasion), N0, M0; or T3, N1, M0; or T1–T4, N0–N1, M1 (distant metastasis)	T1–T4, N0–N1, M1 (distant metastasis)	T1–T4, N0–N1, M1 (distant metastasis)

IVC, inferior vena cava.

palliate the endocrine effects of the tumor. This drug is an isomer of dichlorodiphenyltrichloroethane and not only inhibits steroid production, but also leads to atrophy of adrenocortical cells. Mitotane is associated with numerous side effects, most notably, gastrointestinal and neuromuscular symptoms. In addition, the drug has a relatively narrow therapeutic range, requiring close monitoring of serum levels and provision of exogenous steroid hormone replacement to avoid symptoms associated with adrenal insufficiency due to suppression of the normal contralateral adrenal gland. Other systemic treatment options for patients with unresectable local recurrence or distant metastases include suramin, ketoconazole, and systemic chemotherapy regimens containing cisplatin, etoposide, doxorubicin, or vincristine.

ADRENAL INCIDENTALOMA

With the widespread use of abdominal CT imaging, asymptomatic adrenal lesions are being discovered with increasing frequency. These lesions, termed *incidentalomas*, are seen in up to 4% of routinely performed abdominal imaging studies and in up to 9% of autopsy series. Although most of these lesions are benign adenomas, some are hormonally active, and a small minority represents an invasive malignancy.

All patients identified with an incidental adrenal mass should be screened to rule out a hormonally active adenoma or pheochromocytoma. Evaluation of patients with an incidentally identified adrenal mass includes measurement of serum electrolyte levels, an overnight 1-mg dexamethasone suppression test (described previously), and measurement of plasma metanephrine levels (Fig. 15.2). Any hormonally active lesion, regardless of size, should be resected. Furthermore, surgery is indicated if the adrenal mass shows radiographic characteristics suggestive of malignancy or if the tumor enlarges during follow-up.

If the incidentaloma is nonfunctioning, the risk of malignancy is related to its size and radiographic characteristics. Size is the single best clinical indicator of malignancy in patients who present with an incidental adrenal mass. Adrenal cortical carcinoma accounts for 2%, 6%, and 35% of incidentalomas smaller than 4 cm, 4.1 to 6 cm, and greater than 6 cm in size, respectively. In general, lesions larger than 6 cm should be resected because of the high risk of malignancy. Observation and follow-up is generally recommended for nonfunctioning lesions smaller than 3 cm in diameter, but the management of tumors between 3 and 6 cm is more controversial. Data from our own institution and elsewhere have identified patients with adrenal cortical carcinomas arising in tumors smaller than 5 cm. The majority of these small tumors had CT or MRI characteristics suspicious for carcinoma such as heterogeneity and irregular borders. Based on individual experience and a review of the literature, recent recommendations for resection of nonfunctioning adrenal masses have ranged from 5 cm down to 3 cm. The recent success and advantages of laparoscopic adrenalectomy has led some investigators to suggest operative removal of even small incidentalomas.

At M. D. Anderson, we recommend adrenalectomy for all biochemically confirmed functioning adrenal tumors and those with suspicious radiographic findings, regardless of size. A recent

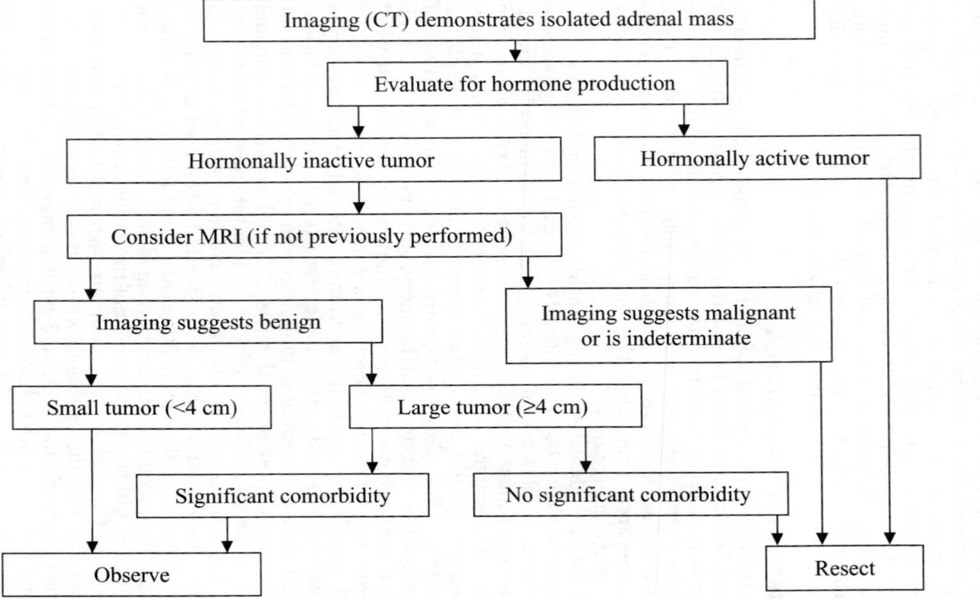

Figure 15.2. Algorithm for the evaluation of patients with isolated, incidentally identified adrenal tumors. CT, computed tomography; MRI, magnetic resonance imaging.

study comparing the incidence of carcinomatosis and local recurrence in patients managed with open versus laparoscopic adrenalectomy identified a much higher rate of carcinomatosis in the laparoscopic group (83%) when compared with open adrenalectomy (8%). Because of the risk of capsular fracture and resultant peritoneal carcinomatosis, we reserve the laparoscopic approach for lesions without worrisome radiographic features on cross-sectional imaging (CT and/or MRI) and for lesions that are less than 4 cm in greatest transverse diameter, while an open transabdominal approach is used for all lesions that do not meet these criteria. Nonfunctioning tumors between 3 and 6 cm in diameter are most appropriately managed on an individual basis with respect to patient age and general health. For example, a 4-cm tumor in an otherwise healthy 40-year-old patient is probably most appropriately managed by adrenalectomy, whereas the same tumor in a 75-year-old patient with multiple comorbidities might be observed. The following may be helpful in evaluating such patients with intermediate-size nonfunctioning adrenal masses: MRI, a more thorough endocrine evaluation, and consideration of age and comorbidity. Figure 15.3 provides an overview of our approach to patients with adrenal incidentalomas.

ADRENAL METASTASES

Metastasis of cancers to the adrenal glands is relatively common. Based on autopsy studies, 42% of lung cancers, 16% of gastric cancers, 58% of breast cancers, 50% of malignant melanomas, and a high percentage of renal and prostate cancers have metastasized to the adrenal glands at the time of death. However, clinical problems related to adrenal metastases, such as adrenal insufficiency, are only rarely encountered. In general, more than 90% of the adrenal gland must be replaced before clinically detectable adrenal cortical hypofunction is appreciated. When adrenal insufficiency does occur, it is usually in the setting of gross enlargement of the adrenal glands as detected by CT.

Surgery for isolated metastases to the adrenal gland may be considered in highly selected patients. These include good-risk individuals in whom there is a prolonged disease-free interval and favorable tumor biology. Evaluation of these patients includes consideration of those who have had a significant progression-free interval, those who have responded to systemic therapy, and those who have a history of isolated metachronous metastases. In particular, a longer disease-free interval from the time of primary cancer therapy to adrenal metastasis is associated with a survival advantage following adrenalectomy. Primary tumor site also appears to affect survival, in that longer median survival times are observed following resection of metastases from primary kidney, melanoma, colon, and lung cancers, and poorer survival in patients with esophageal, liver, unknown primary tumors, and high-grade sarcomas.

Evaluation of the patient with an adrenal mass and a history of malignancy includes an evaluation for hormone production because as many as 50% of these patients will have occult, functioning adrenal tumors unrelated to their prior malignancy (e.g., a pheochromocytoma) (Fig. 15.3). Fine-needle aspiration biopsy may be helpful in selected patients when the results would

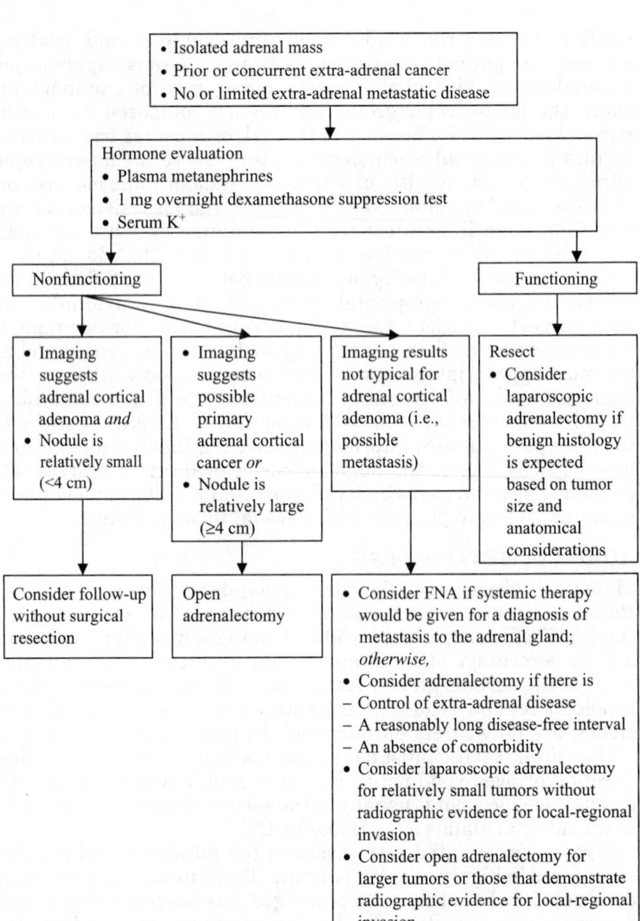

Figure 15.3. Algorithm for the evaluation and surgical treatment of patients with extra-adrenal cancer presenting with an adrenal mass. FNA, fine-needle aspiration.

influence the treatment plan; for example, to confirm a diagnosis of metastasis, particularly in those who are not surgical candidates and in those patients who have not yet had their primary cancer resected. In a study of patients with operable non–small-cell lung cancer and an adrenal mass, 40% had nonfunctioning adenomas by CT-guided biopsy. In selected patients, however, surgical therapy may be planned solely based on the patient's history and on noninvasive studies, and without preoperative needle biopsy. A history of a malignancy that commonly metastasizes to the adrenal glands, with favorable tumor biology, negative biochemical screening for hormone production, and a mass that either fulfills size criteria for surgical excision or is radiographically suspicious for metastasis may be considered for resection without preoperative tissue diagnosis.

At the M. D. Anderson Cancer Center, we investigated the incidence of adrenal metastasis in patients with either a known concurrent extra-adrenal malignancy or a prior extra-adrenal malignancy. One hundred and ninety-six patients were referred for adrenalectomy, and of these, 81 had a prior or concurrent extra-adrenal malignancy. Of the 81 patients, 42 patients (52%) had metastatic disease to the adrenal gland. The three most common primary malignancies were from renal, melanoma, and colorectal primaries. Cross-sectional imaging (CT and/or MRI) was suggestive of metastatic disease in 17 patients (40%), while FNA was used in 18 patients (43%) and supported a diagnosis of cancer in 16 (89%) of these patients. The median actuarial survival of these patients was 3.4 years after adrenalectomy. Therefore, in selected patients with a long disease-free interval, an acceptable performance status, and controlled extra-adrenal disease, long-term palliation may be achieved with adrenalectomy, as seen in patients who undergo metastectomy in other organs.

We emphasize that we do not recommend routine fine-needle aspiration of incidentally identified adrenal tumors in patients without a previous diagnosis of cancer. In the absence of signs or symptoms of a solid tumor malignancy, unilateral adrenal metastases are uncommon. Our recent experience with more than 1,600 patients found that the incidence of metastasis from an occult primary cancer was 0.2% (4 of 1,639). In all four of these patients, malignancy was suspected on the basis of tumor size, bilateral involvement, or symptoms. Therefore, we do not routinely biopsy patients with small nonfunctioning adrenal tumors searching for occult metastatic disease.

LAPAROSCOPIC ADRENALECTOMY

Since the first description of laparoscopic adrenalectomy in 1992, this approach has been expanded and is now considered the standard technique for benign adrenal tumors. Most surgeons have used an anterolateral transperitoneal approach; a posterior or lateral flank retroperitoneal approach has also been reported. A retroperitoneal laparoscopic approach is practical in patients with previous abdominal operations who have relatively small adrenal tumors. Patients who undergo laparoscopic adrenalectomy for relatively small adrenal masses have a more rapid recovery, less discomfort, faster return to preoperative activity level, and better cosmetic results compared with patients who undergo open adrenalectomy. Patients who should be considered for laparoscopic adrenalectomy include those with aldosterone-producing adenomas, other small (<4 cm) functioning cortical neoplasms, those with unilateral, benign-appearing sporadic pheochromocytomas, MEN 2 or VHL patients with a unilateral pheochromocytoma, and selected patients with adrenal metastasis. Bilateral laparoscopic adrenalectomy can be performed in patients with bilateral adrenal hyperplasia; technical considerations suggest that a posterior approach may be simpler than an anterior approach in most of these patients. Laparoscopic cortical-sparing partial adrenalectomy has been successfully performed in patients with bilateral pheochromocytomas in the familial setting; however, we continue to prefer an open anterior approach to maximize the opportunity for adrenal cortical preservation in these patients. We continue to urge caution in the use of laparoscopic adrenalectomy for patients with malignant or potentially malignant primary adrenal tumors. This includes the occasional patient with sporadic pheochromocytoma in whom radiographic imaging raises suspicion for malignancy, patients with hereditary paraganglioma syndrome, and those with cortical neoplasms (functioning or nonfunctioning) 4 cm in size or greater, or those with radiographic evidence of malignancy. It is emphasized that the reason for operating on patients with nonfunctioning adrenal tumors (incidentalomas) is that they are potentially malignant cortical neoplasms. Therefore, we specifically do not recommend laparoscopic adrenalectomy for patients in whom adrenal cortical carcinoma is part of the preoperative differential diagnosis.

Operative Approach

We currently prefer to perform laparoscopic adrenalectomy via a transabdominal intraperitoneal approach. For a left adrenalectomy, the patient is placed in the right lateral decubitus position, with the table appropriately padded and flexed. The abdomen and chest are prepped from the nipple to below the iliac crest, and from the right of the umbilicus to the vertebral column. An infracostal port, 10 to 15 cm anterior to the anterior axillary line, is placed using the open technique, abdominal insufflation achieved, and the 30-degree laparoscope is inserted. Three additional 10-mm trocars are then placed under direct vision. One is placed at the anterior axillary line, one is placed at the posterior axillary line, and one is placed 5 cm posterior to the posterior axillary port, just medial to the left kidney. Dissection begins by mobilizing the splenic flexure of the colon, using gravity to carry it inferiorly and medially. Mobilization of the spleen is performed by incising the peritoneum lateral to the spleen. This incision is developed around to the level of the short gastric vessels. This allows the spleen to rotate medially. It is often helpful to move the laparoscope to the posterior port as dissection proceeds to maximize visualization of the adrenal bed. The adrenal gland is dissected from the retroperitoneal fat; the Harmonic Scalpel (Ethicon Endo-Surgery) works well for this dissection. In contrast to the open approach, technical considerations in laparoscopic adrenalectomy often result in delaying ligation of the adrenal vein to the penultimate step in the procedure, following complete mobilization of the tumor and the adrenal gland, and just prior to specimen removal. Vein division on the left side can be safely accomplished with either the vascular stapler or with two to three titanium clips placed on the proximal side of the vein. The specimen is removed in a sterile plastic retrieval bag through the umbilical port site. Right laparoscopic adrenalectomy is performed with similar positioning in the left lateral decubitus position. Abdominal access is obtained through placement of four 10-mm ports, placed similar to those on the left side. The most medial port is used to assist in retraction of the liver. The surgeon begins the operation through the two lateral ports; the right lateral hepatic attachments and the right triangular ligament of the liver are divided to allow for medial retraction of the liver. The adrenal gland is then dissected inferiorly along the renal vein and medially along the vena cava. The right adrenal vein is usually short and wide, and drains directly into the vena cava. Titanium clips may not adequately secure the vein on the right side; therefore, a laparoscopic vascular stapler is preferred.

RECOMMENDED READING

Primary Hyperaldosteronism

Blumenfeld JC, Sealey JE, Schlussel Y, et al. Diagnosis and therapy of primary hyperaldosteronism. *Ann Intern Med* 1994;121:877.

Lo CY, Tam PC, Kung AWC, et al. Primary aldosteronism: results of surgical treatment. *Ann Surg* 1996;224:125.

Rossi H, Kim A, Prinz RA, et al. Primary hyperaldosteronism in the era of laparoscopic adrenalectomy. *Am Surg* 2002;68:253.

Sawka AM, Young WF, Jr, Thompson GB, et al. Primary aldosteronism: factors associated with normalization of blood pressure after surgery. *Ann Intern Med* 2001;135(4):258–261.

Vallotton MB. Primary aldosteronism. Parts I and II. *Clin Endocrinol* 1996;45:47.

Weigel RJ, Wells SA, Gunnells JC, et al, Surgical treatment of primary hyperaldosteronism. *Ann Surg* 1994;219:347.

Weinberger MH, Fineberg NS. The diagnosis of primary aldosteronism and separation of two major subtypes. *Arch Intern Med* 1993;153:2125.

Young WF, Stanson AW, Thompson GB, et al. Role for adrenal venous sampling in primary aldosteronism. *Surgery* 2004;136(6):1227–1235.

Cushing Syndrome

Lacroix A, Bolte E, Tremblay J, et al. Gastric inhibitory polypeptide-dependent cortisol hypersecretion: a new cause of Cushing's syndrome. *N Engl J Med* 1992;327:974.

Orth DN. Cushing's syndrome. *N Engl J Med* 1995;332:791.

van Heerden JA, Young WF, Jr, Grant CS, et al. Adrenal surgery for hypercortisolism: surgical aspects. *Surgery* 1995;117:466.

Zieger MA, Pass HI, Doppman JD, et al. Surgical strategy in the management of non-small cell ectopic adrenocorticotropic hormone syndrome. *Surgery* 1992;112:994.

Pheochromocytoma

Baghi M, Thompson GB, Young WF, et al. Pheochromocytomas and paragangliomas in Von Hippel-Lindau disease: a role for laparoscopic and cortical-sparing surgery. *Arch Surg* 2002;137:682–689.

Gagner M, Breton JG, Pharand D, et al. Is laparoscopic adrenalectomy indicated for pheochromocytomas? *Surgery* 1996;120:1076.

Jalil ND, Pattou FN, Combemale F, et al. Effectiveness and limits of preoperative imaging studies for the localization of pheochromocytomas and paraganglionomas: a review of 282 cases. *Eur J Surg* 1998;164:23–28.

Lee JE, Curley SA, Gagel RF, et al. Cortical-sparing adrenalectomy for patients with bilateral pheochromocytoma. *Surgery* 1995;120:1064.

Neuman HPH, Bausch B, McWhinney SR, et al. Germ-line mutations in nonsyndromic pheochromocytoma. *N Engl J Med* 2002;346:1459–1466.

Orchard T, Grant CS, van Heerden JA, et al. Pheochromocytoma: continuing evolution of surgical therapy. *Surgery* 1993;114:1153.

Pederson LC, Lee JE. Pheochromocytoma. *Curr Treat Options Oncol* 2003;4:329–337.

Peplinski GR, Norton JA. The predictive value of diagnostic tests

for pheochromocytoma. *Surgery* 1994;116:1101.
Werbel SS, Ober KP. Pheochromocytoma: update on diagnosis, localization, and management. *Med Clin North Am* 1995;79:131.
Yip L, Lee JE, Shapiro S, et al. Surgical management of hereditary pheochromocytoma. *J Am Coll Surg* 2004;198:525.

Adrenocortical Masses and Carcinoma

Baba S, Miyajima A, Uchida A, Asanuma H, Miyakawa A, Murai M. A posterior lumbar approach for retroperitoneoscopic adrenalectomy: assessment of surgical efficacy. *Urology* 1997;50:19–24.
Baba S, Ito K, Yanaihara H, Nagata H, Murai M, Iwamura M. Retroperitoneoscopic adrenalectomy by a lumbodorsal approach: clinical experience with solo surgery. *World J Urol* 1999;17:54–58.
Barnett CC, Varma DG, El-Naggar AK, et al. Limitations of size as a criterion in the evaluation of adrenal tumors. *Surgery* 2000;128:973–982.
Bornstein SR, Stratakis CA, Chrousos GP. Adrenocortical tumors: recent advances in basic concepts and clinical management. *Ann Intern Med* 1999;130:759–771.
Dackiw AP, Lee JE, Gagel RF, Evans DB. Adrenal cortical carcinoma. *World J Surg* 2001;25:914–926.
Demeter JG, De Jong SA, Brooks MH, et al. Long-term results of adrenal autotransplantation in Cushing's disease. *Surgery* 1990;108:1117.
Doppman JL, Reinig JW, Dwyer AJ, et al. Differentiation of adrenal masses by magnetic resonance imaging. *Surgery* 1987;102:1018.
Gagner M, Lacroix A, Bolte E. Laparoscopic adrenalectomy in Cushing's syndrome and pheochromocytoma. *N Engl J Med* 1992;327:1033.
Gonzalez RJ, Shapiro S, Sarlis N, et al. Laparoscopic resection of adrenal cortical carcinoma: a cautionary note. *Surgery* 2005;138:1078.
Graham DJ, McHenry CR. The adrenal incidentaloma: guidelines for evaluation and recommendations for management. *Surg Oncol Clin North Am* 1998;7:749–764.
Herrera MF, Grant CS, van Heerden JA, et al. Incidentally discovered adrenal tumors: an institutional perspective. *Surgery* 1991;110:1014.
Icard P, Chapuis Y, Andreassian BA, et al. Adrenocortical carcinoma in surgically treated patients: a retrospective study on 156 cases by the French Association of Endocrine Surgery. *Surgery* 1992;112:972.
Lee JE, Berger DH, El-Naggar AK, et al. Surgical management, DNA content, and patient survival in adrenal cortical carcinoma. *Surgery* 1995;118:1090.
Lee JE, Evans DB, Hickey RC, et al. Unknown primary cancer presenting as an adrenal mass: frequency and implications for diagnostic evaluation of adrenal incidentalomas. *Surgery* 1998;124:115–122.
Lenert JT, Barnett CC, Kudelka AP, et al. Evaluation and surgical resection of adrenal masses in patients with a history of extra-adrenal malignancy. *Surgery* 2001;130:1060–1067.
Luton JP, Cerdas S, Billaud L, et al. Clinical features of adrenocortical carcinoma, prognostic factors, and the effect of mitotane therapy. *N Engl J Med* 1990;322:1195.
MacFarlane DA. Cancer of the adrenal cortex: the natural history, prognosis and treatment in a study of fifty-five cases. *Ann R Coll Surg Engl* 1958;23:155.
Mercan S, Seven R, Ozarmagan S, Tezelman S. Endoscopic retroperitoneal adrenalectomy. *Surgery* 1995;118:1071–1075, discussion 1075–1076.
Paul CA, Virgo KS, Wade TP, et al. Adrenalectomy for isolated adrenal metastases from non-adrenal cancer. *Int J Oncol* 2000;17(1):181–187.
Pommier RF, Brennan MF, An eleven-year experience with adrenocortical carcinoma. *Surgery* 1992;112:963.

Ross NS, Aron DC. Hormonal evaluation of the patient with an incidentally discovered adrenal mass. *N Engl J Med* 1990;323:1401.

Salem M, Tainsh RE, Bromberg J, et al. Perioperative glucocorticoid coverage: a reassessment 42 years after emergence of a problem. *Ann Surg* 1994;4:416.

Shen WT, Lim RC, Siperstein AE, et al. Laparoscopic vs open adrenalectomy for the treatment of primary hyperaldosteronism. *Arch Surg* 1999;134:628–631, discussion 631–632.

Siren J, Tervahartiala P, Sivula A, et al. Natural course of adrenal incidentalomas: seven-year follow-up study. *World J Surg* 2000;24:579–582.

Siperstein AE, Berber E, Engle KL, Duh QY, Clark OH. Laparoscopic posterior adrenalectomy: technical considerations. *Arch Surg* 2000;135:967–971.

Smith CD, Weber CJ, Amerson JR. Laparoscopic adrenalectomy: new gold standard. *World J Surg* 1999;23:389–396.

Sullivan M, Boileau M, Hodges CV. Adrenal cortical carcinoma. *J Urol* 1978;120:660.

Vassilopoulou-Sellin R, Guinee VF, Klein MJ, et al. Impact of adjuvant mitotane on the clinical course of patients with adrenocortical cancer. *Cancer* 1993;71:3119.

16

Carcinoma of the Thyroid and Parathyroid Glands

Keith D. Amos, Mouhammed A. Habra, and Nancy D. Perrier

THYROID CANCER

Epidemiology

Thyroid cancer is the most common endocrine malignancy and accounts for approximately 1% of all human malignancies, with an estimated incidence in the United States of 25,700 cases in 2005. The majority of cases—approximately 70%—occur in women. Carcinoma of the thyroid gland is considered to be an indolent disease; many affected individuals die of other causes. An estimated 1,500 patients die of this disease each year.

The prevalence of thyroid nodules increases linearly with age, with spontaneous nodules occurring at a rate of 0.08% per year beginning early in life and extending into the eighth decade. Clinically apparent nodules are present in 4% to 7% of the adult population and occur more commonly in women. Most nodules are not malignant. Reported malignancy rates are 5% to 12% in patients with single nodules and 3% in patients with multiple nodules. However, a history of radiation exposure has been reported to increase the risk of malignancy in a nodule to between 30% to 50%.

Risk Factors

Approximately 9% of thyroid cancers are associated with prior radiation exposure. The risk of cancer from radiation increases linearly with doses up to 20 Gy, with thyroid ablation occurring at higher dose levels. The risk of developing thyroid cancer is inversely related to age at exposure. A history of exposure to ionizing radiation in childhood is a major risk factor for thyroid malignancy, almost always of the papillary type. Individuals 15 years of age or older at exposure do not have a demonstrable radiation-dose–dependent risk of thyroid cancer. In general, radiation-induced thyroid cancer is biologically similar to sporadic thyroid cancer and should be treated in the same manner. However, recent information regarding the high incidence of biologically aggressive thyroid cancer in children exposed to radiation after the Chernobyl nuclear disaster suggests that radiation dose and tumor behavior may be linked. The proportions of less well-differentiated papillary thyroid cancers and of solid-variant papillary thyroid cancers were higher among these children than among patients without radiation exposure. Additional evidence of a link between radiation dose and tumor behavior comes from the finding that exposure to different types of radiation results in different patterns of genetic alterations in thyroid tumors.

Aside from radiation exposure, few environmental risk factors have been confirmed for thyroid carcinoma. Hormonal factors and dietary intake of iodine, retinol, vitamin C, and vitamin E have been suggested to play a role in the etiology of thyroid cancer that has yet to be defined.

Associations have been described between thyroid cancer and several other inherited syndromes, including familial polyposis, Gardner syndrome, and Cowden disease (familial goiter and skin hamartoma). In addition, papillary thyroid cancer may occur with increased frequency in some families with breast, ovarian, renal, or central nervous system malignancies. Medullary thyroid cancer occurs with a higher frequency in patients who have Hashimoto thyroiditis. The mechanism underlying these associations is not well understood.

Over the past ten years, significant progress has been made in the identification of genes linked to the pathogenesis of thyroid cancer. Studies of the patterns of genetic alterations present in thyroid tumors suggest that there are differences in the pathogenesis of the different thyroid tumor types, which most likely account for the range in biological behavior observed among thyroid cancers. The *RET* proto-oncogene, which is located on chromosome 10 and encodes a tyrosine kinase receptor, is believed to play a role in the pathogenesis of both hereditary and sporadic medullary thyroid carcinomas (MTCs) and papillary thyroid carcinomas (PTCs). Activating point mutations in the *RET* proto-oncogene of parafollicular C cells have been detected in virtually all hereditary forms of MTC, including familial MTC, multiple endocrine neoplasia 2A (MEN 2A), and MEN 2B, which account for approximately 25% of MTCs. Mutations in the *RET* proto-oncogene have also been found in sporadic MTC, although different codons of the *RET* proto-oncogene are affected. Rearrangements of the *RET* proto-oncogene in thyroid follicular cells are considered to be an early event in the development of PTCs. Nearly all patients with autosomal dominant MEN 2A or MEN 2B will develop MTC; screening for germline *RET* mutations has been invaluable in the early identification of patients who have a genetic basis for their disease. The discovery of the *RET* proto-oncogene has had significant clinical impact, affecting the screening and prophylactic treatment of patients who are members of the MEN kindreds.

Somatic mutations in the *Ras* oncogene have been found in both benign and malignant thyroid tumors, and thus also seem to be an early event in thyroid tumorigenesis, although some reports suggest that *Ras* mutations are more prevalent in follicular thyroid carcinomas (FTCs). The findings of a high prevalence of *p53* mutations in anaplastic carcinomas, but not in well-differentiated thyroid carcinomas, suggest that *p53* mutations play a role later in thyroid tumor pathogenesis—specifically, in the dedifferentiating transition to the anaplastic phenotype. Numerous other genes (e.g., PTEN, TRK, GSP, and the thyroid-stimulating hormone [TSH] receptor gene) have also been implicated in the pathogenesis of thyroid cancer, although their roles still need to be defined. Currently, few of the genetic alterations (e.g., p53, ras, and certain *RET* mutations, including 883 and 918), *RET*/PTC rearrangements found in thyroid tumors, have been shown to have negative implications on prognosis. Much work is still needed to elucidate the molecular biology of thyroid tumors and to translate this knowledge into clinical management.

Pathology

Four tumor types account for more than 90% of thyroid malignancies: PTC, FTC, MTC, and anaplastic thyroid carcinoma (ATC). PTC and FTC are further grouped together and referred to as differentiated thyroid carcinoma (DTC), which accounts for approximately 90% of thyroid carcinomas. Differentiated thyroid cancers more commonly occur in women, whereas an equal gender distribution is seen in both MTC and ATC. PTC, FTC, and ATC are derived from the follicular epithelial cells of the thyroid gland, which produce the thyroid hormones. MTC is derived from the calcitonin-secreting parafollicular C cells. Other less common thyroid carcinomas include Hürthle cell carcinoma (a variant of follicular carcinoma), lymphomas, squamous cell carcinomas, sarcomas, and metastatic carcinomas from other sites, including renal cell carcinoma and melanoma.

PTC is the most common thyroid carcinoma, representing 80% of all cases. Patients with PTC usually present during the third to fifth decades. Females have a higher incidence of this disease than males. PTC occurs as an irregular solid or cystic mass that arises from follicular epithelium. It is nonencapsulated but sharply circumscribed. Microscopically, the hallmark is papillary fronds of epithelium. Rounded calcified deposits (psammoma bodies) are found in 50% of lesions. Multifocality is a prominent feature of PTC and has been documented in up to 80% of patients. Cervical lymph node metastases are quite common at presentation with a reported frequency of between 30% and 80% in most U.S. and European series. PTC is the predominant tumor type found in patients with a history of radiation exposure. The overall prognosis for patients with PTC is very good: 10-year survival rates are 95%.

Follicular thyroid carcinoma is the second most common malignancy of the thyroid gland, comprising 10% to 20% of thyroid cancers. Patients with FTC often present a decade later than patients with PTC, during the fifth and sixth decades. Patients with FTC also tend to have slightly larger tumors at presentation than patients with papillary tumors. Cytologic diagnosis of FTC is often difficult due to the similarities between FTC and benign follicular adenomas. Permanent sections showing capsular or vascular invasion are required to confirm the diagnosis. FTC is usually encapsulated and consists of highly cellular follicles, most of which are single, solid, and noncystic without central necrosis and usually unifocal. Cervical lymph node metastases are uncommon in FTC and are found in approximately 10% of patients at presentation. FTC has a greater tendency to spread hematogenously to distant sites such as lung and bone, and up to 33% of patients have distant metastases at presentation. FTC is often found in association with benign thyroid disorders, such as endemic goiter. A relationship between TSH stimulation and follicular carcinoma has been suggested because of the greater incidence of FTC in iodine-deficient areas. Ten-year survival rates for FTC are 70%

to 95%—slightly worse than those for PTC, which is most likely due to later presentation. When patients are matched by age and tumor stage, there is no significant difference in survival between PTC and FTC.

Hürthle cell carcinomas represent 5% of thyroid cancers and are considered variants of FTC, although Hürthle cell carcinomas and FTC are believed to be distinct pathological entities because of differences in their biological behavior and natural history. As with the diagnosis of FTC, the diagnosis of Hürthle cell carcinomas depends on the presence of vascular or capsular invasion. Hürthle cell carcinomas are characterized microscopically by polygonal, hyperchromatic cells. The incidence of lymph node metastases at presentation is slightly higher in Hürthle cell carcinomas (approximately 25%) than in FTC. Patients with Hürthle cell carcinomas have been reported to have higher tumor recurrence rates and a worse prognosis when compared with patients with PTC and FTC. Hürthle cell tumors concentrate radioactive iodine less avidly than papillary and follicular tumors.

Medullary thyroid carcinomas represent 5% of all thyroid cancers. Eighty percent of tumors are sporadic, and 25% occur as part of an autosomal dominant hereditary syndrome. Sporadic MTC often presents in the fifth decade as a unilateral solitary nodule. Patients with familial MTC more commonly present in the fourth decade with multifocal nodules in the upper poles of both thyroid lobes, where there is the greatest concentration of C cells. Bilateral C-cell hyperplasia is believed to be a precursor to the development of hereditary MTC. Histologically, MTC is an ill-defined, nonencapsulated, invasive mass composed of spindle-shaped or rounded cells separated by fibrous septa and amyloid deposits. Positive immunohistochemical staining for calcitonin, carcinoembryonic antigen, and amyloid aids in the diagnosis of MTC. Medullary carcinomas are slow growing but have a propensity to metastasize early, usually before the primary tumor reaches 2 cm. Fifty percent of patients have regional metastases at the time of diagnosis. Cervical and upper mediastinal lymph nodes are the usual sites involved. Ten-year survival rates for MTC depend on the extent of disease at presentation and are 90% when disease is confined to the thyroid gland, 70% when cervical metastases are present, and 20% when distant metastases are present. The prognosis for patients with MTC falls between that of patients with undifferentiated tumors and patients with well-differentiated tumors. Poor prognostic factors include age greater than 50 years at diagnosis, metastases at the time of diagnosis, and association with MEN 2B. Seventy percent of patients with MEN 2B have metastases at the time of diagnosis of MTC and of these patients, fewer than 50% survive 5 years.

Anaplastic thyroid carcinoma is a rare and highly aggressive tumor that is considered one of the deadliest malignancies. Anaplastic tumors are often inoperable at presentation and account for less than 5% of thyroid cancers. The peak incidence is in the seventh decade, and the incidence is the same in men and women. Patients with ATC usually present with a rapidly growing neck mass, often larger than 5 cm that is fixed to underlying structures and causes symptoms of dysphagia, dyspnea, or dysphonia. On pathological examination, anaplastic tumors are nonencapsulated and often contain areas of extensive necrosis. There are three histologic variants, all of which show high mitotic activity, nuclear pleomorphism, and high vascularity. At the time of diagnosis, 25% of patients have invasion of the trachea, 90% have regional metastases, and 50% have distant metastases—most commonly to the lung. An association between ATC and a history of well-differentiated thyroid cancer has been reported. It has been hypothesized that ATC can develop from within preexisting differentiated thyroid cancer as a result of dedifferentiation of a clone of tumor cells over time. Despite the use of multimodality regimens, treatment rarely results in cure, and 90% of patients succumb within 6 months of diagnosis, often as a result of local progression of disease causing airway obstruction. The 5-year survival rate for ATC is 7%.

Thyroid lymphomas represent fewer than 2% of thyroid cancers. Patients with thyroid lymphomas typically present in the seventh decade. This subtype of thyroid cancer also more commonly affects women and is associated with a history of Hashimoto thyroiditis. The clinical presentation of thyroid lymphoma may be similar to that of UTC, with a rapidly growing neck mass and symptoms of dysphagia and dysphonia. Lymphomas may be primary or secondary; however, non-Hodgkin's B-cell–type lymphomas are the most common primary thyroid lymphomas. Histologically, tumor cells appear monomorphic and noncohesive and stain positive for lymphocyte markers like CD20. It has been reported that 67% of thyroid lymphomas are of mucosa-associated lymphoid tissue (MALT) origin; these tumors are associated with better survival and may be sufficiently treated with radiation therapy alone, instead of the multimodality therapy used for non-MALT lymphomas. Prognosis is related to the extent of disease at the time of diagnosis. When lymphoma is confined to the thyroid gland (stage IE), the 5-year survival rate is 75% to 85%. Patients with disease on both sides of the diaphragm (stage IIIE) or disseminated disease (stage IVE) have a 5-year survival rate of less than 35%.

Diagnosis

Most patients with thyroid cancer have no specific symptoms. These lesions may be identified incidentally during routine carotid ultrasonography and positron emission tomography scanning for other reasons. The most common finding at presentation is a mass or nodule. Less commonly, change in the size of a thyroid nodule or pain from hemorrhage into a nodule will prompt a patient to see a physician. Hoarseness, dysphagia, dyspnea, and hemoptysis are symptoms resulting from invasion of surrounding anatomical structures and are rare in well-differentiated thyroid carcinomas. Occasionally, a patient may present with a palpable cervical lymph node.

A thorough history and physical examination is an important first diagnostic step. Although the history may not be sensitive or specific for detection of a thyroid malignancy, it is important to ascertain whether there is a family history of thyroid cancer, previous radiation exposure, or the presence of symptoms that suggest invasiveness, such as progressive development of hoarseness, dyspnea, and dysphagia. The presence of a single, dominant nodule that is fixed to surrounding tissues and greater than 1 cm in diameter with a hard consistency is suggestive of cancer. The presence of discrete 1- to 2-cm lymph nodes in conjunction with a thyroid nodule is also suggestive of malignancy. Palpable adenopathy is most often found along the middle and lower portions of the jugular vein but may be located lateral to the sternocleidomastoid muscle in the lower portion of the posterior cervical triangle. Other physical findings that suggest invasive malignancy include vocal cord paralysis, fixation of the thyroid nodule, and tracheal deviation or invasion. Cervical spine flexibility should be assessed to ensure adequate hyperextension of the neck can be achieved in case surgery is needed. Examination of the larynx and vocal cords should be performed either indirectly with a mirror or directly with a flexible fiberoptic scope to document the preoperative condition.

Various diagnostic tests are available to help distinguish benign from malignant disease. The ultimate goal is to avoid unnecessary operations on benign lesions whenever possible. The initial evaluation of a patient with a single thyroid nodule consists of laboratory thyroid function studies and fine-needle aspiration (FNA) biopsy. Blood tests, such as the measurement of TSH or thyroglobulin, cannot diagnose thyroid carcinoma. The exception is the measurement of serum calcitonin concentrations that can help identify patients with MTC.

FNA is safe, cost-effective, and the single most useful diagnostic tool in the evaluation of thyroid nodules because it can provide direct information about a lesion. Lesions are classified as benign, malignant, or suspicious for malignancy on the basis of FNA. If an experienced physician performs the FNA and an experienced cytopathologist interprets the cytologic characteristics, the accuracy of FNA in the diagnosis of thyroid cancer can be greater than 90%, with a false-negative rate of less than 5%. Accuracy of FNA is greatest for lesions between 1 and 4 cm; lesions less than 1 cm are difficult to sample, while lesions greater than 4 cm have an increased sampling error as a result of the large area of the lesion. The type of thyroid tumor can also influence the accuracy of FNA. Patients with the diagnosis of follicular neoplasm often require surgical intervention for complete diagnosis. A follicular adenoma cannot be distinguished from a follicular carcinoma by FNA because the presence or absence of capsular or vascular invasion is required to make the diagnosis. Patients with inadequate specimens should undergo repeat FNA or surgery to obtain a tissue diagnosis. Individuals with a finding of benign colloid nodule or thyroiditis by FNA are observed with or without thyroid suppression. Growth of a nodule in a patient receiving thyroid suppression is an indication for surgical intervention. Other specific indications for surgical intervention in thyroid abnormalities are listed in Table 16.1. The incidence of malignancy increases with larger nodule size, male gender, and increasing age. In 15% to 25% of cases, FNA will yield "inadequate diagnostic material," and this necessitates repeat aspiration. The availability of ultrasound guidance has increased the diagnostic yield.

Ultrasonography of the thyroid is an accurate method for determining the character of a thyroid nodule (solid, cystic, or mixed),

Table 16.1. Indications for surgical intervention for thyroid abnormalities

- Fine-needle aspiration (FNA) of thyroid nodule suspicious for carcinoma or follicular neoplasm
- Thyroid mass associated with vocal cord paralysis, regional tissue invasion, cervical lymph node metastasis, or fixation to surrounding tissues
- Thyroid nodule in a patient younger than 20 years or older than 60 years with FNA findings of atypia
- Thyroid nodule in a patient with a history of irradiation exposure to the cervical region
- Hyperfunctioning thyroid nodule in a young patient who (a) fails medical management or (b) refuses medical management or radioactive iodine
- Symptomatic multinodular goiter (dysphagia, difficulty lying supine, or hoarseness)

the number of thyroid nodules, and the status of cervical lymph nodes. Ultrasonography is also useful in guiding an FNA in patients with lesions that are difficult to palpate and also in increasing the yield from aspirations of small or complex lesions. Ultrasonography is also useful in the long-term follow-up of patients with benign thyroid nodules and those treated for thyroid carcinoma. The exact role of ultrasonography in distinguishing benign from malignant nodules is still unresolved. Several ultrasonographic features were proposed to achieve this goal, including the presence of microcalcifications, irregular borders, hypoechogenicity of the nodule, and the absence of surrounding "halo" at the margin of a nodule.

Radionuclide scintigraphy (^{99}Tc-pertechnetate, ^{125}I, or ^{131}I) was previously used as the first diagnostic step in evaluating palpable thyroid masses. Because most thyroid carcinomas and many benign nodules appear cold on scan, the main limitation of radionuclide scanning is that it cannot distinguish between benign and malignant lesions. Approximately 16% of cold (nonfunctioning) nodules and 9% of warm (normal) lesions harbor a malignancy, but rarely do hot (hyperfunctioning) lesions appear malignant. Although a cold lesion has the greatest probability of being malignant, the presence of a hot lesion on a thyroid scan does not exclude malignancy. In general, the use of nuclear thyroid scans has been replaced by FNA for diagnosis, except in the presence of subclinical or clinical hyperthyroidism with a palpable thyroid nodule.

Other diagnostic imaging studies are seldom needed in the initial evaluation of a patient with a thyroid nodule. A chest radiograph should be obtained in certain situations to assess for pulmonary metastases and tracheal deviation. Computed tomography (CT) and magnetic resonance imaging (MRI) are useful in the evaluation of large or recurrent cancers suspected of invasion into the surrounding soft tissue. When indicated by the history and physical findings, CT or MRI of the neck and upper mediastinum may be used to delineate extrathyroidal extension and invasion of the trachea or esophagus, or to determine the presence of significant cervical or mediastinal metastases. The use of four-dimensional CT scanning with 1-mm cuts of the cervical region provides excellent preoperative planning.

Preoperative laboratory assessments should include thyroid function tests and a serum calcium measurement. Although thyroid function tests do not aid in the diagnosis of thyroid cancer, the presence of hypothyroidism or hyperthyroidism is an important factor to take into account in a patient undergoing general anesthesia. Parathyroid function should be assessed by measuring the serum calcium level. The incidence of parathyroid adenomas and other hyperfunctioning anomalies of the parathyroid glands is higher in the presence of thyroid nodules or carcinoma. Thyroid antibody tests are important when thyroiditis is a consideration. Measurement of serum thyroglobulin levels is useful mainly for follow-up studies after treatment of DTC and is not a part of the initial diagnostic evaluation. Serum calcitonin measurements should not be done routinely in nodular thyroid disease because calcitonin measurement can lead to unnecessary thyroidectomy without proven clinical benefit. However, calcitonin should be measured in patients with thyroid nodules who have diarrhea, family history of MTC, or MEN-2 syndrome. Solitary lesions at the junction of the upper one-third and lower two-thirds of the thyroid gland warrant suspicion. Patients who have an increased calcitonin level and a preoperative diagnosis of MTC should be screened for pheochromocytoma with a 24-hour urine collection for vanillylmandelic acid, metanephrine, free catecholamines or plasma metanephrine, and hereditary MTC with *RET* proto-oncogene mutation analysis. Five percent to 7% of patients with apparently sporadic MTC are found to have a mutation consistent with hereditary MTC.

Staging and Prognosis

Several classifications and staging schemes have been proposed for DTC. However, no consensus favoring any one of these systems has emerged. The most commonly used are the AMES (Age, Metastasis, Extent, Size) system, which divides patients into low- and high-risk groups; the TNM (Tumor, Nodes, Metastasis), as used by the American Joint Committee on Cancer; the AGES (Age, Grade, Extent, Size) and MACIS (Metastasis, Age, Completeness of Resection, Invasion, Size) proposed by the Mayo Clinic; the University of Chicago system, which groups patients into four categories—disease limited to the gland (I), lymph node involvement (II), extrathyroidal invasion (III), and distant metastases (IV); and the National Thyroid Cancer Treatment Cooperative Study Registry scheme. The TNM classification stratifies patients into four stages on the basis of tumor size, nodal status, the presence or absence of distant metastases, and age at diagnosis.

The prognosis of patients with stage I well-differentiated thyroid carcinoma is excellent, with 20-year survival rates of nearly 100%. Patients with stage IV disease, in contrast, have a 5-year survival rate of only 25%. Within the group of patients with well-differentiated thyroid cancer are a small number who have more aggressive disease and for whom none of the current staging systems apply. As molecular markers of disease are developed, these patients may be able to be identified at earlier stages and offered additional treatment.

In general, the prognosis for patients with PTC is influenced by age, gender, extent of disease, and volume of the primary tumor. Unlike most solid tumors, age at diagnosis may be the most important predictive factor for survival. The significance of gender as a prognostic factor in thyroid cancer is also greater than that for other solid tumors. The prognostic significance of lymph node metastases in differentiated thyroid cancers continues to be debated; in patients with papillary cancer who are younger than 40 years of age and who frequently have lymph node involvement, the significance of this finding on mortality is negligible, although it increases the recurrence rate. The minimal effect of lymph node metastases on prognosis is reflected in the TNM staging system (Table 16.2), in which lymph node metastases are only factored into the staging of patients older than 45 years of age. The diminished importance of lymph node metastases is based on data suggesting that microscopic metastases are present in up to 90% of lymph nodes examined, yet clinically significant disease develops in only 10% of patients.

The prognosis of patients with FTC is believed to be poorer than that of patients with PTC, perhaps because of the higher incidence of hematogenous metastases. However, treatment decisions and prognosis are based on well-differentiated thyroid malignancies as a group.

Treatment

Controversy continues over the extent of resection necessary in cases of papillary and follicular cancer, the necessity and extent of neck dissection, the role of postresection thyroid hormone suppression, and the appropriate use of postoperative therapeutic radioactive ^{131}I. At this time, no randomized prospective trials have been conducted to clarify these controversies. Certain factors make it unlikely that a prospective trial will be conducted because (a) thyroid cancer is an indolent disease, which would require that patients be followed for long periods of time to detect differences in outcome; and (b) given the low incidence of thyroid cancer, Udelsma et al. reported that between 3,000 and 12,000 patients would need to be randomized to conduct a prospective trial. Thus, the majority of treatment decisions for differentiated thyroid cancer have been made based on data from large retrospective series.

Surgical Resection

The principal treatment for thyroid cancer is surgical resection. Accepted surgical management varies from a thyroid lobectomy and isthmectomy to a total thyroidectomy and a compartment-oriented neck dissection.

The surgical management of well-differentiated thyroid cancer continues to be controversial, with the debate centering on the extent of thyroidectomy. Proponents of total thyroidectomy argue that this operation can be performed safely by experienced surgeons with a less than 2% incidence of permanent recurrent nerve injury or permanent hypoparathyroidism; foci of papillary

Table 16.2. TNM classification system for differentiated thyroid carcinoma

Definition

Primary tumor (T)

TX	Primary tumor cannot be assessed
T0	No evidence of primary tumor
T1	Tumor ≤2 cm, confined to the thyroid
T2	Tumor >2 cm and <4 cm, confined to the thyroid
T3	Tumor >4 cm, confined to the thyroid
T4a	Tumor of any size extending beyond the thyroid capsule to invade subcutaneous soft tissues, larynx, trachea, esophagus, or recurrent laryngeal nerve
T4b	Tumor invades prevertebral fascia or encases carotid artery or mediastinal vessels

Regional lymph nodes (N) (cervical and upper mediastinal)

NX	Regional lymph nodes cannot be assessed
N0	No regional lymph node metastasis
N1	Regional lymph node metastasis N1a metastasis to level VI (pretracheal, paratracheal, and prelaryngeal/Delphian lymph nodes) N1b metastasis in bilateral, midline, or contralateral cervical or superior mediastinal lymph nodes

Distant metastases (M)

MX	Presence of distant metastasis cannot be assessed
M0	No distant metastasis
M1	Distant metastasis

Stages

Papillary and follicular thyroid cancer

	Patient Age <45 Years	Patient Age ≥45 Years
Stage I	Any T, any N, M0	T1, N0, M0
Stage II	Any T, any N, M1	T2, N0, M0
Stage III		T3, N0, M0 T1, N1a, M0 T2, N1a, M0 T3, N1a, M0
Stage IVA		T4a, N0, M0 T4a, N1a, M0 T1, N1b, M0 T2, N1b, M0 T3, N1b, M0 T4a, N1b, M0
Stage IVB		T4b, any N1b, M0
Stage IVC		Any T, any N, M1

(continued)

Table 16.2. (*Continued*)

	Patient Age <45 Years	Patient Age ≥45 Years
Medullary thyroid cancer		
Stage I	T1, N0, M0	
Stage II	T2, N0, M0	
Stage III	T3, N0, M0	
	T1, N1a, M0	
	T2, N1a, M0	
	T3, N1a, M0	
Stage IVA	T4a, N0, M0	
	T4a, N1a, M0	
	T1, N1b, M0	
	T2, N1b, M0	
	T3, N1b, M0	
	T4a, N1b, M0	
Stage IVB	T4b, any N, M0	
Stage IVC	Any T, any N, M1	
Anaplastic thyroid cancer		
Stage IVA	T4a, any N, M0	
Stage IVB	T4b, any N, M0	
Stage IVC	Any T, any N, M1	

carcinoma are found in both thyroid lobes in up to 85% of patients, and 5% to 10% of recurrences occur in the contralateral lobe; the presence of residual thyroid tissue after less than total thyroidectomy hampers the use of thyroglobulin as a marker of persistent or recurrent disease; radioactive iodine can be used to identify and treat residual normal thyroid tissue and recurrent or metastatic disease after total thyroidectomy; there is a lower recurrence rate in patients who have undergone bilateral procedures or total thyroidectomy; and total thyroidectomy minimizes the need for reoperative surgery, which is associated with increased complication rates.

Advocates of more conservative procedures, such as thyroid lobectomy with isthmectomy or near-total thyroidectomy, argue that there is a decreased risk of injury to the recurrent laryngeal nerve and the parathyroid glands with less extensive surgery; it is rare for a total thyroidectomy to remove the entire thyroid gland; occult foci of papillary carcinoma left behind after conservative surgery are rarely of clinical significance; half of clinically significant recurrences after conservative surgery can be safely managed with reoperation; and there is no difference in survival between patients who have undergone more conservative procedures and patients who have undergone total thyroidectomy.

At the M. D. Anderson Cancer Center, we perform a total thyroidectomy and central compartment lymph node excision for all papillary carcinomas. Total thyroidectomy is also our treatment of choice for follicular carcinoma and Hürthle cell carcinoma;

however, these diagnoses often cannot be ascertained by frozen-section examination at the time of surgery. If the diagnosis of follicular or Hürthle cell carcinoma is made postoperatively in a patient treated with a thyroid lobectomy, we suggest that a completion thyroidectomy be performed in high-risk patients (i.e., age >45 years, lesions >1 cm, or distant metastases). Patients who have undergone thyroid lobectomy for other reasons and are found to have an incidental microscopic carcinoma on permanent histologic studies may not require completion thyroidectomy. We combine a therapeutic cervical node dissection with total thyroidectomy in patients with well-differentiated carcinomas and clinical or diagnostic evidence of lymph node metastases. We routinely use preoperative ultrasound to assess the central and lateral compartments of the neck.

Patients with sporadic MTC diagnosed preoperatively undergo a total thyroidectomy with in-continuity central compartment dissection and modified radical neck dissection on the side of the lesion. Patients with palpable cervical lymphadenopathy undergo a bilateral modified radical neck dissection at the time of total thyroidectomy. The goals of our aggressive surgical approach are to maximize locoregional tumor control and survival and to minimize the need for reoperation. Our approach is supported by published reports suggesting that patients who undergo total thyroidectomy with compartment-oriented lymphadenectomy have both improved local-regional disease control and improved survival. Our approach is also supported by our knowledge of the biological behavior of medullary thyroid cancers: these tumors do not concentrate radioiodine, are multifocal, metastasize early, and are not adequately managed with nonsurgical treatments.

Patients who have hereditary MTC as part of the familial MTC or MEN-2 syndromes diagnosed only by positive *RET* mutational analysis undergo total thyroidectomy without lymphadenectomy if preoperative studies show a normal basal calcitonin level and normal findings on a cervical sonogram. Patients who have an increased basal calcitonin level or a thyroid nodule detected on physical examination or sonography undergo total thyroidectomy with central compartment lymphadenectomy and modified neck dissection. Children who are found to carry a hereditary *RET* proto-oncogene mutation should undergo prophylactic total thyroidectomy. Children in families with MEN-2A or familial MTC syndromes should undergo surgery at 5 years of age, while children in families with MEN 2B should undergo surgery as early as possible because invasive MTC has been found as early as at birth in these children.

ATC is an aggressive lesion that is usually diagnosed by FNA. Most anaplastic tumors are unresectable at presentation and are thus managed primarily by combination radiation therapy and chemotherapy. Surgery is rarely indicated other than for tissue sampling or tracheostomy. In the exceedingly rare case, resectable lesions would be treated with total thyroidectomy and wide local excision of adjacent soft tissues followed by postoperative adjuvant chemotherapy and radiation therapy. Although different chemotherapy combinations and radiation therapy regimens have been tried, no therapy has been able to improve the outcome of ATC.

Neck Dissection

An understanding of the lymphatic drainage pattern of the thyroid gland is necessary to ensure the nodal groups at highest risk for metastasis are removed when node dissection is performed. The thyroid gland has an extensive intraglandular network of lymphatic channels that allow for drainage within one lobe and from one lobe to another. The thyroid lymphatics typically drain first into the central compartment (level VI), which contains the pretracheal and paratracheal nodes, and subsequently into the lateral jugular regions (level II–IV). Another route of lymphatic spread for thyroid cancer is along the inferior thyroid artery because it courses behind the common carotid artery to the lower portion of the posterior triangle of the neck (level V). The superior mediastinal nodes also commonly contain metastases and must be closely examined intraoperatively. The submandibular and submental nodes (level I) rarely contain metastases in patients with DTC. The classic radical neck dissection, which consists of lymphadenectomy of levels II to V, as well as removal of the internal jugular vein, sternocleidomastoid muscle, and spinal accessory nerve, is associated with high morbidity and rarely performed. We more commonly perform central compartment node dissection, which removes level VI and superior mediastinal nodes, and compartment-oriented neck dissection, which spares the internal jugular vein, sternocleidomastoid muscle, and spinal accessory nerve, in patients with well-differentiated thyroid cancers.

The necessity and extent of neck dissection, specifically the role of elective node dissection, for differentiated thyroid cancer is another subject of controversy. PTC frequently spreads to cervical lymph nodes, whereas FTC rarely metastasizes to the regional lymph nodes. Although the exact incidence of lymph node metastases in papillary carcinoma is unknown, positive nodes have been found in 30% to 80% of patients who underwent prophylactic neck dissections. Microscopic nodal metastases have been reported in up to 90% of these patients. However, clinically significant nodal disease develops in only approximately 10% of patients with papillary carcinoma. At the heart of the controversy is the issue of whether lymph node metastases have an impact on recurrence or survival. The majority of studies in the literature on DTC have reported that positive nodal status influences local-regional recurrence rates, but not patient survival. The majority of studies have also failed to demonstrate a survival benefit in patients with differentiated thyroid tumors who have undergone extensive, prophylactic (elective) node dissection at the time of initial surgery. Whether elective node dissection reduces local-regional recurrence rates is unclear because there are several conflicting reports in the literature. Of note, though, all studies with patients who underwent extensive cervical lymphadenectomy reported higher complication rates.

For patients with papillary cancer, if a total thyroidectomy is performed, then we also perform an en bloc central compartment dissection. If there are clinically palpable nodes in the lateral regions of the neck, an en bloc modified radical neck dissection on the side containing clinically suspicious disease is also performed at the time of total thyroidectomy. In patients with follicular tumors, because of the low incidence of lymph node metastases, we do not perform central compartment lymphadenectomy at the time of total thyroidectomy, unless there is palpable adenopathy. At M. D. Anderson, the aggressive use of ultrasound, particularly in high-risk patients, has assisted in the preoperative detection of suspicious nodes and the early determination of the need for lymph node dissection.

A poor prognosis is associated with the presence of lymph node metastases in patients with medullary and anaplastic cancers. We therefore perform a central compartment node dissection and a modified radical neck dissection on the side of the primary lesion at the time of total thyroidectomy in patients with sporadic MTC. A bilateral modified radical neck dissection is also performed if the patient presents with palpable adenopathy.

Surgical Technique

Surgical resection of a possible thyroid carcinoma requires meticulous dissection of the ipsilateral thyroid compartment, identification and preservation of the recurrent laryngeal nerve, and complete resection of the affected lobe and thyroid isthmus. Surgery should be performed with general anesthesia. Identification of the ipsilateral parathyroid glands should be attempted, but preservation of the glands may be impossible if there is extensive invasion by cancer or if there are clinical metastases in the paratracheal area. If the diagnosis of thyroid carcinoma is confirmed intraoperatively by frozen-section histologic examination of the surgical specimen, total thyroidectomy is completed by resecting the contralateral lobe with special care taken to identify and spare the parathyroid glands and their blood supply. Once the thyroid gland is removed, the posterior surface is carefully inspected for any possible parathyroid tissue. If suspected parathyroid tissue is identified, a portion is sent for frozen-section examination, with the remnant kept in a cold, sterile, physiological saline solution. If the tissue is confirmed to be parathyroid gland on frozen-section examination, the preserved portion is minced and implanted in a small pocket created in the ipsilateral sternocleidomastoid muscle. Other important structures such as the superior laryngeal nerve, spinal accessory nerve, sternocleidomastoid muscle, esophagus, and trachea should also be preserved unless invasion by tumor is present.

The approach to the thyroid gland itself is through a transverse incision, approximately one or two fingerbreadths above the clavicles. Flaps are elevated superiorly to the level of the thyroid notch and inferiorly to the suprasternal notch in the subplatysmal plane. Separation of the fascia between the strap muscles and the sternocleidomastoid muscles is done to facilitate exposure of the gland and allow inspection of the lower jugular lymph nodes. The strap muscles are separated in the midline and can be divided on the side of the primary tumor if necessary. Portions of the strap muscles adherent to the gland are resected with the specimen. In the reoperative setting, thyroid compartment may be approached laterally along the anterior border of the sternocleidomastoid muscle.

All thyroid vessels are identified and ligated close to the gland. The thyroid lobe is retracted medially and the middle thyroid vein is identified and divided. The dissection is continued medially, allowing for identification, dissection, and preservation of the recurrent laryngeal nerve. A nonrecurrent laryngeal nerve on the right side may be recognized as it originates high from the vagus nerve, or it may be found in proximity to the superior thyroid vessels or the inferior thyroid artery.

The superior pole vessels are then individually transected with a small curved or right-angle hemostat. The superior laryngeal nerve should be identified and preserved between the thyroid vessels as it crosses the constrictor muscle and enters the cricothyroid muscle. The surgeon must exercise caution during dissection of this area as the position of the superior nerve in relation to the vascular pedicle can vary. The fascia that secures the gland (visceral and suspensory ligament) is then meticulously incised and the dissection is continued medially along the posterior aspect of the gland. The ligament of berry is cautiously divided to elevate the gland off the anterior surface of the trachea. The recurrent laryngeal nerve, if not previously located, is identified in the paratracheal groove inferior to the gland and is dissected superiorly. The inferior thyroid artery is then identified and its branches are individually ligated as they enter the thyroid gland, with care taken to avoid injury to the recurrent laryngeal nerve. The anatomical relationship between the nerve and the inferior artery is extremely variable. Also, the nerve may divide into several branches at the level of the inferior thyroid artery. All nerve branches should be preserved during the course of the dissection. Careful dissection is continued up to where the nerve enters the larynx.

Eighty percent of superior parathyroid glands are located within 1 cm of the intersection of the recurrent laryngeal nerve and the inferior thyroid artery, usually within the thyroid fascia. They may be located within the thyroid capsule, and the remainder is in the retropharyngeal or retroesophageal spaces. The location of the inferior parathyroid glands is far more variable. They are usually posterior and lateral to the recurrent laryngeal nerve. Compromise of the blood supply to the parathyroid glands is the most common cause of hypoparathyroidism in the postoperative period. Careful attention to dissection of the inferior thyroid vessels and their branches is warranted to preserve the lateral vascular pedicle. Occasionally, a small portion of thyroid tissue may have to be spared of resection (subtotal resection) to preserve the vascular pedicle to the parathyroid tissue. Meticulous dissection of the parathyroid glands and their vascular supply, as well as autotransplantation of devascularized parathyroid tissue, are important techniques that have contributed to a lower incidence of permanent hypoparathyroidism. All parathyroidlike tissue should be inspected and left attached to individual vascular pedicles. Distinguishing between lymph nodes and parathyroid glands may be difficult. Biopsies should be taken and sent for frozen-section diagnosis if there is any confusion. Histologically confirmed parathyroid glands should be autografted to the ipsilateral sternocleidomastoid muscle. Dissection of the opposite lobe, when indicated, proceeds similarly to the dissection of the involved lobe.

Clinically palpable adenopathy, especially in a high-risk patient, requires that a neck dissection be performed. Most lymphoareolar tissue in the thyroid compartment and upper mediastinum to the level of the innominate vein is accessible through a collar incision. Rarely, because of a patient's anatomy, a sternotomy may be necessary to allow for adequate clearance of upper mediastinal and lower peritracheal nodes. During a central compartment lymphadenectomy, all areolar and lymphatic tissue along the larynx and recurrent laryngeal nerves from the level of the hyoid bone area down to the innominate vessels are removed. Particular attention should be paid to dissecting the tissue posterior to the recurrent laryngeal nerve. The dissection is carried laterally to the internal jugular veins, and the tissue is resected in continuity with the tumor specimen. Attention must be paid to identifying the inferior parathyroid glands, which may be difficult to separate from the mass of nodal and fibrofatty tissue that extends inferiorly off the lower pole of the thyroid gland. When the removal of lateral lymph node metastases is indicated, we perform a compartment-oriented neck dissection, which removes level IIa, III, IV, and V lymph nodes and spares the sternocleidomastoid muscle, internal jugular vein, and spinal accessory nerve.

Although extrathyroidal extension of thyroid carcinoma into surrounding tissues is rare, the tumor extent must be clearly delineated so judicious resection of invaded structures—including resection of laryngeal nerves, tracheal rings, or portions of the larynx—can be performed. Local recurrence is a source of significant morbidity and mortality; therefore, complete surgical extirpation should be performed to optimize local control. Fortunately, locally invasive thyroid carcinoma can often be resected with a much narrower margin than other carcinomas that arise in tissues surrounding the thyroid.

Adjuvant Therapy

Controversy exists over the use of adjuvant treatment in the management of well-differentiated thyroid carcinoma. The goal of treatment is to maximize disease-free survival. Retrospective studies of patient cohorts followed postoperatively for many years (often more than 10–20 years) suggest that multimodality adjuvant therapy can decrease local recurrence and may improve survival. The mainstay of adjuvant treatment for well-differentiated thyroid carcinoma is radioactive ^{131}I treatment and TSH suppression. The use of therapeutic radioactive ablation of remnant thyroid tissue after thyroidectomy is well established, but criteria for the use of this treatment vary from institution to institution.

Our practice after total thyroidectomy for follicular or papillary carcinoma of the thyroid is to delay thyroid hormone replacement for 4 to 6 weeks to maximize iodine uptake during scanning. Patients can receive short-acting thyroid hormone replacement Cytomel to alleviate symptoms of hypothyroidism for approximately 4 weeks after surgery. All thyroid hormone replacement is stopped 2 weeks prior to planned scanning and radioactive thyroid ablation. A tracer dose (2–5 mCi) of radioactive iodine is then administered, and a whole-body scan is performed. This allows scintigraphic staging of disease, and may show the presence and extent of metastases that are minimally recognizable with conventional imaging techniques.

At M. D. Anderson, thyroid remnant ablation is recommended for patients with DTC who are 45 years of age or older, for patients whose primary tumor was greater than 1 cm in diameter or was multifocal, and for patients with extrathyroidal disease due to tissue invasion or metastases. Patients found to have radioiodine uptake in the thyroid bed on the initial postoperative thyroid scan often receive an empiric dose of 30 to 150 mCi of radioactive iodine. However, patients who have evidence of residual disease or metastases on their initial postoperative thyroid scan receive higher doses of ^{131}I, in the range of 150 to 200 mCi. The standard ablative dose of ^{131}I for patients with PTC whose tumor was less than 3 cm in diameter without extrathyroidal invasion and few or no lymph nodes involved is 29 mCi, which can be administered as an outpatient. Remnant ablation in all other patients with well-differentiated thyroid carcinoma is 100 mCi, which requires overnight hospitalization. Higher doses may be administered if subsequent thyroid scans demonstrate recurrent or persistent disease. Radioiodine ablation has been associated with a decrease in local-regional relapse rates of up to 50% and a reduction in disease-specific mortality.

After surgery and subsequent ^{131}I ablation therapy, all patients receive hormonal replacement treatment (levothyroxine sodium) at a dose of 2 μg/kg/d. The dose may vary among patients and is adjusted to reach an appropriate level of TSH suppression for a patient as determined on the basis of the individual patient's disease status and the clinicopathological features of his or her tumor. TSH suppression and radioactive iodine are of no use in the management of medullary and anaplastic thyroid carcinomas because these tumors do not show consistent uptake of radioactive iodine and generally do not contain TSH receptors, making them insensitive to TSH suppression.

The role of external-beam radiation therapy (EBRT) as part of the initial adjuvant treatment regimen for DTC is also controversial. However, several retrospective series have reported that local control can be improved with EBRT, specifically in patients with gross disease following surgical resection or patients considered to be at high risk of relapse (>45 years of age, microscopic residual disease, extensive extrathyroidal invasion). Currently, EBRT is more often used to palliate metastatic or locally advanced disease, such as bone metastases or thyroid bed recurrences. Patients with MTC who are considered to be at high risk for local-regional recurrence because of microscopic residual disease, extraglandular tumor invasion, and lymph node metastasis are also considered for treatment with adjuvant EBRT. Brierley et al. reported a decrease in the local-regional recurrence rate in patients with MTC who have been treated with postoperative adjuvant EBRT.

Overall, cytotoxic chemotherapy has not been very effective in the treatment of thyroid carcinomas. Chemotherapy has limited use in the treatment of DTC, Hürthle cell carcinomas, and MTC. However, chemotherapy, in combination with EBRT and surgery, is more commonly used to treat ATC, for which there is a lack of effective therapies. Small numbers of patients with UTC have had prolonged survival with different regimens of chemotherapeutic agents, most including doxorubicin, and EBRT. Intravenous bisphosphonates can be given in patients with painful bony metastases. Arterial embolization has been used anecdotally to reduce pain in selected cases of metastatic follicular thyroid carcinoma where the lesions are highly vascular.

Surveillance

Most recurrences of well-differentiated thyroid carcinoma occur within the first 5 years after initial treatment, especially in the case of FTC, but recurrences can occur several decades later. Patients with papillary thyroid tumors often recur in the neck, whereas patients with follicular carcinomas more commonly recur at distant sites. Some patients with PTC who have recurrence in the neck die from thyroid cancer. The most common sites of distant metastases for thyroid cancers are the lungs, bone, soft tissues, brain, liver, and adrenal glands. Lung metastases are more common in young patients, whereas bone metastases are more common in older patients.

A coordinated plan of follow-up for thyroid carcinomas must consider the varied presentations possible for recurrent disease. Most patients are seen every 6 months for 1 to 3 years postoperatively and yearly thereafter. Follow-up visits typically include clinical examination and blood tests measuring the serum thyroglobulin, TSH, and free T4 levels and ultrasonography. A chest radiograph is usually obtained on an annual basis. Thyroglobulin values normally drop after thyroidectomy or ablation and serve as a sensitive indicator of recurrent or persistent disease. However, it is important to keep in mind that thyroglobulin production is TSH dependent; therefore, TSH levels can affect the sensitivity of thyroglobulin measurements in detecting disease. Twenty-five percent of patients with differentiated thyroid cancer have antithyroglobulin antibodies, which falsely lower measured thyroglobulin levels. When indicated, a repeat ^{131}I scan is done after temporary (4–6 weeks) cessation of hormonal replacement. Subsequent therapeutic doses of radioactive iodine may be administered. Ultrasonography of the neck may be added to the follow-up regimen, especially in patients who had large tumors or nodal disease. This protocol may vary, depending on the risk group of the patient and special circumstances. Recombinant human TSH (rh TSH) injections can be used instead of thyroid hormone withdrawal to stimulate radioiodine uptake mainly for diagnostic goals and in selected cases for treatment purposes. Serum thyroglobulin can be measured at the time of radioiodine administration after thyroid hormone withdrawal or after rh TSH injections.

Follow-up for medullary carcinoma differs in that no scanning or thyroglobulin measurements are used. Instead, measurement of calcitonin or pentagastrin-stimulated calcitonin levels is used to observe these patients. Similarly, anaplastic carcinoma and lymphoma cannot be followed by thyroid scanning; therefore, patients require regular follow-up physical examination and radiographic or ultrasound studies.

PARATHYROID CARCINOMA

Epidemiology and Etiology

There are approximately 100,000 new cases of primary hyperparathyroidism in the United States each year. Primary hyperparathyroidism can be caused by parathyroid adenoma, hyperplasia, or carcinoma. Carcinoma of the parathyroid gland is a very rare lesion and has been reported to be the cause of primary hyperparathyroidism in only 0.1% to 4% of cases. The incidences of parathyroid carcinoma are equal in men and women, and the tumor is usually diagnosed in the fifth decade. No significant clustering within specific ethnic or income groups or unusual geographic clustering has been observed.

The rarity of parathyroid carcinoma has limited the accumulation of data on its natural history and etiologic factors. Parathyroid carcinoma has been described in association with chronic renal failure and dialysis. It has been proposed that malignant transformation of benign hyperplastic parathyroid tissue occurred in such cases. Associations with familial hyperparathyroidism, including multiple endocrine neoplasia syndromes, and with sporadic hyperparathyroidism have been described. External-beam irradiation has also been associated with parathyroid neoplasms; however, these neoplasms are more frequently adenomas than carcinomas.

Presentation

The majority (95%) of parathyroid carcinomas is functional, and patients with parathyroid carcinoma usually present with severe hypercalcemia. The serum calcium level in parathyroid carcinoma averages more than 14 mg per dL, compared with the lower levels of 10 or 11 mg per dL seen in benign cases of hyperparathyroidism. Intact parathyroid hormone levels in patients with parathyroid carcinoma are at least five times the upper normal limit of 50 to 72 pg per mL. As a result, renal (60%) and skeletal (50%) involvement is significantly more common in parathyroid carcinoma than in patients with benign primary hyperparathyroidism, in which renal and skeletal disease occur in 48% and 20% of patients, respectively. Metabolic abnormalities associated with parathyroid cancer include renal disorders (e.g., nephrolithiasis, renal dysfunction, pyelonephritis), skeletal abnormalities (e.g., osteitis fibrosa cystica), and pancreatitis. Polyuria, polydipsia, or nocturia is observed in 40% of patients and fatigue in 30%. Only 20% of patients diagnosed with parathyroid cancer are asymptomatic compared with up to 80% of patients with benign hyperparathyroidism.

The presence of a palpable neck mass in a patient with hyperparathyroidism should raise the suspicion of parathyroid carcinoma. A palpable neck mass is observed in 40% of patients with parathyroid cancer but is rare for patients with benign hyperparathyroidism. Hoarseness in a patient with hyperparathyroidism also suggests parathyroid cancer, although involvement of the recurrent laryngeal nerve occurs in less than 10% of patients with parathyroid cancer.

Diagnosis

A high index of suspicion of parathyroid carcinoma should be maintained, especially for patients with serum calcium levels higher than 14 mg per dL and a palpable neck mass. Preoperative FNA biopsy is contraindicated for patients with suspected parathyroid cancer because of the risk of local dissemination. Furthermore, distinguishing parathyroid carcinoma from adenoma is extremely difficult, even with histologic examination.

Preoperative localization studies are useful in parathyroid carcinoma. Real-time ultrasound of the neck is effective for localization. Signs of gross invasion and marked irregularity of the tumor margins suggest malignancy.

If the diagnosis has not been suspected before surgery, intraoperative recognition of parathyroid carcinoma is essential. Parathyroid adenomas appear soft, oval, and brownish-red to tan in color. Parathyroid cancer should be suspected in the presence of a gray, firm, adherent parathyroid gland. Fibrosis is not seen in normal or adenomatous glands. Local invasion of adjacent tissues and cervical lymph node metastasis further support the diagnosis of parathyroid carcinoma.

Unless the tumor is clinically aggressive, it is difficult to differentiate benign from malignant tumors by pathological assessment. Invasion of surrounding structures, metastases, or recurrent tumors reflect malignancy. The histologic criteria for a diagnosis of parathyroid malignancy are fibrous capsule or fibrous trabeculae, a trabecular or rosettelike cellular architecture, presence of mitotic figures, and capsular or vascular invasion.

Natural History

Parathyroid carcinoma is a slow-growing, persistent, locally recurrent tumor. Most parathyroid carcinomas are clinically functioning, allowing them to be monitored by measuring intact parathyroid hormone levels. The local recurrence rate has been estimated to range from 36% to 80%, with a wide range in the interval between the initial operation and the manifestation of recurrence (mean 2.6 years; range 1 month to 19 years). Similarly, recurrence after reoperation presents at variable intervals.

In general, recurrent disease should be treated with surgical resection. Although cure after recurrence is rare, some patients will achieve prolonged disease-free intervals by controlling hypercalcemia, which is the major cause of death. Distant metastases tend to occur late, with lung, liver, bone, and pancreas being frequent sites. The overall 10-year survival rate is less than 50%.

There is no American Joint Committee on Cancer TNM staging system for parathyroid carcinoma. The available data on tumor size and lymph node involvement suggest that neither of these factors are important prognostic markers. A multivariate analysis of prognostic factors in parathyroid carcinoma indicated that the extent of surgery when consisting of tumor resection, and en bloc unilateral or bilateral thyroidectomy correlates most strongly with an improved survival and relapse-free period. Hence, it is important to maintain a high level of suspicion for parathyroid cancer during surgery.

Treatment

Surgery is the most effective therapy for carcinoma of the parathyroid glands. Because parathyroid cancer has a propensity for local recurrence and rarely metastasizes to regional nodes, tumors should be resected en bloc with care to preserve the integrity of the parathyroid capsule. En bloc resection requires removal of the ipsilateral central neck contents, including the thyroid lobe and tracheoesophageal soft tissues and lymphatics. Structures such as the recurrent laryngeal nerve, esophageal wall, or strap muscles should be removed if the tumor adheres to them; this will reduce the risk of tumor spillage and local recurrence. The increased local control achieved with resection of the recurrent laryngeal nerve outweighs the complication of vocal cord paralysis, which can be managed, if clinically necessary, with Teflon injection of the paralyzed cord. A prophylactic neck dissection is not necessary at the time of the initial procedure unless clinically positive lymph node metastases are detected or there is extensive soft-tissue invasion.

As previously mentioned, some patients will achieve prolonged disease-free intervals after one or more surgical procedures for recurrent disease in the neck. Similarly, some patients will benefit from resection of lung metastases. Surgical excision of recurrent carcinoma also offers the best control of hypercalcemia, the principal cause of death in these patients.

Localization of metastatic foci is important for treatment of recurrent parathyroid cancer. Thallium chloride scintiscanning and 99m-technetium sestamibi scanning are useful for locating cervical or upper mediastinal recurrence but frequently fail to detect lung metastases. CT is effective for identification and localization of mediastinal or pulmonary metastases. More recently, intraoperative use of a handheld gamma detector after preoperative sestamibi injection has been used to aid in the intraoperative localization of recurrent parathyroid cancer.

Recent reports have challenged the common idea that radiation therapy is not effective in the treatment of parathyroid cancer. This idea was based on anecdotal reports of failure of treatment in patients with advanced unresectable disease. A review of more recent data indicated that radiation therapy might play a role as an adjuvant treatment for patients at high risk for local relapse, such as those with residual microscopic disease and tumor spillage during surgery.

There are no effective chemotherapeutic agents that inhibit parathyroid tumor growth or affect the secretion of parathyroid hormone in parathyroid carcinoma. As a result, medical management is used mainly to control hypercalcemia. Medical therapy is particularly important in patients with unresectable disease or in those with persistent hypercalcemia and negative localization studies. The acute management of severe hypercalcemia includes generous intravenous saline infusion with loop diuretics added later if necessary to increase renal calcium clearance. Mithramycin has been proven to be effective, but toxicity has limited its use. Subcutaneous calcitonin (4–8 units per kg every 6–8 hours) is a safe addition that reduces calcium levels within a few hours, but it is has only a short-term effect. Intravenous bisphosphonates reduce calcium levels by inhibiting osteoclast activity. Pamidronate (30–90 mg intravenously over 1–2 hours) or zoledronic acid (4 mg intravenously) over at least 15 minutes can result in a variable response that may last for a few weeks in selected patients. Calcimimetic agents increase the activity of calcium-sensing receptors and suppress PTH secretion. Cinacalcet is the first U.S. Food and Drug Administration-approved agent of this family in the management of hypercalcemia in patients with parathyroid carcinoma. Other less commonly used approaches include gallium nitrate and, rarely, hemodialysis in very selected patients.

RECOMMENDED READING

Ain KB. Anaplastic thyroid carcinoma: a therapeutic challenge. *Semin Surg Oncol* 1999;16:64.

Anderson BJ, Samaan NA, Vassilopoulou-Sellin R, et al. Parathyroid carcinoma: features and difficulties in diagnosis and management. *Surgery* 1983;94:906.

Austin JR, El-Naggar AK, Goepfert H. Thyroid cancers II: medullary, anaplastic, lymphoma, sarcoma, squamous cell. *Otolaryngol Clin North Am* 1996;29:611.

Brierley JD, Tsang RW. External-beam radiation therapy in the treatment of differentiated thyroid cancer. *Semin Surg Oncol* 1999; 16:42.

Chen H, Udelsman R. Papillary thyroid carcinoma: justification for total thyroidectomy and management of lymph node metastases. *Surg Oncol Clin* 1998;7:645.

Chow E, Tsang RW, Brierley JD, Filice S. Parathyroid carcinoma—the Princess Margaret Hospital experience. *Int J Radiat Oncol Biol Phys* 1998;41:569.

Clayman GL, Gonzalez HE, El-Naggar A, Vassilopoulou-Selin R. Parathyroid carcinoma: evaluation and interdisciplinary management. *Cancer* 2004; 5:900.

Devine RM, Edis AJ, Banks PM. Primary lymphoma of the thyroid: a review of the Mayo Clinic experience through 1978. *World J Surg* 1981;5:33.

Duh QY, Sancho JJ, Greenspan FS, et al. Medullary thyroid carcinoma: the need for early diagnosis and total thyroidectomy. *Arch Surg* 1989;124:1206.

Evans DB, Fleming JB, Lee JE, et al. The surgical treatment of medullary thyroid carcinoma. *Semin Surg Oncol* 1999;16:50.

Gagel RF, Goepfert H, Callender DL. Changing concepts in the pathogenesis and management of thyroid carcinoma. *CA Cancer J Clin* 1996;46:261.

Gimm O. Thyroid cancer. *Cancer Lett* 2001;2163:143.

Goldman ND, Coniglio JU. Thyroid cancers I: papillary, follicular, and Hürthle cell. *Otolaryngol Clin North Am* 1996;29:593.

Hay ID, Grant CS, Taylor WF, et al. Ipsilateral lobectomy versus bilateral lobar resection in papillary thyroid carcinoma: a retrospective analysis of surgical outcome using a novel prognostic scoring system. *Surgery* 1987;102:1089.

Hodgson NC, Button J, Solorzano CC. Thyroid cancer: is the incidence still increasing? *Ann Surg Oncol* 2004;12:1093.

Hundahl SA, Fleming ID, Fremgen AM, et al. Two hundred eighty-six cases of parathyroid carcinoma treated in the U.S. between 1985–1995: a National Cancer Data Base Report. The American College of Surgeons Commission on Cancer and the American Cancer Society [See comments]. *Cancer* 1999;86:538.

Iacobone M, Lumachi F, Favia G. Up-to-date on parathyroid carcinoma: analysis of an experience of 19 cases. *J Surg Oncol* 2004;88:223.

Kebebew E, Clark OH. Differentiated thyroid cancer:

complete rational approach. *World J Surg* 2000;24:942.

Kenady DE, McGrath PC, Schwartz RW. Treatment of thyroid malignancies. *Curr Opin Oncol* 1991;3:128.

Krubsack AJ, Wilson SD, Lawson TL, et al. Prospective comparison of radionucleotide, computed tomographic, sonographic, and magnetic resonance localization of parathyroid tumors. *Surgery* 1989;106:639.

Learoyd DL, Messina M, Zedenius J, et al. Molecular genetics of thyroid tumors and surgical decision making. *World J Surg* 2000;24:922.

Maffioli L, Steens J, Pauwels E, et al. Applications of 99mTc-sestamibi in oncology. *Tumori* 1996;82:12.

Mazzaferri EL, Jhiang SM. Long-term impact of initial surgical and medical therapy on papillary and follicular thyroid cancer. *Am J Med* 1994;97:418.

Mazzaferri EL, Robyn J. Postsurgical management of differentiated thyroid carcinoma. *Otolaryngol Clin North Am* 1996;29:637.

McLeod MK, Thompson NW. Hürthle cell neoplasm of the thyroid. *Otolaryngol Clin North Am* 1990;23:441.

Merino MJ, Boice JD, Ron E, et al. Thyroid cancer: a lethal endocrine neoplasm. *Ann Intern Med* 1991;115:133.

Moley JF, Wells SA. Compartment-mediated dissection for papillary thyroid cancer. *Langenbeck's Arch Surg* 1999;384:9.

Nel CJC, van Heerden JA, Goellner JR, et al. Anaplastic carcinoma of the thyroid: a clinicopathologic study of 82 cases. *Mayo Clin Proc* 1985;60:51.

Niederle B, Roka R, Schemper M, et al. Surgical treatment of distant metastases in differentiated thyroid cancer: indication and results. *Surgery* 1986;100:1088.

Norton JA. Reoperative parathyroid surgery: indication, intraoperative decision-making and results. *Prog Surg* 1986;18:133.

Obara T, Fujimoto Y. Diagnosis and treatment of patients with parathyroid carcinoma: an update and review. *World J Surg* 1991;15:738.

Obara T, Okamoto T, Kanbe M, et al. Functioning parathyroid carcinoma: clinicopathologic features and rational treatment. *Semin Surg Oncol* 1997;13:134.

Pasieka JL. Anaplastic cancer, lymphoma, and metastases of the thyroid gland. *Surg Oncol Clin North Am* 1998;7:707.

Ron E, Saftlas AF. Head and neck radiation carcinogenesis: epidemiologic evidence. *Head Neck Surg* 1996;115:403.

Rosen IB, Sutcliffe SB, Gospodarowicz MK, et al. The role of surgery in the management of thyroid lymphoma. *Surgery* 1988;104:1095.

Samaan NA, Schultz PN, Hickey RC, et al. The results of various modalities of treatment of well differentiated thyroid carcinoma: a retrospective review of 1599 patients. *J Clin Endocrinol Metab* 1992;75:714.

Sandelin K, Auer G, Bondeson L, et al. Prognostic factor in parathyroid cancer: a review of 95 cases. *World J Surg* 1992;16:724.

Sandelin K, Thompson NW, Bondeson L. Metastatic parathyroid carcinoma: dilemmas in management. *Surgery* 1991;110:978.

Shaha AR. Management of the neck in thyroid cancer. *Otolaryngol Clin North Am* 1998;31:823.

Sherman SI. Adjuvant therapy and long-term management of differentiated thyroid carcinoma. *Semin Surg Oncol* 1999;16:30

Sherman SI. Clinicopathologic staging of differentiated thyroid carcinoma. In: Rose B, ed. *UpToDate in Medicine* [CD-ROM]. Wellesley, Mass: UpToDate; 1997.

Sherman SI. Management of differentiated thyroid carcinoma: an overview. In: Rose B, ed. *UpToDate in Medicine* [CD-ROM]. Wellesley, Mass: UpToDate; 1997.

Sherman SI. Radioiodide treatment of differentiated thyroid cancer. In: Rose B, ed. *UpToDate in Medicine* [CD-ROM]. Wellesley, Mass: UpToDate; 1997.

Sherman SI. Surgery for differentiated thyroid carcinoma. In: Rose B, ed. *UpToDate in Medicine* [CD-ROM]. Wellesley, Mass: UpToDate; 1996.

Sherman SI. Toward a standard clinicopathologic staging approach for differentiated thyroid carcinoma. *Semin Surg Oncol* 1999;16:12.

Shortell CK, Andrus CH, Phillips CE, et al. Carcinoma of the parathyroid gland: a 30-year experience. *Surgery* 1991;110:704.

Thomas CG. Role of thyroid-stimulating hormone suppression in the management of thyroid cancer. *Semin Surg Oncol* 1991;7:115.

Vassilopoulou-Sellin R. Management of papillary thyroid cancer. *Oncology* 1995;9:145.

Woolam GL. Cancer statistics, 2000. *CA Cancer J Clin* 2000;50:7.

Wynne AG, van Heerden JA, Carney JA, et al. Parathyroid carcinoma: clinical and pathological features in 43 patients. *Medicine* 1992;71:197.

Hematologic Malignancies and Splenic Tumors

Wayne A.I. Frederick, Jorge A. Romaguera, James A. Reilly, Jr., and Ana M. Grau

Leukemia and lymphoma account for 6% to 8% of adult cancers and approximately 8% of the deaths from malignancy in the United States. In children younger than 15 years, leukemias are the most common malignancies, with non-Hodgkin's lymphoma (NHL) fourth in frequency. Acute leukemias are the leading cause of cancer deaths in patients younger than 35 years.

Leukemia and lymphoma patients are usually referred to a surgeon with a specific request: diagnostic biopsy, vascular access, and therapeutic splenectomy. Surgeons must be familiar with this group of disorders, both to perform the operation appropriately and to know the procedure's probability of success and risks. At times a major procedure is unlikely to achieve the desired result, or the patient's limited life expectancy makes such an operation unwise.

THE LEUKEMIAS

The chronic proliferative diseases appear to be a spectrum of clonal hematopoietic stem cell disorders ranging in increasing severity from polycythemia vera and essential thrombocythemia to myelogenous metaplasia to chronic myelogenous leukemia (CML). Leukemia ultimately develops in a few patients with polycythemia vera and essential thrombocythemia and a larger percentage of patients with myelogenous metaplasia.

Polycythemia Vera and Essential Thrombocythemia

Polycythemia vera is associated with an autonomous expansion of the red blood cell mass and volume with a variable effect on white blood cells (WBCs) and platelets. The most accepted etiologic mechanism involves the existence of a clone with an abnormally high sensitivity to erythropoietin. Essential thrombocythemia is characterized by an increase in the megakaryocyte lineage, with a greatly increased platelet count and a variable effect on erythrocytes and WBCs. In both diseases there is an increased risk of thrombosis and, paradoxically, of hemorrhage. Three-fourths of patients with polycythemia vera have palpable splenomegaly, and about half have hepatic enlargement. Phlebotomy, low-dose chemotherapy, or a combination of these modalities is the primary treatment for patients with polycythemia vera and essential thrombocythemia. The goal is to obtain a hematocrit of 45% or less. Because of the risk of hemorrhage, any operation should be avoided in these patients until the polycythemia is under control. Rapid phlebotomy to a normal hematocrit and fluid replacement should be performed before emergency surgery. Plateletpheresis has been used to control thrombocytosis.

Although splenectomy has little or no role in the treatment of most patients with polycythemia vera or essential thrombocythemia, a condition similar to myelogenous metaplasia develops in a few patients who then require splenectomy. The operative risks are greater and the survival is poorer in this group than in patients with myelogenous metaplasia. Patients with polycythemia vera and essential thrombocythemia should be treated with aggressive nonoperative therapy and offered splenectomy only when pain, anemia, and thrombocytopenia are refractory to other treatment. Splenectomy does not increase the survival rate, but it may improve the quality of life.

Myelogenous Metaplasia

Myelogenous metaplasia is characterized by fibrosis of the bone marrow and extramedullary hematopoiesis, chiefly in the spleen, liver, and lymph nodes. Fibrosis is polyclonal in nature and is thought to be a reactive process to growth factor release from the clonal cells. As the spleen enlarges, the hematopoietic function it serves may be overwhelmed by destructive hypersplenism (excessive destruction of one or more of the blood components, usually by an autoimmune mechanism).

Although some patients are asymptomatic, most present with fatigue, anorexia, and weight loss, or symptomatic splenomegaly. Leukocytosis and thrombocytosis may be present; other hematologic abnormalities such as diminished WBC and platelet counts may result from passive splenic sequestration or active destruction. Active splenic destruction may be humorally mediated (related to specific antibody recognition) or cell mediated (probably by activated macrophages). Peripheral blood smears often demonstrate large platelets, nucleated red cells, anisocytosis, and immature myelogenous elements. The diagnosis is made by bone marrow biopsy. In approximately 5% of cases, myelogenous metaplasia will progress to CML or acute myeloblastic leukemia.

Initial management may include transfusions, steroids, androgens, cytotoxic chemotherapy, and splenic irradiation. If these measures are not effective in treating the complications of hypersplenism, a splenectomy may be indicated. At the University of Texas M. D. Anderson Cancer Center, patients who have myelogenous metaplasia with myelofibrosis are advised to undergo splenectomy under the following conditions: (a) for severe anemia due to hypersplenism when medical management is unsuccessful; (b) for chronically symptomatic splenomegaly; or (c) for the development of worsening congestive heart failure caused by a shunt effect through the spleen. Splenectomy for portal hypertension secondary to increased portal flow associated with splenomegaly has also been reported. Because splenectomy may inadvertently preclude the possibility of performing a splenorenal shunt, it is critical to eliminate hepatic portal hypertension as the cause of the splenomegaly.

Adequate bone marrow activity must be verified before splenectomy is contemplated. If the spleen is the major site of hematopoiesis, splenectomy may result in severe pancytopenia. A bone marrow biopsy and nuclear medicine bone marrow scan may define the hematopoietic productivity of the marrow cavity. Full coagulation studies should be performed and occult disseminated intravascular coagulation should be controlled before surgery.

Splenectomy does not prolong survival but may improve the quality of life. The response rate for anemia varies from 75% to 95% following splenectomy. The morbidity of splenectomy is 35% to 75%, and the mortality rate is 5% to 18%. Low-dose radiation to the spleen may be used in poor candidates for surgery.

Chronic Myelogenous Leukemia

CML, also known as chronic granulocytic leukemia, involves a clonal proliferation of myelogenous stem cells. Approximately 90% of patients will have a translocation of chromosomes 9 and 22; this translocation is called the *Philadelphia chromosome*. The Philadelphia chromosome may be observed clinically to help assess response to therapy.

CML has both a chronic benign phase and a phase of acute blastic transformation. Most patients present with symptoms of the chronic phase, which include fatigue, weakness, night sweats, low-grade fever, and abdominal pain. Splenomegaly may be an isolated finding during physical examination. The WBC and platelet count may be increased; however, the platelets may not function normally. Hypersplenism may result in anemia or thrombocytopenia. Patients with the chronic phase of CML should be evaluated every 3 to 6 months. The median duration of the chronic phase is about 45 months, but some patients may live up to 20 years with this condition. CML will progress from the chronic benign phase to the acute leukemic transformation phase in approximately 80% of patients.

Progressive fatigue, high fevers, increasingly symptomatic splenomegaly, anemia, thrombocytopenia, basophilia, and bone or joint pain may herald the acute or accelerated stage of CML. In addition to the Philadelphia chromosome, other deletions and translocations may be detected. The WBC count may markedly increase and may not be readily controlled by medical means. Increased splenic destruction of blood components may be manifested by more frequent infections or bleeding episodes. Average survival is approximately 6 months, and during this period the disease may become resistant to chemotherapy. Blast crisis is heralded by large numbers of these immature cells in the circulation, with a decrease in other cellular components; this is usually a preterminal event.

Traditional treatment of CML included conventional chemotherapy with hydroxyurea or busulfan. These agents can achieve hematologic remissions, but no significant reduction of Philadelphia chromosome cells has been observed. Interferon alfa (IFN alfa) can achieve hematologic as well as cytogenetic remissions in a significant number of patients and prolong survival in patients who have shown cytogenetic response. Allogenic bone marrow transplant may be curative, but only a limited number of patients qualify for it.

Splenectomy is generally used as palliation for either painful splenomegaly or refractory anemia. Symptoms due to splenomegaly will likely be improved by splenectomy, but the response is variable when splenectomy is performed to correct dyscrasias. Removal of an enlarged spleen before bone marrow transplantation has failed to improve survival or to decrease the relapse frequency. In these patients, though, splenectomy may eliminate a focus of disease or decrease transfusion requirements. Prospective randomized trials will help define the role of splenectomy in the enhancement of bone marrow engraftment. For patients with CML in whom disease becomes resistant to IFN alfa, a splenectomy may improve response to this therapy. Splenectomy does not delay blast transformation, and its effect on survival is controversial. A recent analysis of the M. D. Anderson experience with splenectomy in patients in the accelerated or blastic phase of the disease has shown that although the survival period in these patients may be limited, splenectomy, if indicated, can be performed safely in this phase of the disease and thrombocytopenia can be reliably reversed, minimizing transfusion requirements.

Chronic Lymphocytic Leukemia

Chronic lymphocytic leukemia (CLL) is the most common leukemia in the Western Hemisphere. It is typified by an accumulation of long-lived, mature-appearing but functionally inactive B cells. The median age of onset is in the seventh decade, and the incidence continues to increase beyond that age.

CLL patients may present with enlarged, painless lymph nodes; weakness; weight loss; and anorexia. As the disease progresses, more pronounced lymphadenopathy and splenomegaly may develop. There may be a decrease in red blood cell count due to either bone marrow infiltration with leukemic cells or a Coombs-positive hemolytic anemia. A second malignancy will develop in approximately 20% of patients, most commonly lung cancer, melanoma, or sarcoma. CLL may have either an indolent or an aggressive course, with patient survival ranging from 1 to 20 years. Patients with CLL have a progressive loss of immune function, and infection is the most common cause of death.

Previously, treatment was withheld in the early stages until signs of progression occurred. Currently, at M. D. Anderson, treatment is not generally started in the Rai stage 0 patients (lymphocytosis only), but chemotherapy is used to treat other early stage patients (Rai stage I or II) with poor prognostic signs and all patients with Rai stage III or IV disease (Table 17.1). Fludarabine is used in conjunction with granulocyte-macrophage colony-stimulating factor. Splenectomy may be recommended for patients who are refractory to fludarabine or with symptomatic splenomegaly and for patients with hypersplenism. Experience at M. D. Anderson has shown that splenectomy can provide an excellent hematologic response in patients with either isolated anemia or thrombocytopenia, but this response is relatively poor in patients presenting with both disorders, suggesting that an adequate hematopoietic reserve is required for a significant response. In addition, splenectomy significantly improves survival in selected subgroups of patients with advanced stage CLL when compared with conventional chemotherapy. These subgroups include patients with CLL and hemoglobin levels less than or equal to 10 g/dL or a platelet count less than or equal to 50×10^9L.

Table 17.1. Rai staging of chronic lymphocytic leukemia

Stage	Criteria
0	Lymphocytosis (WBCs >15,000/mL with >40% lymphocytes in the bone marrow)
I	Lymphocytosis with lymphadenopathy
II	Lymphocytosis with enlarged liver or spleen (lymphadenopathy not necessarily present)
III	Lymphocytosis with anemia. Anemia may be due to hemolysis or to decreased production (lymphadenopathy or hepatosplenomegaly need not be present)
IV	Lymphocytosis with thrombocytopenia (platelet count <100,000/μL), anemia, and lymphadenopathy

WBC, white blood cell.

Hairy Cell Leukemia

Hairy cell leukemia (HCL) is a monoclonal lymphoproliferative disorder of mature B cells. It comprises only 2% to 5% of all leukemias, and there is a 3:1 male predominance. The pathognomonic hairy cells are named for their cytoplasmic projections. These cells may be found in both the bone marrow and the peripheral circulation.

Patients with HCL may complain of weakness and fatigue. Splenomegaly is almost universally present. Approximately 10% of patients with HCL will have such mild symptoms that they never require treatment. Most patients will require therapy for neutropenia, splenomegaly, hypersplenism, or bone marrow failure. Infection related to neutropenia is the most common cause of death.

Early efforts to use chemotherapy to treat HCL were unsuccessful because the degree of associated myelosuppression was not tolerable. Splenectomy became the treatment of choice and was associated with increased survival. Since that time, more effective chemotherapeutic agents have become available. At M. D. Anderson, splenectomy is not used in the routine treatment of patients with HCL. Instead, they are treated with IFN alfa, deoxycoformycin, or chlorodeoxyadenosine. The overall response rate to IFN alfa is between 80% and 90%. If relapse occurs, chlorodeoxyadenosine is usually effective in regaining control of the disease. The few patients who relapse after chlorodeoxyadenosine treatment can achieve second remissions with retreatment. Splenectomy may be considered in the rare cases of pure splenic form of the disease.

Acute Lymphocytic and Myelogenous Leukemia

Except in cases of splenic rupture, splenectomy has no role in the treatment of patients with acute lymphocytic or acute myelogenous leukemia during induction chemotherapy or during relapse. In rare cases, patients in complete remission require splenectomy because of persistent fungal granulomas of the spleen.

Splenic Rupture in Leukemia

Splenic rupture is a rare event in leukemic patients and is almost always associated with some form of trauma. There is no increased risk with any particular type of leukemia, but patients with splenomegaly may be more susceptible to splenic trauma. The reported incidence of rupture from four series was 0.72%. Leukemic patients comprise only 3.5% of those with spontaneous splenic rupture.

Signs and symptoms include abdominal tenderness and rigidity, shifting dullness, and tachycardia. The chest radiograph may demonstrate an elevated hemidiaphragm or a pleural effusion. A high index of suspicion is necessary in evaluating patients with splenomegaly and abdominal pain because the precipitating event may have been so minor as to not be remembered.

Survival rates vary with the rapidity of diagnosis and of performance of splenectomy. Patients who survive splenectomy following rupture have a life expectancy similar to that of other patients with the same type of leukemia.

THE LYMPHOMAS

Hodgkin's Disease

The prognosis of patients with Hodgkin's disease (HD) has improved dramatically over the past 20 years. This advancement is due to increased knowledge of the biology of the disease and more effective use of radiation therapy and multiagent chemotherapy. The role of staging laparotomy continues to evolve as nonoperative staging becomes increasingly accurate and as subsets of patients are identified who are unlikely to benefit from the information laparotomy provides.

HD is characterized by the presence of multinucleated Reed-Sternberg (RS) cells or one of their variants. As opposed to NHL, in which a monoclonal population of malignant lymphocytes usually predominates, in HD the malignant cells are a minority population outnumbered by inflammatory cells.

Patients with HD typically present with nontender lymphadenopathy. The cervical nodes are most commonly involved; other regions, which include the axillary, inguinal, mediastinal, and retroperitoneal nodes are less frequently affected at presentation. The presence or absence of B symptoms should be elucidated from the patient's history. B symptoms include any one of the following: unexplained fever with temperature over 38°C, night sweats significant enough to require changing bed clothes, or weight loss of more than 10% of body weight over 6 months. Although classic for HD, the Pel-Ebstein fever, with progressively shortening intervals between fevers, is a relatively rare phenomenon.

The physical examination should include an evaluation of all lymph node–bearing areas, including Waldeyer's tonsillar ring, and palpation for liver or splenic enlargement. Initial workup should include a complete blood cell count with differential count, liver function tests, and a chest radiograph. A bone marrow biopsy is useful to determine the extent of the disease. Excisional biopsy of the largest node that is likely to provide the diagnosis should be performed. Careful selection of the biopsy site is important

Table 17.2. Ann Arbor staging system for Hodgkin's disease

Stage	Criteria
I	Involvement of a single lymph node region (I) or a single extralymphatic organ or site (IE)
II	Involvement of two or more lymph node regions on the same side of the diaphragm (II) or of an extralymphatic organ and its adjoining lymph node site (IIE)
III	Involvement of lymph node sites on both sides of the diaphragm (III) or localized involvement of an extra-lymphatic site (IIIE), spleen (IIIS), or both (IIISE)
IV	Diffuse or disseminated involvement of one or more extralymphatic organs with or without associated lymph node involvement
A	Asymptomatic
B	Fever, night sweats, or weight loss of more than 10%

because some areas, particularly the inguinal region, frequently contain nondiagnostic inflammatory nodes.

Other clinical staging tools include computed tomography (CT), nuclear medicine scans, and bipedal lymphangiography. CT is used to detect mediastinal and abdominal lymphatic enlargement; however, nodes containing HD often are not enlarged. Gallium scans have been useful in detecting residual disease. Bipedal lymphangiography may detect changes in femoral, inguinal, external iliac, and retroperitoneal nodes. Use of lymphangiography has been questioned in terms of the cost-effectiveness. This procedure can identify lymphatic enlargement as well as changes in the architecture of normal-sized nodes caused by neoplastic involvement.

The prognosis of patients with HD depends on the histologic subtype and stage of disease at presentation. The Rye modification of the Lukes-Butler classification of HD identifies four histologic subtypes: lymphocyte predominant, nodular sclerosis, mixed cellularity, and lymphocyte depleted. These subtypes are determined by the specific variant of RS cell, the ratio of these cells to the normal population, and the degree of sclerosis.

The Ann Arbor staging system (Table 17.2) is used for staging HD based on the extent of disease. Clinical staging includes all data from the history and physical examination and nonoperative diagnostic studies. Pathologic staging includes additional information obtained from a staging laparotomy. The Ann Arbor stages are subclassified to reflect lymphatic disease and involvement of extranodal areas designated by *E,* for involvement of an extralymphatic site (i.e., stomach or small intestine), or *S,* for splenic involvement. Disease is further subclassified according to the presence or absence of systemic symptoms of the disease.

Increasing knowledge of the effect of patient characteristics, histologic subtype, and stage of disease have allowed more individualized treatment of patients, with dramatic improvements in survival. Staging laparotomy was first introduced to define disease extent in all presentations of HD. Subsequently, investigators performed staging by laparotomy to determine which patients had early stage disease that could be treated by local irradiation and which had extensive disease requiring systemic therapy. Previously, up to 40% of patients who underwent staging laparotomy had a change in their clinical stage. Both improvements in the accuracy of radiologic diagnostic procedures and more intensive use of chemotherapeutic and radiation treatments earlier in the course of the disease have decreased the number of patients who require staging laparotomy.

Currently at M. D. Anderson, nonoperative staging and prognostic factors are used to guide therapy in almost all the patients. Patients who require chemotherapy with or without radiation therapy because of extensive disease or poor prognostic factors do not benefit from the additional information gained from a staging laparotomy. Most centers have eliminated staging laparotomy in pediatric patients with HD. This approach is supported by failure of long-term follow-up to show a significant difference in survival between clinical and surgical staging.

Components of a Staging Laparotomy

For staging laparotomy of HD, the abdomen is entered through a midline incision from the xiphoid process to below the umbilicus. A thorough exploration is performed to identify palpable abnormalities. This includes bimanual palpation of the liver, examination of the bowel and mesentery, and exploration of the major nodal groups. Lymph nodes containing disease are often normal in size. The areas most likely to contain disease include the spleen and the splenic, celiac, and portal lymph nodes.

Splenectomy and liver biopsies are performed early in the procedure so that ample time is available to ensure hemostasis. The spleen should routinely be removed because it may contain nonpalpable disease. In children, some surgeons advocate performing a partial splenectomy to prevent a lifetime risk of asplenic sepsis. Splenic nodes, along with the distal 3 cm of the splenic artery and vein, should be removed in continuity with the spleen. The ends of the splenic vessels are marked with titanium clips to guide future radiation therapy if it becomes necessary.

A wedge biopsy specimen is obtained from one or both lobes of the liver, and a deeper biopsy with a Tru-cut core needle is done on both lobes. Additional wedge biopsies should be performed on any grossly abnormal areas of the liver.

As each nodal group is dissected, it is sent as a separate specimen in sterile saline to the pathologist, and the area is marked with titanium clips. The gastrohepatic ligament is incised, and lymph nodes along the hepatic artery leading to the celiac axis are removed. The sentinel node at the junction of the portal vein and the duodenum, along with any other nodes along the porta hepatis, are excised. The transverse colon is retracted superiorly, and the small bowel is reflected to the patient's right to visualize the aorta. The retroperitoneum is incised over the aorta from the left renal vein down to the iliac bifurcation. The nodes between the aorta and the inferior mesenteric vein are excised. Nodes along the iliac vessels and within the mesentery seldom contain disease, but they should be sampled and submitted for review. Any lymph nodes that appeared abnormal on the lymphangiogram should also be removed.

If a bone marrow biopsy specimen has not been obtained preoperatively, one should be obtained from the iliac crest while the patient is under general anesthesia. Oophoropexy was once routinely performed in females of reproductive age, but currently its use is limited to patients with suspected iliac nodal involvement. Some surgeons recommend performing appendectomy during the staging procedure.

The morbidity rate is generally less than 10%, and deaths related to staging laparotomy are rare. Complications include wound problems, atelectasis, pneumonia, pulmonary embolus, and infection. Any complications that delay the initiation of needed systemic therapy or radiation therapy are potentially serious. Long-term complications include small-bowel adhesions, asplenic sepsis, and development of secondary leukemia.

Laparoscopic staging of lymphoma is currently being explored as a modality in the treatment of these patients. Case reports and small series of lymphoma patients staged laparoscopically have been reported in the literature. The indications have been the same as those for open staging, and absolute contraindications are portal hypertension and uncorrectable coagulopathy. The components of laparoscopic staging include percutaneous and wedge liver biopsies, lymph node biopsies, and splenectomy. Because the spleen needs to be removed intact to allow complete pathologic evaluation, a 6- to 8-cm midline incision is made to allow removal of the spleen. This midline incision is then used to complete the lymph node dissection under direct vision. Conversion to open procedure has most frequently been secondary to hemorrhage during splenectomy and varies from 0% to 20%. Diagnostic accuracy has been reported to be close to 90%. Laparoscopic staging of lymphoma may result in a shorter hospital stay and recovery time, but the accuracy and morbidity of this technique cannot be known until more experience is available.

Non-Hodgkin's Lymphoma

Patients in the United States with NHL characteristically have a monoclonal proliferation of lymphocytes, with 80% of cases being of B-cell derivation and the remainder originating from T cells. The diagnosis of various subsets of B-cell NHL depends on the identification of histopathologic markers using monoclonal antibodies and on cellular morphology; criteria assessed are a diffuse versus follicular (nodular) pattern of lymph node involvement, small versus large cell type, and cleaved versus noncleaved nuclear morphology. With this information, the lymphoma can be categorized according to the Working Formulation, which is a modification of the Lukes and Collins schema. Although an in-depth discussion of this classification system is beyond the scope of this chapter, the Working Formulation has simplified our understanding of the behaviors of these subtypes by placing them into one of three categories, depending on whether patients have a low, intermediate, or high risk of death due to the disease. The T-cell NHLs are much more difficult to identify precisely and to place into prognostic groups. More recently, the proposed

European-American classification of lymphoid neoplasms uses morphology, phenotype, and cytogenetics to classify these disorders. The clinical relevance of this classification is under study, but it might offer additional information to the Working Formulation.

Most patients with NHL present with superficial adenopathy, most commonly in the cervical lymph nodes. These nodes are generally enlarged and not tender. The Ann Arbor system (Table 17.2) is used to stage these patients, but it is less helpful in NHL than in HD because more than half of NHL patients present with stage III or IV disease and approximately 20% present with B symptoms. Patients with NHL also are more likely to have hematogenous spread versus lymphatic spread as seen in patients with HD.

Because NHLs do not spread in the orderly manner that HD does, the surgeon is generally asked to perform a diagnostic biopsy, to establish vascular access for chemotherapy, or to treat complications of therapy. Staging laparotomy is not indicated in these patients. Splenectomy is necessary, although rarely, for hypersplenism, massive splenomegaly, or a persistent splenic focus of disease, usually in those with low-grade lymphomas. Although primary splenic lymphoma is unusual, splenectomy may be beneficial for patients with isolated splenic disease. This diagnosis is often made only after splenectomy is performed for hypersplenism or splenomegaly. If the lymphoma is localized to the spleen, the prognosis is similar to that of other stage I patients.

Diagnostic Biopsy for Lymphoma

When lymphoma is suspected, proper planning and execution of the biopsy are crucial to enable the pathologist to make a diagnosis. Because preservation of the architecture aids in histologic diagnosis, efforts should be made to avoid traction or cautery. The largest node found on physical examination should be biopsied. If several nodal areas are enlarged, biopsy of the cervical area is preferred to biopsy of an axillary node, which in turn is superior to biopsy of nodes from the inguinal region. In suspected extranodal disease or in the case of matted nodes, it is important to excise as generous an amount of tissue as possible. Communication with the pathologist is important to guarantee that adequate tissue is sent and that it is delivered in an acceptable fashion. In general, the specimen is sent fresh, is sent in saline, or is wrapped in a saline-soaked sponge. It is important that the specimen be sent directly to the pathologist and that there is an indication that the diagnosis of lymphoma is suspected. Needle biopsies rarely provide an adequate amount of tissue, although they may be helpful in ruling out a carcinoma or sarcoma or in suspected relapse of lymphoma when a tissue diagnosis is needed before treatment.

MISCELLANEOUS SPLENIC TUMORS

Splenic Cysts

A splenic cyst may be confused with a neoplastic process when detected as a palpable abnormality or an unexpected radiologic finding. Patients often present with vague symptoms, possibly due to cyst enlargement. Although parasitic cysts are extremely rare in the United States, they are more common outside this country. Parasitic cysts are most commonly due to an echinococcal infection. Nonparasitic cysts comprise 75% of splenic cysts in the United States and are classified as primary if they have a true cellular lining or secondary if they lack this layer. Primary splenic cysts may be congenital, due to an embryologic remnant or neoplastic cyst. The neoplastic cysts include epidermoid cysts, dermoid cysts, lymphangiomas, and cavernous hemangiomas. Secondary cysts are the more common type of nonparasitic cyst and are thought to be the result of splenic injury and resultant hematoma.

Splenic cysts rarely require treatment unless they become infected, hemorrhage, or perforate. Treatment may consist of a partial or total splenectomy; marsupialization or drainage procedures should be avoided.

Inflammatory Pseudotumor

Inflammatory pseudotumor, also known as plasma cell granuloma, has histologic features of inflammation and mesenchymal repair. Such masses can be found in various locations in the body, including the respiratory system, gastrointestinal tract, orbit, and lymph nodes. When a pseudotumor is detected in the spleen, it may be mistaken for lymphoma. Pseudotumors are thought to occur at sites of previous trauma or infection. Unfortunately, the definitive diagnosis can be made only after excision. Immunohistochemical stains and flow cytometry studies of the specimen may be useful to rule out a lymphoproliferative disorder.

Nonlymphoid Tumors

The spleen is involved with various benign and malignant nonlymphoid tumors. Benign vascular tumors include hemangioma, lymphangioma, and hemangioendothelioma. Lipoma and angiomyolipoma are also encountered. Angiosarcoma of the spleen confers a poor prognosis; this tumor has been associated with exposure to thorium dioxide, vinyl chloride, and arsenic. Kaposi's sarcoma may be found as an isolated process in the spleen. Other splenic sarcomas, including malignant fibrous histiocytoma, fibrosarcoma, and leiomyosarcoma, are extremely rare.

Splenic Metastasis

Considering the large percentage of the total blood flow that supplies the spleen, it is a surprisingly rare site for metastasis. In autopsy series of cancer patients, the finding of metastasis involving the spleen ranges from 1.6% to 30%. Splenic metastasis is rarely a clinically relevant problem. Melanoma, breast, and lung cancer are the most frequently detected metastases. Splenomegaly is an unusual finding with solitary metastasis. Several small series have reported the use of splenectomy for an isolated splenic metastasis. Resection with curative intent is rarely possible with splenic metastasis, but splenectomy may be necessary for complications such as perforation, splenic vein thrombosis, and growth into adjacent viscera.

SPLENECTOMY

Splenectomy for Hypersplenism

Anemia, neutropenia, and thrombocytopenia may occur for a number of reasons in patients with hematologic malignancies. Because only patients with excessive destruction of a blood component will benefit from a splenectomy, a careful workup should be done to identify the etiology of the process. Patients with hypersplenism may present with a normal-sized spleen, and others may have massive splenomegaly without hypersplenism.

Infusion of the patient's or normal donor platelets tagged with ^{111}indium is helpful in determining whether the spleen is the site of destruction. Patients with an acquired hemolytic anemia generally have a positive Coombs' test, and the detection of the warm antibody is a good indication that splenectomy will be beneficial. Although chromium-labeled red blood cell scans may be useful in demonstrating decreases in red blood cell survival, they are not as helpful in identifying the site of sequestration. In cases of suspected splenic sequestration, a bone marrow biopsy is important to determine whether adequate precursor cells are available or whether the patient depends on the hematopoietic activity of the spleen.

Splenectomy in patients with CML has been associated with severe bleeding problems. These may be related to impaired clot formation caused by proteases and serases produced by granulocytes. Patients with CML and severe leukocytosis should receive chemotherapy in an attempt to decrease the WBC count to approximately 20,000 cells/mL. Experience at M. D. Anderson suggests that splenectomy is best avoided in patients with CML in whom WBC counts cannot be controlled with chemotherapy. Splenectomy should also be avoided in patients with CML who have had splenic irradiation.

Bleeding and infection are the greatest perioperative risks. Qualitative platelet function should be evaluated rather than relying on a platelet count. The template bleeding time is currently the most widely available laboratory value for identifying adequacy of platelet function. The patient's current and recent medications should be carefully reviewed to identify any drugs that may impair coagulation. Because of potential bleeding problems associated with certain antibiotics, prophylactic coverage must be carefully chosen to avoid increasing the risk of hemorrhage.

Although splenectomy may be performed through either a midline or a subcostal approach, the midline incision is preferred when coagulation defects, thrombocytopenia, or splenomegaly is present. After the splenic pedicle is clamped, thrombocytopenic patients are transfused with fresh single-donor platelets to achieve a platelet count of more than 60,000 cells/mL. Careful hemostasis at the conclusion of the procedure is mandatory. Postoperatively, patients should be monitored closely during the first 48 hours for signs of bleeding. A blood cell count with differential and platelet counts should be obtained every 6 hours for the first 24 hours after the operation. Decreasing platelet and blood counts, despite adequate replacement, suggest an ongoing bleeding process.

Splenectomy for the Massively Enlarged Spleen

Indications for splenectomy in patients with massively enlarged spleens include debilitating symptoms of splenomegaly, excessive destruction of blood components, and concerns of possible splenic rupture. These patients often complain of chronic severe upper abdominal and back pain, impaired respiration, and early satiety. Hypersplenism may be present. Depending on the size of the spleen and the body habitus, the patient may be judged to be at increased risk of splenic trauma.

Preoperatively, it is important to check quantitative and qualitative platelet function values and coagulation studies because hemorrhage is the major complication of splenectomy in this group. Portal venous contrast studies should be performed in patients with possible portal hypertension. If the splenic vein is thrombosed, splenectomy is appropriate, but otherwise it may deprive a patient with portal hypertension of the option of a splenorenal shunt.

Adequate blood products must be available preoperatively. The blood of these patients may be difficult to crossmatch because of numerous past transfusions, and fresh single-donor platelets may be required. Patients should undergo routine bowel preparation, and prophylactic antibiotics should be given.

A midline, rather than subcostal, incision is preferred because the rectus muscles are not severed, which limits bleeding. With increasing size, the spleen becomes more of a midline structure and lends itself to this approach. Before mobilization of the spleen, its vessels should be isolated. The gastrocolic omentum is divided, the lesser sac is entered, and the splenic artery is identified along the posterior-superior surface of the pancreas. The artery is ligated but left intact. The splenic vein is not disturbed yet. The spleen may decrease 20% to 30% in size at this point and allow platelet transfusion without consumption. The splenic flexure of the colon is mobilized, the splenic ligaments are divided, and the spleen is delivered from the splenic fossa. The normally avascular splenic ligaments often contain small vessels in the presence of hematologic malignancies. Dense adhesions between the spleen and the diaphragm may complicate mobilization, and when dissection is particularly difficult, it is better to resect part of the diaphragm with the spleen than to risk hypertrophy of splenic remnants. Such adhesions are formed in areas of splenic infarction and are the most frequent sites of postoperative bleeding in this group of patients.

After the spleen is mobilized, the artery and vein are suture ligated and divided. Liver biopsy may be indicated if involvement by lymphoma is suspected. If an injury to the pancreatic tail is recognized, it should be repaired and drained appropriately. Achieving hemostasis in the splenic bed is crucial and may require suture ligation, cautery, platelet transfusions, and thrombostatic agents. Drains do not reliably warn of postoperative hemorrhage or prevent infection, and except in cases of pancreatic injury, they are not routinely used. Postoperatively, patients should be closely monitored for signs of bleeding or infection.

Laparoscopic Splenectomy

Laparoscopic splenectomy has been used safely in patients with benign hematologic conditions. Recently there has been increasing implementation of this surgical method in splenomegaly in patients with malignant hematologic diseases. The advantages appear to be a quicker recovery and resultant decreased healthcare costs. Prospective randomized trials are required to confirm these observations. To allow adequate pathologic examination of the specimen, the spleen needs to be removed intact through a small incision.

Prophylaxis for Asplenic Sepsis

Patients with hematologic malignancies who undergo splenectomy are at greater risk for asplenic sepsis than are those who have the procedure for other indications. Some patients with hematologic malignancy, especially those with CML and CLL, are at increased risk for sepsis even before splenectomy. The risk of overwhelming postsplenectomy infection (OPSI) is greatest for children. The expected death rate from OPSI in children is one in every 300 to 350 patient-years, and in adults, one in every 800 to 1,000 patient-years. For all patients, the risk is greatest for the first few years following splenectomy, but deaths attributed to OPSI have occurred 30 or more years after splenectomy.

Following splenectomy, there is loss of the opsonins, tuftsin and properdin, a decrease in immunoglobulin M production, impaired phagocytosis, and altered cellular immunity. Poorly opsonized bacteria are best cleared by the spleen, and following the spleen's removal patients are particularly susceptible to the encapsulated bacteria.

Vaccination can decrease the risk of postsplenectomy pneumococcal infection. The 23-valent form of the pneumococcal vaccine should be used. The vaccine is most effective when given several weeks preoperatively. Nevertheless, despite the diminished immunity obtained if the vaccine is given after splenectomy, adequate protection is still achieved in most patients. In patients who are not immunized preoperatively there is no benefit from delaying the immunization for several weeks after surgery, so these patients should be vaccinated without delay. Leukemic patients may not be able to develop antibodies in response to pneumococcal vaccine, but it may still be worthwhile to vaccinate this group. Booster immunizations with the pneumococcal vaccine have no proven benefit, although reimmunization at 3 to 5 years may be required if a decrease in specific antibody levels is documented. Certain subsets of patients are at increased risk of infection with *Haemophilus influenzae* and *Neisseria meningitidis* and, therefore, patients should receive these vaccinations as well. Patients are also instructed to keep a supply of antibiotics such as amoxicillin and Augmentin (amoxicillin; clavulanate potassium) with them, which should be taken at the first sign of a febrile episode. This should also be followed by immediate contact with a physician.

Long-term use of prophylactic oral antibiotics is often recommended in the pediatric population or in patients who may have difficulty reaching a physician. Penicillin is commonly prescribed to these patients. Data have shown benefit of prophylactic penicillin in preventing pneumococcal infection in children with sickle cell disease, but the benefit of this practice has never been proved for other subsets of asplenic patients.

RECOMMENDED READING

Berman RS, Yahanda AM, Mansfield PF, et al. Laparoscopic splenectomy in patients with hematologic malignancies. *Am J Surg* 1999;178:530–536.

Bouroncle BA. Thirty-five years in the progress of hairy cell leukemia. *Leuk Lymphoma* 1994;14:1.

Bouvet M, Babiera GV, Termuhlen PM, et al. Splenectomy in the accelerated or blastic phase of chronic myelogenous leukemia: a single institution, 25-year experience. *Surgery* 1997;122:20.

Brenner B, Nagler A, Tatarsky I, et al. Splenectomy in agnogenic myelogenous metaplasia and postpolycythemic myelogenous metaplasia. *Arch Intern Med* 1988;148:2501.

Canady MR, Welling RE, Strobel SL, et al. Splenic rupture in leukemia. *J Surg Oncol* 1989;41:194.

Carde P, Hagenbeek A, Hayat M, et al. Clinical staging versus laparotomy and combined modality with MOPP versus ABVD in early-stage Hodgkin's disease: the H6 twin randomized trials from the European Organization for Research and Treatment of Cancer Lymphoma Cooperative group. *J Clin Oncol* 1993;11:2258.

Coad JE, Matutes E, Catovsky D. Splenectomy in lymphoproliferative disorders: a report on 70 cases and review of the literature. *Leuk Lymphoma* 193;10:245.

Cortes J, Talpaz M, Kantarjian H. Chronic myelogenous leukemia: a review. *Am J Med* 1996;100:555.

Cusack JC, Seymour JF, Lerner S, et al. The role of splenectomy in chronic lymphocytic leukemia. *J Am Coll Surg* 1997;185:237.

Dawes LG, Malangoni MA. Cystic masses of the spleen. *Am Surg* 1986;52:333.

Edwards MJ, Balch CM. Surgical aspects of lymphoma. *Adv Surg* 1989;22:225.

Farrar WB, Kim JA. Biopsy techniques to establish diagnosis and type of malignant lymphoma. *Surg Oncol Clin North Am* 1993;2:159.

Feldman EJ, Arlin ZA. Modern management of chronic myelogenous leukemia (CML). *Cancer Invest* 1988;6:737.

Fielding AK. Prophylaxis against late infection following splenectomy and bone marrow transplant. *Blood Rev* 1994;8:179.

Flexner JM, Stein RS, Greer JP. Outline of treatment of lymphoma based on hematologic and clinical stage with expected end results. *Surg Oncol Clin North Am* 1993;2:283.

Hagemeister FB, Fuller LM, Martin RG. Staging laparotomy: findings and applications to treatment decisions. In: Fuller L, ed. *Hodgkin's disease and non-Hodgkin's lymphoma in adults and children*. New York: Raven, 1988.

Harris NL. The pathology of lymphomas: a practical approach to diagnosis and classification. *Surg Oncol Clin North Am* 1993;2:167.

Hubbard SM, Longo DL. Treatment-related morbidity in patients with lymphoma. *Curr Opin Oncol* 1991;3:852.

Johnson HA, Deterling RA. Massive splenomegaly. *Surg Gynecol Obstet* 1989;168:131.

Kalhs P, Schwarzinger I, Anderson G, et al. A retrospective analysis of the long-term effect of splenectomy on late infections, graft-versus-host disease, relapse, and survival after allogenic marrow transplantation for chronic myelogenous leukemia. *Blood* 1995;86:2028.

Kantarjian HM, Smith TL, O'Brien S, et al. Prolonged survival in chronic myelogenous leukemia after cytogenetic response to interferon-a therapy. *Ann Intern Med* 1995;122:254.

Klein B, Stein M, Kuten A, et al. Splenomegaly and solitary spleen metastasis in solid tumors. *Cancer* 1987;60:100.

Kluin-Nelemans HC, Noordijk EM. Staging of patients with Hodgkin's disease: what should be done? *Leukemia* 1991;4:132.

Kraus MD, Fleming MD, Vonderhide RH. The spleen as a diagnostic specimen: a review of 10 years' experience at two tertiary care institutions. *Cancer* 2001; 91:11.

Kurzrock R, Talpaz M, Gutterman JU. Hairy cell leukaemia: review of treatment. *Br J Haematol* 1991;79(suppl 1):17.

McBride CM, Hester JP. Chronic myelogenous leukemia: management of splenectomy in a high-risk population. *Cancer* 1977;39:653.

Morgenstern L, Rosenberg J, Geller SA. Tumors of the spleen. *World J Surg* 1985;9:468.

Mower WR, Hawkins JA, Nelson EW. Postsplenectomy infection in patients with chronic leukemia. *Am J Surg* 1986;152:583.

Noordijk EM, Carde P, Mandard AM, et al. Preliminary results of the EORTC-GPMC controlled clinical trial H7 in early stage Hodgkin's disease. *Ann Oncol* 1994;5(suppl 2):107.

Parker SL, Tong T, Bolden S, et al. Cancer statistics 1997. *CA* 1997;47:5.

Pittaluga S, Bijnens L, Teodorovic A, et al. Clinical analysis of 670 cases in two trials of the European Organization for the Research and Treatment of Cancer Lymphoma Cooperative Group subtyped according to the Revised European-American Classification of lymphoid neoplasms: a comparison with the Working Formulation. *Blood* 1996;10:4358.

Pollock R, Hohn D. Splenectomy. In: Roh MS, Ames FC, eds. *Advanced oncologic surgery*. New York: Mosby-Wolfe, 1994.

Shaw JHF, Print CG. Postsplenectomy sepsis. *Br J Surg* 1989;76:1074.

Schrenk P, Wayand W. Value of diagnostic laparoscopy in abdominal malignancies. *Int Surg* 1995;80:353.

Styrt B. Infection associated with asplenia: risks, mechanisms, and prevention. *Am J Med* 1990;88:33N.

Tefferi A, Silverstein MN, Noel P. Agnogenic myelogenous metaplasia. *Semin Oncol* 1995; 22:327.

Wiernik PH, Rader M, Becker NH, et al. Inflammatory pseudotumor of spleen. *Cancer* 1990;66:597.

Cancer of Unknown Primary Site

Gauri R. Varadhachary

Cancer of unknown primary site (CUP) is a heterogeneous group that comprises 3% to 5% of new cancer diagnoses and can be difficult to evaluate and treat. Although chemotherapy is the primary treatment modality in patients with CUP, the surgeon frequently plays an important role in both the diagnosis and the treatment of these patients. In particular, surgeons are often asked to evaluate patients with cancer that has spread to a lymph node, the liver, or the peritoneal cavity.

In this chapter, we define the presentation and clinical features of CUP, outline a practical approach to the diagnostic evaluation of patients with CUP, and discuss the role of surgery in various clinical scenarios.

DEFINITION AND GENERAL CONSIDERATIONS

CUP is defined by the presence of a biopsy-proven cancer for which the anatomical origin of the primary tumor is not revealed after a thorough medical history and physical examination (including breast and pelvic examination in women, and testicular and prostate examination in men), routine laboratory tests, chest X-ray, computed tomography (CT) of the abdomen and pelvis, mammography in women, and prostate-specific antigen (PSA) test in men. This definition of CUP is not always used consistently and varies depending on the extent of the evaluation. The prevailing hypothesis in CUP is that the primary tumor either remains microscopic and escapes clinical detection or disappears after seeding the metastasis, which may be due to angiogenic incompetency of the primary tumor.

These tumors often are grouped according to histologic subtype. The major subtypes include squamous cell cancer, adenocarcinoma, and undifferentiated neoplasms, the name given to a heterogeneous group of tumors of various cell origins. Table 18.1 lists the frequencies of each subtype (adenocarcinoma is the most common).

As found in large series, the most common locations of CUP metastases are the lymph nodes, bones, lungs, and liver. Other metastatic sites include the peritoneum, brain, meninges, pleura, subcutaneous tissues, adrenal glands, kidney, and pancreas.

In most patients, the site of origin of the metastatic disease is never discerned. In others, the primary tumor site from which the metastases are derived is eventually identified through exhaustive search during clinical examinations, surgery, or autopsy. In only 25% of CUP cases is the primary site identifiable during the patient's lifetime; this number is probably lower with sophisticated imaging techniques (where baseline studies have been negative). Metastases from squamous cell cancers typically

Table 18.1. Histopathological subtypes of cancer of unknown primary site

Histopathology	Percentage of CUP Patients
Adenocarcinoma	60
Squamous cell carcinoma	5
Poorly differentiated adenocarcinoma	35
Poorly differentiated carcinoma	
Poorly differentiated neoplasm	
Unclassified neoplasm	

CUP, cancer of unknown primary site.

originate in the head and neck region or the lungs, whereas metastatic adenocarcinomas originate in the lungs, breasts, thyroid gland, pancreas, liver, stomach, colon, or rectum.

The median survival of patients with CUP is 6 to 9 months. Specific subgroups of patients with metastatic CUP have considerably better prognoses than the group as a whole, with appropriate therapy. This includes patients with squamous cell cancer metastatic to cervical lymph nodes, women with metastatic adenocarcinoma in axillary lymph nodes, men with undifferentiated cancer and elevated β-human chorionic gonadotropin (β-hCG) or alpha-fetoprotein (AFP) levels, women with peritoneal carcinomatosis, and patients with neuroendocrine CUP. These subgroups are discussed later in this chapter in more detail.

The therapeutic goal in evaluating patients with CUP is to identify those tumor types for which a cure is possible or adequate disease control and palliation is likely, as well as any symptoms for which localized therapy may be effective.

HISTORY AND PHYSICAL EXAMINATION

In patients with CUP, a complete medical history and physical examination are essential. An individual history of malignancy or a family history of cancer may guide the surgeon in establishing the site of an occult primary tumor. Often, symptoms related to CUP are of relatively recent onset (<3 months), and rapid progression of disease and performance status are crucial factors in individualizing treatment decisions.

During physical examination of a patient with CUP, several anatomical sites warrant particular attention. The head and neck should be examined thoroughly, particularly when a diagnosis of squamous cell cancer has been made. This includes examination of the oropharynx, hypopharynx, nasopharynx, and larynx, typically assisted by indirect or fiberoptic laryngoscopy. The thyroid gland should be examined for enlargement or asymmetry. All nodal basins, including those of the head and neck and the supraclavicular, axillary, and inguinal regions, should be examined for palpable or enlarged lymph nodes.

In women, a careful breast examination and a thorough bimanual pelvic examination should be performed. For men, testicular and prostate examinations are particularly important. All patients should undergo a thorough skin examination and rectal examination.

LABORATORY STUDIES

Routine complete blood cell count, blood chemistry studies, liver function tests, and urinalysis should be performed in all patients, and stool should be checked for occult blood. Beyond these basic tests, the clinical laboratory has limited usefulness in the diagnostic evaluation of patients with CUP, but additional studies should be requested on the basis of histologic and radiologic findings.

RADIOGRAPHIC EVALUATION

Radiographic evaluations of patients with CUP should be focused on identifying the primary tumor and delineating the extent of metastatic disease.

Chest X-ray and Computed Tomography Scan of the Chest

A chest X-ray is indicated for all patients to assess the presence of pulmonary metastases or a primary tumor, as well as for preoperative evaluation. If a patient has pulmonary symptoms, an abnormal chest x-ray, or positive sputum cytologic findings, a CT scan of the chest is indicated. In practice, most physicians order it as part of a body imaging study.

Computed Tomography Scan of the Abdomen and Pelvis

CT scan of the abdomen and pelvis is essential because it can help in locating the primary tumor, evaluating the extent of disease, and selecting the most favorable biopsy site. In a study by Abbruzzese et al. of patients who underwent CT scans of the abdomen and pelvis, a primary tumor was found in 179 of 879 patients (20%). In a retrospective study by McMillan et al., in 21 of 46 patients (46%), a primary tumor was detected on CT scan, and previously unsuspected metastatic disease was detected in 30 (65%) patients. CT was superior to sonography and to contrast studies of the urinary and gastrointestinal tracts in localizing the primary site.

Mammography

Women of childbearing age or older, particularly those with metastatic adenocarcinoma, should undergo mammography. Unfortunately, identifying subtle radiographic abnormalities is difficult in younger women, who often have extremely dense breast tissue. Magnetic resonance imaging (MRI) of the breast is indicated in women who present with isolated axillary adenopathy (if the mammogram and breast sonographic findings are negative).

Magnetic Resonance Imaging

In most cases, MRI is indicated if CT is contraindicated. Its most defined role in CUP is in women who present with isolated axillary lymph node metastases and suspected occult primary breast carcinoma. The results of several studies suggest that MRI of the breast can help with tumor detection in up to 75% of patients. This result can influence surgical management, with a negative breast MRI predicting a low yield at mastectomy.

Positron Emission Tomography

The role of positron emission tomography (PET) scan using 18F-fluoro-2-deoxy-D-glucose (18F-FDG PET) is controversial. PET imaging is recommended in patients with occult primary head and neck cancer (cervical CUP) and in those who present with a solitary potentially resectable CUP lesion. Several recent small studies have described the role of PET in patients who present with cervical CUP. The advantages of locating the primary tumor in patients who present with cervical lymphadenopathy (occult head and neck cancer) are (a) smaller postoperative radiation ports, which can decrease early and late complications; (b) better surveillance for recurrence; and (c) improved prognostic determination. Rusthoven et al. reviewed 16 studies (1994–2003) of 302 patients with cervical lymph node metastases from unknown primary tumors. Conventional workup included either panendoscopy, CT, or MRI, and, in 10 of these 16 studies, both tests were performed before diagnosis. They reported the overall sensitivity, specificity, and accuracy rates of FDG PET in detecting unknown primary tumors as 88.3%, 74.9%, and 78.8%, respectively. Approximately 25% of primary tumors that were not apparent after conventional workup were able to be identified on 18F-FDG PET, as were previously undetected regional or distant metastases in 27% of patients.

In general, an exhaustive search for the primary tumor site in these patients by radiographic evaluation can be expensive, inconvenient, and traumatic for patients and often has no significant effect on patients' therapy or the ultimate course of their disease.

PATHOLOGICAL EVALUATION

Fine-needle aspiration (FNA) biopsy has largely replaced core biopsy as a first pathological test. This can be followed by core biopsy, incisional biopsy, or excisional biopsy as needed for specific histologic types. Good communication between the clinician and the pathologist is important because details of the medical history and physical examination can influence the pathological review and facilitate submission of additional tissue if necessary for an accurate diagnosis.

Light Microscopy

Light microscopy (hematoxylin and eosin staining) is ordinarily sufficient to determine the cell of origin. About 60% of CUPs are found to be adenocarcinoma on light microscopy. An additional 5% are squamous cell carcinoma, and the remaining 35% are diagnosed as poorly differentiated adenocarcinoma, poorly differentiated carcinoma, or poorly differentiated neoplasm. Electron microscopy, which helps identify the ultrastructural features of the cell of origin, is rarely needed. For example, desmosomes and intracellular bridges are associated with squamous cell cancer, whereas tight junctions, microvilli, and acinar spaces are associated with adenocarcinoma. Premelanosomes are associated with melanoma, and neurosecretory granules are associated with small cell or neuroendocrine tumors. Lymphoma is typically characterized by an absence of junctions between the cells on electron microscopy. Electron microscopy can be time-consuming and expensive; therefore, with the availability of immunohistochemical stains, the need for it has diminished.

Immunohistochemical Analysis

Immunohistochemical analyses have become a routine addition to light microscopy, and a broad range of immunohistochemical markers are used to assist in the diagnosis after light microscopy. Common markers used for adenocarcinomas include cytokeratins (CKs) 7 and 20 and thyroid transcription factor (TTF-1). TTF-1, a nuclear protein, can be positive in lung and thyroid cancers. About 65% to 70% of lung adenocarcinomas and 25% of squamous cell lung cancers stain positive for TTF-1, and in patients with CUP, this test is helpful in differentiating between a primary lung tumor and metastatic adenocarcinoma (e.g., in patients presenting with metastatic pleural effusion). The CK marker combination pattern depicted in Figure 18.1 is also helpful.

Breast markers including estrogen receptor (ER), progesterone receptor (PR), Her-2 neu, and gross cystic disease fibrous protein should be checked in women who present with adenocarcinoma, especially isolated axillary adenopathy. Hep-par-1, a hepatocellular carcinoma marker, aids in the diagnosis of hepatocellular

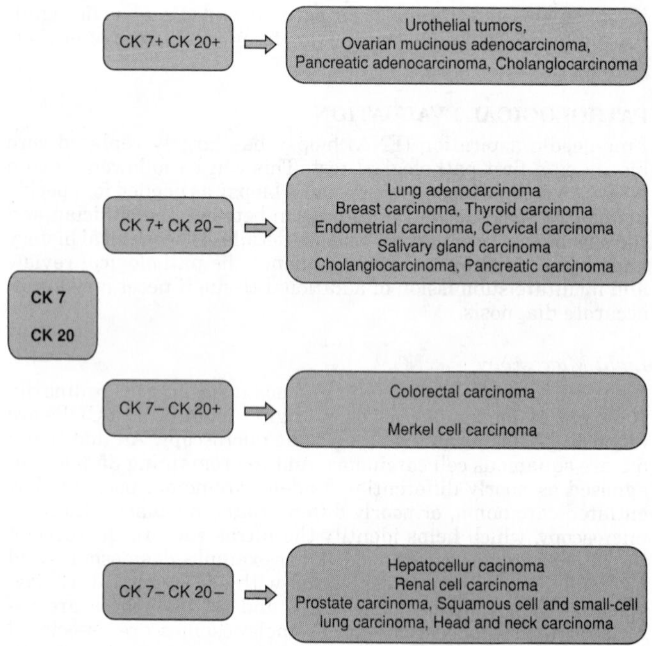

Figure 18.1. Approach to immunohistochemical markers used in cancer of unknown primary site.

cancer, and CK-19 is sometimes used for cholangiocarcinoma. It is sometimes difficult to distinguish metastatic cholangiocarcinoma, metastatic adenocarcinoma, and hepatocellular carcinoma in patients who present with liver-only metastatic disease. Other markers used in a directed fashion on the basis of past microscopy results include prostatic acid phosphatase and PSA for prostate cancer, and neuron-specific enolase and chromogranin for neuroendocrine cancers. Germ cell tumors often stain for β-hCG and AFP.

No immunohistochemical marker is 100% specific, and many of these tests (as well as serum markers) can be confusing and rarely help in the search for a primary tumor or in treatment planning.

Serum Tumor Markers and Cytogenetics

Unfortunately, patients with CUP typically have nonspecific overexpression of many serum tumor markers, including β-hCG, AFP, carcinoembryonic antigen, CA-125, CA 19-9, and CA 15-3. In patients who present with an undifferentiated carcinoma or a poorly differentiated carcinoma (especially with a midline tumor), β-hCG and AFP should be tested to rule out occult germ-line cancers. None of these markers has been found to have adequate specificity or sensitivity to consistently identify a primary tumor, nor the predictive value for either response to chemotherapy or survival.

Motzer et al. presented the molecular and cytogenetic results for 40 patients with CUP with poorly differentiated carcinoma. In 42% of patients (17), the diagnosis was made on the basis of genetic analysis. Thirty percent (12) of patients had cytogenetic changes characteristic of germ cell tumors (isochromosome 12p-I[12p]), increased 12p copy number, or deletion of the long arm of chromosome 12. These patients also responded better to cisplatin-based chemotherapy than did patients with other diagnoses (75% vs. 18%). Pantou et al. studied 20 biopsy specimens from patients with CUP and found that most samples had multiple complex cytogenetic patterns. Table 18.2 lists several common tumor markers and their roles in clinical evaluation of patients with CUP.

SPECIFIC DISEASE SITES

Metastatic Cancer to Cervical Lymph Nodes

Enlarged cervical lymph nodes are often found on biopsy to be positive for metastatic cancer. Patients with squamous cell cancer metastatic to cervical lymph nodes and an unknown primary tumor site have a better prognosis than do patients with CUP overall.

The neck comprises more than 25 nodal basins. These nodes have been grouped into six specific categories to standardize the pathological evaluation of patients. The classification of cervical lymph nodes is shown in Table 18.3. The most common site of metastasis in patients with head and neck squamous cell cancer is the jugulodigastric or level II upper internal jugular chain nodes, followed by the midjugular nodes. Metastasis to the other cervical nodal groups occurs with less frequency.

Table 18.2. Clinical role of selected tumor markers

Tumor Marker	Role in Differential Diagnosis
AFP	Identification of hepatocellular carcinoma or germ cell tumors
β-hCG	Identification of trophoblastic and germ cell tumors
β2-microglobulin	Not very useful
CA 15-3	Identification of possible breast carcinoma, but elevated serum levels also noted in ovarian, lung, and GI carcinomas
CA 19-9	Identification of possible pancreatic cancer or other GI cancer
CA 125	Identification of possible ovarian or uterine cancer, but elevated serum levels may be noted in breast, lung, or GI cancers
Calcitonin	Screening and diagnosis of medullary carcinoma of thyroid
CEA	Distinction of carcinoma from mesothelioma
Cytokeratin	Distinction of carcinoma from lymphoma or melanoma by immunohistochemistry
Epithelial membrane antigen	Distinction of carcinoma from melanoma by membrane immunohistochemistry
LCA	Identification of lymphoma or leukemia by immunohistochemistry
PSA	Identification of prostate carcinoma

AFP, alpha-fetoprotein; β-hCG, β-human chorionic gonadotropin; GI; gastrointestinal; CEA, carcinoembryonic antigen; LCA, leukocyte common antigen; PSA, prostate-specific antigen.

Table 18.3. Classification of cervical lymph nodes

Level	Nodes
I	Submental nodes
II	Upper internal jugular chain nodes
III	Middle internal jugular chain nodes
IV	Lower internal jugular chain nodes
V	Spinal accessory nodes Transverse cervical nodes
VI	Tracheoesophageal groove nodes

In those patients with cervical lymph nodes from an occult squamous cell primary tumor, a careful head and neck examination is particularly important. Adequate lighting and mirrors must be used to visualize the entire oropharynx, hypopharynx, nasopharynx, and larynx. A chest radiograph is always indicated, and a CT scan of the head and neck is usually indicated to determine the primary tumor site and obtain complete staging information.

If no primary tumor is found on physical examination and imaging studies including a CT scan, panendoscopy is a common next step. This is normally performed in the operating room with the patient under general anesthesia. Esophagoscopy, laryngoscopy, bronchoscopy, and nasopharyngoscopy are performed in an attempt to visualize the region and obtain biopsy specimens from the most common sites of occult squamous cell cancer in the head and neck region. Random biopsies of the most probable tumor site locations are performed, on the basis of the location of the adenopathy.

Typical occult primary tumor sites in squamous cell cancer are the nasopharynx, the midbase of the tongue, the pyriform sinus, and the tonsils. Table 18.4 shows the common pattern of cervical metastasis from different squamous cell tumors in the head and neck region. On the basis of the location of the nodal metastases, extrapolation of the likely source of the occult primary tumor is often possible, and the endoscopic examination should be focused on these locations.

If the primary tumor site cannot be identified on endoscopy, the standard approach is a combination of radical neck dissection and postoperative radiation therapy. The role for chemotherapy depends on the presence of bulky nodes (N3 disease), and neoadjuvant chemotherapy has not been well studied. On the basis of large series, the expected 5-year survival in these patients is 32% to 55%, and the overall rate of local control is 75% to 85%. Patients with extranodal extension or lymph nodes larger than 6 cm (N3 disease) have higher rates of both local recurrence and distant metastases.

Table 18.4. Probable sites of primary tumors according to the location of the cervical metastases

Location of Nodes	Primary Tumor Site
Submental	Floor of the mouth, lips, or anterior tongue
Submaxillary	Retromolar trigone or glossopalatine pillar
Jugulodigastric	Hypopharynx, base of the tongue, tonsils, nasopharynx, or larynx
Low jugular	Thyroid, hypopharynx, or nasopharynx
Supraclavicular	Lung (40%), thyroid (20%), GI (12%), or GU (8%)
Posterior triangle	Nasopharynx

GI, gastrointestinal; GU, genitourinary.

Patients with metastatic adenocarcinoma in cervical lymph nodes from an occult primary tumor have a less favorable outcome than do those with squamous cell cancer. Retrospective series have shown that lymphadenectomy and radiation therapy are much less effective in adenocarcinoma than in squamous cell carcinoma; the rate of local recurrence in these cases is nearly 100%, and the 5-year survival rate is 0% to 10%.

Of particular interest is the presence of an enlarged Virchow's (supraclavicular) node, common in patients with metastatic adenocarcinoma. One study retrospectively reviewed 152 FNA biopsy samples of supraclavicular lymph nodes, comparing the sites of primary tumor when the metastasis was in the right versus the left supraclavicular node. Sixteen of 19 primary pelvic tumors metastasized to the left supraclavicular node, and all (6 of 6) primary abdominal malignancies metastasized to the left supraclavicular node. However, thoracic, breast, and head and neck malignancies did not differ in patterns of metastasis to the right and left supraclavicular nodes. On the basis of this information, the search for the primary tumor should be focused on the abdomen and pelvis in patients who present with adenocarcinoma in a left-sided Virchow's node.

Metastatic Cancer to Axillary Lymph Nodes

The histologic type of the tumor should be used to guide the evaluation of patients with cancer metastatic to axillary lymph nodes (lymphoma is not considered a CUP; metastatic melanoma with an unknown primary is discussed separately later in this chapter). Patients with squamous cell cancer metastatic to the axillary lymph nodes should undergo a careful skin examination, a chest X-ray, a thorough head and neck examination, and CT scans of the head, neck, and the chest to look for an occult squamous cell primary tumor.

Men with adenocarcinoma metastatic to an axillary lymph node and CUP should be evaluated for lung, gastrointestinal, and genitourinary primary tumors. Women with adenocarcinoma metastatic to the axillary lymph nodes should be evaluated similarly, although in women the likelihood of an occult breast primary tumor is high. Women with occult breast cancer who present with axillary metastases constitute approximately 0.5% of all women with breast cancer. When many such patients are treated for a presumptive diagnosis of breast cancer, the recurrence and survival results are similar to those of patients with a similar stage of breast cancer and a known primary tumor. A retrospective review of the mastectomy specimens from patients with occult primary tumors showed that in 50% to 65% of cases, the primary tumor was ultimately identified in the surgical specimen. The other tumors were probably too small to be detected by the standard sampling techniques that pathologists use to study breast specimens. Such patients should be examined carefully for breast tumors, and every woman should undergo a mammogram and breast sonography if the mammogram is negative (especially in younger patients with dense breasts). As indicated earlier, MRI of the breast is indicated in most women who present with axillary adenopathy and CUP (with negative mammogram and sonographic findings).

The biopsy specimen from the lymph node should be subjected to routine histologic and immunohistochemical evaluation for ER, PR, and Her-2 neu. Although neither highly sensitive nor highly specific, the presence of ER or PR in this clinical scenario strongly suggests a breast primary tumor.

The treatment for women with adenocarcinoma metastatic to axillary lymph nodes has evolved dramatically over the last decade. The three general approaches are immediate mastectomy, observation, and radiation therapy. Immediate mastectomy is not performed in most patients if the imaging studies are negative because the chances of finding a primary are low. Observation with axillary dissection can result in recurrence in the breast (25%–75%, depending on the study), requiring further therapy. The third approach is breast conservation therapy with locoregional radiation therapy, which has been shown to decrease the local recurrence rate and is the preferred approach for most patients at The University of Texas M. D. Anderson Cancer Center. Our results show that in patients who have undergone axillary lymph node dissection alone, the incidence of local recurrence is 65% at 10 years, whereas a combination of axillary lymph node dissection and radiation therapy reduces the local recurrence rate to 25%. With this treatment, the overall survival rate was no different from that of patients with the same nodal stage of disease who had undergone mastectomy. The addition of adjuvant chemotherapy to surgery and radiation therapy increased the survival rate from 60% to 85% at 10 years. Tamoxifen should be part of the therapy for women of any age whose primary tumor (if identified) or axillary nodal metastases expresses ER or PR.

A retrospective study at M. D. Anderson Cancer Center included 45 women with isolated axillary nodal metastases without a known primary tumor. The median follow-up duration was 7 years. Patients underwent either mastectomy or breast conservation therapy; external-beam radiation therapy was used in 71% of patients, and systemic chemotherapy was used in 73%. No significant difference was found between mastectomy and breast conservation in locoregional recurrence, distant metastases, or 5-year survival rate. Regardless of the surgical treatment used, the number of involved nodes was the only determinant of survival.

Cancer Metastatic to the Inguinal Nodes From an Unknown Primary Site

A relatively infrequent presentation of metastatic CUP is metastases to the inguinal lymph nodes. Excluding melanoma, the two most common histologic types are unclassified carcinoma and squamous cell carcinoma. Adenocarcinoma is rarely observed. In evaluating patients with inguinal metastases, a thorough investigation for the primary tumor should include examination of the skin of the lower extremities, perineum, buttocks, anal canal, and pelvic region. If the inguinal node is the solitary area of presentation, excision followed by local radiation therapy is the next preferred step. For bulky bilateral adenopathy, neoadjuvant chemotherapy followed by surgery, inguinal lymph node dissection, and radiation therapy can be considered if there are no other sites of metastatic disease. These patients are prone to lymphedema after multimodality therapy, so they should be educated regarding the risks and undergo treatment if lymphedema develops.

Peritoneal Carcinomatosis of Unknown Primary Site

Patients with peritoneal carcinomatosis of unknown primary site can present with ascites, bowel obstruction, or nonspecific gastrointestinal symptoms. The two subgroups in this category include (a) patients with mucin-producing adenocarcinoma with and without signet ring cells, and (b) women with primary peritoneal carcinomatosis. Patients with mucin-producing adenocarcinoma often have multiple peritoneal implants, with the primary site most likely being the gastrointestinal tract (i.e., stomach, small bowel, appendix, or colon). Patients in this group have a poorer prognosis and respond poorly to currently available treatment regimens. These patients should undergo an upper endoscopy and colonoscopy to evaluate for a gastrointestinal primary tumor. If CK 20+ and CK 7– on immunohistochemical analysis, the patient may have colon cancer, an aggressive colon cancer regimen should be used because of a higher chance of response and enhanced survival potential.

The second subset is composed of women with primary peritoneal carcinomatosis. A histopathological analysis of these patients reveals cells with serous papillary features and, on occasion, psammoma bodies. These patients may have elevated CA-125 levels but do not have obvious ovarian cancer (on CT pelvis and transvaginal sonography). Several studies have found that women who present with peritoneal carcinomatosis should be treated in a similar fashion to those with known advanced ovarian cancer. This includes maximal surgical cytoreduction at initial laparotomy, followed by platinum-based combination chemotherapy. One study found a prolonged median survival of 13 months in patients who had undergone paclitaxel and carboplatin-based chemotherapy, and 25% of patients had progression-free survival of more than 2 years.

Unknown Primary Tumor With Metastatic Liver Disease

The surgeon is occasionally involved in the evaluation of patients who present with metastatic liver disease from an unknown primary tumor. The liver tumor may be discovered when the patient presents with symptoms on routine physical examination or incidentally on a radiologic study such as an abdominal sonogram or CT scan.

When patients present with metastatic liver disease and CUP, the most common cell type is adenocarcinoma (approximately 60%–65%). However, anaplastic or poorly differentiated carcinoma, small-cell carcinoma, squamous cell carcinoma, neuroendocrine cancer, and unclassified tumors are also found. The likely primary tumors include gastrointestinal cancers (including pancreatic-biliary cancers), followed by a lung or breast tumor.

Most patients undergo a CT scan of the chest, abdomen, and pelvis; mammogram (in women); and an upper endoscopy and colonoscopy if suggested by marker data or symptoms. The overall survival of these patients is usually poor (median, 7 months), although a survival benefit (approximately 12 months) can be seen in patients who have a good performance status and respond to chemotherapy.

A subgroup of patients who present with CUP and liver metastases have low-grade neuroendocrine carcinoma. These may be diagnosed incidentally or when patients complain of hormonal symptoms (diarrhea, flushing, or nausea) or pain. Low-grade neuroendocrine cancers can remain indolent for several years with slow progression and may not need treatment for a long time (hormonal or other). Tumor markers, including serum chromogranin, neuron-specific enolase, and urine 5-HIAA, may be elevated. If a patient has carcinoid symptoms, endocrine therapy alone for hormone-related symptoms with somatostatin analogs should be used. Specific local therapies, such as right hepatectomy or chemoembolization, or systemic therapies, such as chemotherapy with a streptozocin + doxorubicin ± fluorouracil-based regimen, are indicated if the patient is symptomatic with local pain secondary to growth of the metastasis or uncontrolled endocrine symptoms.

CHEMOTHERAPY FOR METASTATIC CANCERS OF UNKNOWN PRIMARY SITE

Data from CUP trials are difficult to interpret because patients with CUP are a heterogeneous group. When chemotherapy is given to unselected groups of patients with metastatic CUP, an overall 5% to 10% 5-year survival rate can be anticipated, with median survival in most studies between 6 and 13 months. Patients with favorable subtypes (e.g., peritoneal carcinomatosis or lymph node-predominant disease) benefit from chemotherapy. Traditionally, cisplatin-based combination chemotherapy regimens have been used to treat patients with CUP. In a phase II study by Hainsworth et al., 55 patients with CUP were treated with paclitaxel, carboplatin, and oral etoposide every 21 days. Most were previously untreated, with only 4 having undergone previous chemotherapy. The overall response rate was 47%, the median overall survival was 13.4 months, and the regimen was well tolerated. Briasoulis et al. found comparable response rates and median overall survival in 77 patients with CUP with paclitaxel and carboplatin and without oral etoposide. In this study, patients with nodal or pleural disease and women with peritoneal carcinomatosis had better response and an overall survival of 13 and 15 months, respectively. A phase II randomized trial by Culine et al. (the French Study Group on Carcinomas of Unknown Primary 01) studied 80 patients who were randomly assigned to receive either gemcitabine + cisplatin (GC) or irinotecan + cisplatin (IC). Seventy-eight patients were assessable for efficacy and toxicity. Objective responses were observed in 21 patients (55%) in the GC arm and in 15 patients (38%) in the IC arm. The median survival was 8 and 6 months in the GC and IC arms, respectively (median follow-up of 22 months).

Patients with poorly differentiated carcinoma, the possible germ cell equivalents, have traditionally undergone a trial of a cisplatin-based regimen. Patients with squamous cell cancer or neuroendocrine cancer have a significantly better response to chemotherapeutic agents than do patients with other tumor types.

The role of second-line chemotherapy in CUP is poorly defined. Hainsworth et al. reported data on 39 patients treated with gemcitabine in a salvage setting (in most patients, disease had failed to respond to a previous regimen containing platinum and a taxane), and only 21% of patients had ever responded to a previous therapy. The overall partial response rate was 8%, and 25% of patients had minor responses or stable disease with improved symptoms. The median time to progression for patients with partial responses or stable disease was 5 months, and the treatment was well tolerated.

Although cure is an unrealistic goal for many patients with metastatic CUP site, surgeons often are involved in the palliative care of such patients, including debulking tumors causing pain or obstruction, placing enteral tubes for decompression, performing thoracentesis for respiratory compromise from pleural effusions, and administering radiation therapy for painful bone metastases. Patients should be offered adequate analgesics to ensure they are comfortable, and both patients and their families should be given adequate emotional support and access to resources that optimize their quality of life.

Trials with targeted agents, including epidermal growth factor receptor antibodies, tyrosine kinase inhibitors, and antivascular endothelial growth factor antibodies (e.g., bevacizumab), in combination with cytotoxic agents, are warranted, and their role in the treatment of CUP will evolve over the next several years. Whenever possible, patients with CUP who do not belong in a defined subgroup should be treated within the context of a clinical trial.

RECOMMENDED READING

Abbruzzese JL, Abbruzzese MC, Hess KR, et al. Unknown primary carcinoma: natural history and prognostic factors in 657 consecutive patients. *J Clin Oncol* 1994;12:1272–80.

Abbruzzese JL, Abbruzzese MC, Lenzi R, et al. Analysis of a diagnostic strategy for patients with suspected tumors of unknown origin. *J Clin Oncol* 1995;13:2094–103.

Briasoulis E, Kalofonos H, Bafaloukos D, et al. Carboplatin plus paclitaxel in unknown primary carcinoma: a phase II Hellenic Cooperative Oncology Group Study. *J Clin Oncol* 2000;18:3101–7.

Bugat R, Bataillard A, Lesimple T, et al. Summary of the Standards, Options and Recommendations for the management of patients with carcinoma of unknown primary site (2002). *Br J Cancer* 89 Suppl 2003;1:S59–66.

Cervin JR, Silverman JF, Loggie BW, et al. Virchow's node revisited. Analysis with clinicopathologic correlation of 152 fine-needle aspiration biopsies of supraclavicular lymph nodes. *Arch Pathol Lab Med* 1995;119:727–30.

Culine S, Kramar A, Saghatchian M, et al. Development and validation of a prognostic model to predict the length of survival in patients with carcinomas of an unknown primary site. *J Clin Oncol* 2002;20:4679–83.

Glover K, Varadhachary GR, Lenzi R, et al. Unknown Primary Cancer, in Abelhoff M (ed): Clinical Oncology (ed 3) (ed third), 2003.

Greco FA, Hainsworth JD: One-hour paclitaxel, carboplatin, and extended-schedule etoposide in the treatment of carcinoma of unknown primary site. *Semin Oncol* 1997;24:S19-101–S19-105.

Hainsworth JD, Burris HA, 3rd, Calvert SW, et al. Gemcitabine in the second-line therapy of patients with carcinoma of unknown primary site: a phase II trial of the Minnie Pearl Cancer Research Network. *Cancer Invest* 2001;19:335–9.

Joshi U, van der Hoeven JJ, Comans EF, et al. In search of an unknown primary tumour presenting with extracervical metastases: the diagnostic performance of FDG-PET. *Br J Radiol* 2004;77:1000–6.

Lassen U, Daugaard G, Eigtved A, et al. 18F-FDG whole body positron emission tomography (PET) in patients with unknown primary tumours (UPT). *Eur J Cancer* 1999;35:1076–82.

Lenzi R, Hess KR, Abbruzzese MC, et al. Poorly differentiated carcinoma and poorly differentiated adenocarcinoma of unknown origin: favorable subsets of patients with unknown-primary carcinoma? *J Clin Oncol* 1997;15:2056–66.

Lenzi R, Raber MN, Frost P, et al. Phase II study of cisplatin, 5-fluorouracil and folinic acid in patients with carcinoma of unknown primary origin. *Eur J Cancer* 1993;29A:1634.

McMillan JH, Levine E, Stephens RH: Computed tomography in the evaluation of metastatic adenocarcinoma from an unknown primary site. A retrospective study. *Radiology* 1982;143:143–6.

Moll R, Lowe A, Laufer J, et al. Cytokeratin 20 in human carcinomas. A new histodiagnostic marker detected by monoclonal antibodies. *Am J Pathol* 1992;140:427–47.

Morris EA, Schwartz LH, Dershaw DD, et al. MR imaging of the breast in patients with occult primary breast carcinoma. *Radiology* 1997;205:437–40.

Motzer RJ, Rodriguez E, Reuter VE, et al. Molecular and cytogenetic studies in the diagnosis of patients with poorly differentiated carcinomas of unknown primary site. *J Clin Oncol* 1995;13: 274–82.

Nystrom JS, Weiner JM, Wolf RM, et al. Identifying the primary site in metastatic cancer of unknown origin. Inadequacy of roentgenographic procedures. *Jama* 1979;241:381–3.

Olson JA, Jr., Morris EA, Van Zee KJ, et al. Magnetic resonance imaging facilitates breast conservation for occult breast cancer. *Ann Surg Oncol* 2000;7:411–5.

Pantou D, Tsarouha H, Papadopoulou A, et al. Cytogenetic profile of unknown primary tumors: clues for their pathogenesis and clinical management. *Neoplasia* 2003;5:23–31.

Pavlidis N, Briasoulis E, Hainsworth J, et al. Diagnostic and therapeutic management of cancer of an unknown primary. *Eur J Cancer* 2003;39:1990–2005.

Randall DA, Johnstone PA, Foss RD, et al. Tonsillectomy in diagnosis of the unknown primary tumor of the head and neck. *Otolaryngol Head Neck Surg* 2000;122:52–5.

Rubin BP, Skarin AT, Pisick E, et al. Use of cytokeratins 7 and 20 in determining the origin of metastatic carcinoma of unknown primary, with special emphasis on lung cancer. *Eur J Cancer Prev* 2001;10:77–82.

Rusthoven KE, Koshy M, Paulino AC. The role of fluorodeoxyglucose positron emission tomography in cervical lymph node metastases from an unknown primary tumor. *Cancer* 2004;101:2641–9.

Schapira D: Cost of diagnosis and survival of patients with unknown primary cancer. *Proc Am Soc Clin Oncol* 13 Abstract, 1994.

Schelfout K, Kersschot E, Van Goethem M, et al. Breast MR imaging in a patient with unilateral axillary lymphadenopathy and unknown primary malignancy. *Eur Radiol* 2003;13:2128–32.

Stoeckli SJ, Mosna-Firlejczyk K, Goerres GW. Lymph node metastasis of squamous cell carcinoma from an unknown primary: impact of positron emission tomography. *Eur J Nucl Med Mol Imaging* 2003;30: 411–6.

Stokkel MP, Terhaard CH, Hordijk GJ, et al. The detection of unknown primary tumors in patients with cervical metastases by dual-head positron emission tomography. *Oral Oncol* 1999;35:390–4.

Tan D, Li Q, Deeb G, et al. Thyroid transcription factor-1 expression prevalence and its clinical implications in non-small cell lung cancer: a high-throughput tissue microarray and immunohistochemistry study. *Hum Pathol* 2003;34:597–604.

Varadhachary GR, Abbruzzese JL, Lenzi R. Diagnostic strategies for unknown primary cancer. *Cancer* 2004;100:1776–85.

Wallack MK, Reynolds B. Cancer to the inguinal nodes from an unknown primary site. *J Surg Oncol* 1981;17:39–43.

Wolff AC, Lange JR, Davidson NE. Occult primary cancer with axillary nodal metastases. In: Singletary SE, Robb GL, Eds. Adjuvant therapy of breast disease. Hamilton, Ontario: BC Decker, 2000.

Genitourinary Cancer

Christopher G. Wood and Colin P. N. Dinney

Global cancer statistics reveal that genitourinary cancers represented approximately 10.4% of new cancers diagnosed worldwide in 2005. These cancers occur in approximately 300,000 patients within the United States each year, and prostate cancer is now the most common malignancy and second leading cause of cancer death in U.S. men. Recognizing these facts, practicing physicians require an essential understanding of the diagnosis and treatment of these diseases. In this chapter, we review the current management of prostate, bladder, renal, and testicular neoplasm.

PROSTATE CANCER

Epidemiology and Etiology

In men, prostate cancer is the most common malignancy and the second leading cause of solid cancer mortality. Average mortality rates (1990–1997) are estimated to be 54.1 per 100,000 in African American males and 23.3 per 100,000 in white males. Prostate cancer screening was introduced in the United States during the mid- to late 1980s. Since this introduction, the pattern of disease incidence has changed. From 1988 to 1992, the annual percent increase of prostate cancer incidence was estimated at 17.5% per year. From 1992 to 1995, the incidence decreased 10.3% per year. This decrease has leveled off and from 1995 to 1997, the average annual decrease in incidence was 2.1%, and the average annual incidence was 149.7 cases per 100,000. These cancer trends are not equivalent between whites and African Americans. Prostate cancer incidence among African Americans has increased an average of 0.7% annually from 1990 to 1997. Furthermore, although the average annual mortality rates have decreased 2.2% per year (1990–1997) overall, African Americans have only experienced an average mortality rate decrease of 1.1% per year throughout 1990 to 1997.

Prostate cancer rarely occurs before age 50 years, and the incidence increases through the ninth decade of life; however, some of this increase may be attributable to an increase in prostate cancer screening in the later decades. It is estimated that 30% to 50% of men older than 50 years have histologic evidence of prostate cancer at autopsy, while at age 75 or older, it is estimated that this figure increases to 50% to 70%.

Many factors have been proposed to be associated with the development of prostate cancer. The presence of an intact hypothalamic-pituitary-gonadal axis and advanced age are the most universally accepted risk factors. Migration studies support a role for environmental influences on prostate cancer. Higher rates of prostate cancer have been found among populations with higher amounts of fat in the diet. Beneficial dietary associations include isoflavonoids, lycopenes, selenium, and vitamin E; however, additional prospective randomized trials are needed to confirm the beneficial effects of these factors. It is unclear whether the increased mortality rate of prostate cancer in African Americans is due to unique racial biological and genetic factors, rather than dietary influences, the existence of confounding medical comorbid conditions, lifestyle differences, and/or access to health care issues. Occupational exposure to cadmium has been associated with increased risk of prostate cancer, but this relationship is not yet proven to be causal.

Evidence has shown that a man with one, two, or three first-degree relatives affected with prostate cancer has a 2, 5, or 11 times greater risk, respectively, of the development of prostate cancer than the general population. A Mendelian pattern of autosomal dominant transmission of prostate cancer accounts for 43% of disease occurring before age 55 years and 9% of all prostate cancers occurring by age 85 years.

Anatomy

The normal prostate gland weighs 15 to 20 g and is divided into three major glandular zones. The *peripheral zone* constitutes 70% of the prostate gland and is the area palpated during digital rectal examination (DRE). The area around the ejaculatory ducts is called the *central zone* and accounts for 25% of the gland. The *transitional zone* comprises 5% of the prostate gland around the urethra. In a pathological review of 104 prostate glands from patients who underwent radical prostatectomy, 68% of the cancers were located in the peripheral zone, 24% in the transitional zone, and only 8% in the central zone. Almost all stage A (nonpalpable) cancers in that study were found in the transitional zone, the area most susceptible to benign prostatic hyperplasia, which can be associated with urinary symptoms of bladder neck obstruction.

Screening

Although good screening methods for prostate cancer are available, controversy surrounds the concept of screening for this disease. It is estimated that less than 10% of men with prostate cancer die because of the disease. This leads to a lack of consensus on the optimal management of early-stage disease and to questions regarding the cost effectiveness of a national screening effort for all men older than 50 years. Currently, the American Cancer Society recommends a DRE and measurement of prostate-specific antigen (PSA) starting at age 50 years. For African American men or men with a family history of prostate cancer, screening should begin at 40 years of age.

Diagnosis

Patients with low-volume, clinically localized prostate cancer are typically asymptomatic; abnormalities are detected by DRE, increased serum PSA level, or both. Advanced prostate cancer can be asymptomatic; present as local symptoms of urinary hesitancy, frequency, and urgency; or present as systemic symptoms of weight loss, fatigue, and bone pain. Rarely, neurologic sequelae of impending spinal cord compression or uremia secondary to bilateral ureteral obstruction can be found in the presentation of advanced cases.

PSA is a serine protease produced by the epithelium of the prostate. PSA is not specific for prostate cancer and can be increased in benign conditions of the prostate such as prostatitis, prostatic infarction, and prostatic hyperplasia. It can also be increased as a consequence of recent ejaculation, and patients should be counseled to abstain from sexual activity for periods of up to 1 week prior to PSA screening. Transurethral resection of the prostate (TURP) and prostatic needle biopsy significantly increase the serum PSA level above baseline for up to 8 weeks. DRE, cystoscopy, and transrectal ultrasound (TRUS) do not alter serum PSA to a clinically significant degree. The positive predictive value of a PSA level greater than 4 ng per mL for the detection of prostate cancer is 34.4%, while the positive predictive value for an abnormal DRE is 21.4%. Detection rates demonstrate that DRE and PSA together (5.8%) are superior to either DRE (3.2%) or PSA (4.6%) alone. Free PSA is a form of PSA not conjugated to protease inhibitors in the serum. Decreased percentage-free PSA (<25%) is associated with prostate cancer, and measurement of free PSA is performed to improve the specificity of PSA testing in the range of 4 to 10 ng per mL and thus eliminate unnecessary biopsies. The primary utility of free PSA is in the patients with a PSA in the 4 to 10 ng per mL range with a history of previously negative prostatic biopsies. In this clinical scenario, the free to total PSA ratio, or alternatively, complexed PSA, can be used to determine the need for repeat biopsies with continued elevation of the serum PSA. A low free to total PSA ratio (<20%) is an indication to repeat TRUS and biopsies of the prostate to rule out the presence of carcinoma.

TRUS is performed using real-time imaging with a 7-MHz transducer, which allows both transverse and sagittal imaging of the prostate gland. Prostate cancer can appear as a hypoechoic region within the prostate, although most experts agree that this is a nonspecific finding. TRUS can also be used to measure the dimensions of the prostate gland to calculate the glandular volume.

Lymphatic metastases can be detected by computed tomography (CT), lymphangiography, and magnetic resonance imaging (MRI). However, the only reliable method for staging pelvic lymph nodes is a pelvic lymphadenectomy.

Radionuclide bone scan remains the most sensitive test to detect skeletal metastases. However, in 1993, Oesterling found the yield of a bone scan was 2% if a patient has a PSA level less than 20 ng per mL and evidence of skeletal metastasis, while no patients had a positive bone scan with a PSA less than 8 ng per mL. Therefore, based on this data, radionuclide bone scans are not necessary for staging prostate cancer patients who have a low serum PSA level (<10 ng per mL) and no skeletal symptoms, particularly in cases of low-grade cancers. When bone metastases are present, 80% are osteoblastic, 15% are mixed osteoblastic-osteolytic, and 5% are osteolytic. A chest radiograph is performed to detect the presence of pulmonary metastases, which are extremely rare.

The diagnosis of prostate cancer is made by the histologic finding of prostate cancer in a prostatic biopsy, in a prostatic needle aspiration, in tissue obtained from prostatectomy for benign disease, or in the biopsy of a suspicious metastatic focus. In the past, sextant biopsies of the prostate were considered adequate in the patient with an elevated PSA, with site-specific biopsies directed at palpable or ultrasonographic abnormalities (hypoechoic regions). More recent data based on whole mount step sectioning of radical prostatectomy specimens suggest that sextant biopsies are inadequate, in favor of 10 or 11 core strategies that include the anterior horns of the prostate and the transition zone bilaterally. Adenocarcinoma is the predominant cell type of prostate cancer and is the only type discussed in this chapter.

Grading and Staging

The Gleason grading system is the most widely used grading system. It recognizes five histologic patterns of prostate cancer, graded on a scale of 1 to 5, from most differentiated to least. The Gleason score is arrived at through the addition of the predominant and secondary grade patterns to yield a range of tumor Gleason scores from 2 to 10. Prostate cancer is well known to be multifocal in nature, so not uncommonly, multiple biopsies from a prostate may be positive, each with a reported Gleason score. The biology of the cancer is frequently dictated by the most aggressive variant found in the prostate.

The biological behavior of the tumor can be further categorized by stage, which accounts for tumor volume and location. Prostate cancer typically spreads to the pelvic lymph nodes, bone, and lungs. The 2002 American Joint Committee on Cancer/International Union Against Cancer TNM staging classification is shown in Table 19.1.

Management of Early Disease

In 1987, the National Cancer Institute published a consensus statement on the treatment of early-stage prostate cancer. The report concluded: "Radical prostatectomy and radiation therapy are clearly effective forms of treatment in the attempt to cure tumors limited to the prostate for appropriately selected patients.... What remains unclear is the relative merit of each in producing lifelong freedom from cancer recurrence.... Properly designed and completed randomized trials that evaluate both disease control and quality of life after modern radiation therapy compared with radical prostatectomy are essential." These criteria have yet to be fulfilled and probably never will; however, there appears to be little difference in clinical and biochemical outcomes between the two modalities when similar patient groups are compared.

Surgery

The surgical excision of prostate cancer by complete removal of the prostate gland, seminal vesicles, and ampullae of the vasa deferentia was first performed in the early 1900s. This procedure, known as a *radical prostatectomy,* can be performed using a perineal or retropubic approach. Newer, minimally invasive surgical techniques such as laparoscopic radical prostatectomy and robot-assisted laparoscopic prostatectomy are now becoming

Table 19.1. Staging systems for prostate cancer

Primary tumor clinical (T)	
TX	Primary tumor cannot be assessed
T0	No evidence of primary tumor
T1	Clinically inapparent tumor not palpable or visible by imaging T1a: Tumor incidental histologic finding in 5% or less of tissue resected T1b: Tumor incidental histologic finding in more than 5% of tissue resected T1c: Tumor identified by needle biopsy because of increased PSA
T2	Tumor confined within the prostate gland T2a: Tumor involves one-half of one lobe or less T2b: Tumor involves more than one-half of one lobe, but not both lobes T2c: Tumor involves both lobes
T3	Tumor extends through the prostate capsule T3a: Extracapsular extension (unilateral or bilateral) T3b: Seminal vesicle invasion
T4	Invasion of bladder neck, rectum, external sphincter, levator muscles, or pelvic side wall
Regional lymph nodes (N)	
NX	Regional lymph nodes cannot be assessed
N0	No regional lymph node metastasis
N1	Metastasis in regional lymph node or nodes
Distant metastases (M)	
MX	Distant metastasis cannot be assessed
M0	No distant metastasis
M1	Distant metastasis M1a: Nonregional lymph nodes M1b: Bone(s) M1c: Other site(s)

PSA, prostate-specific antigen.

more mainstream, with similar oncologic outcomes to open techniques.

In 1994, Zincke et al. reported their experience with radical prostatectomy in 1,143 patients with 10- and 15-year cause-specific survival rates of 90% and 83% and metastasis-free survival of 83% and 77%, respectively. Complication rates are low. Mortality is less than 0.7% and the incidence of severe incontinence is 1.4%. In 1992, Leandri et al. reported on 620 patients and found a 6.9% early complication rate, 1.3% late complication rate, and 0.2% mortality rate. Sexual potency was maintained in

71% in whom a nerve-sparing technique was used, and 5% experienced stress incontinence after 1 year. Factors that predict for postoperative potency include preoperative erectile function, patient age, and number of cavernosal nerve fibers spared. Factors that influence continence results include nerve sparing, patient age, and obesity.

Radiation Therapy

External-beam radiation therapy is used for the definitive treatment of localized and regionally extensive prostatic adenocarcinoma. At M. D. Anderson Cancer Center, 60 to 70 Gy was given to 114 patients with localized prostate cancer as primary therapy. The 5- and 10-year uncorrected survival rates are comparable to radical surgery (89% and 68%, respectively). In this series, there was no difference in survival between patients with stage A and B disease. Skeletal metastases were the most common site of relapse. Serious complications developed in only 1.8% of treated patients. Conformal radiation therapy and intensity modulated radiation therapy are currently used to decrease adverse local side effects of radiation therapy and increase total dosage to the prostate. Larger doses are used in select patients; however, longer follow-up is needed to fully define the role of dose escalation. At M. D. Anderson, we recommend radical prostatectomy for the treatment of early-stage prostate cancer in the patient with minimal comorbidities, less than 70 years of age. Primary radiation therapy is reserved for patients with significant comorbid medical illnesses or patients older than 70 years of age.

Management of Locally Advanced Prostate Cancer/Lymph Node Metastasis

Locally advanced prostate cancer involves areas outside the prostatic capsule, such as fat, seminal vesicles, levator muscles, or other adjacent structures. Locally advanced prostate cancer is associated with a 53% incidence of lymph node metastases and decreased overall survival rate compared with early-stage disease. At M. D. Anderson, locally advanced disease with or without lymph node metastasis is treated with primary radiation therapy and androgen ablation with a 6-year biochemical failure rate of 13%. Longer follow-up is still needed. These patients with locally advanced disease at high risk for relapse are frequently enrolled in clinical protocols that use neoadjuvant systemic therapy in combination with surgical extirpation of the prostate to improve patient outcome. Our experience with locally advanced disease treated with primary radiation therapy demonstrated 5-, 10-, and 15-year uncorrected actuarial survival rates of 72%, 47%, and 17%, respectively. The local control rate was 75% at 15 years of follow-up.

Treatment modalities other than radiation therapy used for locally advanced disease include radical prostatectomy, TURP, and hormonal therapy. Tumor grade, stage, bulk of tumor, and seminal vesicle involvement in locally advanced disease are associated with a decreased interval between radical prostatectomy and disease progression. The actuarial 5-year survival rate for patients with locally advanced disease who have undergone TURP is 64%, making TURP an option for patients with short life expectancies who have significant local symptoms associated with their prostate cancer such as urinary obstruction or intractable hematuria. This strategy may be ideal in the elderly and in those with serious coexisting medical problems.

Systemic Prostate Cancer

Patients with metastatic prostate cancer have a median survival duration of 30 months, with an estimated 5-year survival rate of 20%. The treatment of metastatic prostate cancer is androgen ablation therapy. Trials examining the role of chemotherapy in combination with androgen ablative therapy have not, as yet, demonstrated an additional benefit with regard to progression-free or overall survival when compared with androgen ablation alone. The hypothalamus produces luteinizing hormone-releasing hormone (LHRH) and corticotropin-releasing factor, which stimulate the anterior pituitary gland to release adrenocorticotropic hormone (ACTH) and luteinizing hormone (LH). LH stimulates testosterone production by the testes, and ACTH stimulates the adrenal glands to produce androstenedione and dehydroepiandrosterone, precursors of testosterone and dihydrotestosterone (DHT). Although the testes are the major source of testosterone, the adrenal glands can supply up to 20% of the DHT found in the prostate gland.

Androgen ablation therapy consists of either bilateral orchiectomy or LHRH agonists, which chronically stimulate the pituitary gland, resulting in a decrease in LH release. Direct LHRH antagonists are now also available, but they have not gained widespread acceptance over the agonists that have a more extensive clinical background. Decrease in LH leads to castrate levels of testosterone production by the testes, defined typically as less than 50 ng per mL. Several oral antiandrogens exist that work by blocking uptake or binding of androgen in target tissues. Combination of antiandrogens with either surgical or medical androgen ablation is termed total androgen blockade.

Bilateral orchiectomy and LHRH agonists appear to have equal efficacy when used as monotherapy for metastatic prostate cancer. The Medical Research Council of the United Kingdom performed a randomized prospective trial with 934 patients and found that immediate androgen ablation delays disease progression and decreases pathological fractures. We recommend immediate androgen suppression for select patients. Total androgen ablation with an LHRH agonist plus an antiandrogen is controversial. Many studies have shown no benefit of combined therapy with an antiandrogen versus LHRH agonist monotherapy. Intermittent androgen therapy has been demonstrated to improve quality of life, but its long-term effects on survival are unknown. The median time to hormone refractory prostate cancer in patients with metastatic prostate cancer treated with hormonal therapy is approximately 2 years. The median survival of patients with hormone refractory disease is on the order of 12 to 18 months. Chemotherapeutic regimens are the mainstay of therapy for hormone refractory prostate cancer with taxane-based regimens showing significant activity that includes decreases in

PSA, improved quality of life, objective disease regression, and prolonged survival. Clinical trials continue to be the main and best treatment option for patients; however, some treatment options (primarily taxane-based chemotherapy regimens) now exist that demonstrate objective benefit where none existed previously. Clinical research is now focused on the efficacy of more targeted therapies that act on specific molecular pathways involved in metastatic progression in the management of hormone refractory disease.

BLADDER CANCER

Epidemiology and Etiology

Bladder cancer is the second most common genitourinary malignancy in the United States. It is the fourth most common cancer in men and the tenth most common cancer in women. In 2005, more than 50,000 new cases were reported, and approximately 12,000 deaths were attributed to bladder cancer. The incidence is lowest in African American females (6 per 100,000) and highest in white males (31 per 100,000). White males also have the highest mortality rate: 5.8 deaths per 100,000.

The etiology of urothelial cancers, of which bladder cancer is the most common, is well established. Cigarette smoking has been linked to 30% to 40% of all cases of bladder cancer. The chemicals 1-naphthylamine, 2-naphthylamine, benzidine, and 4-aminobiphenyl have been shown to promote urothelial carcinogenesis. Workers in the textile, leather, aluminum refining, rubber, and chemical industries who are exposed to high levels of these chemicals have an increased incidence of bladder cancer. Other chemicals that have been linked to urothelial cancer are MBUCCA (plastics industry), phenacetin, and the antineoplastic agent cyclophosphamide. In addition, recurrent bladder infections, as well as infections with the parasite *Schistosoma haematobium,* have been associated with squamous cell carcinoma of the bladder.

Pathology

The urinary bladder is a hollow viscus that functions in both the storage and the evacuation of urine. Histologically, the bladder is composed of mucosa, lamina propria, muscularis, and serosa (limited to the dome). Localized bladder cancer is classified as *superficial disease,* which is limited to the mucosa and lamina propria, or *invasive disease,* which extends into the muscularis and beyond. Approximately 70% of newly diagnosed bladder cancers are superficial, whereas the remaining 30% are invasive or metastatic. Once a bladder cancer extends through the basal layer of the mucosa, it may invade blood vessels and lymphatics, thereby providing a route of metastasis. Carcinoma in situ, an aggressive form of superficial disease, is composed of anaplastic cells limited to the mucosal layer.

The World Health Organization (WHO) classifies epithelial tumors of the bladder into four histologic types: transitional cell carcinoma (TCC) (91%), squamous cell carcinoma (7%), adenocarcinoma (2%), and undifferentiated carcinoma (<1%). However, up to 20% of TCCs contain areas of squamous differentiation, and up to 7% contain areas of adenomatous differentiation. The remainder of this section discusses TCC.

Clinical Presentation

Eighty percent of all patients who present with bladder carcinoma have gross or microscopic hematuria, typically painless and intermittent. Approximately 20% of patients complain of symptoms of vesical irritability, including urinary frequency, urgency, dysuria, and stranguria. Other symptoms include pelvic pain, flank pain (from ureteral obstruction), and lower-extremity edema. Patients with systemic disease may present with anemia, weight loss, and bone pain.

Diagnosis

A patient who presents with hematuria or other symptoms of bladder cancer should undergo a thorough urologic evaluation consisting of a history, physical examination, urinalysis, intravenous urogram, cystoscopic examination of the urinary bladder, and voided urine for cytologic examination. A debate continues in the urologic literature as to whether a CT scan of the abdomen and pelvis should replace the intravenous urogram in the workup of hematuria, particularly with the tremendous resolution seen with modern spiral CT scanners. The most useful of these steps is the examination of the bladder using a rigid or flexible cystoscope. Papillary and sessile tumors are easily visualized through the cystoscope; carcinoma in situ, however, can appear as normal mucosa or as erythematous patches throughout the bladder. Fewer than 60% of bladder tumors can be seen on an intravenous urogram, but this examination is obtained primarily to identify other abnormalities that may be present in the upper genitourinary tract. Urine cytology is reported as positive in 30% of patients with grade 1 tumors, 50% of patients with grade 2 tumors, and from 65% to 100% of patients with high-grade tumors or carcinoma in situ (see the next section for definition of grades).

Grading and Staging

The WHO uses a grading system based on the cytologic features of the tumor. Grade 1 represents a well-differentiated tumor; grade 2, a moderately differentiated tumor; and grade 3, a poorly differentiated bladder cancer.

Once a bladder tumor is diagnosed, the urologist must accurately stage the tumor. The initial transurethral resection of the bladder tumor (TURBT), typically done in association with random biopsies of the bladder and prostatic urethra, will determine the histologic depth of invasion of the tumor and the presence or absence of dysplasia or carcinoma in situ. A bimanual examination should be performed at the time of resection to determine whether a mass is present and, if so, whether it is fixed or mobile.

Further workup for detecting metastasis consists of a CT scan, liver function tests, a chest radiograph, and a bone scan (if the alkaline phosphatase level is elevated or the patient's symptoms suggest systemic disease). American Joint Committee on Cancer International Union Against Cancer TNM staging systems are listed in Table 19.2.

Table 19.2. Staging systems for bladder cancer

Primary tumor clinical (T)	
TX	Primary tumor cannot be assessed
T0	No evidence of primary tumor
Ta	Noninvasive papillary carcinoma
Tis	Carcinoma in situ
T1	Tumor invades subepithelial connective tissue
T2	Tumor invades muscle T2a: Tumor invades superficial muscle T2b: Tumor invades deep muscle
T3	Tumor invades perivesical tissue T3a: Microscopically T3b: Macroscopically (extravesical mass)
T4	Invasion of any of the following: prostate gland, uterus, vagina, pelvic wall, or abdominal wall T4a: Tumor invades prostate, uterus, or vagina T4b: Tumor invades pelvic or abdominal wall
Regional lymph nodes (N)	
NX	Regional lymph nodes cannot be assessed
N0	No regional lymph node metastasis
N1	Metastasis in single lymph node 2 cm or less in the largest dimension
N2	Metastasis in single lymph node greater than 2 cm in the largest dimension but less than 5 cm, or multiple lymph nodes, none larger than 5 cm in greatest dimension
N3	Metastasis in a lymph node larger than 5 cm in greatest dimension
Distant metastases (M)	
MX	Distant metastasis cannot be assessed
M0	No distant metastasis
M1	Distant metastasis

Management

Superficial Bladder Cancer

Approximately two-thirds of bladder cancers present as superficial disease (e.g., Ta, T1, or Tis). An estimated 70% of these superficial cancers are Ta and 30% are T1. Ten percent of all bladder cancers present with Tis or carcinoma in situ (CIS). After the initial treatment of superficial bladder cancer, the cancer can be cured, can recur with the same stage and grade, or can recur with progression of stage or grade. Risk factors associated with both disease recurrence and progression include a high tumor grade, lamina propria invasion, dysplasia elsewhere in the bladder, positive urinary cytology findings, tumor diameter larger than 5 cm, vascular or lymphatic invasion, multicentricity, and expression of either epidermal growth factor or transforming growth factor-alpha. Mutations in the P53 gene may also be associated with a significant risk of disease progression.

Initial treatment of superficial bladder cancer focuses on eradication of the existing disease and prophylaxis against disease recurrence or progression. TURBT has been the standard treatment for existing stage Ta and T1 tumors and visible stage Tis tumors. Laser fulguration is another therapeutic option that results in fewer bleeding complications. The advantage of transurethral resection over laser fulguration is that it provides tissue for histologic examination.

Patients with Tis, high-grade Ta or T1 lesions, multiple tumors, recurrent tumors, tumors larger than 5 cm, or persistently positive cytology findings may be candidates for adjuvant intravesical therapy. Intravesical agents can be used as therapeutic, adjuvant, or prophylactic treatment for bladder cancer. Thiotepa, mitomycin C, and doxorubicin are the chemotherapeutic agents used most frequently. Bacille Calmette-Guérin (BCG), a live attenuated tuberculosis organism, has become the most widely used intravesical agent in superficial bladder cancer, either alone or in combination with alpha-interferon. BCG enhances the patient's own immune response against the tumor, providing resistance to disease recurrence and progression. Although specific dose scheduling varies, most treatment regimens include intravesical treatment weekly for 4 to 8 weeks, followed by an optional series of maintenance treatments administered over many months. BCG has been shown to eliminate CIS in 80% of patients at a 5-year follow-up, reduce tumor recurrence rate for patients with T1 disease to 30% at 4 years, and eliminate residual tumor in up to 59% of patients. Maintenance therapy regimens with BCG appear to offer the best outcomes for patients. In 2000, Lamm et al. randomized 384 patients with superficial bladder cancer to receive induction and maintenance BCG or just induction BCG therapy only. Median recurrence-free survival time was longer for those who received induction and maintenance therapy; however, at 5-year follow-up there was no difference in survival.

There is good evidence that T1 high-grade cancer has a high rate of progression and therefore confers a high risk of death. Therefore, we recommend early radical cystectomy for select patients with high-grade T1 bladder cancer. Furthermore, we also recommend cystectomy for patients who recur despite an adequate trial of BCG therapy because these patients have been shown to be at high risk for disease progression if their bladder remains in situ.

Invasive Bladder Cancer

Tumors that have penetrated the muscularis propria are considered invasive. Several options are available for treatment of patients with invasive tumors. A small subset of patients may be eligible for bladder-sparing therapy. In 2001, Herr demonstrated a 76% overall survival rate, with 57% of the patients preserving their bladders in 45 patients treated with aggressive transurethral re-resection of invasive bladder tumors (median follow-up: 61 months). Patients with a muscle-invasive tumor that is primary and solitary, does not have surrounding urothelial atypia, and allows for a 2-cm surgical margin may be candidates for partial cystectomy. At M. D. Anderson, data have shown that approximately 5% of patients are actually suitable for bladder-sparing surgery; 5-year survival rates have been comparable to those achieved with radical cystectomy, when negative margins of resection can be achieved.

Primary external-beam radiation therapy has been used to treat invasive bladder cancer. Treatment protocols advocate doses of 65 to 70 Gy. Five-year survival rates range from 21% to 52% for stage B2 and from 18% to 30% for stage C. Local recurrence occurs in 50% to 70% of these patients. Stage T4 lesions fare worse, with 5-year survival rates consistently less than 10%. Our experience at M. D. Anderson found a 26% 5-year survival rate with primary external-beam radiation. Thus, external-beam radiation therapy may be useful in patients who do not want to have surgery or for whom radical surgery is medically contraindicated; however, the results with radiation therapy, stage for stage, are significantly worse than those seen with radical surgery.

In an attempt to improve survival and bladder preservation rates, multimodality strategies have combined TURBT, chemotherapy, and radiation. In 1997, Kachnic et al. from Massachusetts General Hospital reported on 106 patients with stages T2 to T4 bladder cancers who were treated with TURBT, two cycles of MCV, and 40 Gy radiation therapy plus concurrent cisplatin. Overall 5-year survival was 52%, and overall 5-year survival rate with the bladder intact was 43%. These results are comparable to contemporary radical cystectomy series; however, this regimen involves significant morbidity and patient investment in complex treatment schedules. Moreover, patients are subjected to a considerable risk of eventual cystectomy and superficial bladder cancer recurrence.

Radical cystectomy with pelvic lymphadenectomy is performed with the intent of removing all localized and lymphatic disease. At M. D. Anderson, the 5-year actuarial survival rates for patients with invasive bladder carcinoma after radical cystectomy alone are 79% for stage B, 46% for stage C, 54% for stage D with nodal spread, and 32% for stage D with visceral metastases. The local recurrence rate is 7%, and the operative mortality rate is 1.1%. Fourteen percent of patients undergoing cystectomy with lymphadenectomy are found to have unsuspected metastases to the pelvic lymph nodes. The majority of these cases involve one or two nodes limited to an area below the bifurcation of the common iliac arteries and medial to the external iliac artery.

Once a patient undergoes cystectomy, the ureters must be diverted into an alternate drainage system. The most common urinary diversion used today is the orthotopic urinary diversion with an ileal segment used for bladder substitution. Catheterizable cutaneous reservoirs are also used as methods of urinary diversion in selected patients. Patients who are unable to undergo an orthotopic diversion include patients with elevated serum creatinine, evidence of lymph node metastasis, prostatic urethral invasive TCC or CIS, or inflammatory bowel disease. Furthermore, these patients must be willing and able to undergo a vigorous voiding re-education program. Radiation therapy may render continence difficult; therefore, some patients may not benefit from this type of diversion. In the end, if they are unable to fulfill these criteria, then a cutaneous ileal conduit is recommended.

Metastatic Disease

Cisplatin appears to be the single agent with the greatest activity against TCC of the bladder; however, single-agent therapy response rates are only in the range of 10% to 30%. Traditionally, chemotherapy for bladder cancer included cisplatin, methotrexate, vinblastine, and doxorubicin (M-VAC). In the M. D. Anderson trial of M-VAC, a complete response rate of 35% and a partial response rate of 30% were observed. Other trials have documented similar response rates, with median survival of approximately 1 year. Newer regimens using gemcitabine and cisplatin have demonstrated no significant difference in survival when compared with M-VAC, but adverse side effects and toxicity are less with the newer regimen.

At M. D. Anderson, adjuvant and neoadjuvant chemotherapy is used for select patients with unfavorable disease characteristics. Unfavorable features include resected nodal metastases, extravesical involvement, lymphovascular permeation, or involvement of pelvic viscera. Previously, treatment in select patients with adjuvant chemotherapy at M. D. Anderson resulted in a 70% 5-year survival rate, which is comparable to patients without unfavorable features. Randomized prospective trials are now being completed to confirm these results for neoadjuvant chemotherapy.

RENAL CANCER

Epidemiology and Etiology

Tumors of the renal and perirenal tissues comprise 3% of cancer incidence and mortality in the United States. Renal cell carcinoma (RCC) represents 85% of all renal parenchymal tumors and is the only renal tumor discussed in this chapter. In 2005, an estimated 31,500 people were diagnosed with kidney cancer, and 12,000 people died of this disease. From 1975 to 1995, both the incidence and mortality rates of RCC have increased. The upward trend in mortality rates suggests that the increased incidental diagnosis of early-stage asymptomatic tumors does not fully account for the overall increase in incidence. Males are affected twice as often as females. RCC most frequently occurs in the fifth to sixth decades of life.

Several risk factors have been identified to be associated with RCC. Case-control studies have found strong correlations with smoking and obesity. Hypertension, diabetes mellitus, and diuretic use have also been found to be associated with RCC; however, it is unclear whether this is a causal relationship. RCC can occur either sporadically or genetically. Hereditary RCC tends to occur at an earlier age of onset and tends to be bilateral and multifocal. A well-described familial syndrome is von Hippel-Lindau (VHL) disease, which is characterized by cerebellar hemangioblastoma, retinal angiomata, bilateral RCC, and islet cell tumors of the pancreas. Both sporadic and VHL disease types have a common genetic mechanism that includes loss of a region of chromosome 3. Approximately 70% of clear cell renal cell carcinomas are believed to have loss of the VHL gene either through mutation, deletion, or silence by methylation. Hereditary nonpapillary RCC is an autosomal dominant syndrome associated with the same chromosome 3 abnormalities, while hereditary papillary RCC (type 1) is an autosomal dominant syndrome associated with abnormalities of the *met* gene on chromosome 7. Other genetic RCC syndromes include hereditary papillary RCC (type 2) associated with mutations in the Krebs cycle enzyme fumarate hydratase, and Birt-Hogg-Dube syndrome, which is manifest as bilateral multifocal tumors with both chromophobe RCC and oncocytoma histology. RCC is also associated with polycystic kidney disease, tuberous sclerosis, "horseshoe kidneys," and acquired renal cystic disease.

Pathology

Most RCCs originate in the proximal tubular cells of the kidney. The tumor is multifocal in 6.5% to 10% of cases. The renal capsule and Gerota's fascia surrounding the kidney limit local extension of the tumor. The predominant cell type is clear cell, but granular and spindle-shaped cells also may be present. The tumor cells are typically rich in glycogen and lipid, giving the tumor a clear cell appearance microscopically and a characteristic yellow appearance grossly. Less common pathologies include papillary and chromophobe RCC. Unclassified RCC is a waste basket classification for tumors that do not fit the criteria of the classically described histologies. Sarcomatoid differentiation, once believed to be a separate histologic classification, is now recognized as a dedifferentiation pathway that can occur with any histology, including clear cell, papillary, and chromophobe. Oncocytoma is a benign tumor with no malignant potential that can be problematic to differentiate from chromophobe renal cell carcinoma on needle biopsy.

Clinical Presentation

RCC was traditionally called the "internist's tumor" because of its subtle presentation. Now more than 40% of clinically unsuspected tumors are found incidentally by abdominal imaging done for other reasons. Gross or microscopic hematuria, the most common presenting symptom, is present in more than half of patients with RCC. The classic "too late" triad of hematuria, abdominal mass, and flank pain occurs in approximately 19% of patients. Paraneoplastic syndromes occur in 10% to 40% of cases and consist of pyrexia, anemia, erythrocytosis, hypercalcemia, liver dysfunction (Stauffer syndrome), and hypertension. Other symptoms can include bone pain and central nervous system abnormalities because up to 30% of patients present with bone and brain metastases.

Diagnosis

The workup of a patient with the preceding symptoms should include a history, physical examination, complete blood cell count, serum chemistry panel (including alkaline phosphatase and liver function tests), urinalysis, urine culture, and a contrast-enhanced CT scan. In most cases, the CT scan will define the nature of the mass. If any of the studies obtained suggests involvement of the renal vein or vena cava, an MRI or CT scan with three-dimensional reconstruction should be obtained to assess the extent of the tumor thrombus. In contrast to the management of other renal tumors, RCC may be treated surgically without preoperative histologic diagnosis of the tumor. Biopsy of a renal mass is rarely indicated unless the radiographic characteristics of the mass suggest an etiology other than RCC, such as lymphoma, TCC, or a metastasis from another malignant primary.

If a mass suggests RCC, a metastatic workup consisting of a chest radiograph, CT scan (if not already obtained), and liver function tests should be performed. The most common sites of metastases of RCC in decreasing order are the lung, bone, and regional lymph nodes. If the patient does not have an increased alkaline phosphatase level or skeletal pain, a bone scan is usually not required. A CT scan of the brain can be performed if there is any suspicion of brain metastases; however, this is not done routinely in the absence of symptoms referable to the CNS.

Grading and Staging

The most widely used grading system for RCC is the Fuhrman system, which is based on nuclear and nucleolar morphology, rated on a scale of 1 to 4.

The TNM system is the most commonly used for staging in the United States. Please refer to Table 19.3.

Management

Localized Renal Cell Carcinoma

To date, surgical excision remains the only proven effective treatment of localized RCC. In a radical nephrectomy, the kidney, ipsilateral adrenal gland, and surrounding Gerota's fascia are all resected en bloc. Although no randomized study has proved its benefit over simple nephrectomy, radical nephrectomy has the theoretical advantage of removing the lymphatics within the perinephric fat. Up to 20% of patients can have evidence of regional lymphatic metastases without distant disease, although the incidence of occult nodal involvement is in the range of 3% to 5%. The 5-year survival rates for patients with positive lymph nodes range from 8% to 35%; however, patients with papillary histology and node metastases that undergo aggressive surgical resection can enjoy an extended progression-free and overall survival, in contrast to those patients with nodal metastases from clear cell histology. Extended lymphadenectomy has never been proved to be of benefit in patients who undergo radical nephrectomy, except in the presence of clinically positive lymph nodes, and many surgeons prefer a limited node dissection, which has limited morbidity, for prognostic information. There is clear evidence that all evidence of gross disease should be removed, if feasible, at the time of nephrectomy.

The surgical approach to radical nephrectomy is determined by the size and location of the tumor and the surgeon's preference. A modified flank, midline, or subcostal (chevron) incision can be used. Large upper-pole tumors may be approached through a thoracoabdominal incision for greater exposure. Because the

Table 19.3. Staging systems for renal cell cancer

Primary tumor clinical (T)	
TX	Primary tumor cannot be assessed
T0	No evidence of primary tumor
T1	Tumor 7 cm or less in greatest dimension, limited to the kidney T1a: Tumor $\leq$4 cm, confined to kidney T1b: Tumor >4 cm, $\leq$7 cm, confined to kidney
T2	Tumor >7 cm in greatest dimension, confined to the kidney
T3	Tumor extends into major veins or invades adrenal gland or perinephric tissues (perinephric fat or renal sinus), but not beyond Gerota's fascia T3a: Tumor invades adrenal gland or perinephric tissues, but not beyond Gerota's fascia T3b: Tumor grossly extends into renal vein(s) or vena cava below diaphragm T3c: Tumor grossly extends into vena cava above diaphragm
T4	Tumor invades beyond Gerota's fascia
Regional lymph nodes (N)	
NX	Regional lymph nodes cannot be assessed
N0	No regional lymph node metastasis
N1	Metastasis in single regional lymph node
N2	Metastasis in multiple regional, contralateral, or bilateral nodes
Distant metastases (M)	
MX	Distant metastasis cannot be assessed
M0	No distant metastasis
M1	Distant metastasis

incidence of ipsilateral adrenal metastasis in lower-pole tumors is rare, not removing the adrenal gland at the time of nephrectomy for a lower-pole lesion is accepted.

Approximately 15% to 20% of RCCs invade the renal vein, and 8% to 15% invade the vena cava. Involvement of RCC in the renal vein usually does not pose a significant surgical problem. Vena caval involvement, however, may require additional extensive procedures to completely excise the tumor. Vena caval thrombi have been divided by many authors into three groups. Type 1 thrombi (50%) are completely infrahepatic, type 2 (40%) are intrahepatic, and type 3 (10%) extend up into the right atrium of the heart. In cases with vena caval involvement, it is imperative that the surgeon be familiar with techniques of vascular surgery, and consideration should be given to consulting with a cardiothoracic surgeon, especially for type 3 thrombi. Cardiopulmonary bypass, deep hypothermic arrest, and venovenous bypass have been used in the resection of these locally advanced tumors that extend to the suprahepatic vena cava.

There are situations in which nephron-sparing surgery is indicated for patients with RCC. For example, in cases of bilateral tumor involvement, renal insufficiency, solitary kidney, or VHL, a parenchyma-sparing procedure may be indicated. In this procedure, the renal artery is temporarily occluded, the kidney cooled down, and partial nephrectomy or wedge resection performed. Frozen sections of the surgical margins are typically analyzed to ensure adequacy of resection. After restoration of arterial blood flow, the renal capsule is closed or, alternatively, perirenal fat or biodegradeable hemostatic material is sutured to the defect to promote healing and hemostasis. Five-year survival rates after partial nephrectomy for patients with stage I or II disease are approximately 90% and 70%, respectively. Most urologic oncologists agree that partial nephrectomy has demonstrated oncologic equipoise with radical nephrectomy in patients with anatomically favorable tumors, even those greater than 4 cm.

Although radical nephrectomy remains the standard treatment in patients with localized RCC and a normal contralateral kidney, nephron-sparing surgery for patients with a tumor 4 cm or less (or even larger tumors that are anatomically favorable for a partial nephrectomy approach) yields 5-year cancer-specific survival rates of 92% to 97%. The incidence of tumor recurrence within the renal remnant is reported to be from 0% to 6%. Therefore, nephron-sparing surgery and radical nephrectomy provide equally effective curative treatments for single, small, well-localized tumors.

More recent advances in the surgical therapy of localized RCC have focused on minimally invasive strategies. Laparoscopic radical nephrectomy, performed either through standard or hand-assisted approaches, is rapidly becoming the gold standard for the treatment of patients with localized RCC that is not amenable to nephron-sparing approaches. Laparoscopic partial nephrectomy has also been reported with some success, although hemostasis issues, prolonged renal ischemia times, and increased risk of positive margins have prevented this minimally invasive technique from being widely assimilated. More recent clinical research has focused on energy ablative strategies such as cryotherapy and radiofrequency ablation, either through laparoscopic or percutaneous approaches, as strategies to treat the small (<4 cm) renal mass. These energy ablative strategies still remain investigational and should be used primarily in the setting of a clinical trial or for patients where surgical therapy is contraindicated.

Advanced Renal Cell Carcinoma

Approximately 40% to 50% of patients either present with or develop metastases during the course of the natural history of their disease. The median survival for patients with metastatic RCC is 12 months. Two randomized phase III trials have demonstrated a significant survival benefit for patients who undergo cytoreductive nephrectomy prior to the administration of systemic therapy in those that present with metastatic disease and their primary tumor in situ. The presence of nodal metastases, in the setting of distant metastatic disease, portends a worse prognosis and decreased response to systemic therapy, which may be altered by aggressive surgical resection of the nodes at the time of cytoreductive surgery.

Distant metastatic disease can be categorized as a solitary metastasis or bulky metastatic disease. Several studies have shown higher 3-year survival rates, ranging from 20% to 60%, after radical nephrectomy with removal of a solitary metastasis. Solitary lung metastases appear to be associated with better survival rates than metastases to other organ sites. Multiple metastases or multiple sites of metastases portend a significantly worse prognosis and are usually approached with systemic therapy options, although the benefit of surgical consolidation following maximum response to systemic therapy has been demonstrated in metastatic RCC, in selected patients.

Cytotoxic chemotherapy has been largely ineffective in RCC; the highest objective response rate for single-agent therapy is only 16%. More recently, regimens with gemcitabine and capecitabine have shown significant activity in selected patients. Interleukin-2 (IL-2) has yielded durable response rates of 15% to 19% in various trials, primarily with the use of high-dose bolus intravenous regimens. Subcutaneous IL-2, either alone or in combination with interferon, is believed to be inferior to intravenous IL-2 regimens, but associated with significantly less toxicity. Until recently, IL-2 was the gold standard of therapy for patients with metastatic disease, but recent inroads into the understanding of the molecular pathways associated with renal cell carcinogenesis and progression have resulted in the development of specific molecular targeted therapies that have rapidly replaced IL-2 in the armamentarium of the oncologist. Just this year, two tyrosine kinase inhibitors, sorafenib and sunitinib, received an FDA indication for the treatment of advanced RCC. Preliminary results with these agents demonstrate impressive disease response rates, acceptable toxicity profiles, with significant prolongation of time to disease progression and survival in treated patients. Other targeted therapies that are demonstrating activity in RCC and hold promise for the future include the VEGF inhibitor bevacizumab, CCI-779, and others.

TESTICULAR CANCER

Epidemiology and Etiology

Malignant tumors of the testis are rare. It is estimated that 7,000 cases of testicular cancer were diagnosed in 2005, but only 300 men will die of this disease. Ninety-five percent of these tumors are of germ cell origin. Although testicular tumors can occur at any age, specific tumor types tend to occur at different ages. Choriocarcinomas tend to occur between 24 and 28 years of age, embryonal carcinomas from 26 to 34 years of age, seminomas from 32 to 42 years of age, and lymphomas and spermatocytic seminomas after the age of 50 years.

The most well-known etiologic factor in the development of testicular cancer is cryptorchidism. Between 3% and 11% of all cases of testis cancer occur in cryptorchid testes. Although trauma to the testis has been linked to testis cancer, there is no evidence of a definite relationship. Genetic factors may also play a significant role.

Carcinoma in situ is a precursor of testicular germ cell cancer. Five percent to 6% of men with a unilateral germ cell tumor have CIS in the contralateral testis, and a germ cell tumor will develop in 50% of these men. Other men with a high risk of CIS are individuals with intersex, cryptorchidism, infertility, or an extragonadal germ cell tumor.

Clinical Presentation

Testicular cancer typically presents as a painless testicular enlargement. Advanced disease can present as back pain, flank pain, or systemic symptoms. The differential diagnosis includes varicocele, hydrocele, hematoma, epididymitis, orchitis, and inguinal hernia.

Diagnosis

Although the diagnosis is usually evident at physical examination to an experienced clinician, scrotal ultrasound can be useful in establishing the diagnosis. Any solid testicular mass is considered a testicular tumor until proved otherwise. Patients with testicular enlargement that is believed to be inflammatory in nature (epididymo-orchitis) must be re-examined after the infection has been treated to rule out the presence of an occult testicular mass. Once a testicular tumor is suspected, the patient's levels of the tumor markers alpha-fetoprotein (AFP) and human chorionic gonadotropin (hCG) should be tested. Following this, the patient should undergo a radical (inguinal) orchiectomy. There is no role for fine-needle aspiration or Tru-cut biopsy in the workup of this disease.

After radical orchiectomy, a CT scan of the chest, abdomen, and pelvis should be performed. If they were initially elevated, tumor markers should be reanalyzed following orchiectomy, after allowing the appropriate time for each marker to return to baseline. This would be approximately 1 week for hCG and 5 weeks for AFP.

Staging

The American Joint Committee on Cancer and International Union Against Cancer TNM testicular cancer staging system is outlined in Table 19.4. In terms of biological behavior and therapy, testicular tumors can be categorized as seminomatous or nonseminomatous germ cell tumors (NSGCTs). Seminomas are radiation-sensitive and chemosensitive tumors that undergo lymphatic spread in an orderly fashion. In contrast, NSGCTs are less radiation sensitive and have a higher metastatic potential than seminomas.

Management

Seminomatous Germ Cell Tumors

After radical orchiectomy, stage I and IIA seminomas are typically treated with radiation therapy to the ipsilateral iliac and periaortic areas up to the level of the diaphragm after radical orchiectomy. Using radiation therapy, the cure rate for stage I

Table 19.4. American Joint Committee on Cancer/ International Union Against Cancer Systems for Testicular Cancer

Primary tumor clinical (T)	
pTX	Primary tumor cannot be assessed
pT0	No evidence of primary tumor (scar in testis)
pTis	Intratubular germ cell neoplasia (carcinoma in situ)
pT1	Tumor limited to the testis and epididymis and no vascular/lymphatic invasion Tumor may invade into the tunica albuginea but not the tunica vaginalis
pT2	Tumor limited to the testis and epididymis with vascular/lymphatic invasion or tumor invading into the tunica albuginea with involvement of the tunica vaginalis
pT3	Tumor invades the spermatic cord with or without vascular/lymphatic invasion
pT4	Tumor invades the scrotum with or without vascular/lymphatic invasion
Regional lymph nodes (N)	
NX	Regional lymph nodes cannot be assessed
N0	No regional lymph node metastasis
N1	Lymph node mass 2 cm or less in greatest dimension; or multiple lymph nodes masses, none more than 2 cm in greatest dimension
N2	Lymph node mass, more than 2 cm but not more than 5 cm in greatest dimension; or multiple lymph node masses, any one mass greater than 2 cm but not more than 5 cm in greatest dimension
N3	Lymph node mass more than 5 cm in greatest dimension
Distant metastases (M)	
MX	Distant metastasis cannot be assessed
M0	No distant metastases
M1	Presence of distant metastases M1a: Nonregional nodal or pulmonary metastases M1b: Distant metastases other than to nonregional lymph nodes and lungs

Serum tumor markers

Stage	LDH	hCG (mIU/mL)		AFP (ng/mL)
S0	≤Normal	≤N		≤N
S1	<1.5 × Normal	<5,000		<1,000
S2	1.5–10 × Normal	5,000–50,000		1,000–10,000
S3	>10 × Normal	>50,000		>10,000
Stage 0				
	pTis	N0	M0	S0
Stage I				
IA	T1	N0	M0	S0
IB	T2–T4	N0	M0	S0
IS	Any T	N0	M0	S1–S3
Stage II				
IIA	Any T	N1	M0	S0–S1
IIB	Any T	N2	M0	S0–S1
IIC	Any T	N3	M0	S0–S1
Stage III				
IIIA	Any T	Any N	M1	S0–S1
IIIB	Any T	Any N	M0–M1	S2
IIIC	Any T	Any N	M0–M1	S3

LDH, lactic dehydrogenase; hCG, human chorionic gonadotropin; AFP, alpha-fetoprotein.

disease approaches 100%. Although 10% to 15% of patients with stage IIA disease have relapses, more than half of these respond successfully to salvage therapy, yielding a survival rate of 95% for patients with stage IIA disease.

Stage IIB or III disease is usually treated with cisplatin- or carboplatin-based chemotherapy. Surgery is generally reserved for lymphatic disease that does not respond to chemotherapy or radiation therapy and is rarely performed in the setting of metastatic seminoma following radiation and/or chemotherapy. Using this approach, 5-year disease-free survival rates of 86% and 92% have been obtained for patients with stages IIB and III disease, respectively.

Nonseminomatous Germ Cell Tumors

The optimal therapy for stage I disease is controversial; options include surveillance, retroperitoneal lymph node dissection (RPLND), and primary systemic chemotherapy. Overall, approximately 20% to 30% of patients with stage I disease who undergo surveillance experience relapse. In 1989, Wishnow et al. at M. D. Anderson found that patients with vascular invasion in their tumor, AFP levels greater than 80 ng per mL, or more than 80% embryonal elements in their tumor were at high risk for relapse. High-risk patients have been offered two courses of carboplatin, etoposide, and bleomycin (CEB). Low-risk patients are offered observation. At 30 month's follow-up, no patients treated with CEB experienced relapse.

The recurrence rate after RPLND for low-volume stage II disease is less than 20%. Thus, both RPLND and primary systemic chemotherapy have been used to treat low-volume retroperitoneal disease. Survival rates of 97% or better have been associated with both forms of therapy. At M. D. Anderson, patients with stage II disease are treated with primary chemotherapy, and RPLND is used to remove residual disease.

Because of the high recurrence rates associated with RPLND for stage IIB, IIC, and III NSGCTs, primary systemic chemotherapy is the treatment of choice for this disease. RPLND is used to remove any residual disease that may be present after primary chemotherapy and to determine the need for further therapy. Recent experience with chemotherapy for advanced NSGCT at M. D. Anderson has shown 5-year survival rates of 96% and 76% for low- and high-volume stage III disease, respectively.

Because a majority of NSGCTs produce either AFP or β-hCG, these markers are helpful in monitoring the patient for treatment response and recurrent disease.

Despite the relatively early age of onset of testicular cancer, this disease remains one of the most curable cancers in humans.

RECOMMENDED READING

Prostate Cancer

Ahmed S, Lindsey B, Davies J. Emerging minimally invasive techniques for treating localized prostate cancer. *BJU Int* 2005;96(9):1230–1234.

Ash D. Advances in radiotherapy for prostate cancer. *Br J Radiol* 2005;78:S112–S116.

Berthold DR, Sternberg CN, Tannock IF. Management of advanced prostate cancer after first-line chemotherapy. *J Clin Oncol* 2005;23(32):8247–8252.

Brawn PN, Ayala AG, von Eschenbach AC, et al. Histologic grading study of prostate adenocarcinoma: the development of a new system and comparison of other methods—a preliminary study. *Cancer* 1982;49:525.

Catalona WJ, Partin AW, Slawin KM, et al. Use of percentage of free prostate specific antigen to enhance the differentiation of prostate cancer from benign prostatic disease: a prospective multicenter clinical trial. *JAMA* 1998;297:1542–1547.

Catalona WJ, Richie JP, Ahmann FR, et al. Comparison of DRE and serum PSA in the early detection of prostate cancer. *J Urol* 1994;151:1283–1290.

Chybowski FM, Keller JJ, Bergstralh EJ, et al. Predicting radionucleotide bone scan findings in patients with newly diagnosed untreated prostate cancer: prostate specific antigen is superior to all other clinical parameters. *J Urol* 1991;145:313.

Cooner WH, Mosley BR, Rutherford JR, et al. Prostate cancer detection in a clinical urological practice by ultrasonography, digital rectal examination and prostate specific antigen. *J Urol* 1990;143:1146.

Laufer M, Denmeade SR, Sinibaldi J, et al. Complete androgen blockade for prostate cancer: what went wrong? *J Urol* 2000;164(1):3–9.

Leandri P, Rossignol G, Gautier JR, et al. Radical retropubic prostatectomy: morbidity and quality of life. Experience with 620 consecutive cases. *J Urol* 1992;147:883.

McNeal JE, Redwine EA, Freiha FS, et al. Zonal distribution of prostatic adenocarcinoma. *Am J Surg Pathol* 1988;12:897.

Medical Research Council Prostate Cancer Working Party Investigations Group. Immediate versus deferred treatment for advanced prostate cancer: initial results of the Medical Research Council Trial. *Br J Urol* 1997;79:235.

National Institutes of Health (NIH). *Consensus Development Conference on the Management of Clinically Localized Prostate Cancer (1987: Bethesda, MD)*. NCI monograph no. 7, NIH publication no. 88-3005. Washington, DC: U.S. Government Printing Office; 1988: 3–6.

Oesterling JE. Using PSA to eliminate the staging radionuclide bone scan. Significant economic implications. *Urol Clin North Am* 1993;20(4):671–680.

Osterling JE, Martin SK, Bergstrlh EJ, et al. The use of prostate specific antigen in staging patients with newly diagnosed prostate cancer. *JAMA* 1993;269:57–60.

Petrylak D. Therapeutic options in androgen-independent prostate cancer. Building on docetaxel. *BJU Int* 2005;96:41–46.

Ries LAG, Wingo PA, Miller DS, et al. The annual report to the nation on the status of cancer, 1973-1997, with a special section on colorectal cancer. *Cancer* 2000; 88(10):2398–2422.

Scardino PT, Frankel JM, Wheeler TM, et al. The prognostic significance of post-irradiation biopsy results in patients with prostate cancer. *J Urol* 1986;135:510.

Smith JA, Herrell SD. Robotic-assisted laparoscopic prostatectomy: do minimally invasive approaches offer significant advantages? *J Clin Oncol* 2005;23(32):8170–8175.

Speight JL, Roach M III. Radiotherapy in the management of clinically localized prostate cancer: evolving standards, consensus, controversies, and new directions. *J Clin Oncol* 2005;23(32):8176–8185.

Vogelzang NJ, Scardino PT, Shipley WU, et al. *Comprehensive Textbook of Genitourinary Oncology*. 3rd ed. Philadelphia, Pa: Lippincott Williams & Wilkins; 2005.

Walsh PC. The natural history of prostate cancer: a guide to therapy. In: Walsh PC, Retik AB, Stamey TA, et al., eds. *Campbell's Urology*. 8th ed. Philadelphia, Pa: WB Saunders; 2002.

Zagars GK, Pollack A, von Eschenbach AC. Management of unfavorable locoregional prostate carcinoma with radiation and androgen ablation. *Cancer* 1997;80(4):764–772.

Zagars GK, von Eschenbach AC, Johnson DE, et al. The role of radiation therapy in stages A2 and B adenocarcinoma of the prostate. *Int J Radiat Oncol Biol Phys* 1988;14:701.

Zinke H, Bergstralh EJ, Blute ML, et al. Radical prostatectomy for clinically localized prostate cancer, long term results of 1,143 patients from a single institution. *J Clin Oncol* 1994;12(11):2254–2263.

Bladder Cancer

Cummings KB, Barone JG, Ward WS. Diagnosis and staging of bladder cancer. *Urol Clin North Am* 1992;19:429.

Gillenwater JY, Grayhack JT, Howards SS, et al., eds. *Adult and Pediatric Urology*. 4th ed. Chicago, Ill: Year Book Medical; 2001.

Heney NM, Ahmad S, Flanagan MJ, et al. Superficial bladder cancer: progression and recurrence. *J Urol* 1983;130:1083.

Herr HW. Transurethral resection of muscle invasive bladder cancer. *J Clin Oncol* 2001;19(1):81–93.

Herr HW. Tumour progression and survival in patients with T1G3 bladder tumors: 15 year outcome. *Br J Urol* 1997;80(5):762–765.

Kachnic LA, Kaufman DS, Heney NM, et al. Bladder preservation by combined modality therapy for invasive bladder cancer. *J Clin Oncol* 1997;15:1022.

Kirkali Z, Chan T, Manoharan M, et al. Bladder cancer: epidemiology, staging, grading, and diagnosis. *Urology* 2005;66(6 suppl 1):4–34.

Lamm DL. Long term results of intravesical therapy for superficial bladder cancer. *Urol Clin North Am* 1992;19:573.

Lamm DL, Blumenstein BA, Crissman JD, et al. Maintenance bacillus Calmette-Guérin immunotherapy for recurrent TA, T1 and carcinoma in situ transitional cell carcinoma of the bladder: a randomized Southwest Oncology Group Study. *J Urol* 2000;163(4):1124–1129.

Logothetis C, Swanson D, Amato R, et al. Optimal delivery of perioperative chemotherapy: preliminary results of a randomized, prospective, comparative trial of preoperative and postoperative chemotherapy for invasive bladder carcinoma. *J Urol* 1996;155(4):1241–1245.

Logothetis CJ, Dexeus FH, Finn L, et al. A prospective randomized trial comparing MVAC and CISCA chemotherapy for patients with metastatic urothelial tumors. *J Clin Oncol* 1990;8:1050.

Logothetis CJ, Johnson DE, Chong C, et al. Adjuvant cyclophosphamide, doxorubicin, and cisplatin chemotherapy for bladder cancer: an update. *J Clin Oncol* 1988;6:1590–1596.

Pollack A, Zagars GK, Swanson DA. Muscle-invasive bladder cancer treated with external beam radiotherapy: prognostic factors. *Int J Radiat Oncol Biol Phys* 1994;30:267–277.

Stockle M, Wellek S, Meyenburg W, et al. Radical cystectomy with or without adjuvant polychemotherapy for non-organ-confined transitional cell carcinoma of the urinary bladder: prognostic impact of lymph node involvement. *Urol* 1996;48(6):868–875.

Vogeli TA. The management of superficial transitional cell carcinoma of the bladder: a critical assessment of contemporary concepts and future perspectives. *BJU Int* 2005;96(8):1171–1176.

Vogelzang NJ, Scardino PT, Shipley WU, et al. *Comprehensive Textbook of Genitourinary Oncology*. 3rd ed. Philadelphia, Pa: Lippincott Williams & Wilkins; 2005.

Renal Cancer

Cohen HT, McGovern FJ. Renal cell carcinoma. *N Engl J Med* 2005;353(23):2477–2490.

Couillard DR, deVere White RW. Surgery of renal cell carcinoma. *Urol Clin North Am* 1993;20: 263.

Gillenwater JY, Grayhack JT, Howards SS, et al., eds. *Adult and Pediatric Urology*. 4th ed. Chicago, Ill: Year Book Medical; 2001.

Kletcher BA, Qian J, Bostwick DG, et al. Prospective analysis of multifocality in renal cell carcinoma: influence of histological pattern, grade, size, number, volume, and DNA ploidy. *J Urol* 1995;153:904–906.

Lam JS, Belldegrun AS, Pantuck AJ. Long-term outcomes of the surgical management of renal cell carcinoma. *World J Urol* 2006; Feb 15.

Ries LAG, Kosay CL, Hankey BF, et al., eds. *SEER Cancer Statistics Review, 1973–1995.* Bethesda, Md: National Cancer Institute; 1998.

Wirth MP. Immunotherapy for metastatic renal cell carcinoma. *Urol Clin North Am* 1993;20:283.

Testis Cancer

Albers P, Albrecht W, Algaba F, et al. Guidelines on testicular cancer. *Eur Urol* 2005;48(6):885–894.

Amato R, Banks E, Ro J, et al. Post-orchiectomy adjuvant chemotherapy for patients with stage I non-seminomatous germ cell tumors of the testis (NGCTT) at high risk of relapse (abstract 604). *Proc AUA* 1999;161(suppl):157.

Carver BS, Sheinfeld J. Germ cell tumors of the testis. *Ann Surg Oncol* 2005;12(1):871–880.

Logothetis CJ. The case for relevant staging of germ cell tumors. *Cancer* 1990;65:709.

Sternberg CN. Role of primary chemotherapy in stage I and low-volume stage II non-seminomatous germ-cell testis tumors. *Urol Clin North Am* 1993;20:93.

Vogelzang NJ, Scardino PT, Shipley WU, et al., eds. *Comprehensive Textbook of Genitourinary Oncology.* 3rd ed. Philadelphia, Pa: Lippincott Williams & Wilkins; 2005.

Wishnow KI, Johnson DE, Swanson DA, et al. Identifying patients with low-risk clinical stage I non-seminomatous testicular tumors who should be treated by surveillance. *Urol* 1989;34:339.

20

Gynecologic Cancers

Brian M. Slomovitz, Pamela T. Soliman, and Judith K. Wolf

Surgical oncologists are often consulted by general obstetrician/gynecologists to assist in the management of patients with primary gynecologic malignancies. The surgical oncologist should understand the surgical staging procedures involved with each disease process (i.e., ovarian, fallopian tube, uterine, cervical, vulvar, and vaginal). This chapter discusses the basic principles of gynecologic oncology so appropriate management can occur when these neoplasms are unexpectedly encountered. Emphasis is placed on diagnosis, staging, and surgical management.

OVARIAN CANCER

Ovarian cancer is the deadliest of gynecologic malignancies. In the United States, approximately 20,180 new cases will be diagnosed, and approximately 15,310 women will die in 2006. Ovarian cancers are heterogeneous, and subtypes are defined by histology. The most common, and "typical," is epithelial ovarian cancer. Other less common subtypes are germ cell tumors and sex cord stromal tumors.

Epithelial Ovarian Cancer

Incidence

Epithelial ovarian cancer occurs in 1 in 70 women and constitutes 90% of all ovarian cancers. The median age at diagnosis is 61 years. Approximately 10% of these cases are hereditary, and these are transmitted in an autosomal dominant fashion. Hereditary breast ovarian cancer syndrome (BRCA-1 and BRCA-2 mutations) and Lynch syndrome/hereditary nonpolyposis colorectal cancer (HNPCC) (in which colon, endometrial, ovarian, and other cancers cluster in first- and second-degree relatives) are known hereditary forms of ovarian cancer; other genetic mutations likely remain to be identified.

Risk Factors

Various factors are believed to increase the risk of a woman developing epithelial ovarian cancer. These include increased age (peak age is 70 years), nulliparity, early menarche, late menopause, delayed childbearing, and Ashkenazi Jewish descent. Early studies suggested an association with fertility drugs (i.e., clomiphene and gonadotropin), but more recent studies have not confirmed this link. The use of oral contraceptives for more than 5 years appears to protect against the development of epithelial ovarian cancer.

Pathology

Tumor subtypes are listed in Table 20.1. The incidence of concomitant endometrial carcinoma is 15% to 30% in cases of

Table 20.1. Percentage distribution of epithelial ovarian carcinomas and percentage that are bilateral, by histologic subtype

Histologic Subtype	Percentage Distribution	Bilaterality (%)
Serous	46	73
Mucinous	36	47
Endometrioid	8	33
Clear cell	3	13
Transitional	2	—
Mixed	3	—
Undifferentiated	<2	53
Unclassified	<1	—

endometrioid ovarian carcinoma. Cases of synchronous appendiceal and ovarian mucinous tumors have also been reported, but because it is not unusual for appendiceal cancer to spread to the ovaries, it can be difficult to determine the true site of the primary disease.

Routes of Spread and Sites of Metastasis

Because exfoliated cells tend to assume the circulatory path of the peritoneal fluid and implant along this path, the most common route of metastasis is by seeding. Epithelial ovarian cancer may also metastasize to the lymph nodes, but hematogenous spread is uncommon.

Clinical Features

SYMPTOMS. The interval from onset of disease to diagnosis is often prolonged because of a lack of specific symptoms, and diagnosis is often not made until patients have disseminated disease. Approximately 65% of cases are stage III or IV disease at diagnosis. Symptoms suggestive of ovarian cancer include abdominal fullness, early satiety, weight loss, dyspepsia, urinary frequency, constipation, unexplained pelvic pain, and increased flatulence. Patients with stage IV disease and malignant pleural effusions may present with a cough. It is uncommon for ovarian cancer to be diagnosed by abnormal Papanicolaou (Pap) smear results.

PHYSICAL FINDINGS. An adnexal mass noted on routine pelvic examination and a palpable fluid wave are often found in patients with advanced-stage epithelial ovarian cancer. Five percent of patients with presumed ovarian cancer have another primary tumor that has metastasized to the ovary. The most common primary cancers that metastasize to the ovary are breast, gastrointestinal tract, and other gynecologic cancers.

Pretreatment Workup

Careful physical examination, including pelvic examination with rectovaginal exam, is required. Other components of the pretreatment workup include clinical tests (e.g., complete blood cell count, serum glucose, blood urea nitrogen, creatinine, liver function, serum albumin, CA-125 [which is elevated in approximately 80% of cases]), chest radiography, and mammography. Computed tomography (CT) analysis may help determine the extent of disease. Barium enema is useful in examining the colon and can be particularly helpful in distinguishing between a primary ovarian and primary colon cancer, which may present in the same way.

Staging

The surgical staging schema for epithelial ovarian cancer is outlined in Table 20.2.

Treatment

The initial step in treatment is surgical cytoreduction with appropriate intraoperative staging procedures, including abdominal and pelvic cytologic analysis (or collection of ascites), careful exploration of all abdominal and pelvic structures and surfaces, total abdominal hysterectomy and bilateral salpingo-oophorectomy (except in cases of concern about fertility or of early-stage disease), omentectomy, and selective pelvic and para-aortic lymph node sampling. In patients with a mucinous tumor or an involved appendix, appendectomy should be performed. Primary cytoreduction is a key component in advanced cases because survival is directly correlated to the amount of residual tumor remaining. Optimal tumor reductive surgery is loosely defined as the diameter of the largest residual tumor implant being less than 1 cm. If the residual mass is larger than 1 cm, then cytoreduction is deemed suboptimal.

Although "second-look" laparotomy or laparoscopy was routinely performed in the past, it is no longer performed unless required as part of an investigational trial.

After surgical cytoreduction, patients should be treated with combination platinum- and taxane-based chemotherapy. After six to eight courses of chemotherapy, treatment decisions are based on the presence of persistent disease or the disease-free interval.

In select cases, there may be a role for neoadjuvant ("up-front") chemotherapy followed by an interval cytoreduction procedure. In patients with stage IV disease (i.e., malignant pleural effusions or intraparenchymal liver disease), neoadjuvant chemotherapy may be warranted for those with multiple medical comorbidities that preclude aggressive surgical debulking or extensive disease that cannot be optimally reduced (as determined by CT scan or diagnostic laparotomy or laparoscopy). The effect of this approach on survival, however, is unproven in patients with advanced or bulky disease. A current phase III trial in Europe may determine whether there is a survival advantage to neoadjuvant chemotherapy as first-line treatment.

Prognostic Factors

Prognostic pathological factors include tumor grade (Table 20.3), histologic subtype, tumor grade, and DNA ploidy. Clinical factors of prognostic significance include surgicopathological stage, extent of residual disease remaining after primary cytoreduction (Table 20.3), volume of ascites, patient age, and patient performance status. Patients with poor performance status before

Table 20.2. Surgical staging of epithelial ovarian cancer

Tumor Stage	Description
I	Growth limited to the ovaries
IA	Growth limited to one ovary, no ascites, no tumor on the external surfaces, intact capsules
IB	Growth in both ovaries, no ascites, no tumor on the external surfaces, intact capsules
IC	Stage IA or IB characteristics but with tumor on the surface of one or both ovaries, ruptured capsules, or malignant ascites with positive peritoneal cytologic results
II	Growth involving one or both ovaries with pelvic extension
IIA	Extension and/or metastases to the uterus and/or tubes
IIB	Extension to other pelvic tissues
IIC	Stage IIA or IIB characteristics but with tumor on the surface of one or both ovaries, ruptured capsules, or malignant ascites with positive peritoneal cytologic results
III	Growth involving one or both ovaries with peritoneal implants outside the pelvis and/or positive retroperitoneal or inguinal nodes; superficial liver metastasis equal to stage III; tumor limited to the true pelvis but with histologically proved malignant extension to the small bowel or omentum
IIIA	Tumor grossly limited to the true pelvis with negative nodes but histologically confirmed microscopic seeding of abdominal peritoneal surfaces
IIIB	Tumor involving one or both ovaries with histologically confirmed implants of abdominal peritoneal surfaces $\leq$2 cm in diameter; negative nodes
IIIC	Abdominal implants >2 cm in diameter and/or positive retroperitoneal or inguinal nodes
IV	Growth involving one or both ovaries with distant metastases; positive cytologic results from pleural effusion or pathological confirmation of parenchymal liver metastases

Table 20.3. Five-year survival rates for patients with epithelial ovarian cancer, by tumor stage and grade, amount of residual disease, and disease status

		Survival Rate (%)		
Tumor Stage	All Grades	Grade 1	Grade 2	Grade 3
I				
IA	85	92.5	86	63
IB	69	85	90	79
IC	59	78	49	51
II				
IIA	62	64	65	39
IIB	51	79	43	42
IIC	43	68	46	20
III				
IIIA	31	58	38	20
IIIB	38	73	42	21
IIIC	18	46	22	14
IV	8	14	8	6

	Survival Rate (%)
Amount of residual disease after primary cytoreductive surgery	
Microscopic (residual disease)	40–75
Macroscopic (optimal debulking)	30
Macroscopic (suboptimal debulking)	5
Disease status at second look	
No evidence of disease	50
Microscopic disease	35
Macroscopic disease	5

treatment (Karnofsky score <70%) have significantly shorter survival than do patients with good performance status.

Ovarian Tumors of Low Malignant Potential

These tumors, sometimes referred to as borderline tumors, constitute as many as 5% to 15% of epithelial ovarian malignancies. The highest incidence is among white women, and the mean age at diagnosis is 39 to 45 years (approximately 10 to 15 years younger than that for epithelial ovarian cancer). No risk factors have been identified, and pregnancy and exogenous hormones do not appear to be protective. There is no apparent association with family history.

The most common histologic subtypes of ovarian tumors of low malignant potential (LMP) are serous and mucinous (Table 20.4). Diagnosis requires the absence of frank stromal invasion. Distinct pathological features that may be associated with a more aggressive disease course include micropapillary architecture, microinvasion, and invasive implants.

Patients with ovarian tumors of LMP, as well as those with epithelial ovarian cancers, present similarly. The most common

Table 20.4. Distribution of ovarian tumors of low malignant potential, by tumor stage and histologic type

	Histologic Type (%)	
Tumor Stage	Serous	Mucinous
I	65	89.5
II	14	1
III	20	9
IV	1	0.5

symptoms are lower abdominal pain or discomfort, early satiety, dyspepsia, and a sense of abdominal enlargement. Ovarian tumors of LMP can also be identified as an adnexal mass on routine pelvic examination. The CA-125 levels may be elevated in serous tumors.

Compared with patients with invasive epithelial ovarian cancer, it is more common for patients with ovarian tumors of LMP to be diagnosed with early-stage disease. Recommended treatment for all patients is primary surgery; fertility-sparing procedures should be performed in patients with stage I disease who desire children in the future. There has been no proven benefit to adjuvant therapy in treating this cancer, even in patients with advanced-stage disease. Typically, these tumors have an indolent clinical course and may recur after a long disease-free interval. Tumor stage is the most important predictor of survival (Table 20.5). Secondary cytoreduction can be considered in select patients with recurrent disease.

Ovarian Germ Cell Tumors

Incidence

Germ cell tumors are the second most common type of ovarian tumor. Among persons 20 years of age or younger, 70% of ovarian tumors are of germ cell origin, and one-third of these are malignant. The mean age at diagnosis is 19 years; germ cell tumors rarely occur after the third decade of life. Sixty to 75% of cases are stage I at diagnosis.

Table 20.5. Five-year survival rates for patients with ovarian tumors of low malignant potential, by tumor stage

Tumor Stage	Survival Rate (%)
I	95
II	75–80
III	65–70

Pathology

The histologic subtypes of germ cell tumors and their incidences are listed in Table 20.6.

Routes of Spread and Sites of Metastasis

Germ cell tumors have the same potential as epithelial ovarian tumors to metastasize.

Clinical Features

Germ cell malignancies grow rapidly and are often characterized by pain secondary to torsion, hemorrhage, or necrosis. They may also cause bladder, rectal, or menstrual abnormalities. Dysgerminomas account for 20% to 30% of malignant ovarian tumors diagnosed during pregnancy. Embryonal carcinomas may produce estrogen and cause precocious puberty.

Pretreatment Workup

Careful physical examination, including pelvic examination, is required. Other components of the pretreatment workup include clinical tests (e.g., complete blood cell count, serum glucose, blood urea nitrogen, creatinine, liver function, serum albumin) and chest radiography. Serum markers, including α-fetoprotein, β-human chorionic gonadotropin (β-hCG), and lactic dehydrogenase, should be measured (Table 20.6). The karyotype should be checked in premenopausal women with an ovarian mass because the incidence of dysgenic gonads is increased in patients with these tumors.

Staging

The surgical staging criteria are the same as those for epithelial ovarian cancer (Table 20.2).

Treatment

In general, surgical staging includes unilateral salpingo-oophorectomy (if there is a desire to preserve fertility), peritoneal cytology, omentectomy, and selective biopsies of retroperitoneal lymph nodes and abdominal structures. For patients whose disease is inadequately staged, there are two options: surgical re-exploration and appropriate staging, or initiation of chemotherapy without re-exploration. In most cases, it is imprudent to delay chemotherapy by re-exploration and staging because these tumors are highly chemosensitive.

Chemotherapy is recommended for all patients with germ cell tumors, except those with stage I tumors. Chemotherapy should begin 7 to 10 days after surgical exploration because of rapid tumor growth. The first-line regimen is bleomycin, etoposide, and cisplatin administered for three or four cycles in 21-day intervals. Radiotherapy may have a limited role in treatment of dysgerminomas.

Prognostic Factors

The survival rates for individual ovarian germ cell tumor subtypes are listed in Table 20.7. Dysgerminomas larger than 10 to 15 cm in diameter or with a high mitotic index and anaplasia are

Table 20.6. Clinical features of ovarian germ cell tumors, by histologic subtype

			Tumor Markers		
Histologic Subtype	Incidence (%)	Bilaterality	AFP	β-hCG	LDH
Dysgerminoma	40	10%–15% of cases	−	±	+
Endodermal sinus tumor	22	Rare; dermoids common in contralateral ovary	+	−	±
Immature teratoma	20	Rare; dermoids common in contralateral ovary	±	−	±
Embryonal carcinoma	1–3	Rare	+	+	±
Choriocarcinoma	1–3	Rare	−	+	−
Polyembryonal	1–3	Rare	±	±	±
Mixed tumor	10–15	Varies	±	±	±

AFP, α-fetoprotein; β-hCG, beta subunit of human chorionic gonadotropin; LDH, lactic dehydrogenase; −, negative result; ±, positive/negative result; +, positive result.

Table 20.7. Survival rates for patients with ovarian germ cell tumors, by histologic subtype, tumor stage or grade, and time interval

Histologic Subtype and Tumor Stage or Grade	Interval (y)	Survival Rate
Dysgerminoma	5	
Stage I		90%–95%
All stages		60%–90%
Endodermal sinus tumor	2	
Stages I and II		90%
Stages III and IV		50%
Immature teratoma	5	
Stage I		90%–95%
All stages		70%–80%
Grade 1		82%
Grade 2		62%
Grade 3		30%
Embryonal carcinoma	5	39%
Choriocarcinoma		Low
Polyembryonal		Low
Mixed tumor		Variable; depends on tumor composition

more likely to recur. Prognostic factors for immature teratomas include tumor grade, extent of disease at diagnosis, and amount of residual tumor. The tumor grade of immature teratomas is determined by the presence of immature neural elements. Tumor stage is also an important prognostic factor for all ovarian germ cell tumors (Table 20.8).

Sex Cord Stromal Tumors

Incidence

Sex cord stromal tumors account for 5% to 8% of ovarian malignancies and up to 5% of childhood malignancies. Occurrence before menarche is often associated with precocious puberty.

Table 20.8. Five-year survival rates for patients with ovarian germ cell tumors, by tumor stage

Tumor Stage	Survival Rate (%)
I	72
II	38
III	18
IV	0

Table 20.9. Major classifications of sex cord stromal tumors

Granulosa cell tumors
Adult
Juvenile
Thecomas and fibromas-fibrosarcomas
Stromal tumors with minor sex cord elements
Sertoli stromal cell tumors
Sertoli cell
Leydig cell
Sertoli-Leydig cell
Gynandroblastomas
Sex cord tumors with annular tubules
Unclassified tumors

Pathology

As their name suggests, these tumors are derived from sex cords or stroma. Derivatives include granulosa cells, theca cells, stromal cells, Sertoli cells, Leydig cells, and cells resembling embryonic precursors of these cell types (Table 20.9).

Routes of Spread and Sites of Metastasis

The pattern and sites of metastatic spread are analogous to that of epithelial ovarian cancers.

Clinical Features

GRANULOSA CELL TUMORS. Granulosa cell tumors comprise 1% to 2% of ovarian tumors. Adult-type tumors (90% to 95% of granulosa cell tumors) are characterized by secretion of excess estrogen. Patients may experience menstrual irregularities or postmenopausal bleeding. Five percent of patients present with an acute abdomen caused by tumor hemorrhage. Patients with juvenile-type granulosa cell tumors (5% to 10% of granulosa cell tumors) can also present with menstrual abnormalities, abdominal pain, and (rarely) postmenopausal bleeding. Because granulosa cell tumors produce estrogen, coexisting endometrial pathological processes occur in up to 30% of patients. In rare cases, these tumors may produce testosterone and cause some virilizing features.

THECOMAS. Thecomas are one-third as common as granulosa cell tumors. The mean age at diagnosis is 53 years, and 2% to 3% of these tumors are bilateral. Menstrual abnormalities and postmenopausal bleeding are the most common presenting symptoms. Thecomas also produce estrogen.

FIBROMAS AND FIBROSARCOMAS. Fibromas and fibrosarcomas are the most common sex cord stromal tumors and constitute 4% of ovarian neoplasms. The mean age at diagnosis is 46 years. Ten percent of these lesions are bilateral. Symptoms include ascites in 50% of patients with tumors larger than 6 cm in diameter, increased abdominal girth, Meigs syndrome (right pleural effusion and ascites), and Gorlin syndrome with basal nevi. These tumors are primarily inert but may secrete small amounts of estrogen.

SERTOLI CELL TUMORS. The average age at diagnosis of Sertoli cell tumors is 27 years, but these tumors can occur at any age. Sertoli cell tumors are unilateral. Seventy percent of patients have symptoms related to excess estrogen, whereas 20% exhibit signs of virilization. Rarely, hyperaldosteronemia manifested as hypertension and hyperkalemia may develop. Seventy percent of these tumors produce both estrogen and androgens, whereas 20% produce androgens alone.

LEYDIG CELL TUMORS. Leydig cell tumors occur at an average age of 50 to 70 years but can occur at any age. These tumors are often unilateral. Eighty percent produce androgens and 10% produce estrogen, which often results in hormonally related side effects. Leydig cell tumors are often associated with thyroid disease and may be hereditary.

SERTOLI-LEYDIG CELL TUMORS. Sertoli-Leydig cell tumors occur at an average age of 25 to 40 years but can occur at any age. These tumors are rarely bilateral. Symptoms include amenorrhea, and virilization may occur in up to 50% of patients. Most of these tumors produce testosterone, and some may produce α-fetoprotein.

GYNANDROBLASTOMAS. Gynandroblastomas are unilateral tumors that can occur at any age. Patients may experience estrogenic effects or virilization secondary to the hormone products of these tumors. Histologically, both granulosa cell and Sertoli-Leydig cell components may be present in these tumors. These tumors may produce androgens or estrogen, or they may be inert.

SEX CORD TUMORS WITH ANNULAR TUBULES. The average age of patients with sex cord tumors with annular tubules is 25 to 35 years. These tumors may be associated with Peutz-Jeghers syndrome, and in these cases, 66% are bilateral and most produce estrogen. Among those that occur in women without Peutz-Jeghers syndrome, only 40% produce excess estrogen. These tumors are also associated with endocervical adenocarcinomas.

Pretreatment Workup

Careful physical examination, including pelvic examination, is required. Other components of the pretreatment workup include clinical tests (e.g., complete blood cell count, serum glucose, blood urea nitrogen, creatinine, liver function, serum albumin, CA-125), chest radiography, and mammography. Evaluation of serum concentrations of estradiol, dehydroepiandrosterone, testosterone, 17-OH-progesterone, and hydrocortisone may be helpful in diagnosis. CT and ultrasonography should be performed to evaluate the adrenal glands and ovaries. Although imaging studies may be helpful, they do not often change the planned staging procedure.

Staging

In general, surgical staging of sex cord stromal tumors can be accomplished by unilateral salpingo-oophorectomy (if there is a desire to maintain fertility), peritoneal cytology, infracolic omentectomy, selective biopsies of nodes and abdominal structures, and appropriately targeted biopsies. If a hysterectomy is not performed at the time of surgery, dilatation and curettage

Table 20.10. Five-year survival rates for patients with sex cord stromal tumors, by histologic subtype

Histologic Subtype	Survival Rate
Granulosa cell tumor	
Tumors confined to the ovary	85%–90%
Tumors with extraovarian extension	55%–60%
Sertoli or Leydig cell tumor with poor differentiation	Low
Other tumors of sex cord stromal origin	Consistent with benign processes and low-grade malignancies

and endocervical curettage should be performed to evaluate any coexistent pathological processes. These tumors are surgically staged according to the criteria used for epithelial ovarian cancer (Table 20.2).

Treatment

Tumors of stromal origin (i.e., thecomas and fibromas) and Leydig cell tumors generally follow a benign course; surgery is the only treatment. Sertoli cell or granulosa cell tumors are generally of low malignant potential, tend to recur late, and rarely metastasize. Chemotherapy should be considered for advanced disease. Postoperative adjunctive therapy with bleomycin, etoposide, and cisplatin or other platinum-based chemotherapy should be considered in patients with Sertoli cell or Leydig cell tumors with poor differentiation and heterologous components and in patients with advanced or recurrent stromal tumors; pelvic radiation therapy can also play a role in treatment of these patients. Survival rates are described in Table 20.10.

Management of Incidental Cancers Found at Laparotomy

The finding of an unsuspected ovarian mass at the time of exploratory laparotomy or at laparotomy for an unrelated condition can pose a therapeutic dilemma to the surgeon. Appropriate treatment depends on several factors, including the patient's age, the size and consistency of the mass, possible bilaterality, and gross involvement of other structures. Informed consent is a key component to the decision making. Unless there is a life-threatening situation, a hysterectomy and bilateral salpingo-oophorectomy should be performed only with proper informed consent, especially in women of childbearing age.

OVARIAN MASS IN PREMENOPAUSAL WOMEN. An unsuspected mass in a young patient is most likely benign. The most frequently found benign masses involving the adnexa are functional cysts, which are related to the process of ovulation. These cysts are significant primarily because they cannot be easily distinguished from true neoplasms on clinical grounds alone. If ovulation does not occur, a clear, fluid-filled follicular cyst up to 10 cm in diameter may develop. This follicular cyst usually resolves spontaneously within several days to 2 weeks. Ovulating women can also present with functional ovarian cysts. These are usually asymptomatic but can cause lower abdominal or pelvic pain; signs of an acute abdomen are rare. The corpus luteum, which is formed during ovulation, may become abnormally large if there is hemorrhage within it. A patient with a hemorrhagic corpus luteum may present with an acute abdomen, which necessitates laparotomy. Often the bleeding area may be oversewn without the need for removal of the cyst, fallopian tube, or ovary.

Simple cysts up to 5 cm in diameter may be found incidentally at the time of surgery. These can often be observed safely in women who are in their reproductive years. If it is a functional cyst, it should resolve after the patient's next menstrual period. Resolution can be evaluated with physical examination alone or in conjunction with pelvic ultrasonography. Functional cysts are more common in patients who have anovulatory cycles, such as women who are obese or those who have polycystic ovarian syndrome.

Dermoid cysts, or benign cystic teratomas, are the most common ovarian tumors in women in the second and third decades of life. These cystic masses may be of any size, and up to 15% are bilateral. Torsion is the most frequent complication and commonly occurs in children, young women, and pregnant women. Severe acute abdominal pain is usually the initial symptom, and this condition constitutes an emergency. Treatment is cystectomy and close inspection of the other ovary, and is usually possible even for large lesions.

Other common benign neoplasms that occur in young patients are serous and mucinous cystadenomas. These are treated with unilateral salpingo-oophorectomy if the other ovary appears normal. Endometriomas, which are also called chocolate cysts of endometriosis, can also occur in young women. These patients may have a history of endometriosis or chronic pelvic pain. Often, other endometriosis implants may be seen in the pelvis or abdominal cavity; this finding may be helpful in establishing the diagnosis. The treatment of endometriomas may be cystectomy or unilateral oophorectomy and depends on the degree of the remaining normal-appearing ovarian tissue. Every effort should be made to salvage the normal-appearing portion of ovary.

If ascites is present on opening of the abdomen, it should be evacuated and submitted for cytologic analysis. After careful inspection and palpation, if the ovarian mass appears to be confined to one ovary and malignancy is suspected, unilateral salpingo-oophorectomy is appropriate in most circumstances. If the mass is believed to be benign, ovarian cystectomy may be preferable. The ovarian capsule should be inspected for any evidence of rupture, adherence, or excrescence. Once removed, the ovarian specimen should be sent for frozen-section examination. If malignancy is diagnosed, surgical staging should be performed. This should include biopsies of the omentum, peritoneal surfaces of the pelvis and upper abdomen, and retroperitoneal lymph nodes (including both the para-aortic and the bilateral pelvic regions).

If the contralateral ovary appears normal, random biopsy or wedge resection is probably not indicated because it may interfere with future fertility due to peritoneal adhesions or ovarian failure. If the histologic diagnosis is questionable at the time samples are taken for frozen section, it is always preferable to wait for permanent section results before proceeding with a hysterectomy and bilateral salpingo-oophorectomy in a young patient. General criteria for conservative management include young patients desirous of future childbearing; patient and family consent and agreement to close follow-up; no evidence of dysgenetic gonads; any unilateral malignant germ cell, stromal, or borderline tumor; and stage IA invasive epithelial tumor.

Advances in assisted reproduction have greatly influenced intraoperative management decisions. Traditionally, if a bilateral salpingo-oophorectomy is indicated, a hysterectomy has also been performed. Current technology for donor oocyte transfer and hormonal support, however, allow a woman without ovaries to sustain a normal intrauterine pregnancy. Similarly, if the uterus and one tube and ovary are removed because of tumor involvement, current techniques allow for retrieval of oocytes from the patient's remaining ovary, in vitro fertilization with sperm from her partner, and implantation of the embryo into a surrogate's uterus.

OVARIAN MASS IN POSTMENOPAUSAL WOMEN. The risk of an ovarian mass being malignant begins to increase at 40 years of age and rises steadily thereafter. Therefore, the finding of an unsuspected ovarian mass in a postmenopausal woman is more ominous. The most common malignant neoplasms in this age group are malignant epithelial tumors; germ cell and stromal cell tumors rarely occur. Benign lesions, such as epithelial cystadenomas and dermoid cysts, can still occur in this population, although they do so much less frequently than in younger patients. Treatment of an unanticipated ovarian mass in a postmenopausal patient includes salpingo-oophorectomy and further staging if the frozen section reveals a diagnosis of cancer. Appropriate staging biopsies should also be performed. A gynecologic oncologist should be consulted.

Laparoscopy for the Management of Ovarian Cancer

Laparoscopy has been widely used as the standard surgical approach for benign and suspicious adnexal masses. The role of laparoscopy in the treatment of ovarian cancer is less clear, but some studies have suggested that it can be used safely at the time of second-look surgery or to stage and treat patients with early ovarian cancer. The role of laparoscopy in treating ovarian cancer still needs to be defined, although laparoscopic surgery is associated with significantly less morbidity than laparotomy.

FALLOPIAN TUBE CANCER

Incidence

Fallopian tube cancer accounts for 0.1% to 0.5% of gynecologic malignancies. The average age at diagnosis is 55 years.

Risk Factors

No known risk factors exist for the development of this disease.

Pathology

The most common histologic subtype is adenocarcinoma, and the most common tumors of the fallopian tube are metastatic lesions from other sites. To establish a diagnosis of primary fallopian tube cancer, Hu's criteria must be met: The main tumor must be in the fallopian tube, the mucosa should be involved microscopically and exhibit a papillary pattern, and the transition between benign and malignant tubal epithelium should be demonstrated if the tubal wall is significantly involved with the tumor.

Routes of Spread and Sites of Metastasis

Fallopian tube cancer metastasizes in a manner similar to that of epithelial ovarian cancer. Lymphatic spread tends to play more of a role in fallopian tube cancer, likely because of the presence of particularly extensive lymphatics in the fallopian tubes. One-third of patients with fallopian tube cancer exhibit evidence of nodal metastases.

Clinical Features

The classic triad of primary fallopian tube cancer is watery vaginal discharge, pelvic pain, and a pelvic mass. However, this triad is present in less than 15% of patients. Watery discharge and vaginal bleeding are the most commonly reported symptoms.

Pretreatment Workup

Careful physical examination, including pelvic examination, is required. Other components of the pretreatment workup include clinical tests (e.g., complete blood cell count, serum glucose, blood urea nitrogen, creatinine, liver function, serum albumin, CA-125), chest radiography, and mammography. Imaging studies may be helpful but usually do not change the planned staging procedure. CT may help determine the extent of disease. Barium enema is useful in examining the colon. It can also be particularly helpful in distinguishing a colonic primary in older patients from either fallopian tube or ovarian cancer, which may present with similar symptoms. Intravenous pyelography is also helpful in certain clinical situations.

Staging

There is no official International Federation of Gynecology and Obstetrics (FIGO) staging system for fallopian tube cancer. By convention, the surgical staging criteria used for epithelial ovarian cancer is used (Table 20.2).

Treatment

Treatment of fallopian tube cancer is analogous to that of epithelial ovarian cancer.

Prognostic Factors

It is difficult to determine the prognostic factors specific to fallopian tube cancer because this disease is rare, but they are likely similar to those of epithelial ovarian cancer. The overall 5-year survival rate is estimated to be 40%, which is higher than the 5-year survival rate for patients with epithelial ovarian cancer. This difference in survival is likely related to diagnosis at an earlier stage in fallopian tube cancer than in ovarian cancer.

UTERINE CANCER

Cancers of the uterus are divided into three main categories: those arising from the endometrium (endometrial cancer), those arising from the myometrium or muscle layer (uterine sarcomas), and those associated with pregnancy (gestational trophoblastic disease).

Endometrial Cancer

Incidence

Endometrial cancer is the most common malignancy of the female genital tract and the fourth most common cancer among women in the United States (following breast, lung, and colon cancers). Approximately 40,000 new cases are diagnosed annually, and approximately 7,000 women die yearly from this disease. The median age at onset is 63 years, although up to 25% of patients are premenopausal at the time of diagnosis. Up to 10% of cases of endometrial cancer are hereditary. Lynch syndrome/HNPCC is a hereditary cancer predisposition syndrome characterized by the development of multiple cancers, including endometrial, colorectal, and ovarian cancer.

Risk Factors

Risk factors for endometrial cancer include nulliparity, early menarche, late menopause, obesity, unopposed estrogen therapy, and chronic diseases such as diabetes mellitus and hypertension.

Pathology

Ninety percent of endometrial cancers are endometrioid adenocarcinomas (70% grade 1, 15% grade 2, and 15% grade 3), 5% to 7% are papillary serous carcinomas, and the remaining 3% to 5% are clear cell carcinomas. The latter two histologic subtypes are more aggressive. Although less common than the endometrioid subtype, papillary serous and clear cell carcinomas account for more than 50% of the recurrences and deaths due to endometrial cancer.

Routes of Spread and Sites of Metastasis

Endometrial cancer metastasizes primarily by myometrial invasion and direct extension to adjacent structures, including the cervix, vagina, and adnexa. Lymphatic embolization and hematogenous dissemination can also occur.

Clinical Features

Ninety percent of patients present to their physicians complaining of abnormal uterine bleeding or postmenopausal bleeding; approximately 15% of patients with postmenopausal bleeding have uterine cancer. Patients may also experience pelvic pressure and pelvic pain. Other associated findings include pyometra, hematometra, heavy menses, intermenstrual bleeding, and, in some cases, an abnormal Pap smear result. The presence of atypical glandular cells on a Pap smear requires that an endometrial biopsy be performed to rule out malignancy.

Pretreatment Workup

Careful physical examination, including pelvic examination, is required. Pathological confirmation of the disease by endometrial biopsy or dilatation and curettage is essential. Other components of the pretreatment workup include clinical tests (e.g., complete blood cell count, serum glucose, blood urea nitrogen, creatinine, CA-125), chest radiography, and mammography. Diagnostic tests, including CT, barium enema, proctosigmoidoscopy, cystoscopy, and, in some cases, magnetic resonance imaging (MRI), should be performed as indicated by symptoms or examination findings.

Staging

The surgical staging schema for endometrial cancer is described in Table 20.11. The FIGO grading schema is based on the prevalence of a nonsquamous or nonmorular solid growth pattern (grade 1, 5% or less; grade 2, more than 5% and less than 50%; grade 3, 50% or higher) (Table 20.12).

Table 20.11. Surgical staging of endometrial cancer

Tumor Stage	Description
I	Carcinoma confined to the uterine corpus
IA	Tumor limited to the endometrium
IB	Invasion of half or less of the myometrium
IC	Invasion of more than half of the myometrium
II	Extension of cancer to the cervix but not outside the uterus
IIA	Endocervical glandular involvement only
IIB	Cervical stromal invasion
III	Extension of the tumor outside the uterus but confined to the true pelvis or para-aortic area
IIIA	Tumor invasion of the serosa and/or adnexa, with or without positive cytologic results
IIIB	Metastases to the vagina
IIIC	Metastases to the pelvic and/or para-aortic lymph nodes
IV	Distant metastases or involvement of adjacent pelvic organs
IVA	Tumor invasion of the bowel or bladder mucosa
IVB	Distant metastases, including intra-abdominal and/or inguinal lymph nodes

Table 20.12. International federation of gynecology and obstetrics grading of endometrial cancer

Tumor Grade	Description
1	≤5% a nonsquamous or nonmorular solid growth pattern
2	>5%–50% a nonsquamous or nonmorular solid growth pattern
3	>50% a nonsquamous or nonmorular solid growth pattern

Treatment

Unless a patient has comorbidities that do not allow for surgical intervention, exploratory laparotomy, hysterectomy, and possibly bilateral salpingo-oophorectomy are required for patients with endometrial cancer. Additional surgical staging biopsies, omentectomy, and lymph node dissection are also recommended in certain cases. Up to 20% of patients with endometrial cancer have a synchronous or metastatic ovarian malignancy, so in young patients who want to preserve their ovarian function, the ovaries should be carefully inspected at the time of exploration. After surgical staging, adjuvant chemotherapy, radiation, or both may be indicated. For patients at risk for pelvic or vaginal cancer recurrence, whole pelvic radiotherapy with vaginal brachytherapy has been shown to decrease local recurrence. However, radiation has not been shown to improve overall survival.

For patients with advanced-stage or recurrent disease, chemotherapy is indicated. Chemotherapy is also indicated for patients with high-risk histologic subtypes (papillary serous and clear cell carcinomas). The most active chemotherapeutic agents in the treatment of endometrial cancer are platinum agents, doxorubicin, and taxanes. Administered alone, these agents produce a 30% response rate; combined, the response rate is approximately 50%. Progestin therapy may be used to treat metastatic tumors that express the progesterone receptor; response occurs in 25% to 30% of cases. Hormonal therapy with tamoxifen produces a response in approximately 20% of cases.

Prognostic Factors

Tumor stage is the most important prognostic variable for endometrial cancer (Table 20.13). Other prognostic factors are myometrial invasion, lymphovascular space invasion, nuclear grade, histologic subtype, tumor size, patient age, positive peritoneal cytologic findings, hormone receptor status, and type of primary treatment used (surgery vs. radiation therapy).

Recommended Surveillance

Physical and pelvic examinations should be performed every 3 months in the first year after diagnosis, every 4 months in years 2 and 3, every 6 months in years 4 and 5, and annually thereafter. A Pap smear and chest radiograph should also be obtained annually.

Table 20.13. Five-year survival rates for patients with endometrial cancer, by tumor stage

Tumor Stage	Survival Rate (%)
I	90
II	75
III	40
IV	10

Uterine Sarcomas

Incidence

Uterine sarcomas account for approximately 3% to 5% of uterine cancers.

Risk Factors

Most patients have no known risk factors. A small number of patients have a history of pelvic irradiation.

Pathology

Uterine sarcomas arise from mesodermal derivatives that include uterine smooth muscle, endometrial stroma, and blood and lymphatic vessel walls. The number of mitoses per 10 high-power fields, the degree of cytologic atypia, and the presence of coagulative necrosis are the most reliable predictors of biological behavior. This disease is classified according to the types of elements involved (pure: only mesodermal elements present; mixed: both mesodermal and epithelial elements present) and whether malignant mesodermal elements are normally present in the uterus (homologous: only smooth muscle and stroma present; heterologous: striated muscle and cartilage present) (Table 20.14). Half of endometrial sarcomas are malignant mixed müllerian tumors. Other common histologic subtypes are leiomyosarcomas (40%) and endometrial stromal sarcomas (8%). Less common subtypes are adenosarcomas, pure heterologous sarcomas, and other variants, which together comprise 1% to 2% of uterine sarcomas.

Routes of Spread and Sites of Metastasis

Sarcomas demonstrate a propensity for early hematogenous dissemination and lymphatic spread. Metastasis is exhibited in one-third of patients.

Pretreatment Workup

Careful physical examination, including pelvic examination, is required. Clinical features of uterine sarcomas are listed in Table 20.15. Endometrial biopsy, dilatation and curettage, or both are essential to providing pathological confirmation of disease. Other components of the pretreatment workup include clinical tests (e.g., complete blood cell count, serum glucose, blood urea nitrogen, creatinine, liver function), chest radiography,

Table 20.14. Classification of uterine sarcomas

Tumor Type	Homologous	Heterologous
Pure	Leiomyosarcoma Endometrial stromal sarcoma	Rhabdomyosarcoma Chondrosarcoma Osteosarcoma Liposarcoma
Mixed	Mixed mesodermal (müllerian) sarcoma or malignant mixed mesodermal (müllerian) tumor with homologous components (also called carcinosarcoma)	Mixed mesodermal (müllerian) sarcoma or malignant mixed mesodermal (müllerian) tumor with heterologous components

mammography, and cystoscopy or proctoscopy, depending on the site and extent of the lesion. Preoperative medical clearance is necessary for patients with chronic disease or other appropriate indications.

Staging

No official staging system exists for uterine sarcomas. The FIGO surgical staging schema for endometrial cancer is used instead (Table 20.11).

Treatment

Surgical excision is the only treatment of curative value. Pelvic radiation therapy has a role in local control of the tumor, but because of the propensity of uterine sarcomas for early hematogenous spread, this treatment does not affect outcome. Leiomyosarcomas generally do not respond to radiation therapy. Cisplatin, doxorubicin, and ifosfamide have shown some activity against uterine sarcomas; leiomyosarcomas are more sensitive to doxorubicin. There may be some benefit to hormonal therapy with megestrol acetate; tamoxifen is recommended in cases where hormone receptors have been identified. Hormonal therapy is the treatment of choice for low-grade endometrial stromal sarcomas.

Prognostic Factors

The most important prognostic factor for uterine sarcomas is tumor stage: Diagnosis at stage I has a 5-year survival rate of 50%, whereas diagnosis at any other stage has a 5-year survival rate of 15% or less (Table 20.16). Sarcomatous overgrowth and deep myometrial invasion must be considered in cases of adenosarcoma because they adversely affect prognosis.

Table 20.15. Clinical features of uterine sarcomas and basis for pathological confirmation of the disease, by histologic subtype

Histologic Subtype	Patient's Age	Signs and Symptoms	Pathological Basis for Confirmation of Disease
Endometrial stromal sarcoma	42–53 y	Vaginal bleeding Uterine enlargement Lower abdominal pain or pressure	EMB or D&C
Leiomyosarcoma	45–55 y	Vaginal bleeding Rapid uterine enlargement Lower abdominal pain or pressure	Preoperative diagnosis is difficult: only 15% diagnosed by EMB or D&C
Malignant mixed mesodermal tumor	65–75 y	Several factors in common with endometrial cancer (e.g., nulliparity, obesity, diabetes) Vaginal bleeding Uterine enlargement	EMB or D&C; in up to 50% of cases, the tumor protrudes through the cervix
Adenosarcoma	Any age, but most common in the fifth decade of life	Vaginal bleeding Uterine enlargement	EMB or D&C; in up to 50% of cases, the tumor protrudes through the cervix

EMB, endometrial biopsy; D&C, dilatation and curettage.

Table 20.16. Five-year survival rates for uterine sarcomas, by tumor stage

Tumor Stage	Survival Rate (%)
I	50
II–IV	≤15

Gestational Trophoblastic Disease

Incidence

Gestational trophoblastic disease is characterized by an abnormal proliferation of trophoblastic tissue; all forms develop in association with pregnancy. Because this disease is associated with a gestational event, the age of occurrence spans the entire reproductive spectrum. In the United States, hydatidiform moles occur in 1 in 600 therapeutic abortions and 1 in 1,000 to 2,000 pregnancies; of these, approximately 20% develop malignant sequelae, including invasive moles, placental site trophoblastic tumors, and gestational choriocarcinoma. Choriocarcinoma is estimated to occur in 1 in 20,000 to 40,000 pregnancies. One-half of these cases follow term gestations, one-fourth follow molar gestations, and one-fourth follow other gestational events.

Risk Factors

A number of well-established risk factors are positively associated with hydatidiform mole. These include age younger than 20 years or older than 40 years, previous molar pregnancy (women who have had one molar pregnancy have a 0.5% to 2.5% risk of a second occurrence, and women who have had two molar pregnancies have a 33% risk of a third occurrence), previous spontaneous abortion (the risk increases with each subsequent spontaneous abortion), and Asian race. Black race is negatively associated with hydatidiform mole.

Pathology

Gestational trophoblastic disease is categorized as hydatidiform mole, invasive mole, placental site trophoblastic tumor, and choriocarcinoma. Nonmetastatic disease after molar evacuation may be hydatidiform (invasive) mole or choriocarcinoma. Gestational trophoblastic disease persisting after a nonmolar pregnancy is predominantly choriocarcinoma or, rarely, placental site trophoblastic tumor. Metastatic gestational trophoblastic disease diagnosed in the early months after molar evacuation may be hydatidiform mole or choriocarcinoma. When gestational trophoblastic disease is found remote from a gestational event, it is characteristically choriocarcinoma.

Routes of Spread and Sites of Metastasis

Malignant gestational trophoblastic disease spreads primarily by a hematogenous route. The most frequent site of metastasis is in the lung (80%). Other common sites are the vagina (30%); pelvis (20%); brain (10%); liver (10%); and, bowel, kidney, and spleen (less than 5% each).

Table 20.17. Classification of hydatidiform moles

Feature	Complete Mole	Partial Mole
Hydatidiform swelling of villi	Diffuse	Focal
Trophoblast	Cytotrophoblastic and syncytial hyperplasia	Syncytial hyperplasia
Embryo	Absent	Present
Villous capillaries	No fetal red blood cells	Many fetal red blood cells
Gestational age at diagnosis	8–16 wk	10–22 wk
β-hCG concentration	Usually >50,000 mIU/mL	Usually >50,000 mIU/mL
Proportion that progress to choriocarcinoma	15%–25%	5%–10%
Karyotype	46XX (95%), 46XY (5%)	Triploid (80%)
Uterine size for gestational dates		
Small	33%	65%
Large	33%	10%

β-hCG, beta subunit of human chorionic gonadotropin.

Clinical Features

HYDATIDIFORM MOLE. Vaginal bleeding, uterus size larger than expected for gestational age, and the presence of prominent theca lutein ovarian cysts are characteristic clinical features of hydatidiform mole. Features of partial and complete hydatidiform moles are listed in Table 20.17. Other associated findings include toxemia, hyperemesis, hyperthyroidism, and respiratory symptoms such as dyspnea and respiratory distress. Patients with partial moles may present in the same manner as those with missed or incomplete abortions: vaginal bleeding and the passage of tissue through the vagina.

MALIGNANT GESTATIONAL TROPHOBLASTIC DISEASE. Malignant gestational trophoblastic disease can be categorized as nonmetastatic or locally invasive, or as metastatic. The clinical features of molar pregnancy and the associated incidences of malignant gestational trophoblastic disease are shown in Table 20.18.

Pretreatment Workup for Molar Pregnancy

Careful physical examination, including pelvic examination, is required. Other components of the pretreatment workup include clinical tests (e.g., complete blood cell count, serum glucose, blood urea nitrogen, creatinine, liver function, serum albumin, thyroid function tests, serum β-hCG [in less than 5% of cases, the β-hCG

Table 20.18. Clinical features of molar pregnancy and associated incidences of malignant gestational trophoblastic disease

Clinical Feature	Incidence of Malignant Gestational Trophoblastic Disease (%)
Delayed postmolar evacuation hemorrhage	75
Theca lutein cyst >5 cm	60
Acute pulmonary insufficiency after mole evacuation	58
Uterus large for gestational dates	45
Serum β-hCG concentration >100,000 mIU/mL	45
Second molar gestation	40
Maternal age >40 y	25

β-hCG, beta subunit of human chorionic gonadotropin.

antigen titer may be elevated without clinical or radiographic evidence of disease]), and chest radiography.

Metastatic Workup for Malignant or Persistent Gestational Trophoblastic Disease

Metastatic workup for malignant or persistent gestational trophoblastic disease consists of the tests described for molar pregnancy plus pelvic sonography; CT scan of the abdomen, pelvis, brain, and chest; and MRI of the brain. Metastatic lesions (e.g., a vaginal nodule) should not be biopsied because these lesions are very vascular and patients have exsanguinated from such biopsies.

Staging

The FIGO staging schema of gestational trophoblastic disease is outlined in Table 20.19.

Table 20.19. International federation of gynecology and obstetrics staging of gestational trophoblastic disease

Tumor Stage	Description
I	Confined to the uterine corpus
II	Metastasis to the pelvis and vagina
III	Metastasis to the lung
IV	Distant metastasis to the brain, liver, kidneys, or gastrointestinal tract

Treatment

MOLAR PREGNANCY. Dilation and curettage is the standard treatment for molar pregnancy and is followed by close monitoring of the β-hCG antigen titer. Hysterectomy may be performed if fertility is not an issue.

NONMETASTATIC GESTATIONAL TROPHOBLASTIC DISEASE (FIGO STAGE I). If preserving fertility is not a consideration, a total hysterectomy can be offered. If preserving fertility is desirable, adjuvant single-agent chemotherapy with methotrexate is the most common treatment choice. Chemotherapy should be continued until at least one menstrual cycle beyond normalization of the β-hCG antigen titer. If there is disease resistance (i.e., the β-hCG antigen titer increases or plateaus), the patient should be treated with an alternate single agent, most commonly dactinomycin. If resistance persists, combination chemotherapy with EMA-CO (etoposide, methotrexate, dactinomycin, cyclophosphamide, and vincristine) or MAC (methotrexate, actinomycin, and cyclophosphamide) should be administered.

METASTATIC GESTATIONAL TROPHOBLASTIC DISEASE (FIGO STAGES II TO IV).

Low-risk Disease (World Health Organization Risk Score 0 to 6). For initial treatment, patients generally receive single-agent therapy with methotrexate. If there is disease resistance, the patient should be treated with an alternate single agent, typically dactinomycin. If resistance persists, combination chemotherapy with EMA-CO or MAC should be administered. If there is resistance to EMA-CO and MAC, salvage therapy includes the combination of cisplatin, bleomycin, and vinblastine. Ifosfamide may have a role in refractory cases.

High-risk Disease (World Health Organization Risk Score 7 or Higher). Combination chemotherapy is the treatment of choice. EMA-CO is the initial chemotherapeutic regimen, and cisplatin, bleomycin, and vinblastine are used as salvage treatment.

Special Considerations. Patients with brain metastases may be treated with radiotherapy for local control and prophylaxis against hemorrhage. Patients with residual solitary liver or lung lesions may be candidates for surgical resection.

Prognostic Factors

Factors that may affect a patient's prognosis and response to treatment are outlined in Table 20.20. The cure rate for stage I, II, and III disease is greater than 80%, whereas the cure rate for stage IV disease is approximately 50%.

Recommended Surveillance

Posttreatment surveillance is essentially the same for all cases of gestational trophoblastic disease, except for patients with stage IV disease, who require a longer period of surveillance. β-hCG antigen titers are measured weekly until the level is normal for 3 consecutive weeks and then measured monthly until the level is normal for 12 consecutive months. Patients with stage IV disease are typically followed for 24 months after normalization of β-hCG antigen titer values. Contraception is mandatory throughout the follow-up period.

Table 20.20. Prognostic indicators for patients with gestational trophoblastic disease, by World Health Organization prognostic index score

	World Health Organization Prognostic Index Score			
Prognostic Indicator	0	1	2	4
Age (y)	<39	>39		
Type of antecedant pregnancy	Hydatidiform mole	Abortion	Term	—
Interval between antecedent pregnancy and start of chemotherapy (mo)	<4	4–6	7–12	>12
β-hCG concentration (mIU/mL)	$<10^3$	10^3–10^4	10^4–10^5	$>10^5$
Diameter of largest tumor (cm)		3–5	>5	—
Site of metastasis	Lung, vagina, pelvis	Spleen, kidney	Gastrointestinal tract, liver	Brain
Number of metastases identified	0	1–4	4–8	>8
Prior chemotherapy			1 drug	≥2 drugs

β-hCG, beta subunit of human chorionic gonadotropin.
Low risk 0–6, high risk >6.

Management of Incidental Uterine Masses Found at Laparotomy

The finding of an enlarged or abnormal uterus at the time of exploratory laparotomy or surgery for an unrelated condition can pose a therapeutic dilemma to the surgeon. Uterine fibroids, which are benign tumors of the uterus, are the most common cause of uterine enlargement. In most cases, immediate surgical intervention is unnecessary. Unless the situation is life threatening, hysterectomy and bilateral salpingo-oophorectomy should be performed only after proper informed consent has been obtained, especially in women of childbearing age.

Laparoscopy for the Management of Endometrial Cancer

The use of laparoscopy in the treatment of early-stage endometrial cancer has gained popularity. This approach combines either a laparoscopic-assisted vaginal hysterectomy or a total laparoscopic hysterectomy with a laparoscopic lymphadenectomy. If this approach is used, thorough inspection of the peritoneal cavity, peritoneal washings and appropriate staging biopsies are still important. Laparoscopic surgical staging has not yet been proven to be equivalent in regard to cancer outcome. The Gynecologic Oncology Group is currently evaluating data from a randomized trial of these two approaches.

CERVICAL CANCER

Incidence

Approximately 500,000 women worldwide develop cervical cancer each year. It is the most common cause of cancer-related death among women in underdeveloped countries. In the United States, an estimated 9,710 new cases of cervical cancer and 3,700 deaths due to this disease will occur in 2006.

Risk Factors

Cervical cancer is a sexually transmitted disease. It was the first solid tumor to be linked to a virus: Infection with human papillomavirus, specifically types 16 and 18, is associated with the development of this disease. Other risk factors include early age at first intercourse, multiple sexual partners, multiparity, smoking, and other behaviors associated with exposure to the human papillomavirus. Half of women with newly diagnosed invasive cervical cancer have never had a Pap smear, and another 10% have not had a Pap smear in the previous 5 years.

Pathology

Eighty-five percent of cervical cancers are squamous cell carcinomas, and 10% to 15% are adenocarcinomas, including the less common adenosquamous subtype. Less common histologic subtypes include small cell tumors, sarcomas, lymphomas, and melanomas.

Routes of Spread and Sites of Metastasis

Cervical cancer spreads through various mechanisms. It can directly invade surrounding structures, including the parametria, the corpus, and the vagina. Lymphatic spread commonly occurs in an orderly and predictable sequence involving the parametrial, pelvic, iliac, and finally para-aortic lymph nodes. Hematogenous metastases and intraperitoneal implantation can also occur.

Clinical Features

SYMPTOMS. Discharge and abnormal bleeding, including postcoital, intermenstrual, menorrhagia, and postmenopausal bleeding, are often the first signs of cervical cancer. Frequent voiding and pain on urination can also occur and may indicate advanced disease.

PHYSICAL FINDINGS. Findings on examination vary depending on the site of the lesion (endocervix or ectocervix). Careful inspection and palpation, including bimanual and rectovaginal examinations, are required to determine the size and extent of the lesion.

Pretreatment Workup

Careful physical examination must be performed, including pelvic examination and biopsy of the lesion. Other components of the pretreatment workup include clinical tests (e.g., complete blood cell count, serum glucose, blood urea nitrogen, creatinine, liver function), chest radiography, and mammography.

Cervical cancer is staged by the results of the clinical examination. Therefore, unlike endometrial and ovarian cancer, staging is performed before treatment planning and not at the time of diagnosis. The following studies should be performed for patients with stage IB2 to stage IV cervical cancer: cystoscopy, proctoscopy, intravenous pyelography (or CT of the abdomen or pelvis), and chest X-ray or CT. MRI may be useful, especially in distinguishing endometrial and endocervical lesions.

Staging

The clinical staging scheme for cervical cancer is outlined in Table 20.21. The term microinvasive cervical cancer is sometimes used interchangeably with stage IA lesions. This diagnosis must be made from a cone biopsy or hysterectomy specimen.

Treatment

STAGE IA1. Lesions that satisfy microinvasive disease may be treated conservatively with simple hysterectomy, cervical conization in cases where maintenance of fertility is an issue, or intracavitary radiation therapy for patients who do not qualify for surgery.

STAGE IA2. Lesions that have >3 mm of invasion are significantly more likely to recur when treated conservatively; therefore, radical hysterectomy and lymph node dissection or radiation therapy should be performed.

STAGES IB AND IIA. Surgery or chemosensitizing radiation therapy result in similar cure rates when patients are carefully selected; patients with squamous lesions 4 to 5 cm in diameter and adenocarcinomas smaller than 3 cm in diameter are potential surgical candidates. The standard surgical option is radical hysterectomy with pelvic lymph node dissection. Nonsurgical management may include sensitizing radiation therapy with

Table 20.21. Clinical staging of cervical cancer

Tumor Stage	Description
I	Lesions generally confined to the cervix; uterine involvement is disregarded
IA	Preclinical cervical cancers diagnosed by microscopic analysis alone
IA1	Stromal invasion $\leq$3 mm deep and $\leq$7 mm wide
IA2	Stromal invasion >3 mm but $\leq$5 mm deep and $\leq$7 mm wide
IB	Lesions larger than stage IA lesions, regardless of whether seen clinically
IB1	Clinical lesions $\leq$4 cm
IB2	Clinical lesions >4 cm
II	Extension beyond the cervix but not to the pelvic sidewall or the lower third of the vagina
IIA	No obvious parametrial involvement
IIB	Parametrial involvement
III	Extension to the pelvic wall with no cancer-free space between the tumor and the pelvic wall; tumor involving the lower third of the vagina; hydronephrosis or nonfunctioning kidney unless secondary to an unrelated cause
IIIA	Involvement of the lower third of the vagina; no extension to the pelvic sidewall
IIIB	Extension to the pelvic wall, hydronephrosis, or nonfunctioning kidney
IV	Extension beyond the true pelvis or clinical involvement of the mucosa of the bladder or rectum
IVA	Spread to adjacent organs
IVB	Spread to distant organs

weekly chemotherapy and 40 to 45 Gy external-beam irradiation followed by two intracavitary systems. Among patients who undergo surgery, chemoradiation is used postoperatively in those believed to be at high risk for disease recurrence. Simple hysterectomy after pelvic radiation therapy is indicated primarily for patients whose tumors respond slowly to radiation therapy or when pelvic anatomy precludes optimal intracavitary placement.

STAGES IIB TO IVA. Radiation therapy is the treatment of choice for locally advanced disease. Surgery may be used as adjuvant therapy for stage IVA disease without parametrial involvement and in cases of central disease persisting after radiation therapy.

STAGE IVB. Stage IVB disease is treated primarily with chemotherapy because the disease is disseminated. Cisplatin is the most studied active agent; other options include ifosfamide and mitomycin C. Current clinical trials using vinorelbine (Navelbine) have also demonstrated some activity in cervical cancer.

Table 20.22. Incidence of cervical cancer lymph node metastasis, by tumor stage

	Incidence (%) as Indicated by Lymph Node Metastasis	
Tumor Stage	Pelvic	Para-aortic
I		
IA1	0	0
IA2 (lesion 1–3 mm in diameter)	0.6	0
IA2 (lesion 3–5 mm in diameter)	4.8	<1
IB	15.9	2.2
II		
IIA	24.5	11
IIB	31.4	19
III	44.8	30
IVA	55	40

Radiation therapy may be used in certain cases for local control and palliation of symptoms.

Recurrent Disease

Treatment of recurrent cervical cancer depends on the location of the disease and the type of primary treatment the patient received. Central recurrence may be managed with pelvic exenteration if no contraindicating factors are present. Patients who have had prior radiation therapy and extensive pelvic recurrence or distant metastatic disease are treated with systemic chemotherapy.

Prognostic Factors

The most important prognostic factors for stage I disease include lymphovascular space involvement, tumor size, depth of invasion, and presence of lymph node metastases (Table 20.22). For patients with stage II to stage IV disease, tumor stage, presence of lymph node metastases, tumor volume, age, and the patient's performance status are key prognostic factors. The survival rates for patients with cervical cancer are shown in Table 20.23.

Recommended Surveillance

Physical and pelvic examinations should be performed every 3 months in the first year after diagnosis, every 4 months in years 2 and 3, every 6 months in years 4 and 5, and annually thereafter. A Pap smear and chest radiograph should also be obtained annually.

Among patients who have recurrent cervical cancer, more than 50% are diagnosed with the recurrence within 1 year after primary treatment is completed. Seventy-five percent of patients are diagnosed with their recurrent disease within 2 years, and 95% within 5 years.

Table 20.23. Five-year survival rates for patients with cervical cancer, by tumor stage and histologic subtype

Tumor Stage and Histologic Subtype	Survival Rate (%)
Stage I	
Squamous	65–90
Adenocarcinoma	70–75
Stage II	
Squamous	45–80
Adenocarcinoma	30–40
Stage III	
Squamous	≤60
Adenocarcinoma	20–30
Stage IV (both types)	<15

VULVAR CANCER

Incidence

Vulvar cancer accounts for 3% to 5% of gynecologic malignancies and 1% of malignancies in women. Between 2,000 and 3,000 new cases are diagnosed annually in the United States. The incidence of vulvar cancer tends to be bimodally distributed. Most cases are solitary lesions that occur in postmenopausal women, and the tumors are often associated with chronic vulvar dystrophy. Recently, a subset of tumors has been identified in a younger population; these tumors tend to be multifocal and are associated with human papillomavirus infection.

Risk Factors

The cause of vulvar cancer appears to be multifactorial. Risk factors include human papillomavirus infection (although the association is not as strong as that with cervical cancer), advanced age, low socioeconomic status, hypertension, diabetes mellitus, prior lower genital tract malignancy (e.g., cervical cancer), and immunosuppression.

Pathology

Eighty-five percent of vulvar malignancies are squamous cell carcinomas, and 8% are malignant melanomas. Less common histologic subtypes include basal cell carcinomas, Bartholin gland carcinomas, Paget disease, and adenocarcinomas arising from sweat glands.

Routes of Spread and Sites of Metastasis

Vulvar cancer spreads by direct extension to the vagina, urethra, and rectum. Embolization to regional lymphatics (e.g., the groin) and hematogenous spread to distant sites can also occur.

Clinical Features

SYMPTOMS. Chronic pruritus, ulceration, and nodules on the vulva are the most common presenting symptoms of this disease.

PHYSICAL FINDINGS. Lesions may arise from the labia majora (40%), labia minora (20%), periclitoral area (10%), and perineum or posterior fourchette (15%). Lesions may appear as a dominant mass, warty area, ulcerated area, or thickened white epithelium.

Diagnosis

Five percent of cases are multifocal. Any suspicious area must undergo biopsy, using a Keye punch biopsy and lidocaine without epinephrine for anesthesia.

Pretreatment Workup

Careful physical examination, including pelvic examination and measurement of the lesion, is required. Other components of the pretreatment workup include clinical tests (e.g., complete blood cell count, serum glucose, blood urea nitrogen, creatinine, liver function), chest radiography, mammography, and cystoscopy or proctoscopy, depending on the site and extent of the lesion. Barium enema, CT, and MRI should be performed if indicated. Preoperative medical clearance is necessary for patients with chronic disease or other appropriate indications.

Staging

Since 1988, vulvar cancer has been surgically staged using a system that incorporates TNM (tumor, node, metastasis) classification (Table 20.24). Modifications to the TNM system were added in 1995.

Treatment

STAGE I. Wide local excision should be performed if the lesion has less than 1 mm of invasion into the underlying tissue. Wide radical excision with a traditional 2-cm gross margin (measured with a ruler) and superficial dissection of the ipsilateral groin are appropriate for all other stage I lesions. Bilateral superficial groin dissection should be performed if the lesion is within 2 cm of the midline.

STAGE II. Radical vulvectomy with dissection of bilateral nodes, including superficial and deep inguinal nodes, is the standard approach to stage II disease. The local recurrence rate is similar when the more conservative approach of radical wide excision is used instead of radical vulvectomy. Adjuvant radiation therapy may be indicated if the tumor-free margin of resection is less than 8 mm, the tumor is thicker than 5 mm, or the lymphovascular space invasion is present.

STAGE III. Treatment must be individualized for each patient with stage III disease. Options include surgery, radiation, and a combination of treatment modalities. A modified radical vulvectomy (or a radical wide local excision) with inguinal and femoral node dissection can be performed; pelvic and groin radiation therapy should be administered if positive groin nodes are found. Preoperative radiation therapy (with or without

Table 20.24. Surgical staging of vulvar cancer and corresponding TNM classification

Tumor Stage and Corresponding TNM Classification	Description
I (T1N0M0)	Tumor confined to the vulva and/or perineum; lesion ≤2 cm in diameter; negative nodes
IA	Stromal invasion ≤1 mm
IB	Stromal invasion >1 mm
II (T2N0M0)	Tumor confined to the vulva and/or perineum; lesion >2 cm in diameter; negative nodes
III (T3N0M0, T1N1M0, T3N1M, T2N1M0)	Tumor of any size with adjacent spread to the lower urethra, vagina, or anus, or unilateral regional lymph node metastasis
IV	
IVA (T1N2M0, T3N2M0, TxNxM0)	Tumor invasion of the upper urethra, bladder mucosa, rectal mucosa, or pelvic bone, and/or bilateral regional metastasis
IVB (TxNxM1)	Any distant metastasis, including to the pelvic nodes

Tx, any T; Nx, any N.

radiation-sensitizing chemotherapy) can be given to increase the operability of the lesion and decrease the extent of resection, and is followed by radical excision with bilateral superficial and deep groin node dissection. Radiation therapy alone is an option if the patient is ineligible for radical surgery or the lesion appears to be inoperable.

STAGE IV. Treatment of stage IV disease must also be individualized. Options include radical vulvectomy and pelvic exenteration, radical vulvectomy followed by radiation therapy, preoperative radiation therapy (with or without radiation-sensitizing chemotherapy) followed by radical surgical excision, and radiation therapy (with or without radiation-sensitizing chemotherapy) if the patient is ineligible for surgery or the lesion is deemed inoperable.

Recurrent Disease

Treatment of recurrent disease depends on the site and extent of the recurrence. Options include radical wide excision with or without radiation therapy (depending on prior treatment and extent of recurrence), groin node debulking followed by radiation therapy (depending on prior treatment), and pelvic exenteration. Regional or distant metastasis is difficult to treat, and palliative therapy is often the only option.

Prognostic Factors

The prognostic factors for vulvar carcinoma are various. Inguinal node metastasis appears to be the single most important

Table 20.25. Five-year survival rates for patients with vulvar cancer, by tumor stage

Tumor Stage	Survival Rate (%)
I	95
II	75–85
III	5
IV	
IVA	20
IVB	5

prognostic variable. Other factors include lymphovascular space invasion, tumor stage (Table 20.25), lesion size, lesion site, histologic grade, and depth of invasion.

Recommended Surveillance

Physical and pelvic examinations should be performed every 3 months the first year, every 4 months in years 2 and 3, every 6 months in years 4 and 5, and annually thereafter. A Pap smear should be performed annually.

VAGINAL CANCER

Incidence

Primary vaginal cancer represents 1% to 2% of malignancies of the female genital tract. The average age at diagnosis is 60 years. Most vaginal neoplasms represent metastases from another primary source.

Risk Factors

Risk factors associated with vaginal cancer include low socioeconomic status, history of human papillomavirus infection, chronic vaginal irritation, prior abnormal Pap smear result with cervical intraepithelial neoplasia, prior hysterectomy (59% of patients with primary vaginal cancer), prior treatment for cervical cancer, and in utero exposure to diethylstilbestrol during the first half of pregnancy. Diethylstilbestrol was used from 1940 to 1971 to prevent pregnancy complications such as threatened abortion and prematurity. Clear cell carcinoma of the vagina developed in approximately 1 in 1,000 women exposed to diethylstilbestrol in utero. Since this agent is no longer available, the incidence of this disease has dramatically declined.

Pathology

Eighty-five percent of vaginal cancers are squamous cell neoplasms. Other histologic subtypes include adenocarcinoma (9%), sarcoma (6%), melanoma (<1%), and clear cell carcinoma (<1%).

Routes of Spread and Sites of Metastasis

Vaginal cancer metastasizes via direct extension to adjacent structures. It can also spread through a well-established lymphatic drainage distribution. Lesions of the upper two-thirds of the vagina metastasize directly to pelvic lymph nodes, and lesions of the lower third of the vagina metastasize primarily to the inguinofemoral nodes and secondarily to pelvic nodes. Hematogenous spread is likely a late occurrence because, in most cases, the disease is confined primarily to the pelvis.

Clinical Features

SYMPTOMS. Painless vaginal bleeding and vaginal discharge are the primary symptoms associated with vaginal cancer. Bladder symptoms, tenesmus, and pelvic pain, which are usually indicative of locally advanced disease, are less commonly seen.

PHYSICAL FINDINGS. Lesions are located primarily in the upper third of the vagina, usually on the posterior wall. The appearance of lesions varies. Surface ulceration is usually not present, except in advanced cases. Visualization of lesions identified by Pap smear may require colposcopy.

Pretreatment Workup

Careful physical examination, including pelvic examination with colposcopy, is required unless the lesion is visible. Other components of the pretreatment workup include clinical tests (e.g., complete blood cell count, serum glucose, blood urea nitrogen, creatinine, liver function), chest radiography, mammography, and cystoscopy or proctoscopy, depending on the site and extent of the lesion. Barium enema, CT, and MRI should be performed if indicated. Preoperative medical clearance is necessary for patients with chronic disease or other appropriate indications.

Staging

The clinical staging scheme for vaginal cancers is outlined in Table 20.26.

Table 20.26. Clinical staging of vaginal cancer

Tumor Stage	Description
0	Carcinoma in situ, intraepithelial carcinoma
I	Carcinoma limited to the vaginal wall
II	Carcinoma involving subvaginal tissue but not extending to the pelvic wall
III	Extension to the pelvic wall
IV	Extension beyond the true pelvis, or involvement of the bladder or rectal mucosa
IVA	Spread to adjacent organs and/or direct extension beyond the pelvis
IVB	Spread to distant organs

Table 20.27. Five-year survival rates for patients with vaginal cancer, by tumor stage

Tumor Stage	Survival Rate (%)
I	80
II	45
III	35
IV	10

Treatment

STAGE 0. Stage 0 disease may be treated by surgical excision, laser ablation, and, in some cases, topical 5-fluorouracil.

STAGE I. Lesions of the upper vaginal fornices may be treated with radical hysterectomy and lymphadenectomy or with radiation therapy alone. All stage I lesions (including lesions of the upper vaginal fornices) may be treated with radiation therapy, usually in the form of an intracavitary cylinder.

STAGES II TO IV. External-beam radiation therapy and intracavitary or interstitial radiation therapy are used for stage II to stage IV disease. If the tumor involves the lower third of the vagina, radiation to the groin nodes should be included in the treatment plan.

Recurrent Disease

Treatment of recurrent vaginal cancer depends on the extent of recurrence. Options include wide local excision, partial vaginectomy, and exenteration. Chemotherapy may be given for distant metastatic disease; however, the efficacy of chemotherapy is not well known because of the rarity of the disease.

Prognostic Factors

The most important prognostic factor for vaginal cancer is the tumor stage (Table 20.27).

Recommended Surveillance

Physical and pelvic examinations should be performed every 3 months the first year, every 4 months in years 2 and 3, every 6 months in years 4 and 5, and annually thereafter. A Pap smear should be performed annually.

RECOMMENDED READING

Epithelial Ovarian Cancer

Berek JS, Hacker NF. *Practical Gynecologic Oncology*. 3rd ed. Baltimore, Md: Williams & Wilkins; 2000.

Cannistra SA. Cancer of the ovary. *N Engl J Med* 1993;329:1550.

Dembo AJ, Davy M, Stenwig AE. Prognostic factors in patients with stage I epithelial ovarian cancer. *Obstet Gynecol* 1990;75:263.

Einzig AI, Wiernik PH, Sasloff J, et al. Phase II study and long-term follow-up of patients treated with taxol for advanced ovarian adenocarcinoma. *J Clin Oncol* 1992;10:1748.

Eisenhauer EA, ten Bokkel Huinink WW, Swenerton KD, et al.

European-Canadian randomized trial of paclitaxel in relapsed ovarian cancer: high-dose versus low-dose and long versus short infusion. *J Clin Oncol* 1994;12:2654.

Flam F, Einhorn N, Sjovall K. Symptomatology of ovarian cancer. *Eur J Obstet Gynecol Reprod Biol* 1988;27:53.

Gershenson DM, Mitchell MF, Atkinson N, et al. The effect of prolonged cisplatin-based chemotherapy on progression-free survival in patients with optimal epithelial ovarian cancer: "maintenance" therapy reconsidered. *Gynecol Oncol* 1992;47:7.

Goodman HM, Harlow BL, Sheets EE, et al. The role of cytoreductive surgery in the management of stage IV epithelial ovarian carcinoma. *Gynecol Oncol* 1992;46:367.

Hakes TB, Chalas E, Hoskins WJ, et al. Randomized prospective trial of 5 versus 10 cycles of cyclophosphamide, doxorubicin, and cisplatin in advanced ovarian carcinoma. *Gynecol Oncol* 1992;45:284.

Heintz APM, Hacker NF, Lagasse LD. Epidemiology and etiology of ovarian cancer: a review. *Obstet Gynecol* 1985;66:127.

Hogberg T, Kagedal B. Long-term follow-up of ovarian cancer with monthly determinations of serum CA 125. *Gynecol Oncol* 1992;46:191.

Hoskins WJ. Surgical staging and cytoreductive surgery of epithelial ovarian cancer. *Cancer* 1993;71 (4 suppl):1534.

Hoskins WJ, Bundy BN, Thigpen JT, et al. The influence of cytoreductive surgery on recurrence-free interval and survival in small-volume stage III epithelial ovarian cancer: a Gynecologic Oncology Group study. *Gynecol Oncol* 1992;47:159.

Hoskins WJ, McGuire WP, Brady MF, et al. The effect of diameter of largest residual disease on survival after primary cytoreductive surgery in patients with suboptimal residual epithelial ovarian carcinoma. *Am J Obstet Gynecol* 1994;170:974.

Kohn EC, Sarosy G, Bicher A, et al. Dose-intense taxol: high response rate in patients with platinum-resistant recurrent ovarian cancer. *J Natl Cancer Inst* 1994;86:18.

Krag KJ, Canellos GP, Griffiths CT, et al. Predictive factors for long term survival in patients with advanced ovarian cancer. *Gynecol Oncol* 1989;34:88.

Lynch HT, Watson P, Lynch JF, et al. Hereditary ovarian cancer: heterogeneity in age at onset. *Cancer* 1993;71(2 suppl):573.

Martinez A, Schray MF, Howes AE, et al. Postoperative radiation therapy for epithelial ovarian cancer: the curative role based on a 24-year experience. *J Clin Oncol* 1985;3:901.

McGuire WP, Hoskins WJ, Brady MF, et al. Cyclophosphamide and cisplatin compared with paclitaxel and cisplatin in patients with stage III and stage IV ovarian cancer. *N Engl J Med* 1996;334:1.

Morris M, Gershenson DM, Wharton JT, et al. Secondary cytoreductive surgery for recurrent epithelial ovarian cancer. *Gynecol Oncol* 1989;34:334.

NIH Consensus Conference. Ovarian cancer: screening treatment, and follow-up. *JAMA* 1995;273:491.

Omura GA, Brady MF, Homesley HD, et al. Long-term follow-up and prognostic factor analysis in advanced ovarian carcinoma: the Gynecologic Oncology Group experience. *J Clin Oncol* 1991;9:1138.

Omura GA, Bundy BN, Berek JS, et al. Randomized trial of cyclophosphamide plus cisplatin with or without doxorubicin in ovarian carcinoma: a Gynecologic Oncology Group study. *J Clin Oncol* 1989;7:457.

Pecorelli S, Bolis G, Colombo N, et al. Adjuvant therapy in early ovarian cancer: results of two randomized trials. *Gynecol Oncol* 1994;52:102

Pettersson F. *Annual Report of the Results of Treatment in Gynecologic Cancer*. International Federation of Gynecology and Obstetrics, vol. 20. Stockholm: Panoramic Press; 1988.

Piver MS, Baker TR, Jishi MF, et al. Familial ovarian cancer: a report of 658 families from the Gilda Radner Familial Ovarian Cancer Registry 1981–1991. *Cancer* 1993;71(2 suppl):582.

Piver MS, Malfetano J, Baker TR, et al. Five-year survival for stage IC or stage I, grade 3 epithelial ovarian cancer treated with cisplatin-based chemotherapy. *Gynecol Oncol* 1992;46:357.

Potter ME, Partridge EE, Hatch KD, et al. Primary surgical therapy of ovarian cancer: how much and when? *Gynecol Oncol* 1991;40:195.

Sigurdsson K, Alm P, Gullberg B. Prognostic factors in malignant ovarian tumors. *Gynecol Oncol* 1983;15:370.

Trimble EL, Arbuck SG, McGuire WP. Options for primary chemotherapy of epithelial ovarian cancer: taxanes. *Gynecol Oncol* 1994;55:S114.

van der Burg ME, van Lent M, Buyse M, et al. The effect of debulking surgery after induction chemotherapy on the prognosis in advanced epithelial ovarian cancer. *N Engl J Med* 1995;332:629.

Williams L. The role of secondary cytoreductive surgery in epithelial ovarian malignancies. *Oncology* 1992;6:25.

Young RC, Gynecologic Oncology Group. Phase III randomized study of CBDCA/TAX administered for 3 vs 6 courses for selected stages IA–C and stages IIA–C ovarian epithelial cancer (summary last modified 10/95), GOG-157, clinical trial, active, March 20, 1995.

Young RC, Walton LA, Ellenberg SS, et al. Adjuvant therapy in stage I and stage II epithelial ovarian cancer: results of two prospective randomized trials. *N Engl J Med* 1990;322:1021.

Zaino RJ, Unger ER, Whitney C. Synchronous carcinomas of the uterine corpus and ovary. *Gynecol Oncol* 1984;19:329.

Ovarian Tumors of Low Malignant Potential

Bell DA, Scully RE. Serous borderline tumors of the peritoneum. *Am J Surg Pathol* 1990;14:230.

Casey AC, Bell DA, Lage JM, et al. Epithelial ovarian tumors of borderline malignancy: long-term follow-up. *Gynecol Oncol* 1993;50:316.

de Nictolis M, Montironi R, Tommasoni S, et al. Serous borderline tumors of the ovary. *Cancer* 1992;70:152.

Fort MG, Pierce VK, Saigo PE, et al. Evidence for the efficacy of adjuvant therapy in epithelial ovarian tumors of low malignant potential. *Gynecol Oncol* 1989;32:269.

Gershenson DM, Silva EG. Serous ovarian tumors of low malignant potential with peritoneal implants. *Cancer* 1990;65:578.

Hopkins MP, Kumar NB, Morley GW. An assessment of pathologic features and treatment modalities in ovarian tumors of low malignant potential. *Obstet Gynecol* 1987;70:293.

Koern J, Trope CG, Abeler VM. A retrospective study of 370 borderline tumors of the ovary treated at the Norwegian Radium Hospital from 1970 to 1982. *Cancer* 1993;71:1810.

Kurman RJ, Trimble CL. The behavior of serous tumors of low malignant potential: are they ever malignant? *Int J Gynecol Pathol* 1993;12:120.

Leake JF, Currie JL, Rosenshein NB, et al. Long-term follow-up of serous ovarian tumors of low malignant potential. *Gynecol Oncol* 1992;47:150.

Michael H, Roth LM. Invasive and noninvasive implants in ovarian serous tumors of low malignant potential. *Cancer* 1986;57:1240.

Rice LW, Berkowitz RS, Mark SD, et al. Epithelial ovarian tumors of borderline malignancy. *Gynecol Oncol* 1990;39:195.

Slomovitz BM, Caputo TA, Gretz HF, et al. A comparative analysis of 57 serous borderline tumors with and without a noninvasive micropapillary component. *Am J Surg Pathol* 2002;26:592.

Sutton GP, Bundy BN, Omura GA, et al. Stage III ovarian tumors of low malignant potential treated with cisplatin combination therapy (a Gynecologic Oncology Group study). *Gynecol Oncol* 1991;41:230.

Trimble EL, Trimble CL. Epithelial ovarian tumors of low malignant potential. In: Markman M, Hoskins WJ, eds. *Cancer of the Ovary*. New York, NY: Raven Press; 1993.

Trope C, Kaern J, Vergote IB, et al. Are borderline tumors of the ovary overtreated both surgically and systematically? A review of four prospective randomized trials including 253 patients with borderline tumors. *Gynecol Oncol* 1993;51:236.

Yazigi R, Sandstad J, Munoz AK. Primary staging in ovarian tumors of low malignant potential. *Gynecol Oncol* 1988;31:402.

Ovarian Germ Cell Tumors

Gershenson DM. Update on malignant ovarian germ cell tumors. *Cancer* 1993;71(4 suppl): 1581.

Gershenson DM, Morris M, Cangir A, et al. Treatment of malignant germ cell tumors of the ovary with bleomycin, etoposide, and cisplatin. *J Clin Oncol* 1990;8:715.

Kurman RJ, Norris HJ. Malignant germ cell tumors of the ovary. *Hum Pathol* 1977;8:551.

Morrow CP, Curtin JP, Townsend DE. *Synopsis of Gynecologic Oncology*. 4th ed. New York, NY: Churchill Livingstone; 1993.

Munshi NC, Loehrer PJ, Roth BJ, et al. Vinblastine, ifosfamide and cisplatin (VeIP) as second line chemotherapy in metastatic germ cell tumors (GCT). *Proc Am Soc Clin Oncol* 1990;9:134.

Romero R, Schwartz PE. Alpha-fetoprotein determinations in the management of endodermal sinus tumors and mixed germ cell tumors of the ovary. *Am J Obstet Gynecol* 1981;141:126.

Schwartz PE, Morris JM. Serum lactic dehydrogenase: a tumor marker for dysgerminoma. *Obstet Gynecol* 1988;72:511.

Serov SF, Scully RE, Robin IH. *International Histologic Classification of Tumours, No. 9. Histological Typing of Ovarian Tumours*. Geneva: World Health Organization; 1973.

Slayton RE, Park RC, Silverberg SG, et al. Vincristine, dactinomycin, and cyclophosphamide in the treatment of malignant germ cell tumors of the ovary. *Cancer* 1985;56:243.

Williams S, Blessing JA, Liao SY, et al. Adjuvant therapy of ovarian germ cell tumors with cisplatin, etoposide, and bleomycin: a trial of the Gynecologic Oncology Group. *J Clin Oncol* 1994;12:701.

Williams SD, Birch R, Einhorn LH, et al. Treatment of disseminated germ-cell tumors with cisplatin, bleomycin, and either vinblastine or etoposide. *N Engl J Med* 1987;316:1435.

Williams SD, Blessing JA, Hatch KD, et al. Chemotherapy of advanced dysgerminoma: trials of the Gynecologic Oncology Group. *J Clin Oncol* 1991;9:1950.

Williams SD, Blessing JA, Moore DH, et al. Cisplatin, vinblastine, and bleomycin in advanced and recurrent ovarian germ-cell tumors: a trial of the Gynecologic Oncology Group. *Ann Intern Med* 1989;111:22.

Williams SD, Gershenson DM. Management of germ cell tumors of the ovary. In: Markman M, Hoskins WJ, eds. *Cancer of the Ovary*. New York, NY: Raven Press; 1993.

Williams SD, Gynecologic Oncology Group. Phase II combination chemotherapy with BEP (CDDP/VP-16/BLEO) as induction followed by VAC (VCR/DACT/CTX) as consolidation in patients with incompletely resected malignant ovarian germ cell tumors (summary last modified 10/95), GOG-90, clinical trial, active, September 15, 1986.

Sex Cord Stromal Tumors

Berek JS, Hacker NF. *Practical Gynecologic Oncology*. 3rd ed. Baltimore, Md: Williams & Wilkins; 2000.

Bjorkholm E, Silversward C. Prognostic factors in granulosa-cell tumors. *Gynecol Oncol* 1981;11:261.

Bjorkholm E, Silversward C. Theca cell tumors. Clinical features and prognosis. *Acta Radiol* 1980;19:241.

Evans AT III, Gaffey TA, Malkasian GD, Jr. Clinicopathologic review of

118 granulosa and 82 theca cell tumors. *Obstet Gynecol* 1980;55:231.

Fox H, Agarical K, Langley FA. A clinicopathologic study of 92 cases of granulosa cell tumors of the ovary with special reference to the factors influencing prognosis. *Cancer* 1975;35:231.

Gershenson DM. Management of early ovarian cancer: germ cell and sex cord-stromal tumors. *Gynecol Oncol* 1994;55:S62.

Lappohn RE, Burger HG, Bouma J, et al. Inhibin as a marker for granulosa-cell tumors. *N Engl J Med* 1989;321:790.

Meigs JV, Armstrong SH, Hamilton HH. A further contribution to the syndrome of fibroma of the ovary with fluid in the abdomen and chest, Meig's syndrome. *Am J Obstet Gynecol* 1943;46:19.

Norris HJ, Taylor HB. Prognosis of granulosa-theca tumors of the ovary. *Cancer* 1968;21: 255.

Roth LM, Anderson MC, Govan AD, et al. Sertoli-Leydig cell tumors: a clinicopathologic study of 34 cases. *Cancer* 1981;48:187.

Scully RE. Ovarian tumors: a review. *Am J Pathol* 1977;87:686.

Young RH, Scully RE. Ovarian sex cord-stromal tumors: recent progress. *Int J Gynecol Pathol* 1982;1:101.

Young RH, Scully RE. Ovarian sex cord stromal and steroid cell tumors. In: Roth LM, Czernobilsky B, eds. *Tumors and Tumor-like Conditions of the Ovary*. New York, NY: Churchill Livingstone; 1985.

Young RH, Welch WR, Dickersin GR, et al. Ovarian sex cord tumor with annular tubules. Review of 74 cases including 27 with Peutz-Jeghers syndrome and four with adenoma malignum of the cervix. *Cancer* 1982;50:1384.

Fallopian Tube Cancer

Eddy GL, Copeland LJ, Gershenson DM, et al. Fallopian tube carcinoma. *Obstet Gynecol* 1984;64:156.

Hu CY, Taymor ML, Hertig AT. Primary carcinoma of the fallopian tube. *Am J Obstet Gynecol* 1950;59:58.

Morris M, Gershenson DM, Burke TW, et al. Treatment of fallopian tube carcinoma with cisplatin, doxorubicin and cyclophosphamide. *Obstet Gynecol* 1990;76:1020.

Rose PG, Piver MS, Tsukada Y. Fallopian tube cancer. *Cancer* 1990;66:2661.

Sedlis A. Carcinoma of the fallopian tube. *Surg Clin North Am* 1978;58:121.

Endometrial Cancer

American Cancer Society. *Cancer Facts and Figures*. Atlanta, Ga: American Cancer Society; 1995.

Axelrod JH, Gynecologic Oncology Group. Phase II study of whole-abdominal radiotherapy in patients with papillary serous carcinoma and clear cell carcinoma of the endometrium or with maximally debulked advanced endometrial carcinoma (summary last modified 05/91), GOG-94, clinical trial, closed, February 24, 1992.

Boring CC, Squires TS, Tong T. Cancer statistics, 1991. *Cancer* 1991;41:19.

Burke TW, Munkarah A, Kavanagh JJ, et al. Treatment of advanced or recurrent endometrial carcinoma with single-agent carboplatin. *Gynecol Oncol* 1993;51:397.

Burke TW, Stringer CL, Morris M, et al. Prospective treatment of advanced or recurrent endometrial carcinoma with cisplatin, doxorubicin, and cyclophosphamide. *Gynecol Oncol* 1991;40:264.

Creasman WT. New gynecologic cancer staging. *Obstet Gynecol* 1990;75:287.

Creasman WT, Morrow CP, Bundy BN, et al. Surgical pathologic spread patterns of endometrial cancer: a Gynecologic Oncology Group study. *Cancer* 1987;60:2035.

Gusberg SB. Virulence factors in endometrial cancer. *Cancer* 1993;71(4 suppl):1464.

Hancock KC, Freedman RS, Edwards CL, et al. Use of cisplatin, doxorubicin, and cyclophosphamide to treat advanced and recurrent adenocarcinoma of the endometrium. *Cancer Treat Rep* 1986;70:789.

Homesley HD, Zaino R. Endometrial cancer: prognostic factors. *Semin Oncol* 1994;21:71.

Lanciano RM, Corn BW, Schultz DJ, et al. The justification for a surgical staging system in endometrial carcinoma. *Radiother Oncol* 1993;28:189.

Lentz SS. Advanced and recurrent endometrial carcinoma: hormonal therapy. *Semin Oncol* 1994;21:100.

Marchetti DL, Caglar H, Driscoll DL, et al. Pelvic radiation in stage I endometrial adenocarcinoma with high-risk attributes. *Gynecol Oncol* 1990;37:51.

Morrow CP, Bundy BN, Kurman RJ, et al. Relationship between surgical-pathological risk factors and outcome in clinical stage I and II carcinoma of the endometrium: a Gynecologic Oncology Group study. *Gynecol Oncol* 1991;40:55.

Morrow CP, Curtin JP, Townsend DE. *Synopsis of Gynecologic Oncology*. 4th ed. New York, NY: Churchill Livingstone; 1993.

Nori D, Hilaris BS, Tome M, et al. Combined surgery and radiation in endometrial carcinoma: an analysis of prognostic factors. *Int J Radiat Oncol Biol Phys* 1987;13:489.

Piver MS, Hempling RE. A prospective trial of postoperative vaginal radium/cesium for grade 1–2 less than 50% myometrial invasion and pelvic radiation therapy for grade 3 or deep myometrial invasion in surgical stage I endometrial adenocarcinoma. *Cancer* 1990;66:1133.

Potish RA, Twiggs LB, Adcock LL, et al. Role of whole abdominal radiation therapy in the management of endometrial cancer: prognostic importance of factors indicating peritoneal metastases. *Gynecol Oncol* 1985;21:80.

Quinn MA, Campbell JJ. Tamoxifen therapy in advanced/recurrent endometrial carcinoma. *Gynecol Oncol* 1989;32:1

Roberts JA, Gynecologic Oncology Group. Phase III randomized evaluation of adjuvant postoperative pelvic radiotherapy vs no adjuvant therapy for surgical stage I and occult stage II intermediate-risk endometrial carcinoma (summary last modified 08/95), GOG-99, clinical trial, closed, July 3, 1995.

Rutledge F. The role of radical hysterectomy in adenocarcinoma of the endometrium. *Gynecol Oncol* 1974;2:331.

Seski JC, Edwards CL, Herson J, et al. Cisplatin chemotherapy for disseminated endometrial cancer. *Obstet Gynecol* 1982;59:225.

Slomovitz BM, Burke TW, Eifel PJ, et al. Uterine papillary serous carcinoma (UPSC): a single institution review of 129 cases. *Gynecol Oncol* 2003;91:463.

Uterine Sarcomas

Berek JS, Hacker NF. *Practical Gynecologic Oncology*. 3rd ed. Baltimore, Md: Williams & Wilkins; 2000.

Gershenson DM, Kavanagh JJ, Copeland LJ, et al. Cisplatin therapy for disseminated mixed mesodermal sarcoma of the uterus. *J Clin Oncol* 1987;5: 618.

Harlow BL, Weiss NS, Lofton S. The epidemiology of sarcomas of the uterus. *J Natl Cancer Inst* 1986;76:399.

Hornback NB, Omura G, Major FJ. Observations on the use of adjuvant radiation therapy in patients with stage I and II uterine sarcoma. *Int J Radiat Oncol Biol Phys* 1986;12:2127.

Major FJ, Blessing JA, Silverberg SG, et al. Prognostic factors in early-stage uterine sarcoma: a Gynecologic Oncology Group study. *Cancer* 1993; 71(4 suppl):1702.

Morrow CP, Curtin JP, Townsend DE. *Synopsis of Gynecologic Oncology*. 4th ed. New York, NY: Churchill Livingstone; 1993.

Norris HJ, Taylor HB. Postirradiation sarcomas of the uterus. *Obstet Gynecol* 1965;26:689.

Olah KS, Dunn JA, Gee H. Leiomyosarcomas have a poorer prognosis than mixed mesodermal tumours when adjusting for known prognostic factors: the result of a retrospective study of

423 cases of uterine sarcoma. *Br J Obstet Gynaecol* 1992;99:590.

Omura GA, Blessing JA, Lifshitz S, et al. A randomized clinical trial of adjuvant Adriamycin in uterine sarcomas: a Gynecologic Oncology Group study. *J Clin Oncol* 1985;3:1240.

Omura GA, Blessing JA, Major F, et al. A randomized clinical trial of adjuvant Adriamycin in uterine sarcomas: a Gynecologic Oncology Group study. *J Clin Oncol* 1985;3:1240.

Silverberg SG, Major FJ, Blessing JA, et al. Carcinosarcoma (malignant mixed mesodermal tumor) of the uterus: a Gynecologic Oncology Group pathologic study of 203 cases. *Int J Gynecol Pathol* 1990;9:1.

Sutton GP, Blessing JA, Barrett RJ, et al. Phase II trial of ifosfamide and mesna in leiomyosarcoma of the uterus: a Gynecologic Oncology Group study. *Am J Obstet Gynecol* 1992;166:556.

Sutton GP, Gynecologic Oncology Group. Phase II master protocol study of chemotherapeutic agents in the treatment of recurrent or advanced uterine sarcomas—IFF plus mesna (summary last modified 04/93), GOG-87B, clinical trial, completed, December 28, 1994.

Sutton GP, Gynecologic Oncology Group. Phase III study of IFF and the uroprotector mesna administered alone or with CDDP in patients with advanced or recurrent mixed mesodermal tumors of the uterus (summary last modified 08/95), GOG-108, clinical trial, active, February 15, 1989.

Wheelock JB, Krebs H-B, Schneider V, et al. Uterine sarcoma: analysis of prognostic variables in 71 cases. *Am J Obstet Gynecol* 1985;151: 1016.

Gestational Trophoblastic Disease

Azab M, Droz JP, Theodore C, et al. Cisplatin, vinblastine, and bleomycin combination in the treatment of resistant high-risk gestational trophoblastic tumors. *Cancer* 1989;64:1829.

Bagshawe KD. High-risk metastatic trophoblastic disease. *Obstet Gynecol Clin North Am* 1988;15:531.

Berek JS, Hacker NF. *Practical Gynecologic Oncology*. 3rd ed. Baltimore, Md: Williams & Wilkins; 2000.

Lurain JR. Gestational trophoblastic tumors. *Semin Surg Oncol* 1990;6:347.

Morrow CP, Curtin JP, Townsend DE. *Synopsis of Gynecologic Oncology*. 4th ed. New York, NY: Churchill Livingstone; 1993.

Mutch DG, Soper JT, Babcock CJ, et al. Recurrent gestational trophoblastic disease: experience of the Southeastern Regional Trophoblastic Disease Center. *Cancer* 1990;66:978.

Newlands ES, Bagshawe KD, Begent RH, et al. Results with the EMA/CO (etoposide, methotrexate, actinomycin D, cyclophosphamide, vincristine) regimen in high risk gestational trophoblastic tumours, 1979 to 1989. *Br J Obstet Gynaecol* 1991;98:550.

Surwit EA. Management of high-risk gestational trophoblastic disease. *J Reprod Med* 1987;32:657.

World Health Organization Scientific Group. Gestational trophoblastic diseases. *WHO Tech Rep Ser* 1983;692:1.

Cervical Cancer

Alberts DS, Kronmal R, Baker LH, et al. Phase II randomized trial of cisplatin chemotherapy regimens in the treatment of recurrent or metastatic squamous cell cancer of the cervix: a Southwest Oncology Group study. *J Clin Oncol* 1987;5:1791.

American Cancer Society. *Cancer Facts and Figures*. Atlanta, Ga: American Cancer Society; 2003.

Artman LE, Hoskins WJ, Bibro MC, et al. Radical hysterectomy and pelvic lymphadenectomy for stage IB carcinoma of the cervix: 21 years' experience. *Gynecol Oncol* 1987;28:8.

Coia L, Won M, Lanciano R, et al. The patterns of care outcome study for cancer of the uterine cervix: results of the Second

National Practice Survey. *Cancer* 1990;66:2451.

Coleman RE, Harper PG, Gallagher C, et al. A phase II study of ifosfamide in advanced and relapsed carcinoma of the cervix. *Cancer Chemother Pharmacol* 1986;18:280.

Creasman WF, Fetter BF, Clarke-Pearson DL, et al. Management of stage IA carcinoma of the cervix. *Am J Obstet Gynecol* 1985;153:164.

Creasman WT. New gynecologic cancer staging. *Gynecol Oncol* 1995;58:157.

Dembo AJ, Balogh JM. Advances in radiotherapy in the gynecologic malignancies. *Semin Surg Oncol* 1990;6:323.

Eifel PJ, Burke TW, Delclos L, et al. Early stage I adenocarcinoma of the uterine cervix: treatment results in patients with tumors ≤4 cm in diameter. *Gynecol Oncol* 1991;41:199.

Fletcher GH, Rutledge FN. Overall results in radiotherapy for carcinoma of the cervix. *Clin Obstet Gynecol* 1967;10:958.

Grigsby PW, Perez CA. Radiotherapy alone for medically inoperable carcinoma of the cervix: stage IA and carcinoma in situ. *Int J Radiat Oncol Biol Phys* 1991;21:375.

Hopkins MP, Morley GW. Squamous cell cancer of the cervix: prognostic factors related to survival. *Int J Gynecol Cancer* 1991;1:173.

Morrow CP, Curtin JP, Townsend DE. *Synopsis of Gynecologic Oncology*. 4th ed. New York, NY: Churchill Livingstone; 1993.

Perez CA, Grigsby PW, Nene SM, et al. Effect of tumor size on the prognosis of carcinoma of the uterine cervix treated with irradiation alone. *Cancer* 1992;69:2796.

Rutledge FN, Smith JP, Wharton JT, et al. Pelvic exenteration: analysis of 296 patients. *Am J Obstet Gynecol* 1977;129:881.

Sevin BU, Nadji M, Averette HE, et al. Microinvasive carcinoma of the cervix. *Cancer* 1992;70: 2121.

Stehman FB, Bundy BN, DiSaia PJ, et al. Carcinoma of the cervix treated with radiation therapy: a multivariate analysis of prognostic variables in the Gynecologic Oncology Group. *Cancer* 1991;67:2776.

Thomas G, Dembo A, Fyles A, et al. Concurrent chemoradiation in advanced cervical cancer. *Gynecol Oncol* 1990;38:446.

Vermorken JB. The role of chemotherapy in squamous cell carcinoma of the uterine cervix: a review. *Int J Gynecol Cancer* 1993;3:129.

Vulvar Cancer

Anderson JM, Cassady JR, Shimm DS, et al. Vulvar carcinoma. *Int J Radiat Oncol Biol Phys* 1995;32:1351.

Berek JS, Heaps JM, Fu YS, et al. Concurrent cisplatin and 5-fluorouracil chemotherapy and radiation therapy for advanced-stage squamous carcinoma of the vulva. *Gynecol Oncol* 1991;2:197.

Binder SW, Huang I, Fu YS, et al. Risk factors for the development of lymph node metastasis in vulvar squamous cell carcinoma. *Gynecol Oncol* 1990;37:9.

Boyce J, Fruchter RG, Kasambilides E, et al. Prognostic factors in carcinoma of the vulva. *Gynecol Oncol* 1985;20:364.

Burke TW, Stringer CA, Gershenson DM, et al. Radical wide excision and selective inguinal node dissection for squamous cell carcinoma of the vulva. *Gynecol Oncol* 1990;38:328.

Chung AF, Woodruff JW, Lewis JL, Jr. Malignant melanoma of the vulva: a report of 44 cases. *Obstet Gynecol* 1975;45:638.

Creasman WT. New gynecologic cancer staging. *Gynecol Oncol* 1995;58:157.

Hacker NF, Van der Velden J. Conservative management of early vulvar cancer. *Cancer* 1993;71(4 suppl):1673.

Heaps JM, Fu YS, Montz FJ, et al. Surgical-pathologic variables predictive of local recurrence in squamous cell carcinoma of the vulva. *Gynecol Oncol* 1990;38:309.

Homesley HD, Bundy BN, Sedlis A, et al. Assessment of current International Federation of Gynecology and Obstetrics staging of vulvar carcinoma relative to prognostic factors for survival (a Gynecologic Oncology Group study). *Am J Obstet Gynecol* 1991;164:997.

Homesley HD, Bundy BN, Sedlis A, et al. Prognostic factors for groin node metastasis in squamous cell carcinoma of the vulva (a Gynecologic Oncology Group study). *Gynecol Oncol* 1993;49:279.

Hopkins MP, Reid GC, Morley GW. The surgical management of recurrent squamous cell carcinoma of the vulva. *Obstet Gynecol* 1990;75:1001.

Keys H. Gynecologic Oncology Group randomized trials of combined technique therapy for vulvar cancer. *Cancer* 1993;71 (4 suppl):1691.

Malfetano JH, Piver MS, Tsukada Y, et al. Univariate and multivariate analyses of 5-year survival, recurrence, and inguinal node metastases in stage I and II vulvar carcinoma. *J Surg Oncol* 1985;30:124.

Perez CA, Grigsby PW, Galakatos A, et al. Radiation therapy in management of carcinoma of the vulva with emphasis on conservation therapy. *Cancer* 1993;71:3707.

Podratz KC, Symmonds RE, Taylor WF, et al. Carcinoma of the vulva: analysis of treatment and survival. *Obstet Gynecol* 1983;61:63.

Russell AH, Mesic JB, Scudder SA, et al. Synchronous radiation and cytotoxic chemotherapy for locally advanced or recurrent squamous cancer of the vulva. *Gynecol Oncol* 1992;47:14.

Sedlis A, Homesley H, Bundy BN, et al. Positive groin lymph nodes in superficial squamous cell vulvar cancer: a Gynecologic Oncology Group study. *Am J Obstet Gynecol* 1987;156:1159.

Shimm DS, Fuller AF, Orlow EL, et al. Prognostic variables in the treatment of squamous cell carcinoma of the vulva. *Gynecol Oncol* 1986;24:343.

Stehman FB, Bundy BN, Dvoretsky PM, et al. Early stage I carcinoma of the vulva treated with ipsilateral superficial inguinal lymphadenectomy and modified radical hemivulvectomy: a prospective study of the Gynecologic Oncology Group. *Obstet Gynecol* 1992;79: 490.

Thomas GM, Dembo AJ, Bryson SC, et al. Changing concepts in the management of vulvar cancer. *Gynecol Oncol* 1991;42:9.

Vaginal Cancer

Berek JS, Hacker NF. *Practical Gynecologic Oncology*. 3rd ed. Baltimore, Md: Williams & Wilkins; 2000.

Delclos L, Wharton JT, Rutledge FN. Tumors of the vagina and female urethra. In: Fletcher GH, ed. *Textbook of Radiotherapy*. 3rd ed. Philadelphia, Pa: Lea & Febiger; 1980.

Herbst AL, Robboy SJ, Scully RE, et al. Clear cell adenocarcinoma of the vagina and cervix in girls: analysis of 170 registry cases. *Am J Obstet Gynecol* 1974;119:713.

Kucera H, Vavra N. Radiation management of primary carcinoma of the vagina: clinical and histopathological variables associated with survival. *Gynecol Oncol* 1991;40:12.

Morrow CP, Curtin JP, Townsend DE. *Synopsis of Gynecologic Oncology*. 4th ed. New York, NY: Churchill Livingstone; 1993.

Perez CA, Camel HM, Galakatos AE, et al. Definitive irradiation in carcinoma of the vagina: long-term evaluation of results. *Int J Radiat Oncol Biol Phys* 1988;15:1283.

Stock RG, Chen AS, Seski J. A 30-year experience in the management of primary carcinoma of the vagina: analysis of prognostic factors and treatment modalities. *Gynecol Oncol* 1995;56:45.

Oncologic Emergencies

Jeffrey D. Wayne and Richard J. Bold

True oncologic emergencies are rare, and often do not require surgery, such as superior vena cava (SVC) syndrome, spinal cord compression, and paraneoplastic syndromes. However, surgeons are often asked to consult on how to manage patients with malignancies who have complications from tumor progression, or from cytotoxic therapies. This chapter first describes some of the more common extra-abdominal problems among surgical patients with cancer, and then focuses specifically on the acute abdominal conditions for which surgical consultation is obtained.

EXTRA-ABDOMINAL EMERGENCIES

Superior Vena Cava Syndrome

Obstruction of the SVC results in a constellation of signs and symptoms collectively known as the superior vena cava syndrome (SVCS). Impedance of outflow from the SVC may result from external compression by neoplastic disease, fibrosis secondary to inflammation, or thrombosis. In up to 97% of patients with SVCS, this condition is caused by malignancy. Lung cancer and lymphoma are the most frequent causes. An increasingly common etiology of SVCS is thrombosis secondary to indwelling central venous catheters. The underlying source of obstruction of the SVC must be established, as this information is used to guide therapy and to determine prognosis. In the past, patients with SVCS were emergently treated with mediastinal irradiation. However, because radiation-induced tissue necrosis often frustrates later attempts at tissue diagnosis, empiric radiation therapy is no longer advocated. Therapy based on the specific type of tumor can often provide substantial palliation and even a cure for patients presenting with SVCS.

The SVC is the primary conduit for venous drainage of the head, neck, upper extremities, and upper thorax. This thin-walled, compliant vessel is surrounded by more rigid structures, including the mediastinal and paratracheal lymph nodes, the trachea and right mainstem bronchus, the pulmonary artery, and the aorta. It is therefore susceptible to external compression by any space-occupying lesion. Obstruction of outflow from the SVC results in venous hypertension of the head, neck, and upper extremities, which in turn manifests as SVCS. In most cases, obstruction of the SVC is not an acute event, and the signs and symptoms of SVCS develop gradually. The most common symptoms include dyspnea, which occurs in 63% of patients with SVCS, and facial fullness in 50% of patients. Physical findings commonly associated with SVCS include facial edema, venous engorgement of the neck and chest wall, cyanosis, and plethora. Symptoms worsen when the patient bends forward or reclines. Obstruction of the SVC becomes a true emergency when associated laryngeal edema leads to substantial impedence of the airway, or when intracranial pressure is elevated.

Patients with SVCS should be thoroughly evaluated, beginning with a directed history and physical examination. A history of malignancy, heavy smoking, or symptoms such as cough, fever, and night sweats should be noted. It is important to examine all lymph node basins and to note the presence of a central venous catheter. Chest radiography reveals an abnormality in 84% of patients with SVCS, although the findings are often nonspecific. A computed tomography (CT) scan of the chest is the initial test of choice and will determine whether the obstruction is due to external compression, or to thrombosis. CT scans also provide anatomic detail of tumor masses, and can be used as a guide for percutaneous biopsy. Magnetic resonance imaging (MRI) is an alternative for patients with renal insufficiency or an allergy to contrast. Minimally invasive techniques of tissue diagnosis include sputum cytology, CT-guided percutaneous biopsy, bronchoscopy, lymph node biopsy, and bone marrow biopsy. Invasive procedures, such as mediastinoscopy and thoracotomy, should be considered if all initial measures fail to establish a diagnosis. These invasive procedures can be performed safely in most patients with SVCS. Using these techniques to guide individualized treatment is preferable to proceeding with nonspecific therapy.

When the etiology of SVCS is malignancy, treatment is based on tumor type. Using diuretics and elevation of the head mitigate the symptoms of SVCS, and using steroids reduces inflammation. Only those patients with evidence of impending airway obstruction or elevated intracranial pressure should be considered for emergent radiation therapy. Even in such cases, intubation, mechanical ventilation, and osmotic diuretics can suspend the progression of symptoms for a period sufficient to allow for a tissue diagnosis. Once the diagnosis is made, tumor-specific therapy should be initiated. Small cell lung cancer and lymphoma are best treated with combination chemotherapy; radiation therapy may be used for consolidation. In a series of 56 patients with small cell lung cancer, SVCS was resolved in all 23 patients treated with chemotherapy alone, in 64% of those treated with radiation therapy alone, and in 83% of those treated with combination therapy. Non–small cell lung cancer is most often treated with radiation therapy. One commonly used fractionation schedule provides high-dose treatment (3–4 Gy/day) for 3 days followed by conventional dose fractionation (1.8–2.0 Gy/day) to a total of 50 to 60 Gy. About 70% of patients on such a treatment schedule respond within 2 weeks.

Patients with SVCS secondary to catheter-induced thrombosis may be successfully treated with thrombolytic agents followed by systemic anticoagulation. Thrombolytic agents are most effective when patients are treated within 5 days after the onset of symptoms. Alternatively, catheter removal followed by systemic anticoagulation often results in gradual recanalization of the SVC and resolution of symptoms. For SVCS refractory to such measures, balloon angioplasty and expandable stents are palliative modalities. Surgical intervention consisting of innominate vein-right atrial bypass is generally reserved for patients in whom the SVCS arises from causes other than malignancy.

Spinal Cord Compression

Spinal cord compression is the second most common neurologic complication of cancer, with an estimated 20,000 new cases annually in the United States alone. Autopsy studies suggest that 5% of patients with malignancies have evidence of spinal cord involvement. Early recognition and diagnosis are essential, as spinal cord compression can produce paralysis and loss of sphincter control if left untreated. Patients in whom symptoms present early and in whom neurologic deficits are minimal have the most favorable prognosis. Unfortunately, nearly 80% of patients are unable to walk at the time of presentation.

Spinal cord compression in patients with cancer usually involves extradural metastatic lesions of the vertebral body or neural arch. Tumors expand posteriorly, resulting in anterior compression of the dural sac. Rarely, metastasis can occur in intradural locations without bony involvement. Paraspinal tumors can also cause spinal cord compression by penetrating the intervertebral foramen.

Most of the data on spinal cord compression in malignancy are from animal models. If spinal cord compression develops gradually, decompression can be delayed without impairing the return of neurologic function; however, in cases of rapid compression of the spinal cord, therapeutic intervention must be performed immediately to avoid irreversible neurologic deficits. Spinal cord edema also plays an important role in the development of neurologic injury.

Although spinal cord compression can occur as the initial manifestation of disease, most patients who present with spinal cord compression due to malignancy have been previously diagnosed with cancer. The interval from initial diagnosis to epidural spinal cord compression varies with the type of primary tumor involved. Lung cancer may have an aggressive presentation, with epidural spinal cord compression developing within a few months after diagnosis of the primary lesion. Conversely, patients with carcinoma of the breast have been reported to manifest spinal cord compression up to 20 years after initial presentation of disease.

The incidences of involvement of the three spinal cord segments (cervical, 10%; thoracic, 70%; lumbosacral, 20%) reflect the number of vertebrae in each anatomic segment. More than 90% of patients with spinal cord compression due to malignancy present with localized back pain, which may be exacerbated by movement, recumbency, coughing, sneezing, or straining. The pain due to spinal cord compression can be radicular in distribution. Pain is usually present for several weeks before neurologic symptoms develop. Left untreated, weakness and numbness occur, usually beginning in the toes and ascending to the level of the lesion. Autonomic dysfunction usually occurs late in the disease process. The onset of urinary retention and constipation represents an ominous sign, indicating possible progression to irreversible paraplegia.

Physical examination may reveal tenderness, upon palpation, over the involved vertebrae. Straight leg raise and neck flexion may produce pain at the level of the involved vertebrae. Weakness, spasticity, abnormal reflexes, and extensor plantar response

(Babinski's sign) may be evident on physical examination. A palpable urinary bladder or decreased anal sphincter tone may be present.

Patients with signs of impending neurologic deficits should undergo immediate evaluation and treatment. Depending on the history and physical examination, patients should be treated with dexamethasone 10 mg IV followed by 4 mg IV or PO every 6 hours. Rapid radiographic assessment should be performed simultaneously. In more than two thirds of patients with spinal cord compression, plain films of the spine show evidence of bony abnormalities. Radiographic findings suggestive of a spine metastasis include erosion or loss of vertebral pedicles, partial or complete collapse of vertebral bodies, and paraspinal soft-tissue masses. However, normal spine radiographs do not exclude the possibility that epidural metastases are present. In fact, patients with lymphoma typically have normal spine radiographs even when epidural tumors are present.

Currently, MRI is the study of choice for evaluating patients with suspected spinal cord compression after plain radiographs have been obtained. MRI has several advantages over CT myelogram. Lumbar puncture, which is required for a myelogram, is associated with substantial morbidity in patients who have a space-occupying lesion and with potential bleeding complications in patients who have coagulopathies. MRI is useful in defining the extent of tumor involvement, designing portals for radiation therapy, and planning surgical intervention. MRI also distinguishes extradural from intradural lesions. Gadolinium contrast is usually not required for extradural lesions, but optimal imaging of extramedullary and intramedullary intradural lesions requires the use of this agent. If MRI results in equivocal or negative findings, then CT myelography should be performed.

Early intervention is essential in the management of malignant spinal cord compression. The functional status at the time of presentation clearly correlates with the post-treatment outcome. For example, fewer than 10% of patients who present with paraplegia become ambulatory after treatment. Radiotherapy and/or surgical intervention are the standard treatment modalities. Typically, 3,000 cGy is given in dose fractions of 300 to 500 cGy, with excellent resolution of pain and neurologic symptoms. Laminectomy is effective in managing patients with epidural masses but has limited use if the tumor is growing in a direction anterior to the spinal cord. In select cases, surgical resection may provide symptomatic relief, but careful patient selection is essential. Chemotherapy may help in managing patients with epidural spinal cord compression due to lesions that are sensitive to certain agents; however, a role for chemotherapy as an adjuvant or a primary treatment has not been clearly defined.

Pericardial Tamponade

Tamponade in patients with cancer most often results from malignant obstruction of pericardial lymphatics, leading to the accumulation of fluid within the pericardial sac. While both primary neoplasms of the heart and metastatic lesions can incite the development of pericardial effusions, metastatic disease to the pericardium is the most frequent etiology. Lung cancer, breast cancer, lymphoma, leukemia, and melanoma are the malignancies most commonly implicated in pericardial tamponade. Alternatively, pericardial effusions in the cancer patient can also occur as a result of radiation therapy.

The pericardial sac normally contains 20 mL of fluid at a mean pressure below the values of the right and left ventricular end-diastolic pressures. As pericardial fluid accumulates, this pressure rises until the intrapericardial pressure equals or surpasses the ventricular end-diastolic pressure. At this point, diastolic filling is compromised and cardiac output falls. The development of symptoms depends on the rate of accumulation and the volume of pericardial fluid, as well as on the compliance of the pericardial sac. A pericardial effusion as small as 150 mL may induce hemodynamically significant tamponade. In cases of more gradual accumulation, effusions may reach volumes up to 2 liters.

The symptoms of pericardial tamponade are often vague. Frequent complaints include chest pain, anxiety, and dyspnea. Clinical signs include tachycardia, diminished heart sounds, jugular venous distention, pulsus paradoxus, and ultimately, shock. The electrocardiogram reveals low voltage throughout all leads, with sinus tachycardia. Two-dimensional echocardiography best demonstrates the presence of pericardial fluid and is the test of choice for stable patients with suspected pericardial tamponade.

The treatment of pericardial tamponade is removal of the pericardial effusion, which may be accomplished via needle pericardiocentesis. A drainage catheter may then be inserted into the pericardial space over a guidewire. If readily available, echocardiography will help minimize complications. Removal of a small amount of fluid results in a dramatic and immediate improvement for the patient in extremis. Without additional treatment, malignant pericardial effusions often recur. Thus, a drainage catheter should be left in place so that the rate of fluid accumulation can be monitored. The options for preventing reaccumulation include tetracycline sclerosis, surgery, and radiation therapy. The instillation of 500 to 1,000 mg of tetracycline into the pericardial sac induces an inflammatory response, with subsequent fibrosis and obliteration of the pericardial space. Multiple instillations are usually necessary. Treatment should be repeated until the drainage is less than 25 mL per 24 hours. Successful control of effusions is obtained in 86% of patients who undergo needle pericardiocentesis.

Surgical options to resolve pericardial tamponade include subxiphoid pericardiotomy, window pericardectomy, and complete pericardectomy. The subxiphoid approach is usually preferred, as it avoids the thoracotomy required by the other procedures and can be performed under local anesthesia. Multiple series have documented a recurrence rate of 7% after this technique. Complete pericardiectomy is reserved for patients with radiation-induced effusions. Radiation therapy is useful in stable patients with a malignant effusion secondary to lymphoma; treatment is given in dose fractions of 2 to 3 Gy to a total dose of 20 to 40 Gy.

Outcome after treatment of pericardial tamponade depends in part on tumor type. The median survival times range from

3.5 months for patients with lung cancer to as long as 18.5 months in patients with breast cancer.

Paraneoplastic Crises

Some tumors retain the biochemical characteristics of their cell type of origin and secrete biologically active substances. Other tumors can develop the ability to synthesize and produce hormones that have a wide range of biologic effects. The secretion of these substances is often unregulated, thus disrupting homeostasis. These states have been termed paraneoplastic syndromes. In patients with cancer, these syndromes may cause severe symptoms that require emergent treatment. The full spectrum of paraneoplastic syndromes is extensive; this section describes the more common syndromes, highlighting the physiologic manifestations, pathophysiology, and treatment of each.

Hypercalcemia

Hypercalcemia is the most common metabolic complication of malignancy, occurring in approximately 10% to 20% of cancer patients. Tumors most commonly associated with hypercalcemia include carcinomas of the breast, lung, and kidney, as well as multiple myeloma. Patients with parathyroid carcinoma characteristically present with intractable hypercalcemia. Although more than 80% of patients with hypercalcemia have bone metastasis, there is no correlation between the extent of bone involvement and the degree of hypercalcemia, nor between the presence of bony metastasis and the development of hypercalcemia. Current data suggest that the hypercalcemia of malignancy is mediated by tumor-induced humoral factors. Parathyroid hormone-related protein (PTHRP), osteoclast-activating factor (OAF), prostaglandins, and numerous other cytokines may play a role in the development of hypercalcemia in patients with malignancies.

Calcium homeostasis is normally a tightly controlled process. Parathyroid hormone (PTH), 1,25-dihydroxyvitamin D_3, and calcitonin are the primary regulators of the serum calcium level. These hormones ensure that the net absorption of calcium by the gastrointestinal tract is balanced by the amount excreted by the kidney. Under normal conditions, the serum calcium level is maintained between 8.5 mg/dL and 10.5 mg/dL. Approximately 45% of calcium exists in the ionized, metabolically active form, and the other 55% is protein-bound. Most cases of hormonally mediated hypercalcemia in cancer patients result from the activity of PTHRP, which like PTH, enhances renal tubular resorption of calcium. Unlike patients with hyperparathyroidism, patients with hypercalcemia secondary to PTHRP have impaired production of 1,25-dihydroxyvitamin D_3 and show no evidence of renal bicarbonate wasting. This mechanism is particularly prevalent in solid tumors, especially epidermoid carcinomas.

OAF is responsible for hypercalcemia in patients with multiple myeloma and lymphoma. This osteolytic polypeptide stimulates osteoclast proliferation and the release of lysosomal enzymes and collagenase. Despite the potent osteolytic activity of OAF in vitro, patients with elevated OAF levels do not develop hypercalcemia unless there is associated renal insufficiency. Transforming growth factor, epidermal growth factor, interleukin-1, platelet-derived growth factor, tumor-derived hematopoietic colony-stimulating factors, tumor necrosis factor (TNF) (particularly TNF-β), and lymphotoxin are all potent inducers of bone resorption in vitro and may have a role in the hypercalcemia of malignancy.

Multiple organ systems are involved in the constellation of symptoms caused by hypercalcemia. These symptoms are nonspecific, and their severity is directly related to the degree of calcium elevation. Neuromuscular symptoms often predominate. If left untreated, initial manifestations of fatigue, weakness, lethargy, and apathy can progress to profound mental status changes and psychotic behavior. Nausea, vomiting, anorexia, obstipation, ileus, and abdominal pain are among the gastrointestinal symptoms that may accompany hypercalcemia. Renal tubular dysfunction can occur and is manifested by the development of polydipsia, polyuria, and nocturia. Severe volume contraction occurs, potentiating serum calcium elevation. Without prompt therapy, prolonged hypercalcemia may progress to permanent renal tubular damage.

Because calcium acts as a neurotransmitter, the myocardium is particularly prone to hypercalcemia-induced toxicity. Acute hypercalcemia can slow the heart rate and shorten ventricular systole. With moderate elevation of the calcium level, the QT interval is shortened, and atrial and ventricular arrhythmias may occur. Electrocardiographic changes seen with elevated serum calcium levels include bradycardia, prolonged PR interval, shortened QT interval, and widened T waves. Under extreme circumstances, an acute rise in serum calcium can result in sudden death from cardiac arrhythmias.

Laboratory studies critical in the workup of patients with hypercalcemia include serum calcium, phosphate, alkaline phosphatase, PTH, electrolytes, blood urea nitrogen, total protein, albumin, and creatinine levels. In patients with severe hypoalbuminemia, the ionized calcium level is more accurate than the serum calcium level. Also, abnormal binding of calcium to paraprotein without an elevation in the ionized calcium level can be seen in patients with multiple myeloma. Elevated immunoreactive PTH levels in association with hypophosphatemia suggest ectopic PTH secretion. Hypercalcemia secondary to malignancy usually has an acute onset, a high serum calcium level (>14 mg/dL), a low serum chloride level, and elevated or normal serum phosphate and bicarbonate levels. These laboratory findings help differentiate hypercalcemia caused by cancer from that secondary to hyperparathyroidism, which is associated with an elevated serum calcium level in the presence of decreased serum phosphate and bicarbonate levels.

Prompt identification and treatment of hypercalcemia are essential. Symptomatic patients and those patients with a serum calcium level of 12 mg/dL or greater require urgent treatment. Intravenous hydration with restoration of intravascular volume increases glomerular filtration rate and is the mainstay of initial management. Diuretics that block calcium resorption in the ascending loop of Henle and augment renal calcium excretion (e.g., furosemide) may be helpful after intravascular volume has been repleted. The initial dose of furosemide in patients without renal impairment is 40 mg IV, followed by 40 to 80 mg every 2 to 4 hours as needed.

Bisphosphonates block osteoclastic bone resorption and substantially reduce serum calcium levels. Etidronate disodium was the first biphosphonate approved for use in the United States. A typical dose regimen is 7.5 mg/kg per day IV for several days, followed by 20 mg/kg per day orally. Pamidronate, a "second-generation" biphosphonate, is more effective than etidronate and has the advantage of inhibiting bone resorption caused by osteoclast activity while leaving bone mineralization unimpaired. Furthermore, pamidronate has a faster onset, a longer effect, and a more durable response. The dose of pamidronate is 60 to 90 mg given IV. Patients usually begin to notice relief of symptoms within hours, and the effect usually lasts for 2 to 3 weeks. Maintenance therapy can be given via intermittent IV infusion every 3 to 4 weeks, or continuous oral administration. Oral dosages between 400 and 1,200 mg/day in divided doses have achieved fairly good response rates.

The antibiotic plicamycin (Mithracin), an effective inhibitor of bone resorption, generally induces a decline in serum calcium within 6 to 48 hours. Plicamycin has limited antineoplastic activity; however, when used at doses of 25 mg/kg per day by IV infusion, the drug provides a marked reduction in bone resorption. Toxicities of plicamycin include thrombocytopenia, hypotension, and hepatic and renal insufficiency. These adverse effects are rare when the dosage is restricted to less than 30 mg/kg per day.

Gallium nitrate is another potent inhibitor of bone resorption. Administration of this agent to patients with malignant disease and hyperparathyroidism causes profound reductions in serum calcium. Incorporation of gallium nitrate into bone causes hydroxyapatite to become less soluble and more resistant to cell-mediated resorption. In addition, gallium nitrate impairs osteoclast acidification of bone matrix by decreasing transmembrane proton transport. This agent may also enhance bone formation by stimulating bone collagen synthesis and increasing calcium incorporation into bone. These actions result in a net reduction of serum calcium. When given at a dosage of 100 to 200 mg/kg per day via continuous IV infusion, for 5 to 7 days, normal serum calcium levels are achieved in 80% to 90% of patients. Nephrotoxicity, the dose-limiting factor, may be minimized by pretreatment IV hydration prior to treatment.

Hyponatremia/Syndrome of Inappropriate Antidiuretic Hormone

Considerable neurologic dysfunction can occur when the serum sodium level falls abruptly or decreases to levels below 115 to 125 mg/dL. Mental status changes, seizures, coma, and, ultimately, death may result if therapeutic intervention is not urgently instituted. The syndrome of inappropriate antidiuretic hormone (SIADH) may be associated with cancers of the prostate, adrenal glands, esophagus, pancreas, colon, and head and neck as well as with carcinoid tumors and mesotheliomas. Small cell carcinoma of the lung is the most common malignancy associated with SIADH.

Dilutional hyponatremia is caused by excessive water resorption in the collecting ducts. This increase in intravascular volume leads to increased renal perfusion along with a substantial decrease in proximal tubular absorption of sodium. In the presence of renal insufficiency, there is increased ADH secretion and excessive water reabsorption from the collecting ducts, resulting in dilutional hyponatremia.

Patients with mild hyponatremia frequently complain of anorexia, nausea, myalgia, headaches, and subtle neurologic symptoms. When the onset of hyponatremia is rapid or the absolute serum sodium level falls below 115 mg/dL, patients develop severe neurologic dysfunction. Alterations in mental status can range from lethargy to confusion and can ultimately progress to coma. Seizures and psychotic behavior can occur at low serum sodium levels as well. Physical findings in patients with profound hyponatremia include alterations in mental status, abnormal reflexes, papilledema, and, occasionally, focal neurologic signs.

Laboratory data and diagnostic studies aid clinicians in determining the etiology of hyponatremia. Pseudo-hyponatremia is due to hyperproteinemia, hyperglycemia, or hyperlipidemia. Serum protein electrophoresis, glucose, and lipid determinations can rule this out. The possibility of drug-induced hyponatremia should also be considered. Such chemotherapeutic agents as vincristine and cyclophosphamide, as well as mannitol, morphine and diuretics, may contribute to hyponatremia, as may the abrupt withdrawal of corticosteroids.

A detailed history and physical examination, along with careful evaluation of the patient's fluid intake and output is often sufficient to determine a patient's intravascular volume and can eliminate water toxicity as a possible cause of hyponatremia. Laboratory investigation should include measurement of serum and urine electrolytes and creatinine. A typical finding in patients with SIADH is that the urine sodium concentration is inappropriately high for the level of hyponatremia. Also, the urine osmolality is often greater than the plasma osmolality, and the urine is never maximally diluted. Other findings indicative of SIADH include a low BUN, hypouricemia, and hypophosphatemia, which result from decreased renal proximal tubular resorption. A chest radiograph and head CT scan should be done to exclude unsuspected pathology of the pulmonary or central nervous system (CNS).

Ideally, therapy for SIADH should be directed toward the underlying cause. In the case of small cell lung cancer, effective multi-drug chemotherapy usually results in resolution of hyponatremia. SIADH resulting from CNS metastasis may improve with the use of corticosteroids and radiation therapy. If the etiology of SIADH cannot be identified, then the therapy for patients with severe hyponatremia is water restriction: a restriction of free water to 500 to 1,000 mL/day should correct the hyponatremia within 5 to 10 days. If the serum sodium level does not improve after restriction of free water for this period, demeclocycline should be used. Demeclocycline is an ADH antagonist that produces a dose-dependent, reversible nephrogenic diabetes insipidus. The recommended initial dose of demeclocycline is 600 mg daily (given in two or three divided doses). The potential adverse effect of nephrotoxicity with demeclocycline is usually seen only when extremely high doses are used (1,200 mg/day). Because this agent is secreted in urine and bile, dose adjustments must be made in patients with renal or hepatic insufficiency.

When severe hyponatremia produces seizures or coma, 3% hypertonic saline or normal saline infusion with IV furosemide should be used. The rate of correction of the serum sodium level should be limited to 0.5 to 1.0 mEq per hour to minimize the risk of CNS toxicity.

Hypoglycemia

Insulin-producing islet cell tumors (insulinomas) are the prototypical lesions associated with hypoglycemia. However, other tumors that often result in hypoglycemia include hepatomas, adrenocortical tumors, and tumors of mesenchymal origin. Mesenchymal tumors comprise more than 50% of non-islet cell neoplasms seen in association with hypoglycemia. Of these, mesothelioma, fibrosarcoma, neurofibrosarcoma, and hemangiopericytoma are the most common.

The mechanism of hypoglycemia resulting from insulinomas involves the unregulated and inappropriate secretion of excess insulin. In contrast, the serum insulin level is normal in cases of non-islet cell tumors. Substances with non-suppressible insulin-like activities (NSILAs) have been detected in patients with malignancy-associated hypoglycemia. Two classes of compounds have been isolated based on molecular weight and ethanol solubility. The low-molecular-weight compounds consist of insulin growth factor (IGF)-I, IGF-II, somatomedin A, and somatomedin C. IGF-I and IGF-II have amino acid sequences similar to proinsulin but do not react with anti-insulin antibodies. The metabolic activity of these compounds is only 1% to 2% that of insulin. Approximately 40% of cancer patients with symptomatic hypoglycemia have elevated plasma levels of NSILAs.

Increased glucose use may account for the hypoglycemia seen in association with large tumors. Hepatic glucose production (700 g/day) may fall short of daily glucose requirements in the presence of tumors weighing more than 1 kg, which use 50 to 200 g/day of glucose. Defects in the usual counter-regulatory mechanism of glucose control may also account for malignancy-induced hypoglycemia. Cancer-related hypoglycemia usually develops gradually and does not allow the usual increase in counter-regulatory hormones seen with hypoglycemia arising from nonmalignant etiologies.

Symptoms of hypoglycemia include excessive fatigue, weakness, dizziness, and confusion. In malignancy-associated hypoglycemia, neurologic symptoms usually predominate and may progress to seizures and coma if left untreated. These more severe neurologic complications are usually associated with serum glucose levels below 40 to 45 mg/dL.

Before cancer is determined to be the etiology of hypoglycemia, all other potential causes must be excluded. Exogenous insulin or oral hypoglycemic agents, adrenal insufficiency, pituitary insufficiency, ethanol abuse, and malnutrition are among the common causes of hypoglycemia. In cases of cancer, measurement of fasting serum glucose and insulin levels will aid in determining whether hypoglycemia is due to an islet cell tumor or to a non-islet cell tumor. Patients with insulinomas have increased insulin levels, with fasting glucose levels below 50 mg/dL. In contrast, cases of non-islet cell tumors are marked by a normal or low insulin level associated with hypoglycemia. Also, because insulinomas produce large amounts of proinsulin, they tend to have an elevated proinsulin-to-insulin ratio.

Under ideal circumstances, complete extirpation of the tumor is the optimal therapeutic intervention for hypoglycemia secondary to solid tumors. In cases of an insulinoma, simple enucleation or subtotal pancreatectomy frequently provides a cure. About 90% of these tumors are benign. Diazoxide may benefit patients with insulin-secreting tumors by inhibiting insulin secretion. This drug is not effective in the treatment of non-islet cell tumors. In some cases, radiation therapy reduces tumor bulk and provides palliation of hypoglycemia. Diet modification should be used as the second line of therapy, i.e., when resection is not possible. Frequent feedings can reduce hypoglycemic attacks. Corticosteroids and growth hormone may provide temporary relief. Subcutaneous glucagon injections can also be used to aid in glucose regulation.

Tumor Lysis Syndrome

Tumor lysis syndrome is a critical complication of cytotoxic therapy that requires a team approach in the intensive care unit to prevent the sequelae of permanent renal failure and death. The syndrome is triggered by rapid cell turnover and increased release of intracellular contents into the bloodstream, and is characterized by hyperuricemia, hyperkalemia, hyperphosphatemia, and hypocalcemia. Occasionally, this syndrome occurs spontaneously in patients with lymphomas and leukemia; however, it is more common after cytotoxic chemotherapy-induced rapid cell lysis. The rapid release of intracellular contents can overwhelm the excretory ability of the kidneys, and electrolyte levels can become dangerously elevated. Patients with large, bulky tumors that are sensitive to cytotoxic chemotherapy are particularly prone to this syndrome, as are patients undergoing treatment for Burkitt's or non-Hodgkin's lymphoma, acute lymphoblastic leukemia, acute nonlymphoblastic leukemia, or chronic myelogenous leukemia in blast crisis. Tumor lysis syndrome can also occur after treatment of small cell lung cancer, metastatic breast cancer, and metastatic medulloblastoma. Tumor lysis syndrome occurs not only with cytotoxic chemotherapy but also following radiation therapy, hormonal therapy (e.g., tamoxifen), and cryotherapy of primary and metastatic tumors of the liver.

Metabolic abnormalities associated with tumor lysis syndrome include hyperuricemia, hyperkalemia, and hyperphosphatemia with hypocalcemia. The pathologic processes seen with this syndrome are due to the propensity of uric acid, xanthine, and phosphate to precipitate in the renal tubules. This precipitation can impair renal excretory function and cause further elevation of these metabolites in the serum. Renal insufficiency typically does not develop from the metabolic derangements alone; a combination of low urine flow rates and elevated serum metabolites is usually required to precipitate renal dysfunction. Thus, oliguric patients are at significantly higher risk of developing renal failure during rapid cellular lysis.

Hyperkalemia results from the release of intracellular contents and is further perpetuated by renal insufficiency. Potassium elevation can have life-threatening consequences and requires immediate intervention. Cardiac toxicity is evidenced by the characteristic electrocardiographic changes seen with potassium levels above 6 mEq/dL. These changes include loss of P waves, peaked T waves, a widened QRS complex, and depressed ST segments. Heart block and diastolic cardiac arrest may result if hyperkalemia is left untreated.

Rapid tumor lysis can also cause hyperphosphatemia, which is usually accompanied by hypocalcemia. Hypocalcemia in tumor lysis syndrome is thought to be due to the formation of calcium-phosphate salts that precipitate in soft tissues. Hyperphosphatemia is further exacerbated by the formation of these calcium-phosphate complexes in renal tubules, causing progressive renal insufficiency.

Preventive measures can be taken to minimize the toxicities of tumor lysis. Patients should undergo vigorous IV hydration before treatment with potentially toxic chemotherapeutic agents is begun. Another important preventive measure is to alkalinize the urine during the first 1 to 2 days of cytotoxic treatment. These measures counteract hyperuricemia by increasing the solubility of uric acid. Allopurinol has also been shown to effectively decrease the formation of uric acid and to reduce the incidence of uric acid nephropathy. In patients with large, bulky tumors that are known to have a high growth fraction, allopurinol should be administered before planned chemotherapeutic intervention.

An electrocardiogram should be obtained in all patients with hyperkalemia or hypocalcemia, and continuous cardiac monitoring should be instituted. Hyperkalemia should be treated with the standard measures for acutely lowering the serum potassium level. These measures include IV administration of insulin and glucose, loop diuretics, and sodium bicarbonate. Calcium should be given to stabilize the myocardium. Regardless of measures used to acutely lower the serum potassium, a sodium-potassium exchange resin should be given to lower the total body potassium load (15 g sodium polystyrene sulfonate [Kayexalate] orally or by rectum every 6 hours). If there is evidence of worsening renal function with poor resolution of the metabolic abnormalities, hemodialysis should be considered.

Central Venous Catheter Sepsis

The use of indwelling vascular access catheters is widespread in modern cancer care. Catheter-based infection is a major source of morbidity. When catheter infection is suspected, the access site should be carefully examined. Erythema, induration, and suppuration are signs of site infection, which require immediate catheter removal. Bacteremia and sepsis from catheter infection should be documented by drawing blood cultures from both the catheter and peripheral sites. Coagulase-negative staphylococci are the most common pathogens isolated in catheter-based infection, although numerous gram-positive, gram-negative, and fungal species may also be responsible. More than 80% of catheter-based infections can be treated effectively with a 10- to 14-day course of IV antibiotics. Antibiotic therapy should be given through the infected catheter and rotated between ports when multilumen catheters are present. Persistence of positive blood cultures or signs of systemic sepsis, particularly in neutropenic patients, necessitates immediate catheter removal. In patients with vascular grafts or implanted prostheses, immediate catheter removal is indicated once an infection has been documented.

ABDOMINAL EMERGENCIES

Intestinal Obstruction

Bowel obstruction continues to be a considerable source of morbidity and mortality in patients with cancer. The decisions regarding the timing and the extent of surgery remain difficult, and few studies offer much guidance. Approximately two thirds of patients with ovarian cancer present with at least one episode of bowel obstruction, and nearly all patients with carcinomatosis suffer some sort of intestinal complication. In up to one third of all patients with a history of cancer who present with a bowel obstruction, the cause of the obstruction is a benign source (e.g., adhesions, hernias, and radiation enteritis). In the other two thirds of these patients, either primary or metastatic disease is the source of their intestinal obstruction. The intra-abdominal malignancies most often associated with obstruction of the gastrointestinal tract are carcinomas of the ovary, colon, and stomach. Extra-abdominal malignancies may metastasize to the peritoneal cavity and cause obstruction; in such cases, the most common sources are carcinomas of the lung, breast, and melanoma.

Functional obstruction of the bowel without a mechanical cause (colonic "pseudo-obstruction" or Ogilvie's syndrome) is a common problem in patients with cancer. Narcotic analgesics, electrolyte abnormalities, radiation therapy, malnutrition, and prolonged bedrest may all contribute to delayed intestinal motility. The treatment consists of correcting the underlying cause and decompressing the bowel with a nasogastric tube. Colonoscopic decompression should be considered when the size of the cecum reaches 10 cm. Surgery is indicated if the degree of intestinal dilatation progresses to the point of impending perforation or if the patient shows any evidence of peritonitis. Tube cecostomy is the procedure of choice in these often-debilitated patients, with resection and ileostomy formation reserved for cases of frank perforation. Another measure that has been recently described involves the administration of neostigmine (2.0–2.5 mg IV). This therapy has shown promise in a number of small series, but should only be considered for patients in a closely monitored setting.

The evaluation of intestinal obstruction in patients with cancer should be similar to that in patients with benign disease. After a complete history, physical examination, and evaluation of laboratory and radiologic data, the degree and site of obstruction should be delineated. Immediate laparotomy is indicated for those patients who have signs or symptoms of intestinal ischemia, necrosis, or frank perforation (abdominal tenderness, leukocytosis, fever, or tachycardia). Nearly 10% of patients will have concurrent small- and large-bowel obstruction. To exclude the possibility of colonic obstruction before laparotomy, a Gastografin enema may be obtained, particularly in patients with multiple sites of intra-abdominal tumor. Either an upper gastrointestinal series with small-bowel follow-through or enteroclysis may be useful in patients with recurrent partial small-bowel obstructions. Finally, a CT scan of the abdomen and pelvis using oral and rectal contrast may help identify the location and etiology of the obstruction. Before laparotomy, all patients should undergo standard resuscitation including IV fluid administration, correction of electrolyte abnormalities, and placement of a nasogastric tube.

In patients with a partial small-bowel obstruction, a trial of medical management is worthwhile. Up to 50% of patients respond to conservative treatment, which may require up to 2 weeks of intestinal decompression. Surgery is advocated for patients who do not respond to medical management or whose condition progresses to complete obstruction. Medical management is rarely successful in patients with a complete obstruction at any level, and these patients should undergo exploration. The goal of surgery is to provide relief of the obstruction, although this goal cannot always be accomplished. The surgeon should fully explore the abdomen and attempt to identify the cause of the obstruction. Benign adhesions should be lysed with care. In cases of radiation enteritis, gentle handling of the bowel is essential. Resection may be adequate for short segments of intestine but long segments are best treated by internal bypass. A similar approach should be taken in relieving bowel obstruction caused by malignancy, although occasionally the extent of the malignant disease is too extensive to allow for any of these options. In such cases, placement of a venting gastrostomy for symptomatic relief is all that is indicated. A gastrostomy provides considerable relief from continued emesis and avoids the need for prolonged placement of a nasogastric tube.

Exploration related to a malignant bowel obstruction is associated with substantial morbidity and mortality. Almost 10% of patients die because of surgery, and another 30% suffer operative complications. Furthermore, patients have a mean survival of only about 6 months following laparotomy for a malignant bowel obstruction. Bowel obstruction from benign disease is rare in patients with known residual or recurrent intra-abdominal tumor. Therefore, bowel obstruction in patients with documented intra-abdominal disease can be viewed as a premorbid event, with prolonged survival unlikely despite any intervention. Given such a poor prognosis, it is often more appropriate to pursue nonsurgical options (e.g., placement of a percutaneous endoscopic gastrostomy tube).

Another recently employed management strategy for malignant obstruction of the rectum is the use of self-expanding metal stents. These stents may be used either as a definitive measure or as an adjunct to allow for bowel decompression and cleansing in preparation for surgery. While colonic perforation is a potential complication, these devices may allow patients with near-complete obstructions to avoid an ostomy and thus enjoy better quality of life.

Intestinal Perforation

Perforation of the gastrointestinal tract in patients with cancer may occur at nearly any time in the course of the disease. Indeed, the condition may be the presenting sign of cancer, such as in cases of perforated primary colorectal carcinoma. The perforation may occur during treatment (either chemotherapy or radiation therapy), or it may be the result of metastatic tumor later in the course of the disease. Most perforations of the gastrointestinal tract of cancer patients are from benign causes (e.g., peptic ulcer disease, diverticulitis, and appendicitis) and should be treated according to standard surgical principles. Surgery is associated with significant morbidity and mortality but is often the only therapeutic option available for this life-threatening complication. Patients must be well informed of the risks of surgery and must understand that an ostomy is a possibility before an emergency laparotomy. Nonsurgical treatment, comfort care, or both may be appropriate, depending on the patient's wishes, prognosis, and overall medical status.

Intestinal perforation is the presenting symptom of disease in a small group of patients with undiagnosed colorectal carcinoma. However, on further questioning, these patients usually state that they have had some symptoms, whether related to obstruction or to bleeding, attributable to the tumor. The perforation may be the result of full-thickness colonic involvement with the tumor and subsequent necrosis of a region of the intestinal wall. A carcinoma that nearly or completely obstructs the lumen of the colon may also present with perforation proximal in the intestinal tract, usually the cecum. In general, patients who present with either perforated or obstructing colorectal cancer have a poorer overall prognosis, stage for stage, than do patients without these presentations. Furthermore, the operative mortality rate associated with emergency laparotomy for perforated colorectal cancer approaches 30%.

Perforation of the gastrointestinal tract following chemotherapy for metastatic solid tumors is a potentially fatal complication. The rate of operative mortality has been reported to be as high as 80% for an emergency laparotomy in patients with metastatic cancer receiving chemotherapy. Factors associated with a high rate of complications include chemotherapy-induced myeloid toxicity, protein malnutrition, and immunosuppression. Furthermore, traditional signs of an acute surgical abdomen may be masked in these patients, leading to a delay in diagnosis. Finally, because the prognosis of these patients is poor, the decision to proceed with exploratory laparotomy is difficult and is often made late in the clinical course.

Most cases of gastrointestinal perforation related to malignant disease are caused by hematologic malignancies, with solid tumors, such as ovarian carcinoma, being an extremely uncommon cause. Lymphoma with intestinal involvement is the malignancy most likely to lead to gastrointestinal perforation following systemic chemotherapy. In such cases, perforation is often related to transmural involvement of the intestine, resulting in full-thickness necrosis following chemotherapy. Furthermore, because of the extensive involvement of the gastrointestinal tract by lymphoma and the relative chemosensitivity of this neoplasm, perforation is not uncommon following chemotherapy. Conversely, metastases from solid organ tumors are often limited to the serosal surface and therefore do not lead to full-thickness necrosis following chemotherapy.

Radiation therapy directed at the abdomen may damage the gastrointestinal tract. The extent of injury depends on the dose of radiation delivered, the radiation fields utilized, the energy of the ionizing radiation, and the use of adjunctive methods to shield the intestines. Immediate effects include damage and subsequent sloughing of the mucosal layer of the intestinal tract. Most of the immediate effects lead to substantial nausea and vomiting, which are usually temporary. Most patients can be managed as outpatients, and oral agents can be used to palliate symptoms. However, a small but significant fraction of patients require hospitalization for intravenous administration of fluid and antiemetics. Finally, in its severest form, radiation-induced injury leads to full-thickness injury of the intestinal tract with subsequent perforation. Such an injury usually occurs later in the course of the radiation therapy or follows the completion of treatment. Once the diagnosis is made, the management of this condition is similar to that of any intestinal perforation.

Upon abdominal exploration, the area of perforation should be resected, if possible. A conservative approach to reestablishing gastrointestinal continuity should be used, especially for patients with poor nutritional status, altered host immune response or impending shock. Ostomies should be used liberally and may be reversed at a subsequent procedure, if appropriate. Furthermore, strong consideration should be given to the placement of gastrostomy and feeding jejunostomy tubes. Such devices obviate the need for prolonged nasogastric intubation and allow for early enteral feeding.

Biliary Obstruction

Biliary obstruction by metastases to the hilum of the liver or portal lymph nodes is an uncommon but troublesome problem in patients with cancer. Such obstructions may be caused by a variety of tumor types, including lymphoma, melanoma, and carcinoma of the breast, colon, stomach, lung, or ovary. Obstruction of the biliary tree due to primary carcinomas of the common bile duct and pancreas is discussed elsewhere. Evaluation is best performed with CT scan, which provides information on the site of obstruction, reveals the degree of biliary obstruction, allows evaluation of the remainder of the abdomen, and often gives clues as to the cause of obstruction. When necessary, endoscopic ultrasound or CT-guided fine-needle aspiration can be performed in this region to obtain a tissue diagnosis.

The prognosis for patients with biliary obstruction from metastatic disease is poor. In one published series of 12 patients with biliary obstruction from metastases, 11 patients had disease either in other intra-abdominal sites or in extra-abdominal locations. The 60-day mortality rate in this group has been reported to be as high as 67%. Thus, treatment should aim to palliate jaundice and to prevent cholangitis. Endoscopic retrograde cholangiopancreatography and stent placement best accomplish drainage of the biliary tree. If this approach is unsuccessful, percutaneous transhepatic drainage is indicated. External-beam irradiation, with or without chemotherapy, may also provide substantial palliation, especially in cases of obstruction due to primary biliary or pancreatic carcinoma. Surgery should be reserved for patients who are at low-risk–that is patients for whom the risk of metastatic disease is low and the chance for long-term survival is high.

Neutropenic Enterocolitis

The terms neutropenic enterocolitis, typhlitis, necrotizing enteropathy, and ileocecal syndrome have all been used to describe a clinical entity characterized by febrile neutropenia, abdominal distension, right-sided abdominal pain, tenderness, and diarrhea. The syndrome most often occurs in patients undergoing chemotherapy for a hematologic malignancy, but may also occur in patients with solid tumors. Signs and symptoms characteristically develop after neutropenia lasting 7 days or more. The initial presentation consists of right-sided abdominal pain, tenderness, and fever and may mimic appendicitis. The diagnosis is made clinically, often by exclusion of other pathologic causes. Serial examinations by the same examiner are critical for proper diagnosis and treatment. Abdominal films characteristically reveal a nonspecific ileus pattern with some dilation of the cecum. Pneumatosis is an inconsistent finding. The CT findings for neutropenic enterocolitis are also nonspecific, consisting mainly of bowel-wall thickening and edema. However, CT scans are invaluable to rule out other pathologic conditions. Complete workup should include stool cultures for bacteria and *Clostridium difficile* toxin.

The severity of neutropenic enterocolitis varies, and therapy must be individualized. Medical management, which includes bowel rest, nasogastric suction, broad-spectrum antibiotics, and IV hyperalimentation, is successful in most cases. Although granulocyte transfusion has never been proven to be effective, granulocyte colony-stimulating factors, which shorten the neutropenic period, likely improve outcome. Surgical intervention is indicated in cases of perforation, uncontrolled hemorrhage, sepsis, and progression of symptoms on medical therapy. Right hemicolectomy with or without ileostomy is the surgery of choice in most cases.

Hemorrhage

Malignant tumors are rarely the source of significant intra-abdominal hemorrhage, even in patients with known cancer. Peptic ulcer disease and gastritis, the most common causes of bleeding in unselected series, are the leading etiologies in 54% to 75% of patients with cancer. Gastrointestinal lymphomas and metastatic tumors are the lesions that most commonly initiate massive hemorrhage. Because spontaneous hemorrhage caused by tumors rarely occurs, individuals with cancer should receive the same systematic approach to diagnosis and treatment as do those without malignant disease. While resuscitation with crystalloid and blood products is under way, the diagnostic workup to define the site and etiology of bleeding should begin. Bleeding proximal to the ligament of Treitz is marked clinically by hematemesis or blood per nasogastric aspirate. Upon the finding of such signs, upper endoscopy should be performed promptly.

Bright red blood per rectum should initiate investigation of a colonic or rectal source. In such cases, either proctoscopy or sigmoidoscopy serves as an expedient initial diagnostic maneuver. Angiography and nuclear red cell scans are often useful to localize bleeding sites in the colon and small bowel. Mild blood loss due to a colonic neoplasm can usually be treated endoscopically with electrocautery or placement of topical hemostatic agents if the lesion is within the rectum. Some patients require urgent surgical resection of a colonic neoplasm for continued bleeding, but this procedure can usually be delayed to allow for localization of the site of bleeding and until the bowel has been mechanically cleansed to allow for a primary anastomosis. If the bleeding cannot be localized and the hemorrhage is massive, immediate exploration with intraoperative endoscopy should be considered. Exploration, endoscopy, or both may allow localization of the bleeding site so that surgical resection may be directed; however, total abdominal colectomy may be needed if the hemorrhage cannot be precisely localized. Small-bowel tumors rarely present with massive gastrointestinal hemorrhage, although gastric carcinoma may occasionally present with acute bleeding. The evaluation and treatment approaches are nearly identical to those for similar conditions arising from a colonic source, with endoscopy as the first line of treatment and surgical resection reserved for a more elective setting.

Extraluminal, intra-abdominal hemorrhage should be suspected when there is significant blood loss without hematemesis, melena, or hematochezia. The retroperitoneum is the most frequent site of occult intra-abdominal hemorrhage. If this condition is suspected, CT scan is the best method of evaluation. Therapy for intra-abdominal hemorrhage is initially directed at resuscitation and correction of any existing coagulopathy. A history of aspirin or nonsteroidal anti-inflammatory use within 1 week must raise suspicion of platelet dysfunction, and a bleeding time should be obtained. After the site and source of bleeding have been identified, specific therapy is instituted. Under controlled conditions, invasive therapies, such as angiographic embolization, may be attempted. The timing of surgical intervention is based on the rate and volume of blood loss, the underlying pathology, and the patient's overall prognosis.

RECOMMENDED READING

Arrambide K, Toto RD. Tumor lysis syndrome. *Semin Nephrol* 1993;13:273–280.

Aurora R, Milite F, Vander Els NJ. Respiratory emergencies. *Semin Oncol* 2000;27:256–269.

Camunez F, Echenagusia A, Simo G, et al. Malignant colorectal obstruction treated by means of self-expanding metallic stents: effectiveness before surgery and in palliation. *Radiology* 2000;216:492–497.

Chen HS, Sheen-Chen SM. Obstruction and perforation in colorectal adenocarcinoma: an analysis of prognosis and current trends. *Surgery* 2000;127:370–376.

Ciezki JP, Komurcu S Macklis RM. Palliative radiotherapy. *Semin Oncol* 2000;27:90–93.

Chisolm MA, Mulloy AL, Taylor AT. Acute management of cancer-related hypercalcemia. *Ann Pharmacother* 1996;30:507–513.

Hoegler D. Radiotherapy for palliation of symptoms in incurable cancer. *Curr Probl Cancer* 1997;21:129–183.

Ibrahim NK, Sahin AA, Dubrow RA, et al. Colitis associated with docetaxel-based chemotherapy in patients with metastatic breast cancer. *Lancet* 2000;355: 281–283.

Lefor AT. Perioperative management of the patient with cancer. *Chest* 1999;115[5 suppl]:165S–171S.

Makris A, Kunkler IH. Controversies in the management of metastatic spinal cord compression. *Clin Oncol* 1995;7:77–81.

Miller M. Inappropriate antidiuretic hormone secretion. *Curr Ther Endocrinol Metab* 1997;6:206–209.

Nussbaum SR. Pathophysiology and management of severe hypercalcemia. *Endocrinol Metab Clin North Am* 1993;22:343–362.

Ostler PJ, Clarke DP, Watkinson AF, et al. Superior vena cava obstruction: a modern management strategy. *Clin Oncol* 1997;9:83–89.

Ponec RJ, Saunders MD, Kimmey MB. Neostigmine for the treatment of acute colonic pseudo-obstruction. *N Engl J Med* 1999;341:137–141.

Reed CR, Sessler CN, Glauser FL, et al. Central venous catheter infections: concepts and controversies. *Intensive Care Med* 1995;21:177–183.

Reyes CV, Thompson KS, Massarani-Wafai R, et al. Utilization of fine-needle aspiration cytology in the diagnosis of neoplastic superior vena cava syndrome. *Diagn Cytopathol* 1998;19:84–88.

Schindler N, Vogelzang RL. Superior vena cava syndrome. Experience with endovascular stents and surgical therapy. *Surg Clin North Am* 1999;79:683–694.

Tang E, Davis D, Silberman H. Bowel obstruction in cancer patients. *Arch Surg* 1995;130:832–836.

Theriault RL. Hypercalcemia of malignancy: pathophysiology and implications for treatment. *Oncology* 1993;7:47–50.

Wade DS, Nava HR, Douglass HO Jr. Neutropenic enterocolitis. *Cancer* 1992;69:17–23.

Biological Cancer Therapy

Daniel Albo, Thomas N. Wang, and
George P. Tuszynski

INTRODUCTION

Biological therapy is cancer treatment that produces antitumor effects primarily through the manipulation of natural defense mechanisms of the host. Biological therapy induces, uses, or modifies the host's immune system to efficiently recognize and destroy cancer cells. Biological therapy has emerged as an important fourth modality for the treatment of cancer, joining surgery, radiation therapy, and chemotherapy in our armamentarium against cancer. The increasing application of biological therapy is the result of a better understanding of the basic concepts of host defense mechanisms. Basic science research on the immune system has taken biological therapy out of its infancy and into clinical trials. Although several types of biological therapies targeting cytokines, vaccines, cellular therapies, monoclonal antibodies (MAbs), and gene therapies have shown promise in the treatment of human cancers, it is in the field of antiangiogenic therapies where some of the better understood and more promising agents are being developed. Because detailed description of all available biological cancer therapies is not feasible in only one chapter, we focus primarily on antiangiogenic therapies.

Angiogenesis, or the formation of new blood vessels from preexisting ones, is a complex process that normally occurs in adults only under specific conditions such as wound healing, inflammation, and development of the corpus luteum in the menstrual cycle. Although small numbers of tumor cells can potentially survive without stimulating angiogenesis, tumor size is limited, and in this situation, growth is balanced by apoptosis. Further growth of the tumor requires an "angiogenic switch," such that the tumor induces the growth of a blood supply from existing vessels. There are at least four potential mechanisms by which tumors can stimulate angiogenesis. The first hypothesis, put forth by Judah Folkman in the 1970s, suggested that tumors stimulate the sprouting of new blood vessels, by secreting proangiogenic growth factors such as vascular endothelial growth factor (VEGF), basic fibroblast growth factor (bFGF), transforming growth factor-beta (TGF-β), and others. The second mechanism suggests that tumors can co-opt existing vasculature. Third, the regulation of angiogenesis may, in part, be contributed to by circulating hematopoietic precursors. The fourth potential mechanism is known as vascular mimicry, a process by which aggressive tumor cells form a pattern of vasculogeniclike networks in three-dimensional culture, with concomitant expression of vascular-associated cell markers.

Tumor angiogenesis begins by mutual stimulation between tumor cells and endothelial cells by paracrine mechanisms. Angiogenesis requires tumor cells or stromal cells to release stimulatory factors and endothelial cells to respond to them such that endothelial cells can release proteolytic enzymes to degrade the extracellular matrix for migration and proliferation. Endothelial proliferation typically occurs at the leading edge of the migration at potentially hundreds of times that observed in quiescent vasculature. This is followed by lumen formation and stabilization of the new vessel. A new basement membrane is created and support cells (including pericytes and smooth muscle cells) are recruited. Cell adhesion proteins called integrins regulate the invasion, migration, and proliferation of endothelial cells. Changes in expression of certain integrins on the newly formed sprouts are critical for the formation of new vessels. The resulting chaotic tumor vasculature is tortuous and dilated with heterogeneous flow and permeability.

Understanding angiogenesis and its unique characteristics in tumor growth has provided insight into numerous ways to interrupt this process. Since the mid-1990s, research on antiangiogenic agents has exploded, along with public interest in its potential. We now have a clearer understanding of the process of tumor angiogenesis, including key cytokines, differences between normal and immature tumor vasculature, and endogenous inhibitors, along with methods to quantify angiogenesis. As a result of this, numerous antiangiogenic agents are currently in both preclinical and clinical trials. However, no clear "silver bullet" has yet emerged from the agents investigated thus far. In this chapter, we review the different types of angiogenesis inhibitors available for cancer treatment and prevention, and how they have fared in clinical trials. Furthermore, we analyze the potential pitfalls in trial design and interpretation of trial results, as well as potential future directions in this exciting research field.

ANGIOGENESIS INHIBITORS

With respect to their target, angiogenesis inhibitors can be subdivided into two classes: direct and indirect. Direct angiogenesis inhibitors, such as endostatin, target the microvascular endothelial cells that are recruited to the tumor bed. Direct angiogenesis inhibitors prevent vascular endothelial cells from proliferating, migrating, or avoiding cell death in response to a spectrum of proangiogenic proteins (i.e., VEGF, bFGF) (Table 22.1). Direct angiogenesis inhibitors are the least likely to induce acquired drug resistance because they target genetically stable endothelial cells rather than unstable mutating tumor cells.

Indirect angiogenesis inhibitors generally prevent the expression of or block the activity of a tumor protein that activates angiogenesis or the expression of its receptor on endothelial cells (Table 22.2). Many of these tumor cell proteins are the products of oncogenes that drive the angiogenic switch. Targeting oncogene products not only affects cancer cell proliferation and cell death, but also disrupts the production of angiogenic factors. Reactivation of tumor suppressors such as p53 can also inhibit angiogenesis by different mechanisms.

It is important for clinical researchers to recognize that anticancer drugs that target an oncogene product can inhibit angiogenesis because this can affect drug dose and schedule. A drug that inhibits angiogenesis indirectly might be discontinued prematurely because of "resistance," which is determined by

Table 22.1. Direct inhibitors of angiogenesis in clinical trials

Drug	Mechanism	Trial
Direct-acting inhibitors of endothelial cells/receptor antagonists		
Thalidomide	Decrease TNFα, bFGF, VEGF	Phase I malignant glioma, melanoma Phase II melanoma, ovarian, metastatic prostate, colorectal, lymphoma, gynecologic sarcomas, liver, CLL Phase III non–small-cell lung, prostate, multiple myeloma, renal cell
SU6668	Blocks VEGF-R2, FGF-R, PDGF-R	Phase I advanced solid tumors
Squalamine	Inhibits sodium-hydrogen exchanger (NHE3)	Phase I advanced solid tumors Phase II non–small-cell lung, ovarian, brain
ZD1839	EGF-R inhibitor	Phase III non–small-cell lung
Erbitux (C225)	Monoclonal antibody against EGF-R	Phase II advanced solid tumors Phase III advanced solid tumors
IMC-1C11	VEGF-R2 inhibitor	Phase I metastatic colorectal
Angiozyme	Inhibits VEGF-R2 and VEFG-R2	Phase II breast, colorectal
Endostatin	Glypican, tropomyosin, $\alpha_v\beta_3$ integrin, MMP	Phase II neuroendocrine tumors, metastatic melanoma
Angiostatin	ATP synthase, Angiomotin, $\alpha_v\beta_3$ integrin	Phase I advanced solid tumors

TNFα, tumor necrosis factor-α; bFGF, basic fibroblast growth factor; VEGF, vascular endothelial growth factor; MMP, matrix metalloproteinase; ATP, adenosine triphosphate.

increased tumor angiogenesis. Instead, a second inhibitor could be added to the therapeutic regimen. For example, trastuzumab, an antibody that blocks ERBB2 (also known as HER2/neu) receptor tyrosine kinase signaling, suppresses cancer cell production of angiogenic factors such as TGF-β, angiopoietin-1 and plasminogen-activator inhibitor-1 (PAI1), and possibly also VEGF. If the tumor, however, begins to express a different angiogenic protein, such as bFGF or IL-8, the tumor under treatment might seem to have become "resistant" to trastuzumab, and the therapy will be discontinued. But this practice might not be

Table 22.2. Indirect inhibitors of angiogenesis in clinical trials

Drug	Mechanism	Trial
Indirect-acting/growth factor inhibitors		
Rhu Mab VEGF	Monoclonal antibody against VEGF	Phase II head and neck, metastatic renal cell, advanced colorectal, metastatic breast, non-Hodgkin lymphoma, hematologic malignancies, metastatic prostate, inflammatory breast, cervical, non–small-cell lung Phase III non–small-cell lung, metastatic colorectal, metastatic breast
MMP inhibitors		
BMS-275291	Synthetic MMP inhibitor	Phase I Kaposi sarcoma, non–small-cell lung, brain
COL-3	MMP-2, MMP-9 inhibitor	Phase II Kaposi sarcoma, brain
Neovastat	Natural MMP inhibitor	Phase II multiple myeloma Phase III renal cell, non–small-cell lung
Inhibitors of adhesion molecules/integrins signaling		
Vitaxin	Monoclonal antibody against $\alpha_v\beta_3$	Phase I/II irinotecan-refractory advanced colorectal cancer
EMD121974	Small molecule blocker of integrin (anti-$\alpha_v\beta_3$)	Phase I Kaposi sarcoma Phase III anaplastic glioma
Unknown or nonspecific mechanism of action		
Interferon α-2a	Decrease bFGF, VEGF	Phase I/II advanced solid tumors
Panzem (2-ME)	Unknown	Phase I/II advanced solid tumors
Celecoxib	COX-2 inhibitor	Phase I prostate, cervical Phase II cervical, basal cell, metastatic breast
IL-12	Upregulation of interferon γ	Phase I/II Kaposi sarcoma
CAI	Inhibitor of calcium influx	Phase I solid tumors Phase II ovarian, metastatic renal cell
IM862	Unknown	Phase II metastatic colorectal, ovarian

VEGF, vascular endothelial growth factor; MMP, matrix metalloproteinase; bFGF, basic fibroblast growth factor.

prudent for a drug with significant antiangiogenic activity. It might be more effective to add a second antiangiogenic drug to the regimen.

With respect to how they function, angiogenesis inhibitors can be subdivided into several categories, such as (a) agents that inhibit vascular endothelial activation; (b) agents that inhibit vascular endothelial migration, proliferation, and/or survival; (c) agents that inhibit degradation of extracellular matrix; and (d) agents that inhibit integrin activation, among others.

Agents That Inhibit Vascular Endothelial Activation: Vascular Endothelial Growth Factor

One of the key stimulatory factors for endothelial cells found to be highly upregulated in angiogenesis is the pivotal cytokine VEGF. VEGF is particularly notable as a growth factor for endothelial cells because it is relatively endothelial cell specific and will promote the growth of most tumor cells only due to paracrine effects from endothelial cells. Overexpression of VEGF has been reported to occur in the majority of clinically important human tumors examined.

The endothelial cell specificity of VEGF is due to the nearly exclusive expression of its receptors Flt-1 (VEGFR1) and Flk-1/KDR (VEGFR2) on endothelial cells. Activation of the Flk-1/KDR receptor is considered most closely associated with signals for proliferation, migration, permeability, and tube formation. This information led to the search for and the development of compounds to inhibit the tyrosine kinase activity of the receptor or antibodies to block receptor activity. A small molecule tyrosine kinase inhibitor, SU5416 (Pfizer, New York, NY), which is membrane permeable and inhibits the VEGF-dependent phosphorylation of tyrosine residues on the Flk-1 receptor, is currently in phase I/II and III trials. Another related small molecule tyrosine kinase inhibitor (SU6668) currently in phase I clinical trials has been shown to have significantly greater effect on mouse tumor and endothelial cell apoptosis than SU5416 with a corresponding decrease in liver metastases of CT-26 colon cancer cells. Both SU5416 and SU6668 inhibit tumor endothelial cell proliferation and decrease tumor vascularization. In other studies, orally or intraperitoneally administered SU6668 demonstrated antitumor activity without toxic effect in mice with xenografts of various cancer cell lines. Because inhibition of VEGF may be required on a chronic basis, the development of oral inhibitors such as SU6668 and ZD4190 (an inhibitor of both the Flk-1 and Flt-1 receptors) may prove valuable.

Inhibition of the VEGF Flk-1/KDR receptor and decreased tumor growth has also been demonstrated using MAbs. In addition to antibodies against the VEGF receptors, the MAb A.4.6.1 against VEGF protein has inhibited tumor growth and metastases in preclinical studies. RhuMAb VEGF (Genentech, South San Francisco, CA), a humanized form of the antibody, has been studied in preclinical trials, where it has been well tolerated, and is currently being used in phase II and III clinical trials.

In addition to preclinical and clinical trials to evaluate VEGF and VEGF receptor inhibition, trials combining these antiangiogenic agents with other traditional cytotoxic strategies have been initiated. A preclinical mouse study combining *anti*-VEGF receptor antibody with the chemotherapeutic agents cyclophosphamide, vinblastine, Taxol, or doxorubicin demonstrated that combined treatment potentiates the antitumor effect of either drug alone. A phase I/II trial combining SU5416, a VEGF-receptor inhibitor, with paclitaxel, a chemotherapy agent affecting both microtubules and angiogenesis, is ongoing in patients with advanced malignancies. In addition, combination *anti*-VEGF therapy has also been suggested for patients undergoing androgen ablation therapy or in combination with external-beam radiation.

Agents That Inhibit Vascular Endothelial Migration, Proliferation, and/or Survival

TNP-470 (AGM-1470)

TNP-470 (TAP Pharmaceuticals, Lake Forest, IL) is a potent analog of the antibiotic fumagillin and is currently in phase II clinical trials on various solid tumors. It inhibits endothelial migration, proliferation, and tube formation, as well as the growth and metastasis of numerous human xenografts and murine tumors. It has demonstrated little toxicity in patients and has been associated with partial responses such as disease stabilization or tumor flattening in some (18%) Kaposi sarcoma patients, disease stabilization of some cervical cancer (33%) patients, and decreased prostate-specific antigen level in 1 of 32 prostate cancer patients. Treatment with TNP-470 has been shown to be more effective at limiting the growth of micrometastases than limiting the growth of established primary tumors. The effect of TNP-470 as an antiangiogenic agent used in combination with other antiangiogenic agents, other chemotherapeutic agents, and ionizing radiation is also currently being investigated.

Thalidomide

Thalidomide (Celgene Corporation, Summit, NJ), originally prescribed as an oral sedative that produced stunted limb growth when used in the first 2 months of pregnancy, has been found to inhibit angiogenesis. When used in nonpregnant adults, it has been associated with few side effects. It is currently being used routinely to treat lepromatous leprosy and to inhibit the growth of solid tumors in preclinical and clinical trials (phase II). The specific mechanism by which thalidomide inhibits angiogenesis is currently unknown. As thalidomide blocks angiogenesis induced by both bFGF and VEGF, it may target multiple pathways. It has also been hypothesized that it may downregulate v3 integrin receptors. Thalidomide may also disrupt later-stage events in angiogenesis and has been shown to induce fenestrations in blood vessels of treated animals that are not observed in control animals. Although thalidomide has minimal antitumor effects when used alone, its apparent ability to increase efficacy of treatment in combined therapy (i.e., with Cytoxan, Adriamycin, or 5-FU) studies is intriguing.

Angiostatin and Endostatin

Angiostatin is a fragment of human plasminogen, and endostatin is a fragment of collagen XVIII that is 30 times more potent than angiostatin. Both agents have been shown to block endothelial proliferation, migration, and tube formation in vitro, and angiogenesis and metastasis in vivo. Concerns that angiostatin therapy may require high dosages, repeated injections, and long-term therapy have made it less attractive for clinical trials.

A very different and much more optimistic potential for the use of angiostatin is its potential use in combination with external-beam radiation. Experimental data provide support for combining ionizing radiation with angiostatin to improve tumor eradication without increasing deleterious effects, suggesting that angiostatin may be most effective in clinical trials when used in combination therapy, rather than as primary therapy.

Endostatin is currently in phase I clinical studies of solid tumors. In studies in which the efficacy of endostatin has been compared with angiostatin, endostatin appeared more effective in inhibiting tumor growth at several stages of growth. However, the combination of endostatin with angiostatin has proven more effective than endostatin or angiostatin alone in preclinical studies.

Agents That Inhibit Degradation of Extracellular Matrix

For new vessels to develop, degradation of the basement membrane by proteolytic enzymes is necessary for tumor invasion, metastasis, growth, and angiogenesis. In addition, this degradation releases growth factors or inhibitors from the extracellular matrix (ECM). ECM proteolysis occurs by the activity of two types of proteolytic enzymes, plasmin and the matrix metalloproteinases (MMPs). Increased expression of MMPs has been linked to invasive behavior and metastatic potential, and increased expression of MMPs has been documented in numerous human cancers. Several inhibitors are now in advanced clinical trials and include marimastat (phase I/II/III) and AG3340 (phase II/III).

Marimastat

Marimastat is a second-generation, peptidomimetic MMP inhibitor with oral bioavailability developed from batimastat. Like batimastat, marimastat is relatively nonspecific, inhibiting the activity of MMP-1, -2, -3, -7, and -9. In preclinical studies, marimastat inhibited tumor metastasis. There were dose-limiting toxicities, including musculoskeletal side effects (severe inflammatory polyarthritis) in all the studies, particularly of the arms and hands. Despite some early discouraging results, a recent phase III clinical trial has shown a survival benefit for patients with metastatic gastric cancer treated with marimastat. The greatest benefit was observed in patients that had previously received chemotherapy (5-FU–based). In addition, a phase II clinical trial of glioblastoma patients showed a survival advantage for patients treated with marimastat and temozolomide combination therapy. These trials showed that MMP inhibitors can act synergistically with other chemotherapeutic and/or biological agents. In addition, a phase III clinical trial of pancreatic cancer patients showed that the effect of marimastat was comparable to that of the toxic chemotherapeutic agent gemcitabine. The results of these clinical trials are indeed very promising because they represent the first clear indication that antiangiogenic agents can offer a significant survival advantage in cancer patients. Furthermore, these trials only included patients with advanced disease (disseminated metastasis), not the ideal target population for these type of agents. Therefore, using these agents in patients with less advanced disease could yield potentially even better results.

AG3340

AG3340 (Agouron Pharmaceuticals, Inc., San Diego, CA) is a hydroxaminic acid derivative MMP inhibitor based on MMP X-ray crystallography. AG3340 potently inhibits MMP-2, -9, -3, -13, and -14. AG3340 decreases tumor angiogenesis and has significant antimetastatic and antitumor activity. The large magnitude of inhibition by AG3340 is in contrast to the modest inhibition by other MMP inhibitors. Combination therapy of MMP inhibition with cytotoxic chemotherapy may prove more effective than either modality used alone. This agent is currently in phase II/III studies, including combination studies with Taxol and carboplatin.

Agents That Inhibit Integrin Activation

Integrins are heterodimeric transmembrane proteins responsible not only for cell-extracellular matrix adhesion, but also for the regulation of entry into and withdrawal from the cell cycle. Appropriate integrin activation on endothelial cells is required for maturation of angiogenic vessels because blockade of certain integrins during angiogenesis may result in apoptosis of endothelial cells on newly formed vascular sprouts with decreased angiogenesis. One of these integrins, the v3 receptor, is able to bind numerous extracellular matrix proteins via an arg-gly-asp (RGD) sequence. Intense research has been focused on this receptor because it is expressed only at low levels on quiescent vascular, intestinal, and uterine smooth muscle cells but is highly activated on cytokine-stimulated endothelial cells and smooth muscle cells, particularly those on newly formed vessels around tumors. Experimental data show that this receptor plays a significant role in tumor angiogenesis and tumor progression.

Vitaxin (IXSYS, Inc., Lajolla, CA), the humanized form of the MAb v3 inhibitor LM609, is now in phase II clinical trials in cancer patients. Vitaxin induced either stable disease or tumor shrinkage in 8 of 14 patients with no apparent toxicity at all dose levels.

In addition to the MAb LM609, cyclic RGD peptides have been developed that specifically inhibit the v3 receptor, including EMD121974 (Merck & Co., Inc., Whitehouse Station, NJ), a cyclic pentapeptide currently in phase I trials. Such small cyclic peptides are easily synthesized, are resistant to proteolysis, and have only weak immunogenicity. Cyclic RGD peptides synergize with antibody-cytokine fusion proteins to eradicate primary tumors and metastasis in syngeneic mouse models. For this strategy, inflammatory cells that are activated and directed to the tumor microenvironment by tumor-specific antibody-IL-2 fusion proteins mediate the tumor cell-specific therapy. The antiangiogenic treatment may suppress micrometastases-induced neovascularization and thus preclude enlargement of metastatic foci. This would facilitate eradication of micrometastases by tumor-directed therapies, which are optimally effective in the minimal residual disease setting. The simultaneous targeting of the vascular and tumor compartments proved very effective in these models; it combined a decrease in tumor cell nourishment with the active destruction of tumor cells, leading to a regression of primary tumors and the eradication of distant metastases. The results suggest that combinations of specific antiangiogenic and tumor cell-targeted therapies may frequently synergize in regression of primary tumors and eradication of micrometastases.

ANTIANGIOGENIC AGENTS: CHEMOPREVENTION

The potential to block tumor growth in the early stages of tumor development by inhibiting neoangiogenic processes represents an intriguing approach to the treatment of cancer. The high proliferation rate in the tumor deprived of proper vascularization would be balanced by cell death due to lack of diffusion of nutrients and oxygen. Antiangiogenic agents can prevent the further growth of micrometastases. Increasing evidence indicates that the "angiogenic switch," defined as the point at which a tumor induces angiogenesis, occurs very early in tumorigenesis in both murine models and human tumors, and that early intervention can curtail tumor growth.

Cancer chemoprevention is the use of agents to slow or inhibit the progression of carcinogenesis with the aim of lowering the risk of developing invasive or clinically significant disease. Several agents shown to have chemopreventive activity in experimental test systems or clinical trials also show significant antiangiogenic activities. The antiangiogenic activity of many chemopreventive compounds, or "angioprevention," may actually be a common and critical effect for the inhibition of cancer by these agents through blocking or retarding the development of the tumor vasculature. Various substances proposed as possible cancer chemopreventive agents show antiangiogenic properties when tested in in vitro and in vivo angiogenesis models. We briefly review several diverse chemically unrelated chemopreventive agents that apparently share common mechanisms to exert antiangiogenic activity.

Thiols

Modulation of extracellular and intracellular thiols is being investigated as a promising strategy in cancer prevention. In preclinical studies, *N*-acetyl-L-cysteine (NAC), a free oxygen radical scavenger that also inhibits COX-2 expression and COX-1-mediated activation of carcinogens, has been shown to inhibit initial tumor take, tumor cell invasion in vitro, and metastasis formation in vivo. NAC is able to cause inhibition of secreted MMP-2 and MMP-9, the type IV collagenases typically overexpressed by tumors, and activated endothelial cells involved in invasion and angiogenesis. NAC could also affect angiogenesis by modulating VEGF expression by tumor cells.

Polyphenolic Compounds

Flavonoids are the most abundant polyphenols in our diet. They are natural estrogenic compounds derived from soybeans, tea, fruits, and vegetables that have been proposed to act as chemopreventive agents. The isoflavone genistein, a polyphenol found in soy products, is a potent inhibitor of tyrosine kinases and, along with flavonoids such as kaempferol and apigenin, is an inhibitor of topoisomerases I and II, enzymes crucial to cellular proliferation. Genistein has been shown to inhibit tumor cell invasion through inhibition of MMP-9 expression in in vitro and in vivo models of breast cancer progression. In addition, it has also been shown to inhibit angiogenesis by decreasing vessel density and levels of VEGF and TGF-β1. The beneficial effects of green tea and its active components have been abundantly documented in the literature, and include cancer chemoprevention; inhibition of tumor cell growth, invasion, and metastasis; and antiviral and anti-inflammatory activities. Green tea contains numerous polyphenols, most of which are flavonols commonly known as catechins. Epigallocatechin-3-gallate (EGCG), the main flavonol found in green tea extracts, appears to act as a direct inhibitor of MMP-2 and, with slightly lower efficacy, of MMP-9. A recent study demonstrated that this compound also inhibits in vivo growth and angiogenesis of tumors derived by the colon carcinoma HT29 cell line by blocking the induction of VEGF.

NSAIDs

NSAIDs are effective colon cancer chemopreventive agents that might also be useful in preventing other types of cancer. Recent reports indicate that NSAIDs inhibit tube formation by endothelial cells in in vitro models of angiogenesis. The antiangiogenic effect of the selective COX-2 inhibitor celecoxib has been demonstrated in a rat model of angiogenesis. Inhibition of angiogenesis by NSAIDs apparently follows more than one pathway, prostaglandin dependent and independent. Early angiogenic stimuli also use the MAP kinase pathway, which in turn can lead to activation of nitric oxide synthase (NOS). Although the inhibitory effects of NO on tumorigenesis have been associated with an antiangiogenic effect, the importance of the different isoforms of NOS for tumor vascularization is not yet clear. Many angiogenic molecules also stimulate NOS activity; endothelial NOS has been shown to play an essential role in VEGF-induced angiogenesis.

PPARγ Ligands

A member of the steroid hormone receptor superfamily, PPARγ, is activated by eicosanoids, including the natural ligand 15-deoxy-delta12, 14-prostaglandin J2 (15D-PGJ2), a prostanoid derived from the cyclooxygenase product PGD2, and by antidiabetic agents such as thiazolidinediones. PPARγ is a key transcription factor involved in adipogenesis and monocyte differentiation. The role of PPARs in cancer chemoprevention has recently been reviewed. PPARγ, activated by 15D-PGJ2 or by new antidiabetic agents (BRL49653 and ciglitazone), showed a potent antiangiogenic activity by inhibiting differentiation of HUVEC cells into tubelike structures in a tridimensional collagen matrix. In addition, 15D-PGJ2 and cyclopentenone prostaglandins have been shown to inhibit the NF-κB–dependent transcription of target genes, including COX-2, by directly blocking IκB kinase in a PPARγ-independent manner. Again, blockade of NF-κB signaling inhibits angiogenesis of ovarian cancer by suppressing the expression of VEGF and IL-8. Because the NF-κB signaling pathway appears to be a key regulatory pathway in inflammation and angiogenesis, this novel mechanism could enhance the antiangiogenic activity of COX-2 inhibitors.

Protease Inhibitors

Because an altered equilibrium of the protease/protease inhibitor activity ratio is at the base of tumor invasion and extravasation and is associated with other diseases characterized by excessive angiogenesis, an increasing number of selective protease inhibitors, including synthetic MMP inhibitors, are currently under clinical investigation.

Experimental evidence suggests that MMP-7 (matrilysin) plays an essential role in much earlier stages of intestinal tumorigenesis. Matrilysin is detected in a high percentage of preinvasive lesions, in contrast to its absence in most normal tissues, and is expressed by the epithelial-derived tumor cells. Manipulating levels of this enzyme in vitro results in cell lines with enhanced tumorigenic potential, while ablating the gene in vivo leads to a significant reduction in tumor number in two different animal models of intestinal tumorigenesis. In addition, regulation of matrilysin gene expression appears to be under the control of genetic pathways that are activated early in the tumor development sequence. Although the precise mechanism by which matrilysin activity contributes to tumor formation is not yet clear, it has been proposed that MMP inhibitors may be of benefit as chemopreventive agents, in addition to their therapeutic potential for metastatic disease.

Protease inhibitors with potential use in angiogenesis/tumor chemoprevention include the free oxygen radical scavenger *N*-acetyl-L-cysteine and flavonoids, such as EGCG. *N*-acetyl-L-cysteine is able to reduce the invasive and metastatic potential of melanoma cells and to inhibit endothelial cell invasion by direct inhibition of MMP activity. EGCG, a flavonoid from green tea that possesses chemopreventive activity in experimental and epidemiologic studies, is a potent inhibitor of MMP-2 and MMP-9.

Miscellaneous

Other chemopreventive agents not mentioned in this chapter, including natural or synthetic retinoids, steroid hormone antagonists, peroxisome proliferator-activated receptor, and vitamin D, might also have antiangiogenesis as an important mechanism of action, a novel concept termed "angioprevention." The "angiogenic" switch is an early event in carcinogenesis, making angioprevention an optimal target for cancer prevention.

ANTIANGIOGENIC AGENTS: TRIALS AND TRIBULATIONS

Presently, a multitude of clinical trials exist that test the efficacy of antiangiogenic agents (Tables 22.1 and 22.2). Most of these agents are in phase I or II trials. At least 12 antiangiogenic agents have entered or completed phase III trials. The growing interest in the use of antiangiogenic agents in the treatment of cancer lies in the theoretical advantages of this molecularly targeted modality of chemotherapy. Delivery of antiangiogenic agents is not complicated by having to penetrate large bulky masses but, instead, have easy access to tumoral endothelial cells. Antiangiogenic drugs may not cause cytopenias and thus will avoid many of the unwarranted toxicities of standard chemotherapeutic agents. Because they act directly on nascent endothelial cells, antiangiogenic agents may avoid tumor resistance mechanisms. If antiangiogenic agents are successful, they might be applicable to many tumor types and not be dependent on cell type or growth fraction of cells within a tumor. However, there remain several important obstacles with regard to using antiangiogenic drugs in clinical trials with which we must contend in order to accurately determine the efficacy of these agents.

Dosage

Because these agents do not result in the usual toxicities seen with chemotherapy agents (i.e., bone marrow or gastrointestinal tract), the appropriate dose that confers optimal antiangiogenic activity may be difficult to determine. A dose-limiting toxicity may not be reached with these agents. It is likely that the optimal biological dose is not the maximally tolerated dose. The best way to determine appropriate biological doses is to have reliable biological correlates. Because these have yet to be optimally discerned, the dosing problem remains a challenge. Many clinical trials have been discontinued because tumors have not decreased in size by radiologic measurements. However, this approach may not be accurate because many of these agents induce disease stabilization. There is also evidence in preclinical studies with angiostatin and endostatin that the onset of the antiangiogenic effect may take days to weeks. It may be reasonable to continue therapy for months unless a biological correlate demonstrates that the drug has no antiangiogenic activity in vivo before this time period.

Scheduling of Drugs

Because antiangiogenic therapy is considered to be long-term, chronic therapy for suppression of primary tumor growth and metastases, the optimal scheduling of these drugs needs to be determined. However, many of these studies lack pharmacokinetic information. It is necessary to measure levels of the drug or its metabolites in the blood and to determine the best route and form of delivery based on chronic maintenance of effective therapeutic concentrations. This information may vary from patient to patient, as well as from one disease state to another. Therefore, more pharmacokinetic data of new antiangiogenic drugs from preclinical studies is necessary on entry to clinical trials. Design of phase I trials should include measurement of drug levels in the blood because it is so critical for these agents to maintain a consistent therapeutic drug level for chronic suppression of angiogenesis and tumor growth.

Biological End Points

The biological end points for antiangiogenic therapy remain controversial. Determining the antiangiogenic activity of inhibitors in patients is challenging, in part, because tumor tissue may not be easily available for immunohistochemical and gene expression studies. Some investigators are now studying endothelial cell shedding from tumor vasculature as a correlate for antiangiogenic activity of drugs. Methods are currently being developed to detect endothelial cells in the circulation of patients. Other methods to determine angiogenesis in vivo include imaging strategies to evaluate perfusion, angiography, sonography, and magnetic resonance visualization of tumor vasculature. The use of fluorodeoxyglucose and positron emission tomography imaging was used to monitor regional blood flow in tumors of patients participating in a recent phase I trial of endostatin. Evaluation of tumor-free progression, time to progression, and disease stabilization may be the best way to assess new inhibitors in clinical trial. Because most of these inhibitors may be blocking new angiogenic growth of tumors, regression of disease may be difficult to achieve. The goal of this type of treatment is to prevent any further growth of tumors.

Optimal Clinical Settings

How best to use antiangiogenic agents in cancer therapy is not known. Many phase I trials have entered patients with metastatic disease after failure of standard therapies. However, it may not be the best way to incorporate these drugs into clinical trials. To gain insight into the effectiveness of these agents on inhibition of angiogenesis in vivo, it may be best to incorporate them initially in patients who have been successfully treated and deemed free of disease (i.e., the adjuvant setting). The nature of the neovessels in advanced disease may be heterogeneous and more difficult to treat with antiangiogenic agents compared with microscopic or early-stage disease, where there may be a more uniform nascent vasculature. This approach may prevent a useful antiangiogenic drug from being prematurely discarded, especially if it does not show activity in advanced disease.

Combination Therapy

How to use these antiangiogenic agents with other modalities or other biological agents has not been determined. Because some chemotherapeutic drugs have antiangiogenic activity, perhaps there may be synergistic antitumor effects. With regard to combining angiogenesis inhibitors with radiation, perhaps they may work as radiation sensitizers. In mouse models, Paris et al. showed that microvascular endothelial cells are a primary target of radiation damage. There is also evidence that radiation therapy delivered to tumors in mice can be enhanced if mice are treated with angiostatin. Therefore, angiogenesis inhibitors could be used for enhancing the local effects of radiotherapy and perhaps leading to lower regional recurrence rates. The use of antiangiogenic agents can also be envisioned in combination therapies with biological agents that have already been approved for cancer.

Individualized Therapies

It has been shown that early in tumor development, one or several angiogenic factors are secreted by a tumor. With further progress of the tumor, there are other angiogenic factors that are added. With this knowledge, it may be envisioned that antiangiogenic therapy could be customized, depending on the angiogenic profile of a patient's tumor and blood. Therefore, it may be that anti-VEGF monoclonal antibody could be effective in early stages, but that in advanced stages, it may be best to combine this antibody with a tyrosine kinase inhibitor that could interfere with signaling mediated by other growth factors. Genomic and proteomic arrays of tumor tissue could help identify various highly expressed angiogenic factors and lead to customized therapy.

FUTURE DIRECTIONS

Molecular Profiling: Treatment Tailored to the Individual Patient

The concept of employing tumor characteristics, such as histologic features, to predict the best treatment for an individual patient has long been part of the practice of oncology. A significant refinement of this histology-based approach to selection of treatment has been the application of molecular markers, an approach best exemplified in the use of markers in the treatment of human leukemias. For solid tumors, the development of tumor markers for the prediction of therapeutic response has generally been much slower. However, the *HER2/neu* gene is an impressive positive example of a tumor marker useful in solid tumors. The *HER2/neu* gene encodes a 185-kD protein belonging to the transmembrane type I tyrosine kinase receptor family, which also includes the EGF receptor, HER3, and HER4. Clinical studies demonstrated that HER2 amplification or overexpression is a marker of poor prognosis for patients with lymph node-positive breast cancer. A major question, however, has been whether this poor prognosis is irrevocable or can be bypassed by some intervention. In 1994, the Cancer and Leukemia Group B (CALGB) demonstrated that the poor clinical outcome of patients with lymph node-positive breast cancer with HER2 overexpression can be overcome by adequate dose-intensive regimens of cyclophosphamide, doxorubicin, and 5-FU. The HER2-negative group, however, experienced no benefit from the dose escalation. These data raised the possibility that the adverse effects of HER2 overexpression can be specifically overcome by effective doses of doxorubicin. The most definitive test of the HER2–doxorubicin interaction was seen in two studies: the reanalysis of the National Surgical Adjuvant Breast and Bowel Project trial B-11, and the 10-year follow-up of the analysis of the complete cohort in CALGB trial 8541. Important in the analysis was that the HER2 determination was rigorously validated through concurrent analysis by immunohistochemistry, differential polymerase chain reaction (PCR), and fluorescent in situ hybridization. Patients with HER2-positive tumors responded with improved overall survival when treated with dose-intensive cyclophosphamide, doxorubicin, and 5-FU chemotherapy, whereas HER2-negative patients showed no benefit with dose escalation. Although the mechanism of this interaction and putative resistance is unclear, there is evidence that inhibition of HER2 signaling is associated with a decreased ability of the cell to repair DNA damage such as is seen after exposure to chemotherapy.

HER2 is an example of how the molecular profile of a cancer may allow prediction of its response to standard chemotherapeutic agents. In most cases, the mechanism for oncogene-associated relative resistance or sensitivity of a tumor to chemotherapy is uncertain. However, many markers may themselves be suitable targets for molecularly based therapeutics. Given the surface location of HER2 on cells and the overexpression that occurs mainly in cancerous states, the HER2 oncoprotein represented one such attractive target for Ab-directed therapies. One such Ab, 4D5, suppressed cancer cell growth in both in vitro and in vivo animal studies. When coupled with standard chemotherapeutic agents, 4D5 showed additive and potentially synergistic antiproliferative effects. The humanized form of the murine 4D5 Ab (Herceptin) was developed for clinical applications. Based on a phase II clinical trial that showed improvement in response rates in patients receiving Herceptin, a phase III study was conducted in which individuals with metastatic breast cancer were randomly assigned to chemotherapy alone or chemotherapy plus weekly Herceptin. The results showed that patients treated with chemotherapy and Herceptin exhibited an improvement in all measures: response rate (49% vs. 32% with chemotherapy alone), median duration of response (9.3 vs. 5.9 months with chemotherapy alone), and time to progression (7.6 months vs. 4.6 months with chemotherapy alone). Thus, as predicted in the in vitro investigations, the combination of chemotherapy and Herceptin led to a more favorable outcome.

Because oncogenes are signaling molecules that rely on protein–protein interactions to conduct their signals, interruption of these interactions was predicted to disrupt critical pathways that maintain the cancerous state. Inhibition of the enzymatic activity of certain oncogenes, such as the genes encoding ras proteins and kinases, with small chemically derived molecules has been both an attractive and ultimately successful approach. Some of the most notable clinical successes have been in the treatment of leukemias. There is currently a rich developmental pipeline for these kinase inhibitors, with many potential agents being tested (or soon to be ready for testing) in the clinical setting. The targets include the ras proteins PDGF and EGF and the VEGF receptors. The number and diversity of targets make molecular profiling a necessary adjunct to therapeutic decision making. Thus, a comprehensive approach for target detection will no longer remain solely of academic interest but is predicted to become a clinical necessity.

Postgenome Challenge for Molecular Medicine

The recently completed sequencing of the entire human genome will have incalculable effects on science and society. The data on gene expression and putative gene functions inferred from sequence similarities and motif analysis will provide a powerful means of assessing the transcriptional activity of the genome in the cells and tissue before, during, and after the development of disease. However, completion of the human genome sequence is just the beginning. The current challenge is to generate a comprehensive understanding of the software and the hardware of the cell and the organism. Less than 2% of the noninfectious human disease burden is monogenic in nature. The rest (98%) is polygenic (caused by multiple genes at once) or epigenic (caused by nongenetic or postgenetic alterations in cellular molecules). Consequently, fully elucidating the causal mechanisms driving carcinogenesis and cancer progression will require analysis tools ranging from direct DNA sequencing, to mRNA expression monitoring, to protein sequencing and protein localization studies, to metabolic or physiological profiling.

A further essential phase will be a description of the normal range of human polymorphisms (base variations in the genome), which may provide a starting point for correlating genetic variance with disease states. The final physiological state is further complicated because biological diversity causally associated with disease may be due to posttranslational processes regulated by the cellular environment. These changes cannot be inferred from known DNA variance. Thus, a complete understanding of the molecular basis of cancer will depend on a multidisciplinary approach combining genetics, pathology, protein structure and function analysis, cell biology, and clinical medicine.

Finding the expressed human genes is a different task from sequencing the genome itself. This is because the actual expressed genes and their regulatory elements comprise only a small proportion of the genome. The number of expressed human genes may be 100,000. However, at any point in time, for any individual cell in any given tissue, the number of genes in use may be as few as 10,000. Of this 10,000, only a proportion may be susceptible to the influence of carcinogenic events. Thus, an important goal for molecular profiling of cancer is to identify a subset of expressed genes that is correlated with or causally related to the development and progression of cancer. Setting aside hereditary susceptibility, it is likely that the majority of cancers originate in tissue that starts with a completely normal genome and that carcinogenic events produce heritable genetic alterations that expand in microscopic premalignant states, such as hyperplasia and dysplasia, before frank malignant cancer ensues. Identification of the important genetic derangements and the causally important genes and proteins will depend on direct analysis of actual human cancer tissues, combined with insights gained using animal and cell culture methods. The massive profiling of genes associated with cancer progression is now possible using new technology for microdissection and array hybridization.

In response to this challenge, investigators in both the public and the private sectors have been perfecting complementary DNA (cDNA) arrays (so-called gene chips) that can be used to survey patterns of gene expression. Changes in the pattern can then be correlated with histomorphology, clinical behavior, or response to treatment. Typically, the cDNA arrays take the form of rows and rows of oligonucleotide strands lined up in dots on a miniature silicon chip, glass slide, or sheet of nitrocellulose. The microarrays work as follows. First, the RNA is extracted from the tumor tissue, amplified, and labeled with a fluorescent or radioactive probe. This of course assumes that the highly labile RNA is preserved when the tissue is extracted. The labeled total RNA, containing the mRNA of the expressed genes, is applied to the surface of the chip or sheet. After appropriate hybridization, the relative intensity of the signal for each spot on the chip corresponds to the abundance of its matching mRNA species and hence reflects the expression level for its gene. With appropriate pattern recognition software, it is possible to assemble a global score for the gene study set represented on the substratum. Tremendous progress has been made in the use of cDNA arrays to analyze gene expression patterns in human cancer cell lines and human cancer tissue.

Once a putative marker (or set of markers) is identified by cDNA array analysis of cancer tissue samples, the next step is to validate these markers in a large population of human tumors. This exhaustive process has now been telescoped into a high-throughput miniaturized tissue array. The array consists of 1,000 cylindrical tissue biopsies, each from a different patient, all distributed on a single glass slide. Tumor arrays are ideal for comparing large numbers of solid tumor samples. Full automation of tumor array creation and screening is envisioned as a means to expeditiously correlate marker levels over large study sets of tumors.

Molecular analysis of pure cell populations in their native tissue environment will be an important component of the next generation of medical genetics. Accomplishing this goal is much more difficult than just grinding up a piece of tissue and applying the extracted molecules to a panel of assays. This is because tissues are complicated three-dimensional structures composed of large numbers of different types of interacting cell populations. The cell subpopulation of interest may constitute a tiny fraction of the total tissue volume—for example, one goal may be to analyze the genetic changes in the premalignant cells or malignant cells, but these subpopulations are frequently located in microscopic regions occupying less than 5% of the tissue volume. Culturing cell populations from fresh tissue is one means of reducing contamination. However, cultured cells may not accurately represent the molecular events taking place in the actual tissue from which they were derived. Assuming the tissue cells of interest can be successfully isolated and grown in culture, the gene expression pattern of the cultured cells will be influenced by the culture environment and may be quite different from the gene expression pattern in the native tissue state. This is because the cultured cells are separated from the tissue elements that regulate gene expression, such as soluble factors, extracellular matrix molecules, and cell–cell communication. Thus, the problem of cellular heterogeneity has been a significant barrier to the molecular analysis of normal and diseased tissue. This problem can now be overcome by new developments in the field of tissue microdissection. Laser-capture microdissection (LCM) has been developed to provide scientists with a fast and dependable method of capturing and preserving specific cells from tissue, under direct microscopic visualization. With the ease of procuring a homogeneous population of cells from a complex tissue using LCM, the approaches to molecular analysis of pathological processes are significantly enhanced. The mRNA from microdissected tumors has been used as the starting material to produce cDNA libraries, microarrays, differential display, and other techniques used to find new genes or mutations. The development of LCM allows investigators to determine specific gene expression patterns from tissues of individual patients. Pure populations of cells can be obtained, and RNA can be extracted, copied to cDNA, and hybridized to thousands of genes on a cDNA microarray. In this manner, an individualized molecular profile can be obtained for each histologically identified pathological subtype. Using such multiplex analysis, investigators will be able to correlate the pattern of expressed genes with etiology, premalignant progression, and response to treatment. A patient's risk for disease and appropriate choice of treatment could, in the future, be personalized based on the profile. A growing clinical database of such results could be used to develop a minimal subset of key markers that will lead to a revolutionary approach for early detection and accurate diagnosis of disease.

Beyond Functional Genomics to Cancer Proteomics

Although DNA is an information archive, proteins do all the work of the cell. The existence of a given DNA sequence does not guarantee the synthesis of a corresponding protein. The DNA sequence is also not sufficient to describe protein structure, function, and cellular location. This is because protein complexity and versatility stems from context-dependent posttranslational processes such as phosphorylation, sulfation, and glycosylation. Moreover, the DNA code does not provide information about how proteins link together into networks and functional machines in the cell. In fact, the activation of a protein signal pathway causing a cell to migrate, die, or initiate division can occur immediately, before any changes occur in DNA/RNA gene expression. Consequently, the technology to drive the molecular medicine revolution into the third phase is emerging from protein analytical methods. An important goal will be to apply this knowledge at the level of human tissue itself.

The term *proteome* denotes the proteins expressed by a genome. Proteomics is proclaimed as the next step after genomics. A goal of investigators in this exciting field is to assemble a complete library of all human proteins. Only a small percentage of the proteome has been catalogued in 2002. Because PCR for proteins does not exist, sequencing the order of the up to 20 possible amino acids in a given protein remains relatively slow and labor-intensive work compared with nucleotide sequencing. Although a number of new technologies are being introduced for high-throughput protein characterization and discovery, the mainstay of protein identification continues to be two-dimensional gel electrophoresis. When a mixture of proteins is applied to the two-dimensional gel, individual proteins in the mixture are separated out into signature locations on the display, depending on their individual size and charge. Each signature is a spot on the gel that can constitute a unique single-protein species. The protein spot can be procured from the gel, and a partial amino acid sequence can be read. In this manner, known proteins can be monitored for changes in abundance with treatment, or new proteins can be identified. An experimental two-dimensional gel image can be captured and overlaid digitally with known archived two-dimensional gels. In this way, it is possible to immediately highlight proteins that are differentially abundant in one state versus another (e.g., tumor vs. normal or before and after hormone treatment). The use of LCM in combination with proteomics allows for studying protein expression of specific subpopulations of cells within a tumor. This approach allows for studying these cells in their normal microenvironment and avoids the problems of tissue heterogeneity and contamination.

Using a protein biochip that classified protein populations into molecular weight classes, Paweletz et al. showed distinct protein patterns of normal, premalignant, and malignant cancer cells microdissected from human tissue. Furthermore, they reported that different histologic types of cancer and normal tissue (ovarian, esophageal, prostate, breast, and hepatic) exhibited distinct protein profiles. Such a means to rapidly display a pattern of expressed proteins from microscopic tissue cellular populations will potentially be an important enabling technology for pharmacoproteomics, molecular pathology, and drug intervention. Proteomic array technologies of the future will be used to rapidly generate displays of signal pathway profiles. Investigators will be able to assess the status of defined pathways that control mitogenesis, apoptosis, survival, and a host of other physiological states. The information flow through these circuits, separately or through cross-talk, may dictate clinical behavior and susceptibility to therapy.

CONCLUSION

Biological cancer therapies hold enormous promise; many different forms of biological therapy, from cytokines to vaccines, have been shown to induce tumor regression in many human clinical trials. Although the response rates are not high, they are encouraging because the best results in trials in animals have been in small-volume disease and prevention, not in the treatment of established large cancers. Because most biological therapies rely on the induction of host immune responses, patients with end-stage, bulky disease and poor nutritional status may not respond optimally. Therefore, most biological modalities may not have been adequately tested clinically to date. Furthermore, more specific and possibly more potent therapies are just now entering clinical trials. Advances in biotechnology offer the promise of even more sophisticated therapeutics. The next generation of biological therapies will most likely consist of multimodality biological treatments targeting both humoral and cellular immunity against multiple tumor antigens.

Angiogenesis plays a crucial role in tumor development and tumor progression. Therapies targeting tumor angiogenesis are rapidly emerging and hold great promise. These tumor-directed therapies target endothelial cells, a more phenotypically stable target than rapidly mutating tumor cells. Toxicity profiles are more favorable than standard chemotherapeutic regimens. Moreover, antiangiogenic therapy shows great potential in combination with chemotherapy and radiation therapy. Antiangiogenic therapy, however, has not provided the "magic bullet" for cancer treatment that many have predicted it would be. Issues about trial design, scheduling and mode of delivery of drugs, proper biological end points, and adequate surrogate markers for efficacy of therapy, among others, need to be further delineated. Clearly, more work is necessary to further advance this field and tap into its enormous potential.

RECOMMENDED READING

Boehm T, Folkman J, Browder T, O'Reilly MS. Antiangiogenic therapy of experimental cancer does not induce acquired drug resistance. *Nature* 1997;390: 404–407.

Bramhall SR, Rosemurgy A, Brown PD, et al. Marimastat as first-line therapy for patients with unresectable pancreatic cancer: a randomized trial. *J Clin Oncol* 2001;19:3447–3455.

Bramhall SR, Schulz J, Nemunaitis J, et al. A double-blind placebo-controlled, randomised study comparing gemcitabine and marimastat with gemcitabine and placebo as first line therapy in patients with advanced pancreatic cancer. *Br J Cancer* 2002;87: 161–167.

Browder T, Butterfield CE, Kraling BM, et al. Antiangiogenic scheduling of chemotherapy improves efficacy against experimental drug-resistant cancer. *Cancer Res* 2000;60: 1878–1886.

Chung AS, Yoon SO, Park SJ, Yun CH. Roles of matrix metalloproteinases in tumor metastasis and angiogenesis. *J Biochem Mol Biol* 2003;36: 128–137.

Clark JI, Weiner LM. Biologic treatment of human cancer. *Curr Probl Cancer* 1995;19:185.

Clark JW. Biological response modifiers. *Cancer Chemother Biol Response Modif* 1996;16: 239.

DeVita VT, Hellman S, Rosenberg SA, eds. *Biologic Therapy of Cancer*. 2nd ed. Philadelphia, Pa: Lippincott; 1995.

Eatock MM, Schatzlein A, Kaye SB. Tumour vasculature as a target for anticancer therapy. *Cancer Treat Rev* 2000;26:191–204.

Eberhard A, Kahlert S, Goede V, et al. Heterogeneity of angiogenesis and blood vessel maturation in human tumors: implications for antiangiogenic tumor therapies. *Cancer Res* 2000;60:1388–1393.

Fidler IJ, Ellis LM. The implications of angiogenesis to the biology and therapy of cancer metastasis. *Cell* 1994;79:185.

Folkman J. Angiogenesis in cancer, vascular, rheumatoid and other disease. *Nat Med* 1995;1:27.

Folkman J. Anti-angiogenesis: new concept for therapy of solid tumors. *Ann Surg* 1972;175: 409–416.

Folkman J. Incipient angiogenesis. *J Natl Cancer Inst* 2000;92:94–95.

Folkman J. Tumor angiogenesis: therapeutic implications. *N Engl J Med* 1971;285:1182–1186.

Gasparini G. The rationale and future potential of angiogenesis inhibitors in neoplasia. *Drugs* 1999;58:17–38.

Gradishar WJ. An overview of clinical trials involving inhibitors of angiogenesis and their mechanism of action. *Invest New Drugs* 1997;15:49–59.

Groves MD, Puduvalli VK, Hess KR, et al. Phase II trial of temozolomide plus the matrix metalloproteinase inhibitor, marimastat, in recurrent and progressive glioblastoma multiforme. *J Clin Oncol* 2002;20:1383–1388.

Hanahan D, Folkman J. Patterns and emerging mechanisms of the angiogenic switch during tumorigenesis. *Cell* 1996;86:353–364.

Harris SR, Thorgeirsson UP. Tumor angiogenesis: biology and therapeutic prospects. *In Vivo* 1998;12:563–570.

Kakeji Y, Teicher BA. Preclinical studies of the combination of angiogenic inhibitors with cytotoxic agents. *Invest New Drugs* 1997;15:39–48.

Kerbel R, Folkman J. Clinical translation of angiogenesis inhibitors. *Nat Rev Cancer* 2002;2:727–739.

Kerbel RS. Clinical trials of antiangiogenic drugs: opportunities, problems, and assessment of initial results. *J Clin Oncol* 2001;19:45S-51S.

Kerbel RS. Inhibition of tumor angiogenesis as a strategy to circumvent acquired resistance to anti-cancer therapeutic agents. *Bioessays* 1991;13:31–36.

Kerbel RS. Tumor angiogenesis: past, present and the near future. *Carcinogenesis* 2000;21:505–515.

Kerbel RS, Viloria-Petit A, Okada F, Rak J. Establishing a link between oncogenes and tumor angiogenesis. *Mol Med* 1998;4:286–295.

Keshet E, Ben-Sasson SA. Anticancer drug targets: approaching angiogenesis. *J Clin Invest* 1999;104:1497–1501.

Kleiner DE, Stetler-Stevenson WG. Matrix metalloproteinases and metastasis. *Cancer Chemother Pharmacol* 1999;43(suppl): S42–S51.

Klohs WD, Hamby JM. Antiangiogenic agents. *Curr Opin Biotechnol* 1999;10:544–549.

Li WW. Tumor angiogenesis: molecular pathology, therapeutic targeting, and imaging. *Acad Radiol* 2000;7:800–811.

Liotta LA, Steeg PS, Settler-Stevenson WG. Cancer metastasis and angiogenesis: an imbalance of positive and negative regulation. *Cell* 1991;64:327.

Molema G, Meijer DK, de Leij LF. Tumor vasculature targeted therapies: getting the players organized. *Biochem Pharmacol* 1998;55:1939–1945.

Stetler-Stevenson WG. Matrix metalloproteinases in angiogenesis: a moving target for therapeutic intervention. *J Clin Invest* 1999;103:1237–1241.

Stetler-Stevenson WG. The role of matrix metalloproteinases in tumor invasion, metastasis, and angiogenesis. *Surg Oncol Clin N Am* 2001;10:383–392.

Teicher BA, Sotomayor EA, Huang ZD. Antiangiogenic agents potentiate cytotoxic cancer therapies against primary and metastatic disease. *Cancer Res* 1992;52:6702–6704.

Tosetti F, Ferrari N, De Flora S, Albini A. Angioprevention: angiogenesis is a common and key target for cancer chemopreventive agents. *FASEB J* 2002;16: 2–14.

van Hinsbergh VW, Collen A, Koolwijk P. Angiogenesis and anti-angiogenesis: perspectives for the treatment of solid tumors. *Ann Oncol* 1999;10(suppl 4):60–63.

Wojtowicz-Praga SM, Dickson RB, Hawkins MJ. Matrix metalloproteinase inhibitors. *Invest New Drugs* 1997;15:61–75.

23

Pharmacotherapy of Cancer

Judy L. Chase and Chad M. Barnett

A basic understanding of cancer pharmacotherapy and related toxicities is mandatory for the full integration of the surgical oncologist into a multidisciplinary cancer care program. To intelligently discuss surgical options with patients, knowledge of the available treatment regimens and their potential for toxicity is essential.

This chapter includes a discussion of basic principles of chemotherapy, an overview of the mechanisms of drug action and drug resistance, a tabular listing of the drugs available and their common toxicities, and a tabular listing of approved biological agents used in oncology. Finally, a summary of cancer pain management and the treatment of chemotherapy-induced emesis (CIE) is included.

The reader should be aware that a complete discussion of cancer chemotherapy is beyond the scope of this brief overview. The drug and dosage regimens listed are representative examples only and do not constitute a listing of all available protocols. For specific prescribing information, the practitioner is advised to consult individual manufacturer package inserts or one of the referenced texts.

BASIC PRINCIPLES OF CHEMOTHERAPY

Cancer chemotherapeutic agents are the result of drug design and, largely, empiricism. Their use has developed based on an understanding of tumor growth characteristics, the cell cycle, drug mechanisms of action, and drug resistance. It is hoped that new techniques and advances in molecular biology will allow improvements in drug design to extend the possibility of complete chemotherapeutic response and possibly the cure of patients currently deemed beyond salvage.

Tumor Growth and Kinetics

Kinetic aspects of tumor growth have been well described. Two concepts that underscore our knowledge of the kinetics of tumor growth are Skipper's laws and Gompertzian growth. Skipper's laws apply to cells in the proliferating compartment of a tumor. First, the doubling time of proliferating cells is constant, creating a straight line on a semilog plot. Second, cell kill by a particular drug at a given dose is constant, irrespective of body burden. In most solid tumors, however, only a portion of cells within the tumor—the growth fraction—is proliferating at any given time. This partially accounts for the refractory nature of many solid tumors to chemotherapy.

Human tumors follow a pattern of Gompertzian, rather than straight line, growth. Gompertzian growth describes a cell population decreasing as a result of cell death and increasing because of proliferation. Also, cell subpopulations may have ceased to proliferate but have not died, further swaying the growth curve from a straight semilog plot. The normal Gompertzian growth curve is sigmoid in shape. Maximum tumor growth rate occurs at approximately 30% of maximum tumor volume, where nutrient and oxygen supply to the greatest number of tumor cells is optimized. This portion of the curve is also where drug efficacy against a particular tumor may best be estimated.

The cell cycle is an important fundamental concept to understand when designing chemotherapeutic agents and treatment regimens. The cell cycle is divided into five components. The resting or nonproliferating cell is in the G0 phase. Upon entering the active portion of the cycle following stimulation, DNA synthesis occurs during the S phase and is followed by the postsynthetic G2 phase. Mitosis occurs during the M phase, which precedes the postmitotic G1 phase.

The cell cycle becomes important in drug selection because cells in the growth fraction are more susceptible to certain agents. In a broad sense, antineoplastic agents may be classified on the basis of their activity in relation to the cell cycle. Most antimetabolites, etoposide, hydroxyurea, vinca alkaloids, and bleomycin are cell cycle-specific agents that are most effective against tumors with a high growth fraction. In contrast, alkylating agents, antineoplastic antibiotics, fluorouracil, floxuridine, and procarbazine exert their effect independent of the cell cycle, and generally show more activity against slow-growing tumors.

Drug Mechanisms and Therapeutics

Knowledge of the basic mechanisms of action of chemotherapeutic agents is critical in selecting drugs for an effective chemotherapy combination regimen, minimizing toxicity and drug interactions, and preventing emergence of drug-resistant clones. Agents may damage the DNA template by alkylation, cross-linking, double-strand cleavage by topoisomerase II, intercalation, and blockage of RNA synthesis. Spindle poisons may arrest mitosis. Antimetabolites block enzymes necessary for DNA synthesis. Hormonal agents and their antagonists may influence cellular signal transduction, and biological response modifiers may influence the host's immune response to the tumor alone or in the context of concomitantly administered drugs. Antibody-based therapeutics have revolutionized the care of some cancer patients, including those with colon cancer, breast cancer, and certain leukemias and lymphomas. These therapies explicitly target cancer cells based on structural and biological properties that differ from normal cells. They include unconjugated antibodies or antibodies that have toxic materials attached that can deliver radiation or immunotoxins directly to cancer cells. Unconjugated antibodies, such as rituximab and trastuzumab, exert their cytotoxicity by invoking immune responses against the targeted cells. Conjugated antibodies, such as Zevalin and Bexxar, deliver toxic compounds directly to tumor sites, thus resulting in cell death. In addition to antibody-based therapies, orally available small molecule targeted therapies have been created, such as imatinib mesylate, gefitinib, and erlotinib. Imatinib mesylate is a protein tyrosine kinase inhibitor of bcr/abl, an abnormality found in some patients with chronic myelogenous leukemia. Gefitinib and erlotinib are small molecule tyrosine kinase inhibitors that target the epidermal growth factor receptor.

Combination chemotherapy is frequently used in an effort to forestall the development of drug resistance to antineoplastic agents and to achieve synergism with reduced toxicity. The Goldie-Coldman hypothesis assumes that at the time of diagnosis, most tumors possess resistant clones. Multiple mechanisms of drug resistance develop during cancer progression. The most well studied of these involves the *mdr* gene, which codes for membrane-bound P-glycoprotein. P-glycoprotein serves as a channel through which cellular toxins (i.e., chemotherapeutic agents) may be excreted from the cell. Additional mechanisms of drug resistance are decreased drug transport into cells, reduction of drug activation, drug metabolism enhancement, development of alternative metabolic pathways, drug inhibition of enzyme targets overcome by gene amplification, and impairment of drug binding to a target. A single drug may be subject to one or more mechanisms.

Interestingly, normal human cells never develop drug resistance. As a result, several caveats of combination chemotherapy have emerged. Drugs shown to be active as single agents should be chosen, and drugs selected for combined use should have different mechanisms of action. Ideally, drugs with different dose-limiting toxicities should be administered together, although toxicity overlap may necessitate dose reduction, as with myelosuppression. Finally, drug combinations with similar patterns of resistance should be avoided.

Different patterns of chemotherapy administration are used in particular settings with specific goals. Induction chemotherapy is usually high dose and given in combination to induce complete remission. Consolidation is a repetition of an induction regimen in a complete responder to prolong remission or increase the cure rate. Chemotherapy given with an intent similar to that of consolidation but with higher doses than induction or with different agents at high doses is known as intensification. Maintenance regimens are low-dose, long-term protocols intended to delay tumor cell regrowth after complete remission. Induction, consolidation, intensification, and maintenance usually apply to hematologic malignancies but may also describe solid tumor regimens.

Neoadjuvant treatment in the preoperative or perioperative period is used more commonly with solid tumors, such as locally advanced breast carcinoma, soft-tissue sarcomas of the extremities, and, more recently, rectal carcinoma and squamous cell carcinoma of the head and neck. It is often given in combination with radiation therapy to improve survival, resectability, and organ preservation.

Palliative chemotherapy may be given to control symptoms or, if the toxicity profile is favorable, prolong life for incurable patients. Salvage chemotherapy involves the use of a potentially curative, high-dose protocol in patients failing or recurring after different standard treatment plans have been attempted.

Adjuvant chemotherapy is administered following curative surgery or radiation therapy as a short-course, high-dose regimen to destroy a low number of residual tumor cells. Several factors determine the effectiveness of adjuvant regimens, including tumor burden, drug dose and schedule, combination chemotherapy, and drug resistance. The drug(s) must be active locally against residual cells and distantly against clinically occult metastatic deposits. Extensive literature supports the use of adjuvant chemotherapy for breast, colon, rectal, and anal carcinomas and for ovarian germ cell tumors, osteosarcoma, and pediatric solid tumors. No definitive benefit has been reported yet for pancreatic, gastric, and testicular carcinomas or for cervical cancer and melanoma, although investigative adjuvant therapy protocols are ongoing and open for patient enrollment in these disease sites.

Most chemotherapeutic agents exhibit very steep dose–response profiles and have low therapeutic indices, making a high-dose, short-term administration desirable. This can be accomplished through regional dose intensification. One example is intraperitoneal chemotherapy for ovarian cancer with high risk of peritoneal recurrence or for primary tumors that manifest as intraperitoneal disease, such as pseudomyxoma peritonei and peritoneal mesothelioma. Another type of regional dose intensification is intra-arterial therapy, which requires regional tumor confinement and a unique tumor blood supply and is most commonly used in hepatic artery infusion for primary or metastatic liver tumors that are surgically unresectable. Intra-arterial chemotherapy has also been used for gliomas of the brain and some head and neck tumors. Isolated perfusion of a specific anatomical site, usually the extremities, is one more type of regional dose intensification that allows for the delivery of very high doses of chemotherapy to the involved site with little systemic toxicity; it is often combined with hyperthermia. The largest body of literature discusses its use in all stages of melanoma, although limb perfusion for extremity sarcoma has been reported.

CHEMOTHERAPEUTIC AGENTS

Fundamental knowledge of the drugs available for cancer treatment, their mechanisms of action, general dose ranges, dominant toxicities, and indications for use is important to the general surgeon caring for cancer patients. Table 23.1 lists the available agents and their mechanisms of action, doses, and toxicities. Table 23.2 lists the available biological agents, as well as their U.S. Food and Drug Administration (FDA) indications and dosages. Table 23.3 lists commonly used combination chemotherapeutic regimens.

MANAGEMENT OF CANCER PAIN

The vast majority of patients with advanced cancer, and as many as 60% of patients with any stage of disease, experience significant pain. However, cancer pain is frequently undertreated for a multitude of reasons and fears that are largely unfounded. Effective management of cancer pain is achieved best with a multidisciplinary approach, including pain specialists, oncologists, nurses, pharmacists, physiatrists, physical and occupational therapists, psychologists, psychiatrists, primary care physicians, social workers, clergy, and hospice caregivers. Open lines of communication are of paramount importance to the successful management of cancer pain.

(*Text continues on page 625.*)

Table 23.1. Cancer chemotherapeutic agents: Mechanisms, doses, and toxicities

Drug	Dose and Schedule	Toxicity
Alkylating agents		
Altretamine (hexamethylmelamine, Hexalen)	260 mg/m^2 PO in divided doses × 14–21 d	Nausea and vomiting, myelosuppression, paresthesias, CNS toxicity
Busulfan (Myleran)	4–8 mg PO daily	Myelosuppression, pulmonary fibrosis, aplastic anemia, skin hyperpigmentation
Carmustine (BCNU, BiCNU)	150–200 mg/m^2 IV every 6–8 wk	Delayed myelosuppression, nausea and vomiting, hepatotoxicity
Chlorambucil (Leukeran)	0.1–0.2 mg/kg/d PO × 3–6 wk (average 4–10 mg/d)	Myelosuppression, pulmonary fibrosis, hepatotoxicity
Carboplatin (Paraplatin)	300–360 mg/m^2 IV every 4 wk or Target area under the curve (AUC) of 4–6 mg/dL every 4 wk	Myelosuppression, nausea and vomiting, peripheral neuropathy, ototoxicity
Cisplatin (Platinol, Platinol-AQ)	40–120 mg/m^2 IV every 3–4 wk 20 mg/m^2/d IV × 5 d every 3–4 wk	Nephrotoxicity, nausea and vomiting, peripheral neuropathy, myelosuppression, ototoxicity
Cyclophosphamide (Cytoxan, Neosar)	40–50 mg/kg IV in divided doses over 2–5 d 1–5 mg/kg/d PO	Myelosuppression, hemorrhagic cystitis, immunosuppression, alopecia, stomatitis, SIADH

Dacarbazine (DTIC-Dome)	2.0–4.5 mg/kg/d IV × 10 d 250 $mg/m^2/d$ IV × 5 d (melanoma) 150 $mg/m^2/d$ IV × 5 d 375 mg/m^2 IV every 15 d (Hodgkin disease)	Myelosuppression, nausea and vomiting, flulike syndrome, hepatoxicity, alopecia, seizures
Ifosfamide (Ifex)	1.2 g/m^2 IV daily × 5 d every 3 wk	Myelosuppression, hemorrhagic cystitis, somnolence, confusion
Lomustine (CCNU, CeeNU)	130 mg/m^2 PO every 6 wk	Delayed myelosuppression, nausea and vomiting, hepatotoxicity, neurotoxicity, nephrotoxicity
Mechlorethamine (Nitrogen mustard, Mustargen)	0.4 mg/kg IV single dose or in divided doses of 0.1–0.2 mg/kg/d	Myelosuppression, nausea and vomiting, phlebitis, gonadal dysfunction
Melphalan (Alkeran)	2–6 mg PO daily × 14–21 d 10 mg PO daily × 7–10 d 16 mg/m^2 IV every 2 wk	Myelosuppression, stomatitis, nausea and vomiting, gonadal dysfunction
Procarbazine (Matulane)	1–6 mg/kg/d PO daily 100 $mg/m^2/d$ PO × 14 d	Myelosuppression, nausea and vomiting, lethargy, depression, paresthesias, headache, flulike syndrome
Streptozocin (Zanosar)	500 $mg/m^2/d$ IV × 5 d 1,000–1,500 mg/m^2 IV weekly	Renal toxicity, nausea and vomiting, diarrhea, altered glucose metabolism, liver dysfunction
Thiotepa (Thioplex)	0.3–0.4 mg/kg IV every 1–4 wk	Myelosuppression, nausea and vomiting, mucositis, skin rashes
Antimetabolites		
Azacitidine (Vidaza)	75–100 mg/m^2 SC × 7 d every 4 wk	Nausea and vomiting, myelosuppression, pyrexia, diarrhea, constipation, fatigue, ecchymosis

(*continued*)

Table 23.1. (*Continued*)

Drug	Dose and Schedule	Toxicity
Capecitabine (Xeloda)	2,000–2,500 mg/m^2/d PO × 14 d every 21 d	Diarrhea, stomatitis, nausea and vomiting, hand-foot syndrome, myelosuppression
Cladribine (Leustatin)	0.09–0.1 mg/kg/d IV continuous infusion × 7 d every 4 wk	Myelosuppression, fever, rash
Clofarabine (Clolar)	52 mg/m^2 IV × 5 d every 2–6 wk	Nausea and vomiting, diarrhea, myelosuppression, pruritis, rigors, dermatitis, abdominal pain, infection
Cytarabine (Ara-C, Cytosar, DepoCyt)	100–200 mg/m^2/d IV infusion × 5–7 d 3 g/m^2 IV every 12 h × 4–12 doses	Myelosuppression, nausea and vomiting, diarrhea, hepatotoxicity, fever, conjunctivitis, CNS toxicity
Fludarabine (Fludara)	25 mg/m^2/d IV × 5 d every 4 wk	Myelosuppression, nausea and vomiting, fever, malaise, pulmonary infiltrates
Floxuridine (FUDR)	0.1–0.6 mg/kg/d × 5–14 d continuous arterial infusion	Hepatotoxicity, gastritis, nausea and vomiting, diarrhea
5-Fluorouracil (5-FU, Adrucil)	300–500 mg/m^2/d IV × 3–5 d 10–15 mg/kg IV weekly 200–300 mg/m^2/d IV continuous infusion	Stomatitis, myelosuppression, diarrhea, nausea and vomiting, cerebellar ataxia
Gemcitabine (Gemzar)	1,000–1,250 mg/m^2 IV weekly	Myelosuppression, fever, flulike syndrome, rash, mild nausea and vomiting
Hydroxyurea (Hydrea)	80 mg/kg PO every 3 d 20–30 mg/kg PO daily	Myelosuppression, nausea and vomiting, rash

6-Mercaptopurine (6-MP, Purinethol)	1.5–2.5 mg/kg/d PO (average 100–200 mg/d)	Myelosuppression, nausea and vomiting, anorexia, diarrhea, hepatotoxicity
Methotrexate (MTX, Mexate, Rheumatrex)	2.5–5.0 mg PO daily (low dose) 50 mg/m^2 IV every 2–3 wk (low dose) 1–12 g/m^2 IV every 1–3 wk (high dose) 5–10 mg/m^2 (max 15 mg) intrathecal every 3–7 d	Mucositis, myelosuppression, pulmonary fibrosis, hepatotoxicity, nephrotoxicity, diarrhea, skin erythema
Pemetrexed (Alimta)	500–600 mg/m^2 IV every 21 d	Myelosuppression, fatigue, nausea and vomiting, diarrhea, rash, infection
Pentostatin (Nipent)	4 mg/m^2 IV every other wk	Nephrotoxicity, CNS depression, myelosuppression, nausea and vomiting, conjunctivitis
6-Thioguanine (6-TG, Tabloid)	2 mg/kg PO daily	Myelosuppression, hepatotoxicity, stomatitis
Natural products		
Antitumor antibiotics		
Bleomycin (Blenoxane)	10–20 U/m^2 IV, IM, or SC once–twice weekly	Pneumonitis, pulmonary fibrosis, fever, hypersensitivity, hyperpigmentation, alopecia
Dactinomycin (Actinomycin D, Cosmegen)	0.5 mg/day IV × 5 d max 0.012–0.015 mg/kg/d IV × 5 d max (children)	Stomatitis, myelosuppression, anorexia, nausea and vomiting, diarrhea, alopecia
Daunorubicin (Cerubidine)	30–45 mg/m^2/d IV × 3 d 40 mg/m^2 IV every 2 wk (liposomal)	Myelosuppression, cardiotoxicity, mucositis, alopecia, nausea and vomiting

(*continued*)

Table 23.1. (*Continued*)

Drug	Dose and Schedule	Toxicity
Doxorubicin (Adriamycin PFS, Adriamycin RDF)	40–75 mg/m^2 IV every 21 d 20–30 mg/m^2/d IV × 3 d, every 3–4 wk 20–50 mg/m^2 IV every 3–4 wk (liposomal)	Myelosuppression, cardiotoxicity, stomatitis, alopecia, nausea and vomiting
Epirubicin (Ellence)	100–120 mg/m^2 IV every 3–4 wk	Myelosuppression, nausea and vomiting, cardiotoxicity, alopecia
Idarubicin (Idamycin)	12 mg/m^2/d IV × 3 d every 3 wk	Myelosuppression, nausea and vomiting, stomatitis, alopecia, cardiotoxicity
Mitomycin C (Mutamycin)	20 mg/m^2 IV every 6–8 wk	Myelosuppression, nausea and vomiting, anorexia, alopecia, stomatitis
Mitoxantrone (Novantrone)	12 mg/m^2/d IV × 3 d 12–14 mg/m^2 IV every 3 wk	Myelosuppression, cardiotoxicity, alopecia, stomatitis, nausea and vomiting
Mitotic inhibitors		
Estramustine (Emcyt)	10–16 mg/kg PO daily	Myelosuppression, ischemic heart disease, thrombophlebitis, hepatotoxicity, nausea and vomiting
Docetaxel (Taxotere)	60–100 mg/m^2 IV every 21 d	Myelosuppression, fluid retention, hypersensitivity, peripheral neuropathy, onycholysis, alopecia
Paclitaxel (Taxol)	135–175 mg/m^2/d IV infusion every 3 wk 80 mg/m^2 IV infusion weekly	Myelosuppression, peripheral neuropathy, alopecia, mucositis, anaphylaxis, onycholysis

Vinblastine (Velban)	3–18.5 mg/m^2 IV every 1–2 wk	Myelosuppression, paralytic ileus, alopecia, nausea, stomatitis
Vincristine (Vincasar)	0.03–1.4 mg/m^2 IV weekly (2.0 mg/wk max)	Peripheral neuropathy, paralytic ileus, SIADH, myelosuppression
Vinorelbine (Navelbine)	25–30 mg/m^2 IV weekly	Peripheral neuropathy, myelosuppression, nausea and vomiting, hepatic dysfunction
Topoisomerase inhibitors		
Etoposide (VP–16, VePesid)	35–100 mg/m^2/d IV × 3–5 d 100 mg/m^2/d PO × 5 d	Myelosuppression, nausea and vomiting, diarrhea, fever, hypotension with infusion, alopecia
Irinotecan (CPT-11, Camptosar)	125 mg/m^2 IV weekly 350 mg/m^2 IV every 3 wk	Myelosuppression, diarrhea, nausea and vomiting, anorexia
Teniposide (Vumon)	60 mg/m^2/d IV × 5 d every 3 wk 50–100 mg/m^2 IV once weekly	Myelosuppression, nausea and vomiting, alopecia, hepatotoxicity, hypotension with infusion
Topotecan (Hycamtin)	1.25–1.5 mg/m^2/d IV × 5 d	Myelosuppression, fever, flulike syndrome, nausea and vomiting
Enzymes		
Asparaginase	6,000 IU/m^2 IM 3 × wk 1,000 IU/kg/d IV × 10 d	Allergic reactions, nausea and vomiting, liver dysfunction, CNS depression, hyperglycemia
Pegaspargase (Oncaspar)	2,500 IU/m^2 IM every 14 d	Hypersensitivity reactions, hepatotoxicity, fever, nausea and vomiting
Hormonal agents		
Adrenocorticoids		
Dexamethasone (Decadron)	0.5–4.0 mg PO, IV, IM daily	Fluid retention, hyperglycemia, hypertension, infection

(*continued*)

Table 23.1. (*Continued*)

Drug	Dose and Schedule	Toxicity
Methylprednisolone (Depo-Medrol, Medrol, Solu-Medrol)	4–200 mg/d PO, IV daily	Fluid retention, hyperglycemia, hypertension, infection
Prednisone (Deltasone)	5–100 mg/d PO	Same as above
Estrogens		
Diethylstilbestrol (DES)	1–15 mg/d PO	Fluid retention, feminization, uterine bleeding, nausea and vomiting, thromboembolism
Estradiol (Climara, Estrace)	0.6–30 mg PO daily	Same as above
Progestins		
Medroxyprogesterone (Provera, Depo-Provera)	400–1,000 mg IM weekly	Weight gain, fluid retention, feminization, cardiovascular effects
Megestrol (Megace)	40–320 mg/d PO	Same as above
Antiestrogens		
Tamoxifen (Nolvadex)	20–40 mg/d PO	Hot flashes, nausea and vomiting, altered menses
Toremifene (Fareston)	60 mg PO daily	Same as above
Fulvestrant (Faslodex)	250 mg IM monthly	Nausea and vomiting, constipation, diarrhea, headache, back pain, hot flushes, pharyngitis
Aromatase inhibitors		
Aminoglutethimide (Cytadren)	250 mg PO bid–qid	Rash, hot flushes, fever, drowsiness, nausea, anorexia
Anastrozole (Arimidex)	1 mg PO daily	Same as above
Exemestane (Aromasin)	25 mg PO daily	Same as above
Letrozole (Femara)	2.5 mg PO daily	Same as above

Androgens		
Testosterone (Androderm, Depo-Testosterone)	200–400 mg IM every 2–4 wk (long acting)	Masculinization, amenorrhea, gynecomastia, nausea, water retention, changes in libido, skin hypersensitivity, hepatotoxicity
Methyltestosterone (Android, Testred)	50–200 mg PO daily	Same as above
Fluoxymesterone (Halotestin)	10–40 mg PO daily	Same as above
Antiandrogens		
Bicalutamide (Casodex)	50 mg PO daily	Hot flashes, decreased libido, impotence, diarrhea, nausea and vomiting, gynecomastia, hepatotoxicity
Flutamide (Eulexin)	250 mg PO tid	Same as above
Nilutamide (Nilandron)	150–300 mg PO daily	Same as above
LHRH analogs		
Leuprolide (Lupron Depot)	1 mg SC daily 7.5 mg IM monthly, 22.5 mg IM every 3 mo, or 30 mg IM every 4 mo 22.5 mg IM every 3 mo	Hot flashes, menstrual irregularity, sexual dysfunction, edema
Goserelin (Zoladex)	3.6–10.8 mg implant SC every 1–3 mo	Same as above
Triptorelin (Trelstar Depot, Trelstar LA)	3.75 mg IM monthly (Depot) or 11.75 mg IM every 84 d (LA)	Same as above
Abarelix (Plenaxis)	100 mg IM on days 1, 15, 29, and every 4 wk thereafter	Same as above

PO, orally; CNS, central nervous system; IV, intravenously; SIADH, syndrome of inappropriate antidiuretic secretion; SC, subcutaneously; IM, intramuscularly; bid, twice daily; qid, four times daily; tid; three times daily; LHRH, luteinizing hormone-releasing hormone.

Table 23.2. Biological agents used in oncology

Cytokine	Indications	Dose and Schedule	Toxicity
Interferon-alfa (Roferon-A, Intron A)	Melanoma, hairy-cell leukemia, Kaposi sarcoma, chronic hepatitis B and C	2–50 million IU/m^2/d or 3 × per wk	Flulike syndrome, anorexia, depression, fatigue
Interleukin-2 (Aldesleukin, Proleukin)	Renal cell carcinoma, metastatic melanoma	600,000–720,000 IU/kg every 8 h × 14 doses	Chills, fever, edema, hepatotoxicity, nephrotoxicity, hypotension, mental status changes, anemia, thrombocytopenia, diarrhea, nausea and vomiting
Interleukin-11 (Oprelvekin, Neumega)	Thrombocytopenia	50 μg/kg SC once daily	Fluid retention, peripheral edema, dyspnea, tachycardia, atrial arrhythmias, dizziness
Filgrastim (G-CSF, Neupogen)	Nonmyeloid malignancy, neutropenia	5–10 μg/kg IV or SC daily	Hypersensitivity, bone pain, fever, malaise
Pegfilgrastim (pegylated G-CSF, Neulasta)	Nonmyeloid malignancy, neutropenia	6 mg SC once per chemotherapy cycle 24 h after chemotherapy	Bone pain, nausea and vomiting, fever, fatigue

Sargramostim (GM-CSF) (Leukine)	Acceleration of myeloid recovery BMT failure or engraftment delay Induction for acute myelogenous leukemia Mobilization after autologous peripheral blood progenitor cells	250 μg/m^2/d IV or SC	Rash, fluid retention, bone pain, cardiac arrhythmia, dyspnea, hypersensitivity
Epoetin alfa (Erythropoietin; Epogen, Procrit)	Anemia associated with chronic renal failure, cancer chemotherapy, or AIDS treatments Reduction of blood transfusions in surgery patients	Initial dose: 50–300 U/kg IV or SC 3 × per wk or 40,000–60,000 U SC weekly	Hypertension, hypersensitivity, fever, tachycardia, nausea, thrombotic events
Darbepoetin (Aranesp)	Anemia associated with chronic renal failure and cancer chemotherapy	Initial dose: 2.25–4.5 μg/kg SC weekly or 200–300 μg SC every 2 wk	Same as above
Monoclonal antibody			
Bevacizumab (Avastin)	Colorectal cancer	5–10 mg/kg IV infusion every 2 wk	Infusion-related reactions, nausea and vomiting, hypertension, proteinuria, gastrointestinal perforation, wound healing complications, thrombotic events
Bortezomib (Velcade)	Multiple myeloma	1.3 mg/m^2 IV twice weekly for 2 wk followed by a 10 d rest period (21 d cycle)	Fatigue, pyrexia, nausea and vomiting, thrombocytopenia, anemia, hypotension, diarrhea, constipation, peripheral neuropathy

(continued)

Table 23.2. (*Continued*)

Cytokine	Indications	Dose and Schedule	Toxicity
Cetuximab (Erbitux)	Colorectal cancer	400 mg/m^2 IV infusion (loading dose), then 250 mg/m^2 IV infusion weekly	Infusion-related reactions, skin rash, fever, nausea and vomiting, constipation, diarrhea
Rituximab (Rituxan)	Non-Hodgkin lymphoma	375 mg/m^2 IV infusion weekly × 4–8 doses	Hypersensitivity, infusion-related fever and chills/rigors, hypotension
Trastuzumab (Herceptin)	Breast cancer	Initial dose: 4 mg/kg IV infusion Maintenance dose: 2 mg/kg IV infusion weekly	Infusion-related fever and chills; cardiac dysfunction, including dyspnea, cough, peripheral edema; nausea and vomiting; hypersensitivity; diarrhea
Alemtuzumab (Campath)	B-cell chronic lymphocytic leukemia	Initial dose: 3 mg/d IV infusion, if tolerated increase to 10 mg/d IV, if tolerated increase to 30 mg/d IV 3 × per wk	Infusion-related fever, chills, rash, nausea, hypotension, shortness of breath, opportunistic infections, neutropenia, thrombocytopenia
Gemtuzumab ozogamicin (Mylotarg)	Acute myeloid leukemia	9 mg/m^2 IV infusion every 14 d × 2 doses	Chills, fever, nausea, vomiting, headache, hypotension, myelosuppression

Immunotoxin			
Denileukin diftitox (Ontak)	Cutaneous T-cell lymphoma	9 or 18 μg/kg/d IV × 5 d, repeat every 21 d	Acute hypersensitivity, including hypotension, dyspnea, rash, chest pain, tachycardia; vascular leak syndrome; confusion; nausea and vomiting; diarrhea
Radiopharmaceutical			
Tositumomab and Iodine 131/ Tositumomab (Bexxar)	Non-Hodgkin lymphoma	Dosimetric step: Tositumomab 450 mg IV followed by iodine I-131 tositumomab (5 mCi iodine I-131, 35 mg tositumomab) IV Therapeutic step: Tositumomab 450 mg IV followed by iodine I-131 tositumomab (iodine I-131 to deliver 75 cGy and 35 mg tositumomab) IV	Myelosuppression, asthenia, fever, chills, cough, pain, infection, nausea and vomiting, human-antimurine antibodies, secondary malignancies
Ibritumomab tiuxetan (Zevalin)	Non-Hodgkin lymphoma	Dosimetric step: Rituximab 250 mg/m^2 IV followed by Indium-111 ibritumomab tiuxetan (5 mCi) IV Therapeutic step: Rituximab 250 mg/m^2 IV followed by yttrium-90 ibritumomab tiuxetan 0.4 mCi/kg (maximum 32 mCi) IV	Myelosuppression, asthenia, infusion-related reactions, nausea and vomiting, cough, secondary malignancies

(*continued*)

Table 23.2. (*Continued*)

Cytokine	Indications	Dose and Schedule	Toxicity
Growth factor receptor inhibitors			
Erlotinib (Tarceva)	Non–small-cell lung cancer	150 mg PO daily	Rash, diarrhea, fatigue, cough, nausea and vomiting, conjunctivitis, increased hepatic transaminases
Gefitinib (Iressa)	Non–small-cell lung cancer	250 mg PO daily	Rash, diarrhea, fatigue, interstitial lung disease, nausea and vomiting, diarrhea, conjunctivitis, increased hepatic transaminases
Imatinib (Gleevec)	Chronic myeloid leukemia, gastrointestinal stromal tumors	400–800 mg PO daily	Fluid retention, muscle cramps, nausea and vomiting, diarrhea, fatigue, hepatotoxicity, myelosuppression

SC, subcutaneously; IV, intravenously; BMT, bone marrow transplant.

Table 23.3. Commonly used combination chemotherapeutic regimens

Acronym	Cancer Use	Agents
ABH	Melanoma	Dactinomycin, carmustine, hydroxyurea
ABV	Hodgkin lymphoma	Doxorubicin, bleomycin, vinblastine
ABVD	Hodgkin lymphoma	Doxorubicin, bleomycin, vinblastine, dacarbazine
AC	Breast, sarcoma, neuroblastoma	Doxorubicin, cyclophosphamide
ACE, CAE	Small-cell lung	Cyclophosphamide, doxorubicin, etoposide
AP	Ovarian, endometrial	Doxorubicin, cisplatin
BEACOPP	Hodgkin lymphoma	Bleomycin, etoposide, doxorubicin, cyclophosphamide, vincristine, procarbazine, prednisone, filgrastim
BEAM	Bone marrow transplant	Carmustine, etoposide, cytarabine, melphalan
BEP	Testicular	Bleomycin, etoposide, cisplatin
BHD	Melanoma	Carmustine, hydroxyurea, dacarbazine
Bold-IFN	Melanoma	Bleomycin, vincristine, lomustine, dacarbazine, interferon alfa 2b
BOP	Testicular	Bleomycin, vincristine, cisplatin
BuCy	Bone marrow transplant	Busulfan, cyclophosphamide
CABO	Head and neck	Cisplatin, methotrexate, bleomycin, vincristine
CAF	Breast	Cyclophosphamide, doxorubicin, fluorouracil
CAMP	Non–small-cell lung	Cyclophosphamide, doxorubicin, methotrexate, procarbazine
CAP	Non–small-cell lung	Cyclophosphamide, doxorubicin, cisplatin
CAVE	Small-cell lung	Cyclophosphamide, doxorubicin, vincristine, etoposide
CEF	Breast	Cyclophosphamide, epirubicin, fluorouracil
CF	Head and neck	Cisplatin, fluorouracil

(*continued*)

Table 23.3. (*Continued*)

Acronym	Cancer Use	Agents
CGI	Bladder	Cisplatin, gemcitabine, ifosfamide
CHOP	Non-Hodgkin lymphoma	Cyclophosphamide, doxorubicin, vincristine, prednisone
CHOP-Bleo	Non-Hodgkin lymphoma	Cyclophosphamide, doxorubicin, vincristine, prednisone, bleomycin
CMF	Breast	Methotrexate, fluorouracil, cyclophosphamide
COMLA	Non-Hodgkin lymphoma	Cyclophosphamide, vincristine, methotrexate, leucovorin, cytarabine
COPE	Small-cell lung	Cyclophosphamide, vincristine, cisplatin, etoposide
COPP	Hodgkin lymphoma	Cyclophosphamide, vincristine, prednisone, procarbazine
CVD	Prostate	Cyclophosphamide, vincristine, dexamethasone
CVD	Melanoma	Cyclophosphamide, vincristine, dacarbazine
CVD + IL-21	Malignant melanoma	Cisplatin, vinblastine, dacarbazine, aldesleukin, interferon-α
CYVADIC	Sarcoma (bone or soft tissue)	Cyclophosphamide, vincristine, doxorubicin, dacarbazine
Cy-TBI	Bone marrow transplant	Cyclophosphamide, total body irradiation
DCTER	Acute myelogenous leukemia, myelodysplastic syndrome	Daunorubicin, cytarabine, thioguanine, etoposide
DI	Soft-tissue sarcoma	Doxorubicin, ifosfamide
EAP	Gastric, small bowel	Etoposide, doxorubicin, cisplatin
EC	Lung	Etoposide, carboplatin
ECF	Esophageal	Epirubicin, cisplatin, fluorouracil
EFP	Gastric, small bowel	Etoposide, fluorouracil, cisplatin
ELF	Gastric	Etoposide, leucovorin, fluorouracil

(*continued*)

Table 23.3. (*Continued*)

Acronym	Cancer Use	Agents
EOX	Esophageal	Epirubicin, oxaliplatin, capecitabine
EP	Testicular, lung	Etoposide, cisplatin
ESHAP	Non-Hodgkin lymphoma	Methylprednisolone, etoposide, cytarabine, cisplatin
FAC	Breast	Fluorouracil, doxorubicin, cyclophosphamide
FAM	Gastric, pancreas	Fluorouracil, doxorubicin, mitomycin
FAMTX	Gastric	Methotrexate, fluorouracil, leucovorin, doxorubicin
FAP	Gastric	Fluorouracil, doxorubicin, cisplatin
FEC	Breast	Fluorouracil, epirubicin, cyclophosphamide
FOLFIRI	Colorectal	Irinotecan, fluorouracil, leucovorin
FOLFOX	Colorectal	Oxaliplatin, fluorouracil, leucovorin
FU/LV	Colorectal	Fluorouracil, leucovorin
GTX	Pancreatic	Gemcitabine, docetaxel, capecitabine
HyperCVAD	Acute lymphocytic leukemia	Cyclophosphamide, doxorubicin, vincristine, dexamethasone
IFL	Colorectal	Irinotecan, fluorouracil, leucovorin
ITP	Bladder	Ifosfamide, paclitaxel, cisplatin
KAVE	Prostate	Ketoconazole, doxorubicin, vincristine, estramustine
MACOP-B	Non-Hodgkin lymphoma	Methotrexate, leucovorin, doxorubicin, prednisone, cyclophosphamide, vincristine, bleomycin
MAID	Soft-tissue sarcoma	Mesna, doxorubicin, ifosfamide, dacarbazine
m-BACOD	Non-Hodgkin lymphoma	Methotrexate, leucovorin, doxorubicin, cyclophosphamide, vincristine, bleomycin, dexamethasone
MICE (ICE)	Sarcoma, lung	Ifosfamide, carboplatin, etoposide, mesna
MBC	Head and neck	Methotrexate, bleomycin, cisplatin

(*continued*)

Table 23.3. (*Continued*)

Acronym	Cancer Use	Agents
MOPP	Hodgkin lymphoma	Mechlorethamine, vincristine, procarbazine, prednisone
MP	Multiple myeloma	Melphalan, prednisone
MP	Prostate gland	Mitoxantrone, prednisone
M-VAC	Bladder	Methotrexate, vinblastine, doxorubicin, cisplatin
PAC	Ovarian, endometrial	Cisplatin, doxorubicin, cyclophosphamide
PVB	Testicular, adenocarcinoma	Cisplatin, vinblastine, bleomycin
R-CHOP	Non-Hodgkin lymphoma	Rituximab, cyclophosphamide, doxorubicin, vincristine, prednisone
SMF	Pancreas	Streptozocin, mitomycin, fluorouracil
TAC	Breast	Docetaxel, doxorubicin, cyclophosphamide
TCF	Esophageal	Paclitaxel, cisplatin, fluorouracil
TIP	Head and neck, esophageal, testicular	Paclitaxel, ifosfamide, mesna, cisplatin
TEC	Prostate	Paclitaxel, estramustine, carboplatin
TEE	Prostate	Paclitaxel, estramustine, etoposide
TMP	Bladder	Paclitaxel, methotrexate, cisplatin
VAC	Sarcoma	Vincristine, dactinomycin, cyclophosphamide
VAD	Multiple myeloma, acute lymphocytic leukemia	Vincristine, doxorubicin, dexamethasone
VB	Testicular	Vinblastine, bleomycin
VC	Non–small-cell lung	Vinorelbine, cisplatin
VIP	Testicular, genitourinary, lung	Etoposide, cisplatin, ifosfamide, mesna
XELIRI	Colorectal	Irinotecan, capecitabine
XELOX	Colorectal	Oxaliplatin, capecitabine
5 + 2	Acute myelocytic leukemia	Cytarabine, daunorubicin or mitoxantrone
7 + 3	Acute myelocytic leukemia	Cytarabine, daunorubicin or mitoxantrone

Cancer pain may be due to direct tumor involvement of bone, nerves, viscera, blood vessels, or mucous membranes and can occur postoperatively, after radiation therapy, or after chemotherapy. Narcotic use should follow the basic principles of cancer pain management, beginning with an agent that has the potential to provide relief; individualization of the agent, route, dose, and schedule; titration to efficacy; and provision of relief for breakthrough pain. Side effects should be anticipated and treated. Change from one route of administration to another should be done with equianalgesic doses, and the oral route should be used whenever possible. In cancer patients receiving chemotherapy, combination analgesics employing an acetaminophen component may not be the best choice for treatment of chronic pain secondary to the risk of masking a neutropenic fever and the risk of acetaminophen toxicity if large doses are required. In addition, combination products using an aspirin component are discouraged secondary to the antiplatelet and antipyretic effects. The nonsteroidal anti-inflammatory agents are a useful adjunct to the treatment of cancer pain but must be used with caution secondary to the antiplatelet effects. The practitioner should be aware of various adjuncts to pain management, including steroids, antidepressants, anxiolytics, and neuroleptics, as well as neuroablative, neurostimulatory, and anesthetic procedures.

Table 23.4 is a compilation of various nonnarcotic and narcotic analgesic agents for treating cancer pain and includes dose ranges and expected toxicities.

MANAGEMENT OF CHEMOTHERAPY-INDUCED EMESIS

Because many surgical patients receive neoadjuvant and adjuvant chemotherapy, the surgeon may be called on to treat CIE, which is often a dose-limiting toxicity that may lead patients to refuse further therapy. Three physiological areas are included in the pathogenesis of CIE: (a) the emetic center in the lateral reticular formation of the medulla, (b) vagal and splanchnic afferents from the gastrointestinal tract to the central nervous system, and (c) the chemoreceptor trigger zone in the area postrema of the medulla. Chemotherapeutic agents and their metabolites may trigger the latter two directly.

Three patterns of emesis tend to occur in association with chemotherapy. Acute emesis occurs within 24 hours of chemotherapy. Delayed emesis occurs more than 24 hours after the cessation of chemotherapy administration and is predisposed by female gender, high-dose cisplatin, and prior episodes of acute emesis. Anticipatory emesis may occur before retreatment in patients whose prior episodes of emesis were poorly controlled, occurring in up to 25% of patients who received prior chemotherapy. Younger age and history of motion sickness also predispose to CIE.

Table 23.5 lists the emetogenic potential of many of the individual chemotherapeutic agents. As chemotherapeutic agents are combined, the combination will have a higher emetogenic potential than the individual agents, and appropriate prevention of nausea and vomiting will be required. It is often helpful to identify the overall emetogenicity of multiple chemotherapy agents given concomitantly. The first step is to identify the emetogenicity level

(*Text continues on page 630.*)

Table 23.4. Nonnarcotic and narcotic analgesic agents used for treating cancer pain

Drug	How Supplied	Dose and Schedule	Toxicity
Nonnarcotics			
Acetaminophen (Tylenol)	Various tablets, liquid, and suppository strengths	650–1,000 mg PO every 6 h	Hepatic and renal impairment
Celecoxib (Celebrex)	Capsules: 100 and 200 mg	100–400 mg PO daily	Dyspepsia, heartburn, nausea, gastrointestinal bleeding, renal dysfunction
Ibuprofen (Advil, Motrin)	Tablets: 50, 100, 200, 400, 600, and 800 mg Suspension: 100 mg/5 mL	200–400 mg PO every 4–6 h	Same as above
Ketorolac (Toradol)	Injection: 15 and 30 mg/mL Tablets: 10 mg	15–30 mg IV/IM every 6 h 10 mg PO every 6 h (limit therapy to 5 d)	Same as above
Nabumetone (Relafen)	Tablets: 500 and 750 mg	100–2,000 mg PO daily	Same as above
Naproxen (Naprosyn)	Tablets: 125, 220, 250, 275, 375, 500, and 750 mg Suspension: 125 mg/5 mL	250–500 mg PO twice daily	Same as above
Tramadol (Ultram, Ultracet)	Tablets: 50 mg Tablets: 37.5 mg with acetaminophen	50–100 mg PO every 4–6 h	Dizziness, nausea, constipation, headache

Narcotics			
Codeine	Tablets: 15, 30, and 60 mg Oral solution: 15 mg/5 mL Tablets: 15, 30, and 60 mg with acetaminophen Injection: 30 and 60 mg	15–60 mg PO, IM, IV, or SC every 4–6 h 50–100 mcg IM/IV every 1–2 h	Sedation, constipation, nausea, respiratory depression; occurs with all narcotic analgesics
Fentanyl (Duragesic, Sublimaze)	Lozenges: 200, 300, 400, 600, 800, 1,200, and 1,600 mcg Transdermal patch: 25, 50, 75, and 100 μg/h Injection: 50 mcg/5 mL	200–400 mcg PO every 2–3 h Apply one patch (25–300 mcg/h) every 72 h	Same as above
Levorphanol (Levo-Dromoran)	Tablets: 2 mg Injection: 2 mg/mL	2–4 mg PO/IV/IM every 4–6 h	Same as above
Hydrocodone (Lortab, Vicodin)	Tablets: 5, 7.5, and 10 mg with acetaminophen Oral elixir: 2.5 mg with acetaminophen/5 mL	5–10 mg PO every 4–6 h	Same as above
Hydromorphone (Dilaudid)	Tablets: 1, 2, 4, and 8 mg Injection: 1, 2, 4, and 10 mg/mL Oral liquid: 5 mg/5 mL Suppository: 3 mg	2–4 mg PO every 3–4 h 0.5–2 mg IV/IM every 3–4 h	Same as above
Methadone (Dolophine)	Tablets: 5, 10, and 40 mg Oral solution: 1, 2, and 10 mg/mL Injection: 10 mg/mL	2.5–20 mg PO every 3–4 h 5–15 mg IV/IM every 3–4 h	As above: Delayed toxicity, accumulation

(*continued*)

Table 23.4. *(Continued)*

Drug	How Supplied	Dose and Schedule	Toxicity
Meperidine (Demerol)	Tablets: 50 and 100 mg Oral syrup: 50 mg/5 mL Injection: 25, 50, 75, and 100 mg/mL	50–150 mg PO every 3–4 h 25–100 mg IV/IM every 3–4 h	As above: Seizures from normeperidine metabolite accumulation
Morphine (MSIR, MS Contin)	Tablets: 10, 15, and 30 mg Oral solution: 10, 20, and 100 mg/5 mL	10–30 mg PO every 3–4 h	As above
	Extended-release tablets/capsules: 15, 20, 30, 60, 90, 100, 120, and 200 mg	30–200 mg PO every 8–24 h	
	Injection: 0.5, 1, 2, 4, 8, 10, 15, 25, and 50 mg/mL	2–10 mg IV/IM every 3–4 h	
	Suppositories: 5, 10, 20, and 30 mg		
Oxycodone (Percocet, Tylox, OxyContin)	Tablet/capsule: 5, 15, 30 mg Oral solution: 1 and 20 mg/mL Tablets: 2.5, 5, 7.5, and 10 mg with acetaminophen	5–10 mg PO every 4–6 h	As above
	Controlled-release tablets: 10, 20, 40, 80, and 160 mg	20–160 mg PO every 8–12 h	
Propoxyphene (Darvon, Darvocet N-100)	Tablets: 65 mg (as HCl) Tablets: 50 and 100 mg with acetaminophen	65 mg PO every 4 h 50–100 mg PO every 4 h	As above

PO, orally; IM, intramuscularly; IV, intravenously; SC, subcutaneously.

Table 23.5. Emetogenic potential of individual chemotherapeutic agents

Frequency of Emesis[a]	Agents	
High emetic risk, Level 5 (>90% frequency of emesis)	Altretamine (oral)	Dactinomycin
	Carmustine > 250 mg/m^2	Mechlorethamine
	Cisplatin ≥ 50 mg/m^2	Melphalan (IV)
	Cyclophosphamide > 1,500 mg/m^2	Procarbazine (oral)
	Dacarbazine	Streptozocin
Moderate emetogenic risk, Level 4 (60%–90% frequency of emesis)	Carboplatin	Cytarabine > 1 g/m^2
	Carmustine ≤ 250 mg/m^2	Doxorubicin > 60 mg/m^2
	Cisplatin < 50 mg/m^2	Methotrexate > 1,000 mg/m^2
	Cyclophosphamide 750–1,500 mg/m^2	
Moderate emetogenic risk, Level 3 (30%–60% frequency of emesis)	Arsenic trioxide	Idarubicin
	Cyclophosphamide ≤ 750 mg/m^2	Ifosfamide
	Cyclophosphamide (oral)	Methotrexate 250–1,000 mg/m^2
	Daunorubicin	
	Doxorubicin 20–60 mg/m^2	Mitoxantrone
		Oxaliplatin
	Epirubicin ≤ 90 mg/m^2	
	Gemcitabine	Topotecan
Low emetogenic risk, Level 2 (10%–30% frequency of emesis)	Anastrozole	Mitomycin
	Capecitabine	Paclitaxel
	Cetuximab	Pemetrexed
	Docetaxel	Pentostatin
	Etoposide	Temozolomide
	5-Fluorouracil	Teniposide
	Irinotecan	Thiotepa
	Methotrexate 50–250 mg/m^2	Trastuzumab
Minimal emetogenic risk, Level 1 (<10% frequency of emesis)	Alemtuzumab	Hydroxyurea
	Asparaginase	Interferon Alfa
	Bicalutamide	Interleukin-2
	Bleomycin	6-Mercaptopurine
	Busulfan	Melphalan (oral)
	Chlorambucil (oral)	Methotrexate ≤ 50 mg/m^2
	Cladribine	Rituximab
	Denileukin diftitox	Tamoxifen
	Erlotinib	Thioguanine (oral)
	Fludarabine	Vinblastine
	Gemtuzumab ozogamicin	Vincristine
	Imatinib mesylate	Vinorelbine

[a]Proportion of patients who experience emesis in the absence of effective antiemetic prophylaxis.

Adapted from: Ettinger DS, Bieman PJ, Bradbury B, et al. NCCN Antiemesis Clinical Practice Guidelines in Oncology. Version 1.2006, National Comprehensive Cancer Network, 2006. The University of Texas M.D. Anderson Cancer Center. Antiemetic Guidelines for Chemotherapy-Induced Nausea and Vomiting (CINV). 2006.

Table 23.6. General recommendations for treatment of acute and delayed chemotherapy-induced emesis

Emetogenicity Level	Acute Emesis	Delayed Emesis
Level 5	5-HT3 antagonist + corticosteroids ± aprepitant ± lorazepam	5-HT3 antagonist + corticosteroids ± aprepitant ± lorazepam
Levels 3 and 4	5-HT3 antagonist + corticosteroids ± lorazepam ± aprepitant	5-HT3 antagonist **OR** metoclopramide ± diphenhydramine **OR** corticosteroids ± lorazepam ± aprepitant
Level 2	Corticosteroids **OR** prochlorperazine **OR** metoclopramide ± diphenhydramine ± lorazepam	No prophylaxis recommended
Level 1	No prophylaxis recommended	No prophylaxis recommended

Adapted from: Ettinger DS, Bieman PJ, Bradbury B, et al. NCCN Antiemesis Clinical Practice Guidelines in Oncology. Version 1.2006, National Comprehensive Cancer Network, 2006. The University of Texas M.D. Anderson Cancer Center. Antiemetic Guidelines for Chemotherapy-Induced Nausea and Vomiting (CINV). 2006.

of each agent in the regimen (Table 23.5). Identify the most emetogenic agent in the regimen, and assess the relative contribution of the other agents. Level 1 agents do not contribute the emetogenicity of the regimen. Adding one or more level 2 agent(s) increases the emetogenicity of the regimen by one level greater than the most emetogenic agent in the combination. Adding a level 3 or 4 agent increases the emetogenicity of the combination by one level per agent. Once the total level of emetogenicity is determined, the recommended agents for prevention of acute and delayed emesis for the chemotherapy combination can be ascertained from available antiemetic guidelines (Table 23.6). The emetogenic potential of many agents is dose dependent. Therefore, additional antiemetic prophylaxis/treatment may be required with higher chemotherapy dosages.

The treatment of CIE underwent a veritable revolution with the introduction of the first selective serotonin antagonist, ondansetron. Currently, there are four FDA-approved selective serotonin antagonists available for the treatment and prevention of CIE (ondansetron, dolasetron, granisetron, and palonosetron). Palonosetron is the only selective serotonin antagonist FDA approved for the prevention of acute and delayed nausea and vomiting. These agents have also found great utility in the prevention

(*Text continues on page 633.*)

Table 23.7. Antiemetic agents for chemotherapy-induced emesis

Drug	Class/Mechanism	Dose and Schedule	Toxicity
Ondansetron (Zofran)	Selective serotonin receptor antagonist	8–32 mg IV daily 4–8 mg PO every 8 h	Headache, constipation, diarrhea, dizziness, ECG changes
Granisetron (Kytril)	Selective serotonin receptor antagonist	1–2 mg IV daily 2 mg PO daily	Same as above
Dolasetron (Anzemet)	Selective serotonin receptor antagonist	100 mg IV or PO daily	Same as above
Palonosetron (Aloxi)	Selective serotonin receptor antagonist	0.25 mg IV day 1 of chemotherapy	Same as above
Aprepitant (Emend)	Substance P/Neurokinin 1 receptor antagonist	125 mg PO day 1, 80 mg PO daily days 2 and 3	Fatigue, hiccups, diarrhea, increased hepatic enzymes
Metoclopramide (Reglan)	Other—dopamine antagonist	0.5–2 mg/kg IV every 3–4 h for highly emetogenic agents 20–40 mg PO every 4–6 h for less emetogenic agents	Diarrhea, dystonia, akathisia, extrapyramidal effects, sedation, ECG changes
Haloperidol (Haldol)	Other—dopamine antagonist	1–3 mg IV or PO every 3–6 h	Dystonia, akathisia, hypotension, sedation, extrapyramidal effects
Droperidol (Inapsine)	Other–dopamine antagonist	0.5–2.0 mg IV every 4 h	Same as above

(continued)

Table 23.7. (*Continued*)

Drug	Class/Mechanism	Dose and Schedule	Toxicity
Prochlorperazine (Compazine)	Phenothiazine—dopamine antagonist	10 mg PO or IV every 4–6 h 25 mg PR every 6 h	Dystonia, extrapyramidal effects, sedation, anticholinergic effects (dry mouth, dizziness, blurred vision, etc.)
Chlorpromazine (Thorazine)	Phenothiazine—dopamine antagonist	25–50 mg PO every 4–6 h	Same as above
Dexamethasone (Decadron)	Other—corticosteroid	10–20 mg IV daily 4 mg PO every 6–12 h 4 mg PO every 6–12 hours	Hyperglycemia, euphoria, insomnia, psychosis, gastrointestinal upset
Methylprednisolone (Depo-Medrol, Medrol, Solu-Medrol)	Other—corticosteroid	250–500 mg IV daily	Same as above
Lorazepam (Ativan)	Other—benzodiazepine	1–2 mg IV/PO/SL every 4–8 h	Sedation, amnesia, confusion
Diphenhydramine (Benadryl)	Antihistamine/anticholinergic	25–50 mg IV or PO every 6 h	Sedation, anticholinergic effects (dry mouth, dizziness, blurred vision, etc.)
Dronabinol (Marinol)	Other—cannabinoid	5–10 mg/m^2 PO every 4–6 h	Drowsiness, dizziness, euphoria, dysphoria, hypotension, hallucinations

IV, intravenously; PO, orally; ECG, electrocardiogram; PR, as needed; SL, sublingually.

of postoperative nausea and vomiting and radiation therapy-induced nausea and vomiting. Intravenous (IV) administration is not necessary in most cases of noncisplatin-induced emesis because efficacy by oral administration is comparable. The exception to this is palonosetron, which is only available by IV administration. They also have the advantage of not causing sedation, and therefore can be safely administered in combination with other agents. High-dose IV metoclopramide has been found effective in treating CIE, although less so than ondansetron, but its extrapyramidal side effects can be a significant problem. These extrapyramidal side effects may occur with any of the antidopaminergic agents, including metoclopramide, haloperidol, droperidol, and the phenothiazines. The extrapyramidal side effects can be treated/prevented by coadministration or pretreatment with an anticholinergic such as benztropine or diphenhydramine. Standard phenothiazines are less effective but serve as useful adjuncts in the treatment of CIE. Corticosteroids, especially dexamethasone and methylprednisolone, act via a mechanism that is still unclear. In combination with other agents, corticosteroids dramatically improve antiemetic efficacy and may reduce the incidence of unwanted side effects by permitting dosage reduction. Corticosteroids are especially useful in treating/preventing delayed emesis. Aprepitant is an orally administered substance P/neurokinin (NK) 1 receptor antagonist. It is FDA-approved for prevention of acute and delayed CIE with initial and repeated courses of highly emetogenic chemotherapy, and must be used in combination with a serotonin receptor antagonist and a corticosteroid. Aprepitant is not indicated as treatment for breakthrough nausea or emesis. Due to interactions with the CYP450 system, aprepitant has a potential to interact with many medications, including chemotherapy. Lorazepam, a benzodiazepine, is useful in the prevention of anticipatory emesis and may reduce the incidence of dystonic reactions to metoclopramide. Most important, combinations of these agents, specifically ondansetron, dexamethasone, lorazepam, and metoclopramide, increase antiemetic efficacy and reduce troublesome side effects through presumed synergistic activity.

Table 23.7 lists available and commonly used antiemetic agents with their dose ranges and the known major side effects.

RECOMMENDED READING

Abramowicz M, ed. Drugs of choice for cancer chemotherapy. *Med Lett Drugs Ther* 1993;35:43.

Burnham T, ed. *Drug Facts and Comparisons*. 55th ed. St. Louis, Mo: Facts and Comparisons, Wolters Kluwer; 2001.

Chang HM. Pain and its management in patients with cancer. *Cancer Invest* 2004; 22(5):799–809.

DeVita V, Hellman S, Rosenberg S, eds. *Cancer: Principles and Practice of Oncology*. 7th ed. Philadelphia, Pa: Lippincott; 2004.

Ettinger DS, Bieman PJ, Bradbury B et al. *NCCN Antiemesis Clinical Practice Guidelines in Oncology*. Version 1. 2006. National Comprehensive Cancer Network, 2006. Available at: URL: http://www.nccn.org.

Krakoff I. Cancer chemotherapeutic

and biologic agents. *CA Cancer J Clin* 1991;41:264.

McEvoy G, ed. *AHFS Drug Information*. Easton, Md: American Society of Hospital Pharmacists; 2001.

Pazdur R, ed. *Cancer Management: A Multidisciplinary Approach*. 8th ed. Melville, NY: PRR, Inc.; 2004.

Perry M, ed. *The Chemotherapy Source Book*. 3rd ed. Philadelphia, Pa: Lippincott Williams & Wilkins; 2001.

Reconstructive Surgery in the Cancer Patient

Jules A. Feledy, Jr., Matthew M. Hanasono, and Geoffrey L. Robb

INTRODUCTION

Reconstructive surgery in the cancer patient endeavors to restore form and function following ablative surgery. The partition of oncologic ablation from plastic surgery reconstruction facilitates resection of a cancer lesion independent of the steps required for restoration. Reconstructive strategies balance the requirements of the resulting wound defect, including the overall size, functional priorities, and constitutive vital requisites of the patient with the available donor sources and the consequent additional morbidities associated with tissue harvest. Successful reconstructive surgery achieves restoration of function and form with minimal donor site deformity and consequent enhancement of quality of life.

GENERAL PRINCIPLES

Wound defects are assessed based on size, location, physical components, and functional requirements. The defect may originate following tumor resection or as a result of tumor necrosis, and may be complicated by infection or exposure of vital structures. The physiological function of a bodily region may be impaired and the quality of life compromised. An evaluation for the components of tissue that will be required to repair a region is made, including components of skin, mucosa, muscle, nerves, fascia, and bone. For example, an anterior base of skull defect may require coverage of dura, cranium, and exposed blood vessels, in addition to closure of the oral mucosa and external skin, while a perineal wound may require reconstruction of the pelvic floor, genital structures, and coverage of the external skin.

Selection of the appropriate reconstructive technique is based on several factors. The patient's medical and functional condition must be assessed relative to the anticipated reconstructive goals. The ability to tolerate a lengthy operative procedure and the postoperative physiological stresses are important preoperative considerations. In addition, the role of reconstruction in the overall oncologic treatment plan must be determined. Reconstructive surgery optimally does not interfere with the administration of adjuvant therapy. Furthermore, the lifestyle and personal considerations of the patient often factor into the decision to proceed with specific reconstructive options. Finally, local wound defect considerations, such as previous radiation therapy and incisional scar patterns, may influence the choice of procedure.

Reconstructive surgery can be performed in the immediate or delayed setting. The timing of reconstructive surgery is influenced by the tumor pathology, extent of resection, adjuvant therapy, surgical expertise, and patient preference. Immediate defect wound coverage is necessitated for coverage of vital structures, including brain and dura, major organ and vascular structures, and spine and joints. Immediate reconstruction is generally preferred following tumor extirpation because dissected tissue planes are available, pliable skin and soft-tissue coverage are maximally preserved, and nonfibrosed tissues are accessible. Scar tissue formation and contracture may preclude later restoration of anatomically critical structures, and preservation of these structures may necessitate immediate reconstruction.

Delayed reconstruction, in contrast, necessitates exposure through fibrosed and often irradiated tissue fields. There is generally a greater requirement for the replacement of overlying skin and subcutaneous tissues. Donor tissue for transfer and their accompanying vessels are likely to have reduced capacity for delayed transfer, and potential recipient vessel dissection for microvascular transfer may be complicated by circumferential encasement in scar tissue and vessel wall friability. Delayed reconstruction is indicated when the oncologic surgical team is unable to determine the extent of surgical resection based on surgical tumor margins, when extensive necrosis is complicated by infection, or in circumstances when immediate reconstruction will delay adjuvant chemotherapy.

The choice of a reconstructive procedure balances reconstruction of a specific wound defect with the available donor sources and consequent additional morbidities associated with tissue harvest. A flexible paradigm of a "reconstructive ladder" provides a starting point from which to consider the various options available for wound closure. Options are considered in increasing order of complexity for a specific defect: Primary closure is generally considered as the first choice, when possible, followed by skin grafts, local flaps, regional flaps, and distant flaps. Multiple different options may exist for a defect, and surgical options are often based on the quality of the anticipated reconstruction. A complex microvascular procedure may be selected over a simpler procedure when it will produce a superior reconstructive result. Moreover, alternative therapies, including tissue expansion and vacuum-assisted coverage, may represent viable options. The restoration of function and form often requires integration of multiple steps in a complex reconstructive strategy.

RECONSTRUCTIVE OPTIONS

The reconstruction of wound defects, aside from primary closure, is fundamentally dependent on tissue transfer from one bodily region to another. A broad armamentarium has been established consisting of different tissue categories, and optimal reconstruction depends on reliable design and transfer of these tissues.

Grafts consist of nonvascularized tissue that is separated from a donor site and depends on the growth of new vessels at the recipient site. Grafts undergo regulated stages of maturation, which begin with the diffusion of oxygen and nutrients across a wound interface followed by an intermediate phase of neovascularization and then later matrix remodeling and stabilization. The most common grafts used for reconstruction include partial- or full-thickness skin, cartilage, nerve, and cortical or cancellous bone. The success of the grafting procedure depends on there being vascularized recipient wound tissue, which is often devitalized because of hypoxia, infection, or previous radiation therapy.

Flaps are tissues that are transferred with an intact blood supply and represent the fundamental method of tissue transfer used in reconstruction. The preservation and incorporation of the blood supply is the salient feature of flaps, allowing for transfer of composite tissues. Each flap has distinct features based on its inherent anatomical characteristics, including pattern of circulation, blood supply, component tissues, thickness, and function. Complex reconstruction is based on manipulation of the properties of different flaps to achieve an engineered result.

The most useful classifications of flaps are those based on the vascular anatomy, component parts, and proximity to the wound defects. The vascular pattern for each flap is divided into random pattern, indicating circulation that depends on the tributaries of the plexus at the attached base, or axial pattern, specifying the presence of a dominant central blood supply. A complex classification based on the blood supply to each flap is used to harvest and inset donor tissues. Flaps are also classified by the tissue components incorporated in the flap; thus, there are skin, fasciocutaneous, muscle, musculocutaneous, osseous, osteocutaneous, and osteomyocutaneous flaps. The attributes of the various flaps enable the surgeon to select the best flap to match the wound defect to achieve complex reconstruction. The distance from the wound defect is characterized as local, indicating transfer from an adjacent area; regional, specifying flaps that originate from a separate part of the body but that have a sufficient arc of rotation to reach a wound defect without division of the blood supply; and distant, implying that the flap exists beyond the reach of the wound defect.

Tissue expansion is a common flap modification based on staged expansion of regional tissue and delayed transfer. It optimizes the use of local tissues but requires placement of a prosthetic device.

Microvascular tissue transfer is a specific application of flap transfer. This technique entails elevation of a composite tissue flap followed by division of the blood supply and re-establishment of the circulation to a recipient blood supply within proximity to the wound defect. Anastomosis is usually performed with the assistance of a microscope or loupe magnification. Flap choice is based on the vascular pedicle length, tissue components, and ability to provide a stable reconstructive result. The main advantage of this approach is the recruitment of tissues from another region of the body.

HEAD AND NECK RECONSTRUCTION

The goals of head and neck reconstruction are to protect vital structures, preserve function, restore contour, and maximize aesthetic appearance. The challenge is achieving these requirements in this complex region.

Scalp

Reconstructive options for the scalp must be considered in the context of the cause of the defect. The restoration of ablative defects involves matching the defect with the available tissue. Local rotation flaps are preferred for small defects; multiple broadly based flaps, augmented with galeal scoring, can often close most small (<3 cm) defects. For larger defects, large rotation flap advancement with skin grafting of the exposed donor site or microvascular flap coverage can be performed. Ablative control often necessitates composite resection of involved calvarial bone, so reconstruction may also require the use of alloplastic materials, such as titanium mesh or methyl methacrylate, or of vascularized bone flaps, such as vascularized rib flaps. Scalp defects resulting from irradiation injury, however, preclude the use of local flaps, and reconstruction in such cases instead involves the debridement of devitalized tissues and then autologous flap coverage.

Facial Skin

Although most facial defects are small, they tend to be located in aesthetically and functionally difficult regions, such as the nasal tip or in proximity to the eyelid. Small superficial defects of the facial skin are treated primarily with skin grafts and local flaps. If local tissue can be mobilized, then local tissue closure is preferable. For example, small random flaps or regional axial flaps can be rotated into a defect. Alternatively, full-thickness skin grafts can be harvested from areas with skin of similar thickness, color, and quality as that of the face. Preauricular, postauricular, and cervical skin sites provide superior matches for facial skin defects. Larger defects, however, may require advanced procedures with complex rotation flaps or, in rare cases, microvascular flap transfer.

Neck

The neck is often treated with radiation for potential or clinically detectable nodal disease in cancer. Following neck dissection, irradiated neck skin may be unable to provide sufficient coverage of the major vessels of the neck, resulting in their prolonged exposure and the risk of hemorrhage. In some circumstances, the sternocleidomastoid muscle can be rotated to cover the vessels; however, the muscle is limited by a segmental blood supply. Therefore, nonirradiated autologous tissue is generally recruited, which will enable minimally restricted neck movement. The most commonly used flap is a pedicled pectoralis major muscle flap rotated on the thoracoacromial axis and covered with an overlying skin graft. Alternative options for neck coverage include free tissue transfer with musculocutaneous flaps, such as a latissimus dorsi flap supplied by the thoracodorsal vessels, or with fasciocutaneous flaps, such as a radial forearm flap supplied by the radial artery, an anterolateral thigh flap based on the descending branch of the lateral circumflex femoral artery, or a scapular flap supplied by the circumflex scapular vessels to available neck vessels.

Nose

The nose is typically reconstructed with local and regional flaps. In general, such flaps result in cosmetic results superior to those attainable by skin grafts. Full-thickness defects must be repaired with an inner lining, a framework, and an exterior cover. The nasal lining is usually replaced with local flaps taken from the nasal mucosa. Cartilage grafts from the ear or rib can be used to replace the cartilaginous framework. When possible, entire subunits of the nose, including the dorsum, sidewalls, ala, tip, columella, and soft triangles, are replaced for the best aesthetic results. For larger defects, the nasolabial flap, which may be based on the angular artery inferiorly or the dorsal branch of the ophthalmic artery superiorly, or the paramedian forehead flap, which is based on the supratrochlear artery, are used. The paramedian forehead flap may be used to resurface the entire exterior nasal skin. Note that the pedicles of the nasolabial and paramedian forehead flaps are left intact for approximately 2 weeks before division.

Lips

Defects involving approximately one-third or less of the width of the upper or lower lip can be repaired by primary closure. For full-thickness defects wider than this, local flaps are needed. Lip switch flaps, in which pedicled tissue is transferred from the upper lip to the lower lip or vice versa, are used for defects that are approximately one-third to two-thirds of the width of the upper or lower lip. Larger defects require bilateral rotation or advancement flaps. In addition, total lip defects can be reconstructed with fasciocutaneous free flaps, such as the radial forearm flap, folded on themselves to re-create the inner and outer surfaces of the lip.

Ear

Most partial ear reconstructions can be performed by using local tissues, as in primary closure of wedge-type resections, rearrangement of the remaining auricle, and coverage by pedicled skin flaps from the postauricular area. For larger defects, the cartilaginous framework of the auricle can be re-created by using cartilage grafts obtained from the ribs and covered with the superficial temporal fascia, also known as the temporoparietal fascia, which derives its blood supply from the superficial temporal artery. Split-thickness skin grafts will survive on the superficial temporal fascia. Some surgeons have also had success with alloplastic frameworks covered by the superficial temporal fascia and a skin graft. Alternately, prosthetic ears can be manufactured for total or near-total defects and secured with osteointegrated implants.

Oral Cavity

The oral cavity includes the tongue, floor of mouth, alveolar ridges, retromolar trigone, palate, and buccal mucosa. Defects in any of these structures can compromise speech, chewing, swallowing, and breathing, and multiple sites may be involved. In addition, resection of higher-stage cancers that invade maxillary or mandibular bone can result in composite defects. The pedicled pectoralis major flap has long been used for such situations. However, in many cases, the pectoralis flap's bulk, lack of pliability, and limited reach still make it a second choice behind free flaps in oral cavity reconstruction.

The radial forearm free flap is an excellent option for reconstructing thin mucosal defects, such as those in the floor of mouth, buccal area, and palate, and for reconstructing partial glossectomy defects. The lateral arm flap, which is supplied by the posterior radial collateral vessels, and the anterolateral thigh flap may also be appropriate choices for patients with a thin layer of sufficient subcutaneous fat in the extremities. In full-thickness cheek defects, the radial forearm flap or other fasciocutaneous flaps can be folded on themselves to provide an internal and external lining. Total and near-total glossectomies require bulky flaps to potentially restore swallowing; for example, the rectus abdominus and anterolateral thigh flaps can provide adequate bulk for reconstructing large defects of the tongue.

Mandible

The most common indication for mandibular reconstruction remains ablative surgery for neoplastic processes of the oral cavity and oropharynx. The functional losses and aesthetic deformity that occur with mandibular defects depend on the size and location of the segmental mandibular defect. Defects in the posterior body or ramus are better tolerated, while anterior defects are associated with significant deformity and loss of function. Mastication and deglutition are compromised as structural support for the tongue and larynx is lost. Airway compromise necessitating tracheostomy may result from the loss of airway stability and tongue support. Malocclusion may develop from mandibular shifts from resection. Functional and aesthetic goals are important considerations, and reconstruction following ablative surgery optimally preserves these functions, restores lower facial aesthetics, and allows for later dental rehabilitation.

The functional and aesthetic results obtained with microvascular tissue transfer are superior to those obtained with nonvascularized bone grafts or pedicled tissue transfers. Although smaller bony defects may be reconstructed with nonvascularized grafts and metal plates, these defects represent only a small percentage of cases. Most cases involve either a larger segmental bony resection or the involvement of internal oral lining or external skin. Free tissue transfer allows for sufficient bony and soft-tissue transfer with a reliable vascular supply. In general, vascularized bone flaps are used to reconstruct mandibular defects greater than 5 to 6 cm or composite defects. Bone union rates are high for vascularized bone flaps because they heal by primary bone healing, similarly to fractures, in contrast to nonvascularized bone grafts, which heal by osteoconduction.

The mainstay of mandibular reconstruction is the fibula flap. Up to 25 cm of bone can be harvested, which provides sufficient length to reconstruct any defect from mandibular angle to mandibular angle. The bony shape is relatively consistent, and osteotomies can be made at intervals to conform the bone to a locking reconstruction plate modeled after the resected mandible. A skin paddle can be harvested to provide soft-tissue coverage. Harvest of the central fibula is well tolerated if 5 cm of proximal and distal fibula are preserved in situ for tibial stability. The pedicle length and caliber are sufficient for reanastomosis in the neck. The fibula flap is based on the peroneal artery and vein; therefore, its use requires adequate distal lower limb perfusion by either the anterior or the posterior tibial vessels. If distal perfusion is in doubt, an angiogram should be obtained preoperatively.

Secondary flap sources for mandible reconstruction include the iliac crest flap, the scapula flap, and the radial forearm flap.

Maxilla

The maxilla is the predominant bony structure in the midface and contains or contributes to the palate, superior alveolar ridge, lateral nasal wall, orbital floor, and malar eminence. Previously, many maxillary defects were not reconstructed. Instead, defects resulting from a maxillectomy were lined with skin grafts or allowed to re-epithelialize spontaneously so they could be better monitored for tumor recurrence. Historically, prosthetic obturators were used in lieu of autologous tissue to isolate the oral cavity from the maxillary cavity and sometimes to restore contour to the midface. Prior to the introduction of contemporary imaging modalities, there was concern that autologous tissue transfer could make the detection of early recurrences difficult. Now, with the improved ability to detect tumor recurrence by imaging studies, the plastic surgeon can perform autologous reconstruction, which provides midfacial contour, oronasal competence, and support for the orbit. However, the optimal tissue to use for reconstruction in this area is controversial and depends on the specific defect. Muscle or musculocutaneous free flaps such as the rectus abdominis, fasciocutaneous free flaps such as the anterolateral thigh flap and the radial forearm flap, and osseous or osteocutaneous free flaps such as the fibula and iliac free flaps have all been used for reconstruction of this area.

Pharynx and Esophagus

Reconstruction of the pharynx and proximal esophagus is challenging. The goal is to restore swallowing and speech functions. Further complicating reconstructive efforts is that most patients will receive radiation therapy.

Traditional methods of reconstruction, including tubed deltopectoral flaps, gastric pull-up procedures, and colonic interposition placement, have given way to current microvascular transfers with jejunal segment, radial forearm, and anterolateral thigh flaps. Microvascular flaps are associated with greater success in restoration of swallowing and speech functions. A tracheoesophageal puncture for speech is generally performed after the immediate reconstruction. Abdominal procedures involve an additional laparotomy and bowel anastomosis. Microvascular transfer with the anterolateral thigh flap has been shown to have a slightly better functional outcome than the jejunal flap. Although the free jejunum flap offers the benefit of a secretory surface, which can help reduce symptoms of xerostomia, swallowing is often interrupted from disordered peristalsis within the flap, and speech tends to be less robust and understandable. The rates of stricture formation and fistula formation are similar, both being superior to nonmicrovascular alternatives.

BREAST RECONSTRUCTION

The goals of breast reconstruction are the restoration of the form and contour of the female breast and symmetry with the contralateral breast. Salient challenges include matching the appropriate technique with the particular needs of the patient and incorporating the reconstructive approach chosen into the overall treatment plan.

Initial considerations for deciding which reconstructive method to use include the type of breast defect, the status of the contralateral breast, the overall health of the patient, any history of previous irradiation or smoking, and the preferences of the patient.

Patients with partial mastectomy defects as a result of breast conservation therapy tend to be reconstructed based on the relative size of the partial defect in relation to the overall breast size. Options for reconstruction include local tissue rearrangement, breast reduction, and pedicled flap transposition. Our preference is for immediate reconstruction when possible.

Implant-based reconstruction techniques use an internal prosthesis to provide breast volume and form. Breast implants contain a silicone-elastomer shell filled with either saline or silicone gel. Common indications for the use of implants include a thin habitus woman with insufficient donor tissue for autologous reconstruction, a small breast volume, and minimal ptosis. Previous radiation treatment of the breast represents a relative contraindication to expander/implant reconstruction.

A staged reconstruction consisting of tissue expansion followed by permanent implant placement is most commonly performed. This procedure involves placing an expander under the mastectomy skin in the subpectoralis muscle either immediately after mastectomy or as a delayed procedure. After allowing the overlying incisions to heal, aliquots of saline are injected transcutaneously on an interval basis until the desired final volume size is achieved. A second-stage operation is then performed to remove the breast expanders and place the permanent breast implant. The advantages of this method of reconstruction include its simplicity, its requirement of less operating room time, and its suitability for women who are not able to undergo autologous reconstruction. The disadvantages include potential local complications, development of capsular contracture, and rupture of the implant.

A second implant-based technique uses a latissimus dorsi flap with an implant. A pedicled musculocutaneous flap based on the thoracodorsal vascular supply is rotated anteriorly to the breast and is used to cover the implant. The implants used are generally the same as those used after tissue expansion. The skin paddle may be included with the muscle to facilitate coverage of the mastectomy wound. The primary advantage of the latissimus dorsi flap procedure is that sufficient tissue for coverage of the implant is available without tissue expansion and a staged approach is not required. Another key advantage is that vascularized tissue can be transferred to the breast in a predictable manner. Two major drawbacks are that a donor site scar is created and that some resultant weakness of upper torso strength may be realized. This approach does, however, represent a viable option for women with a thin habitus or insufficient pannus who are not candidates for an abdominal flap or for women who have previously failed other types of reconstruction.

Reconstructive techniques that use autologous tissue transfer skin, fat, and muscle from one area of the body to the chest and generally eliminate the need for a supplemental prosthesis. The transverse rectus abdominus myocutaneous (TRAM) flap procedure is the most common technique for autologous reconstruction and uses the lower abdominal fat supplied by epigastric vascular perforators through the rectus abdominis muscle. A large volume of well-vascularized skin and subcutaneous tissue can be transferred to the chest to reconstruct the mastectomy site. A pedicled TRAM flap procedure involves rotation of the lower abdominal pannus through a subcutaneous tunnel from the abdomen to the chest along the arc of the upper rectus muscle that protects the superior epigastric blood supply.

A variation of this method uses a microvascular free TRAM flap. The free TRAM flap maximizes the blood supply to the lower abdominal pannus by using the deep inferior epigastric blood vessels, which provide greater blood flow than do the superior epigastric vessels. The deep inferior epigastric vessels are divided from the iliac blood vessels and then anastomosed in the chest under microscopic magnification to, most commonly, the internal mammary or thoracodorsal blood vessels. The advantages of the TRAM are the relatively large skin and fill volumes available for reconstruction of a projecting breast. Some refinements to this technique include the muscle-sparing TRAM flap procedure, in which a selective blood supply from either the medial or the lateral row of deep inferior epigastric perforators (DIEPs) to the flap is harvested along with a strip of muscle, while a portion of the rectus muscle and its corresponding fascia and the perforator flaps is preserved. With the DIEP flaps, for example, one or several perforators to the flap are dissected away from the muscle in a way that preserves the entire muscle and fascia.

Alternative autologous flaps can be harvested from other sites, including the buttocks, with either a superior gluteal or inferior gluteal blood supply, and the flank with a deep circumflex iliac blood supply (Rubens flap). These alternative flaps are reserved for circumstances in which the abdomen is not available as a donor site. Overall, autologous tissue reconstruction produces the best long-term results. These operations are of greater magnitude, have longer postoperative recuperation times, and have a small but definitive risk of failure.

Nipple-areolar reconstruction is performed as a separate procedure after the reconstructed breast has had time to attain its final shape and position. A nipple position on the breast mound is determined, and a nipple is constructed from local flaps. An areola is tattooed around the central nipple flap.

TRUNK AND PERINEUM RECONSTRUCTION

Chest Wall and Sternum

The principles of chest wall reconstruction are to restore the dynamic stability of the chest, protect the thoracic viscera, and maintain the respiratory and cardiac physiological functions. Contour considerations are addressed after functional requirements are met. Large defects can result from tumor resection for local or metastatic control and are often complicated by radiation injury or the development of infection, invariably in compromised tissue fields. Skeletal stabilization with prosthetic materials is performed for resections involving either four or more rib segments or chest wall cavities greater than 6 cm in diameter to reduce the risk of flail chest.

The majority of these defects can be repaired with local and regional musculocutaneous flaps. Muscle flap options for sternal wound coverage include the pectoralis major muscle, either as a pedicled flap based on the thoracoacromial vessels or as a turnover flap based on perforators from the internal mammary vessels, and the rectus abdominis muscle based on the superior epigastric vessels. Options for axillary coverage include the pectoralis major and the latissimus dorsi flaps. Coverage of the posterior thorax can be provided by the latissimus dorsi flap, the trapezius flap, paraspinous muscle flaps, or different large design flaps, such as a hemiback rotation advancement flap, depending on the specific location of the defect. In rare circumstances, the omentum can be transferred outside the abdomen through a tunnel to provide vascularized wound coverage. In the absence of local tissue options, microvascular transfer of distant tissues may be required to provide coverage.

Abdomen

After oncologic surgery of the abdomen, abdominal wall reconstruction is required to protect the abdominal viscera and restore abdominal fascial continuity. Local tissue techniques include component separation, in which the layers of the abdominal wall musculature are separated and advanced; fascial partition release, which consists of parallel parasagittal relaxing incisions into the abdominal wall musculature; and tissue expansion. Fascial integrity can be restored with fascial sheet grafts from the tensor fascia lata, prosthetic mesh, or flap recruitment. Pedicled musculocutaneous flaps from the hip and thigh can be rotated to the lower abdomen. Microvascular transfer of distant tissue is required to reconstruct large defects.

Perineum

The principles of perineal reconstruction are to maximize wound healing, provide durable coverage when possible, and facilitate early patient rehabilitation. Most patients with perineal defects after oncologic surgery have received radiation treatment. Our experience has shown that immediate reconstruction substantially reduces postoperative complications, such as infection, fistula formation, small bowel obstruction, and delayed wound healing. Myocutaneous flaps provide both well-vascularized tissues to fill the lower pelvic space and healthy tissues for wound closure. Local pedicled flaps can often be rotated from the abdomen or the thigh.

Penile and scrotal surface coverage or vaginal reconstruction is frequently required with perineal reconstruction. The requirements of mobility and durability must be balanced with considerations of coital ability and body habitus. For superficial defects of the penis and scrotum, partial- and full-thickness skin grafts may provide adequate coverage, although larger defects may require rotational muscle flaps. Testicular preservation may necessitate temporary coverage in the subcutaneous anterior thigh region. Partial vaginal defects can be restored with local random flaps from the vulvar region or smaller pedicled flaps from the thigh, such as the gracilis or anterolateral thigh, while larger defects usually require flap rotation from the thigh or abdomen. Circumferential neovaginal reconstruction is a complex procedure requiring a pedicled flap with a large skin paddled for rolling on itself such as provided by a rectus abdominis or anterolateral thigh flap, or a combination of two smaller flaps to provide the large skin surface area from either bilateral posterior thigh flaps or gracilis flaps.

EXTREMITIES

The goal of extremity reconstruction is limb salvage rather than amputation. Reconstructive surgery after extirpative surgery to manage cutaneous malignancies in the extremities generally involves primary closure, skin grafts, and local or regional cutaneous and musculocutaneous flaps. Soft-tissue and bony neoplasms are much less common but generally require reconstruction with microvascular free flaps. Adjuvant therapy often results in decreased tumor size and facilitates sparing of the limb; however, the use of adjuvant modalities may have a strong negative impact on wound healing and may necessitate covering the wound with nonirradiated tissue to facilitate healing and provide coverage of the nerves, vessels, and bone required to maintain a useful limb.

The need to replace various tissues, including bone, nerves, muscle, soft tissues, and skin, must be anticipated before reconstruction. Bony defects can be corrected by limb shortening, with or without later bone transport for lengthening, allografts, bone grafts, or vascularized bone flaps. Free and pedicled muscle transfers not only can provide well-vascularized wound coverage, but can also be neurotized and used for functional muscle transfer. Fasciocutaneous flaps, musculocutaneous flaps, and muscle flaps covered with split-thickness skin grafts are used for replacement of soft tissue and skin. Nerve repair can be performed by using microsurgical techniques to restore motor and sensory functions. Primary nerve repair performed at the time of tumor resection results in the best functional outcome. If the nerve deficit is too large to perform a tension-free repair, nerve grafting can be used. The sural nerve, which provides sensation to the lateral foot, is typically chosen as the donor nerve and can provide as much as 30 to 40 cm of nerve from one leg with minimal morbidity.

Limb sparing, however, must be weighed against performing an adequate oncologic resection. Also, leaving a patient with a limb that is nonfunctional, insensate, or painful provides little if any benefit over amputation. Indications for amputation include major neurovascular or extensive muscle involvement of the limb by the tumor, which would result in a nonfunctional limb; infection and fractures, which could compromise reconstruction and delay adjuvant therapy; poor nutrition and other serious medical conditions; a lack of patient motivation for rehabilitation; and the need for multiple surgeries. Patients must be warned before reconstructive surgery that poor functional outcomes, infections and other wound complications, and tumor recurrence may ultimately lead to amputation.

Upper Extremity

As in other locations, flap coverage is indicated for upper-extremity defects to reconstruct wounds with extensive tissue loss or to protect exposed vital structures, such as bone, tendons, nerves, or major vessels, when skin grafts would be unlikely to adhere or provide durable coverage or would lead to significant scarring and decreased function. For example, scar contracture of incisions placed parallel to the axis of the limb across joints can result in a decreased range of motion and may require lengthening with z-plasty procedures or interposition of a pliable flap. Similarly, not only are tendons stripped bare of paratenon-poor recipients for skin grafts, but their function can also be compromised, if adherence occurs, by the prevention of free gliding movement.

There are several local flaps used in hand surgery, including advancement, rotation, transposition, and cross-finger flaps. In the case of an amputation of a digit or limb, fillet flaps, in which the bone has been partially or totally removed, can be used to cover the distal stump with well-vascularized tissue.

A pedicled radial forearm flap based on the radial artery and its venae comitantes (i.e., paired veins intimately associated with the artery) is the main flap used to provide fasciocutaneous tissue to the forearm and elbow. An Allen's test should be performed prior to surgery to document patent ulnar and radial blood flow to the hand. If single vessel flow is inadequate to perfuse the hand, vein grafting can be performed to re-establish blood flow, as needed. A lateral arm flap can be used in the upper arm and can reach the acromion and posterior axilla.

Upper limb wounds can also be covered with pedicled flaps from the trunk and pelvis. After neovascularization of the flap at its recipient site, the donor pedicle is divided. These flaps generally require 2 to 3 weeks (or more) of immobilization. Such distant pedicled flaps include the groin flap, supplied by the superficial circumflex iliac vessels; the anterior chest wall flap, supplied by the intercostal or thoracoepigastric vessels; and the epigastric or abdominal flaps, supplied by the superficial inferior epigastric vessels or a random-pattern blood flow. The pectoralis major flap, based on the thoracoacromial vessels, is used for anterior shoulder wounds or amputation coverage. The latissimus dorsi flap, based on the thoracodorsal vessels, is used for shoulder, axillary, and upper arm wounds; this flap can reach beyond the olecranon or antecubital fossa in many cases and can be used for functional muscle transfer to restore elbow flexion or extension.

Many free muscle, musculocutaneous, and fasciocutaneous flaps used elsewhere for reconstruction are also useful in the upper extremity. Specifically, the rectus abdominus, latissimus dorsi, serratus anterior, and gracilis (often the flap of choice for innervated functional reconstruction) muscle flaps and the radial forearm, ulnar forearm, lateral arm, anterolateral thigh, dorsalis pedis, and scapular/parascapular fasciocutaneous flaps have all been successfully used for upper-extremity reconstruction. The temporoparietal fascia flap, based on the superficial temporal artery and covered by a skin graft, can reconstruct the dorsal hand and provide a suitable gliding surface for underlying tendons. In addition, the first and second toes have been successfully transferred to replace the thumb, and the fibula and iliac crest osseous flaps have been used to reconstruct the long bones of the upper limb. Angiography may be indicated before the harvesting of a fibular flap if distal perfusion to the foot is in question.

Adequate sensory and motor function of the limb, hand, or digit in question must be present, or reconstruction may be more of a hindrance than a benefit to the patient's quality of life. Primary or nerve graft repairs are often needed to preserve adequate function. Epineural or interfascicular repairs are typically performed, depending on the nerve and location. Tendon transfers in which functionally expendable muscle/tendon units are rerouted to replace functionally critical units can also be performed. At a minimum, the goal of functional upper limb reconstruction requires having a stable shoulder joint, restoring elbow flexion, and ensuring median nerve sensibility.

Lower Extremity

Defects in the groin and proximal medial or anterior thigh can often be closed by using a pedicled rectus abdominus flap supplied by the deep inferior epigastric vessels. Large defects in other areas of the thigh are typically reconstructed with adjacent muscles, including the rectus abdominus or latissimus dorsi muscle, or free tissue transfer with musculocutaneous flaps. The femoral and deep femoral vessels are usually good recipients for these flaps. End-to-side anastomoses are commonly performed in the lower extremity to preserve the distal blood flow.

Tumors of the knee, distal femur, or proximal tibia usually require reconstruction with an allograft or endoprosthesis. The medial or lateral heads of the gastrocnemius can be separated and used as pedicled muscle flaps, or both heads can be used to provide muscle flap coverage of the knee, the upper third of the lower leg, or the first 15 cm of the thigh above the knee. This pedicled flap receives its blood supply from the sural artery and vein, which are branches of the popliteal vessels. If both heads are used, the soleus muscle must be left intact to preserve plantar flexion of the foot. Flaps from the soleus muscle can also be used to reliably cover defects of the middle third of the leg. As with the gastrocnemius, the soleus can be split down its median raphe, and the medial and lateral heads can be used separately. If the soleus is used for reconstruction, then the gastrocnemius must be left intact to preserve plantar flexion. Alternatively, one head of the soleus and one head of the gastrocnemius can be used for reconstruction, which spares plantar flexion of the foot. Finally, reconstructing the distal third of the leg with local or regional muscle flaps is, for the most part, not an option. Generally, all but the smallest wounds in this region require free fasciocutaneous or muscle/musculocutaneous flap coverage because local tissues lack laxity.

Reconstruction options for small defects of the foot include the use of skin grafts and local flaps. Larger defects require microvascular free tissue transfer reconstruction. Free muscle flaps, such as gracilis muscle or serratus anterior muscle flaps covered by a skin graft, provide coverage that conforms well to many defects.

The largest defects may require rectus abdominus or latissimus dorsi flaps covered by a skin graft. The design of muscle flaps used for foot reconstruction must take into account the expected atrophy of the muscle with time; too much flap bulk is usually unfavorable for ambulation and may necessitate revision, special orthotic footwear, or both. Fasciocutaneous flaps, such as a radial forearm flap, are also used for foot reconstruction and can be designed to include sensory innervation. Muscle and fasciocutaneous flaps are susceptible to pressure ulceration and so must be vigilantly monitored for the breakdown of skin and soft tissue.

Re-establishing plantar sensation after nerve resection is critical in lower limb reconstruction. Without protective sensation, the lower limb is prone to ulceration and injury that can lead to infection and, ultimately, the need for amputation. Good extremity management may allow a patient to otherwise maintain a "bioprosthesis." Proximal nerve resection and repair yield poorer functional restoration than does distal reconstruction. In addition, postoperative immobilization after nerve repair is necessary for approximately 7 to 10 days. Reinnervation usually occurs no faster than 1 mm per day and can be detected by testing for advancing Tinel sign and performing nerve conduction studies. Muscle stimulation to maintain motor end-plate function can be attempted when reinnervation is expected to take longer than 12 to 18 months.

Free tissue transfer and bony reconstruction of the lower extremity usually require a period of bedrest with elevation of the extremity. The prevention of deep venous thrombosis is important during this time. After 5 to 7 days, the patient can dangle the extremity for short periods of 15 to 30 minutes at a time. Standing and crutch-assisted ambulation with gradual weight bearing is then allowed with the flap gently wrapped with an elastic bandage to prevent venous pooling and to help contour the flap.

RECOMMENDED READING

Head and Neck

Ariyan S. The pectoralis major myocutaneous flap for reconstruction in the head and neck. *Plast Reconstr Surg* 1979;63:73–81.

Burget GC, Menick FJ. Nasal reconstruction: seeking a fourth dimension. *Plast Reconstr Surg* 1986;78:145–157.

Hidalgo DA. Fibula free flap: a new method of mandible reconstruction. *Plast Reconstr Surg* 1989;87:71–78.

Newman MI, Hanasono MM, Disa JJ, et al. Scalp reconstruction: a fifteen-year experience. *Ann Plast Surg* 2004;52:501–506.

Robb GL, Lewin JS, Deschler DG, et al. Speech and swallowing outcomes in reconstructions of the pharynx and cervical esophagus. *Head Neck* 2003;25:232–244.

Breast

Bostwick J. *Plastic and Reconstructive Breast Surgery*. 2nd ed. St. Louis, Mo: Quality Medical Publishing; 2000.

Kroll SS, Reece GP. *The Well-informed Patient's Guide to Breast Reconstruction*. Houston, Tex: The University of Texas M. D. Anderson Cancer Center; 2002.

Kroll SS, Schusterman MA, Reece GP, et al. Choice of flap and incidence of free flap success. *Plast Reconstr Surg* 1996;98:459–463.

Kronowitz SJ, Robb GL, Youssef A, et al. Optimizing autologous breast reconstruction in thin patients. *Plast Reconstr Surg* 2003;112:1768–1778.

Miller MJ, Rock CS, Robb GL. Aesthetic breast reconstruction using a combination of free transverse rectus abdominis musculocutaneous flaps and breast implants. *Ann Plast Surg* 1996;37:258–264.

Tran NV, Evans GR, Kroll SS, et al. Postoperative adjuvant irradiation: effects on transverse rectus abdominis muscle flap breast reconstruction. *Plast Reconstr Surg* 2000;106:313–317.

Trunk and Perineum

Arnold PG, Pairolero PC. Chest wall reconstruction: an account of 500 consecutive patients. *Plastic Reconstr Surg* 1996;98:804–810.

Buchel EW, Finical S, Johnson C. Pelvic reconstruction using vertical rectus abdominis musculocutaneous flaps. *Ann Plast Surg* 2004;52:22–26

Chang RR, Mehrara BJ, Hu QY, et al. Reconstruction of complex oncologic chest wall defects: a 10-year experience. *Plastic Reconstr Surg* 2004;52:471–479.

McCraw JB, Papp C, Ye Z, et al. Reconstruction of the perineum after tumor surgery. *Surg Oncol Clin N Am* 1997;6:177–189.

Extremity

Barwick WJ, Goldberg JA, Scully SP, Harrelson JM. Vascularized tissue transfer for closure of irradiated wounds after soft tissue sarcoma resection. *Ann Surg* 1992: 216;591–595.

Brennan MF. Management of extremity soft-tissue sarcoma. *Am J Surg* 1989;158:71–78.

Cordeiro PG, Neves RI, Hidalgo DA. The role of free tissue transfer following oncologic resection in the lower extremity. *Ann Plast Surg* 1994;33:9–16.

Evans GRD, Goldberg DP. Principles of extremity microvascular reconstruction. In: Schusterman MA, ed. *Microsurgical Reconstruction of the Cancer Patient*. Philadelphia, Pa: Lippincott-Raven; 1997: 233–247.

Gidumal R, Wood MB, Sim FH, Shives TC. Vascularized bone transfer of limb salvage and reconstruction after resection of aggressive bone lesions. *J Reconstr Microsurg* 1987;3:183–188.

Hidalgo DA, Carrasquillo IM. The treatment of lower extremity sarcomas with wide excision, radiotherapy, and free-flap reconstruction. *Plast Reconstr Surg* 1992;89:96–101.

Reece GP, Schusterman MA, Pollock RE, et al. Immediate versus delayed free-tissue transfer salvage of the lower extremity in soft tissue sarcoma patients. *Ann Surg Oncol* 1994;1:11–17.

Robb GL, Reece GP. Lower extremity reconstruction. In: Schusterman MA, ed. *Microsurgical Reconstruction of the Cancer Patient*. Philadelphia, Pa: Lippincott-Raven; 1997: 289–322.

Index

Page numbers followed by f indicate figure; those followed by t indicate table.